MCAT

SUCCESS

2003

Stefan Bosworth, Ph.D. ■ Marion A. Brisk, Ph.D.
Ronald P. Drucker, Ph.D. ■ Denise Garland, Ph.D.
Edgar M. Schnebel, Ph.D. ■ Rosie Soy, M.A.

THOMSON
PETERSON'S

Australia • Canada • Mexico • Singapore • Spain • United Kingdom • United States

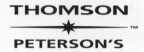

About The Thomson Corporation and Peterson's

With revenues of US$7.2 billion, The Thomson Corporation (www.thomson.com) is a leading global provider of integrated information solutions for business, education, and professional customers. Its Learning businesses and brands (www.thomsonlearning.com) serve the needs of individuals, learning institutions, and corporations with products and services for both traditional and distributed learning.

Peterson's, part of The Thomson Corporation, is one of the nation's most respected providers of lifelong learning online resources, software, reference guides, and books. The Education Supersite^{SM} at www.petersons.com—the Internet's most heavily traveled education resource—has searchable databases and interactive tools for contacting U.S.-accredited institutions and programs. In addition, Peterson's serves more than 105 million education consumers annually.

For more information, contact Peterson's, 2000 Lenox Drive, Lawrenceville, NJ 08648; 800-338-3282; or find us on the World Wide Web at www.petersons.com/about.

ISBN 0-7689-0986-4

Printed in the United States of America

10 9 8 7 6 5 4 3 2 1   05 04 03

CONTENTS

Unit 3 Writing Sample

Unit 4 Biological Sciences

HOW TO PREPARE FOR THE MEDICAL COLLEGE ADMISSION TEST (MCAT)

WHO TAKES THE MCAT AND WHEN IT IS GIVEN

Virtually all students who plan to enroll in medical school in the United States or Canada take the MCAT. In addition, many schools of veterinary medicine and podiatry either require or recommend taking the MCAT. The MCAT is used as a tool in evaluating whether to consider a student for admission. Medical schools also review grades, letters of reference, and medical school application essays before deciding which candidates should be called for interviews for medical school admission. Success on the MCAT greatly enhances your chances of being accepted to medical school.

The MCAT is given twice a year, once in April and once in August. Application forms are available at the premed office in your school or you can write to the MCAT Program Office at P.O. Box 4056, Iowa City, IA 52243-4056. You may take the MCAT as many times as you like. Nevertheless, scores from previous MCATs are furnished to the medical schools to which you apply and could affect your chances of being accepted. If you want to take the exam more than three times, you must request permission in writing from the American Association of Medical Colleges. The MCAT score you receive is good for five years, after which you are required to take the exam again. Some medical schools will not accept scores that are more than two or three years old. You need to check with the particular medical or podiatric schools in which you are interested. Most students take the MCAT during the spring of their junior year or at the beginning of their senior year; however, you may take the MCAT at any time during your academic career.

FORMAT AND SCORING THE MCAT

The MCAT exam is divided into four sections: Physical Science, 77 questions that you are allowed 100 minutes to answer; Verbal Reasoning, 60 questions that you are allowed 85 minutes to answer; Writing, two questions that you are allowed 60 minutes to answer; and Biological Science, 77 questions that you are allowed 100 minutes to answer. You will be given a 10-minute break between the Physical Science section and Verbal Reasoning section, a 60-minute lunch break between the Verbal Reasoning section and the Writing section, and another 10-minute break between the Writing section and the Biological Science section.

The scoring on the Physical Science, Verbal Reasoning, and Biological Science sections is based on a scale of 1 to 15, with 1 being the lowest and 15 being the highest possible scores. The scores on the Writing section are converted to an alphabetical score with J being the lowest and T being the highest possible scores. The letter scores represent the sum of two individual gradings.

For further information about the MCAT, it is recommended that you purchase the MCAT Student Manual available at most college bookstores or directly from the American Association of Medical Colleges.

HOW TO USE THIS BOOK TO STUDY FOR THE MCAT

Take Practice Exam I

Start your MCAT preparation by taking Practice Exam I, on page 565. Do not take this exam in sections. Take the exam as if it were the actual exam. Set aside a whole day to take the exam. Use a stopwatch to make sure that you follow the time limits exactly. If you finish a section of the exam early, use the extra time to go over your answers. Do not begin another section of the exam until the time for the previous section is up. The more closely you adhere to the timetable of the actual exam, the more meaningful your pretest score will be. This means that you may not use a calculator during the exam, and that you may not eat or drink except during the breaks.

Your pretest score is a fairly accurate assessment of where you would be if you took the exam without studying. This score gives you an idea of your strengths and weaknesses. From this information, you can begin to design a study plan. Your study plan should take into account how much time is left before the exam and any other activities that you must accomplish during this time period, including school, work, and household responsibilities. The plan you develop should have week-by-week objectives. Without these objectives, it is easy to put off studying until the last minute. Plan to spend more time on sections on which you did poorly and less time on sections on which you did well. You should, however, plan to review every section as you prepare for the test.

After you have completed the practice test, check your answers with the explanations that follow the test. Concentrate first on the explanations of the questions that you answered incorrectly. Next, go over the questions that you answered hesitantly, and then look over the questions that you answered correctly by guessing. Finally, go over the explanations for the questions you answered correctly. By studying all the explanations, you may gain new insights into choosing the correct answers, and you may pick up new and useful information.

Try to discover whether you tend to miss certain types of questions more often than other types of questions. Even on topics you did well, look for subsections within the topics where you were less successful in getting correct answers. For instance, it might be that in the Physical Science section, you missed problems that used conversion factors more than other types of problems. Or, in the Verbal Reasoning section, you may have missed questions that required inference more than questions that simply required recalling knowledge. This information will help you to fine-tune your study plan.

List the topics on which you were weak in each subject area. When you design your study schedule, set aside extra time for each topic on which you did not do well. This assures that when you study, you will be sure to spend your study time in the most fruitful way.

Set Up a Study Place

Before you begin to study for the MCAT exam, pick a quiet spot with good light and a clear workspace. Assemble all the tools you'll need: review books, text-books, reference books, class notes, computer, a calculator (note: you cannot use a calculator on the actual MCAT exam), pencils, pens, paper, and so on. Valuable study time is lost when you cannot find things that you need while you are studying. Minimize interruptions so that you are not forced to go over material that you have already reviewed. This loss of concentration can be particularly damaging when studying the sciences. Eliminate as many distractions as possible (such as the radio, television, CD player, telephone, and pagers). It is a good idea to unplug the telephone or turn it off, because this is the only way you can control incoming calls completely. If you just turn on the answering machine, you will still be distracted by the ring of the telephone.

Create a Time Schedule

After you have taken your first practice exam and before you begin to study, establish a time schedule. Include in the schedule the time you must spend studying your course work, time you must spend at work, time you must spend doing household chores, the time you spend traveling to and from school, and any other activities that you are involved in on a regular basis. This schedule should include what you regularly need to accomplish, as well as time for studying the MCAT. Adjust your schedule every week to reflect changes in what you need to accomplish each week.

Schedule your MCAT studying, particularly your science studying, in one- to two-hour blocks of time every day. Although you should not study more than two hours at a time for the MCAT, that does not mean that you should not study more than two hours a day. As long as you intersperse your study activity with other activities, such as eating or watching television, you can and should study more than two hours a day. It is also possible to study for more than two hours at a time as long as you change the subject you are studying.

When you set up your study schedule, be specific. Do not simply write that you are going to study chemistry from 8:00 p.m. to 10:00 p.m. on Monday. Instead, write down the topic you are actually going to study and what you are going to do. For example, you might write Stoichiometry problem solving—8:00 p.m. to 10:00 p.m. The more specific you are, the less time you will waste.

You should not study two science subjects at the same time. Set aside separate weeks for studying each science subject. However, you can study for the Verbal Reasoning and Writing sections while studying a science subject.

Study for the Exam a Section at a Time

After you have gone over your Practice Exam I and reviewed the test carefully, which should take at least one week and probably longer, begin to review material one section at a time. You can expect to spend two to three weeks studying each section of the exam. The amount of time you spend on each section depends on how well you did on that section of the practice exam and how much time you have left before the MCAT exam is to be given. Be sure to spend at least two weeks studying each section of the exam, even the ones on which you did well in the practice test. When students ignore sections on which they did well when taking the practice test, their scores on the actual exam often turn out to be lower than they were on the practice exam.

At the end of each Review Section, you will find a sample exam for that section. After you review a section, take the sample exam to evaluate how effective your studying has been and to identify areas in which you are still weak. When you take the section exam, be sure to pace yourself so that you have time to answer every question. Since there is no penalty for a wrong answer on the MCAT exam, blind guessing is worthwhile. Usually, however, you can do better than blind guessing. With multiple-choice questions, it is often possible to eliminate several incorrect choices even if you do not know the correct choice. Often, you know part of an answer even if you do not know the whole answer and can therefore eliminate answers that do not agree with the information you already have. On the science sections, estimating answers can help you reduce the number of answers that might be correct, thus improving your chances of guessing correctly. Answer every question. Put a mark by those questions you need more time to think about, and go back to them if you have time. You should be able to complete the section exam in the allotted time because you have been studying since you took the first practice exam. One of your goals in taking practice exams, either section exams or the whole exam, is to increase your speed.

Don't be discouraged if you do not know the answers to several questions. When you have finished the exam, you should have time to go over problems that you did not understand or the questions you could not answer, and you may be able to answer some of these questions the second time around. In addition, it is assumed that you will not know all the answers to the questions, and the test is graded accordingly. Just guess at the questions you don't know, and you will soon come to questions that you can answer. If you have studied well, you should be fully prepared for the exam and should be confident enough to avoid the anxiety of not knowing the answers to a few questions.

Take Practice Exam II

After studying each section and taking the practice section exams, you should be ready to take Practice Exam II. Once again, plan to take the practice exam in one sitting, just as you'll have to in the actual MCAT.

Read the test instructions carefully. Students often read only part of the test instructions and make serious mistakes because they do not fully understand what they are being asked to do. Read every question completely and carefully. Make sure you fully understand each question. Read each of the answers before choosing one. Remember that on multiple-choice questions, there are often at least two answers that appear to be correct. Only after carefully reading all of the answers will you be able to make the correct choice. Also, even when you don't know which answer is correct, by reading all the answers you should be able to eliminate a number of incorrect answers and thus improve your success at guessing. In the science sections, you should practice estimating what the answer should look like. This technique can save you time and improve your test score. One useful text on this subject is *Estimation In Problem Solving In Chemistry, 1989* (by Green and Garland).

If you finish any section of the practice MCAT exam before the time is up, use the extra time to go over your answers. If the time is running out and you know you are not going to be able to complete a section, spend the final few minutes guessing at answers. Do not leave any answer blank. As previously stated, there is no penalty for guessing on the MCAT exam. When taking the practice exam, mark the point where you started guessing, and then proceed to answer by guessing the answers to whatever questions are left. This gives you a more accurate practice test score. If you are unable to complete a section of the exam within the allotted time, either you must learn to pace yourself better or you do not know the material well enough. Pacing improves as you take more practice exams and your knowledge improves as you review more extensively.

When you have completed the exam, check your answers with the correct answers that follow the exam. Your scores on the second practice exam should be a good indication of the kind of progress that you are making. The exam should also tell you whether your studying is effective. If there is no improvement on the second exam, be honest with yourself as you answer the following questions: How much time have you really spent studying? Did you go over the questions you missed carefully? Have you gone over your class notes? Have you reviewed your science textbooks, especially in your areas of weaknesses? Have you developed a detailed study plan and have you followed the plan?

Regularize Your MCAT Study

Set aside a regular time for your MCAT studying. You should choose a time that does not interfere with other studying that you have to do. If your MCAT studying conflicts with your school studying, one or the other or both will probably suffer. In addition to setting aside study time for the MCAT, you should set aside time at least once a week for either a practice section exam or a practice test. This will guarantee that you get sufficient practice taking exams like the MCAT to improve your test-taking skills.

Use Study Groups

The use of study groups can be effective in preparing for the MCAT exam. Study groups can help to provide the discipline you need to keep to your study schedule and can also be another important resource for MCAT study.

A good size for a study group is from three to six members. This group size provides enough diversity of information and knowledge to be helpful when studying without being so large that the group becomes hard to control. The pooling of different academic strengths can compensate for the weaknesses of individual members.

Study groups should meet at least once a week and for at least two hours at a time. It's best to schedule these weekly meetings at the end of the week as a culmination of the week's studying. Each member of the study group should be assigned a topic that he or she is responsible for going over with the group. Assigning responsibilities helps to ensure that every member of the group can be held accountable and therefore encourages each member of the group to do his or her fair share. Study groups succeed when everyone in the group takes responsibility for a part of the work that has to be completed. However, study groups do not work well when one or several members of the group fail to do their fair share of the work.

Study groups also can help you practice for the exam. Study group members can quiz each other, thus helping each member of the group to increase the pace at which he or she answers questions. It is a good idea to have each member of the study group come to each session with a prepared set of questions on the topic that he or she has been assigned, to explain to the rest of the group. These questions can be used to test what you know on a subject, and when you don't know something, the person who made up the question can explain the answer.

Study groups are also helpful in improving your writing skills for the essay section of the exam. Members of the group can pick writing topics on which to quiz each other and can be very helpful in correcting each other's essays. It is hard to evaluate your own writing, but other people can give you an accurate appraisal of your work. In addition, editing other members' writing can help you improve your own writing skills.

Take Practice Exam III

Even if you believe that you are fully prepared for the MCAT exam, you should keep on practicing. The more you study in a systematic manner, the better you will do on the examination. The more familiar you are with the material, the less likely you are to make careless mistakes on the exam. Remember that on the MCAT, you not only need to know the material, but you also need to be able to recall the information rapidly because you have only a very limited time to read and answer each question.

Reserve the final two to four weeks to eliminate any remaining weaknesses. This is the time to take Practice Exam III. This exam should give you a last-minute evaluation of where you are still weak and where you are strong. By now, you should be able to complete each section of the exam in the allotted amount of time and your score should be close to where you want it to be.

After grading the exam, go over the results carefully. As before, you need to know what sections on which you did not do well and what types of questions you missed. If your score is not anywhere near what you had hoped it would be, perhaps you should consider postponing the test to the next available date. It is better to postpone the exam and do well than to take the exam sooner and do poorly. If you have been studying for several weeks, using both the review sections and the practice exams, your score should show substantial improvement from earlier practice exams. There may, however, still be some areas in which your score was not what you had hoped it would be. These are the areas that you need to focus on during the final two to four weeks before the exam.

Score Yourself

Use the scoring guide on the following page to give yourself some indication as to how well you have done on the practice exams. The guide should help you to identify your areas of weakness so that you can direct your study where it will do you the most good. You might also want to highlight your score on each successive practice exam to keep track of your increasing expertise on the MCAT. Do be aware, however, that this guide is only an approximation. This is not the actual scoring mechanism used on the MCAT. The range of raw scores contributing to each scaled score is adjusted with each administration of the MCAT to take into account variations in difficulty of questions.

Physical Sciences		Verbal Reasoning		Biological Sciences	
Raw Score	Scaled Score	Raw Score	Scaled Score	Raw Score	Scaled Score
0–9	1	0–6	1	0–8	1
10–17	2	7–14	2	9–17	2
18–28	3	15–21	3	18–29	3
29–34	4	22–28	4	30–34	4
35–39	5	29–34	5	35–40	5
40–45	6	35–38	6	41–46	6
46–49	7	39–43	7	47–51	7
50–56	8	44–48	8	52–58	8
57–61	9	49–53	9	59–64	9
62–65	10	54–56	10	65–68	10
66–69	11	57–59	11	69–70	11
70–72	12	60–61	12	71–72	12
73–74	13	62–63	13	62–63	13
75–76	14	64	14	74–76	14
77	15	65	15	77	15

THE FOUR SECTIONS OF THE MCAT EXAM REQUIRE DIFFERENT TYPES OF STUDYING

The four sections of the MCAT exam are quite different from each other. There are two science sections: one for the physical sciences (general chemistry and physics) and one for biological sciences (general biology and organic chemistry). Both the Biological and Physical Science sections are problem-based. This means that although the answers are in multiple-choice format, to answer the questions you must solve problems in the physical and biological sciences. You will also need to review mathematical skills through pre-calculus, as these skills will be needed in both the physical and biological sections of the MCAT exam. (When preparing for the MCAT exam Physical and Biological Science sections, be sure to do all mathematical calculations without a calculator because calculators are not allowed when taking the MCAT exam. Do not assume that you know how to do these calculations. Remember, it may have been a long time since you worked without a calculator.)

Physical Sciences

The Physical Sciences section includes inorganic chemistry and physics. The knowledge required for this section of the exam includes the basic concepts covered in the first year of general chemistry and the first year of physics. Knowledge acquired beyond this level is not required to be successful on this part of the exam. No math beyond pre-calculus is required to solve problems on this section of the exam. However, some knowledge of basic statistics is needed for both the Physical and Biological Sciences sections.

The test contains 10 or 11 problem sets based on written passages with 4 to 8 questions on each problem set. The Physical Science section also contains an additional 15 independent questions. The total number of questions in the section is 77. The questions are designed to test your knowledge of basic concepts and may include graphs, charts, and tables. You will be given 1 hour and 40 minutes to answer these questions, which means you have approximately 1 minute and 14 seconds to spend on each question in this section.

The specific concepts covered include the following: acids/bases, atomic and nuclear structure, bonding, electrochemistry, electronic circuits, electrostatic and electromagnetism, electronic structure and the periodic table, equilibrium and momentum, fluids and solids, force and motion, gravitation, light and geometrical optics, phases and phase equilibria, rate processes in chemical reactions, kinetics and equilibrium, solution chemistry, sound, stoichiometry, thermodynamics and thermochemistry, translational motion, wave characteristics and periodic motion, and work and energy. Although these are the main areas covered in physical science, other areas may also be touched.

To be successful on this section of the exam, you must be able to use key formulas and equations that you learned in your first-year chemistry and physics courses. It is important not only to know these formulas and equations, but also to be able to use them quickly and easily. Many of the key formulas and equations you need to know are covered in a later section of this book, but it is also a good idea to review your textbook and class notes before taking the MCAT exam.

Verbal Reasoning

The Verbal Reasoning section consists of nine articles ranging in length from 500 to 600 words, taken from the sciences, social sciences, and humanities. Each article is followed by six to ten questions for a total of 60 questions to be answered in 85 minutes. No prior knowledge of subject material is needed for this section.

Although this section does not require specific subject knowledge, it does require both effective reading and comprehension abilities. The questions require not only the ability to remember information that you have just read, but also the ability to interpret the information and draw conclusions that go beyond the scope of the article. Many students will feel that they are already effective readers and therefore do not need to study for this section of the exam. Taking the pretest will probably prove most of them wrong. Other students will recognize that they might not do well on this kind of exam, but will be convinced that there is no way to study for this exam. Using the material in the Verbal Reasoning section of this book will prove them wrong too. Practice with Verbal Reasoning questions can and will improve your performance on this section of the exam.

The Verbal Reasoning section of the MCAT exam tests a number of specific skills. You may be asked to recognize information that supports a writer's thesis and to evaluate additional information that does not support the writer's argument. You may be asked to evaluate the strengths and weaknesses of a particular author's arguments or to use information given in a passage to solve problems that are not directly included in the passage. You may be asked what effect new information might have on the conclusions of specific passages and how broad conclusions, explanations, and hypotheses can be applied.

In addition to using the material in this book, you should also get into the habit of reading scientific and other scholarly periodicals. Ask yourself what the article was about, what information could be gathered directly from the article, and what information was implied by or could be inferred from the article. Be sure when you use the review section in this book to answer the practice questions under the pressure of time. It's a good idea to use a stopwatch. Remember that you are not only being asked to read for accuracy and understand complicated arguments, but also to answer questions on the articles in 40 seconds per question.

Writing Sample

The writing sample on the MCAT exam is based on the experimental writing section that has been used on previous MCAT exams. The section consists of two 30-minute essays on specific topics presented in the test. Each writing sample item consists of a statement followed by three writing tasks. The first task is to explain the statement. The second task is to provide an example illustrating a viewpoint opposite to the statement given. The third is to discuss how the conflict between these two opposing statements might be resolved.

Your essays will be read by two readers who are looking for your ability to organize an answer, explain the statement, develop a central concept, synthesize conflicting concepts and ideas, and express yourself clearly and correctly.

The essay topics will not be controversial subjects such as religion or politics, nor will they be medical topics or topics requiring prior knowledge. The essays are scored on a scale of J to T. J is the lowest possible score and T is the highest. Failure to respond to any one of the three writing tasks will reduce your score by three points. Any school to which you send your MCAT scores will receive your writing score. Copies of your essays will be sent to those medical schools that request them.

Don't assume that you will be successful on this section because you have been a good writer in the past. The nature of the topics and the fact that you will be writing under the pressure of time should convince you of the need for extensive essay-writing practice to succeed on this section of the exam.

Studying for the written part of this exam means spending a lot of time writing. If you are a science major, your writing skills are likely to be rusty. After taking your practice test, go over your essays. If possible, ask a teacher or friend who has strong writing skills to go over your essays. On the MCAT exam, it is expected that you can write at the college level. Even though you are writing under pressure of a time limit, you are expected to produce a cohesive, well-organized, and grammatically correct essay.

Biological Sciences

The Biological Sciences section tests biological concepts covered in the first year of general biology (some genetic concepts may be included that may not have been covered in your first-year biology course), as well as concepts covered in the first year of organic chemistry. Topics in cellular and molecular biology are likely to be stressed, as are other topics that could have potential medical applications. It's a good idea to review general statistical concepts, particularly as they pertain to genetics and environmental concepts. The biology section of this book highlights information that is important for the MCAT exam.

The Biological Sciences section focuses on the following specific topics in biology: molecular biology (biological molecules, proteins as enzymes, cellular metabolism, nucleic acids, protein synthesis), cellular biology (eukaryotic cells, cell membranes and membrane transport, cell reproduction, eukaryotic tissues), microbiology (prokaryotic cells, bacteria, viruses, fungi), vertebrate organ systems (integumentary, skeletal, muscle, nervous, sensory, endocrine, circulatory, lymphatic and immune, respiratory, digestive, excretory, reproductive, embryology and development), genetics, and evolution. Specific topics in organic chemistry include molecular structure of organic molecules (sigma and pi bonds, multiple bonding, stereochemistry), hydrocarbons (saturated/alkanes, unsaturated/alkenes, aromatic compounds), oxygen-containing compounds (alcohols, aldehydes, ketones, carboxylic acids, common acid derivatives, ethers, phenols), amines (description, principles, reactions, quaternary ammonium salts), biological molecules (amino acids and proteins, carbohydrates, lipids, phosphorus compounds), spectroscopy (nuclear magnetic resonance, infrared), separations, and purifications (distillation, crystallization, extraction, chromatography). These topics will be emphasized, but others may also be included.

The Biological Sciences problem-solving section includes 10 to 11 problem sets, each consisting of a written passage followed by 4 to 8 multiple-choice questions. This section also includes 15 independent multiple-choice questions, for a total of 77 questions. You will be given 1 hour and 4 minutes to answer these questions, which amounts to approximately 1 minute and 14 seconds for each question.

Unit One

PHYSICAL SCIENCES

INTRODUCTION

The Physical Science section of the MCAT exam tests your knowledge and understanding of important topics of general chemistry and physics. In the following sections, the important aspects of each of these topics are presented followed by multiple-choice questions to help you assess your mastery of the material. Answers to these questions are provided along with explanations. As indicated in the Introduction to the Biological Sciences, your knowledge will be tested in a variety of formats. However, keep in mind that a thorough understanding of important chemical and physical principles is required regardless of the format of questions or problems presented. In addition, knowledge of basic mathematical skills is required. These are listed below for you.

Examples of passages and independent questions in the Physical Science section are provided in the Sample Questions and Practice Exams. These examples will not only serve as a review but will acquaint you with the various passage formats you will encounter on the exam.

REQUIRED MATH SKILLS

1. Arithmetic Operations
   - proportion
   - ratio
   - percentage
   - estimation of square root

2. Math skills at the level of a second-year algebra High School course
   - exponentials (base 10 and natural logarithms)
   - scientific notation
   - solutions of quadratic and simultaneous equations
   - graphical representation of data and functions including associated terminology (e.g., abscissa, ordinate, slope or rate of change)
   - reciprocals
   - various scales (arithmetic, semilog vs. arithmetic, log vs. log)

3. Basic trigonometric functions
   - values of sine and cosine of 0°, 90°, and 180°
   - relationship between length of sides of a right triangle containing 30°, 45°, and 60° angles
   - understanding of the inverse of the trigonometric functions

4. Units and Their Manipulation
   - common metric units and their conversion factors (Memorization of conversion factors between the metric and English system is not required.)
   - balance equations with physical units

5. Experimental Error
   - relative magnitude of experimental error
   - effect of propagation of error
   - reasonable estimates
   - significant figures of a value

6. Mathematical calculation of the probability of an event at an elementary level

7. Vectors
   - addition
   - subtraction
   - right hand rule (dot and cross product not required)

8. Simple statistical concepts
   - arithmetic mean
   - range of a set of data
   - standard deviation as a measure of variability
   - general concepts of statistical correlation and association (calculations not required)

CHAPTER 1

Chemistry

1.1 STOICHIOMETRY

Stoichiometry is the branch of chemistry that treats mass relationships in chemical reactions. Important tools for solving problems in stoichiometry include the concepts of molecular formula, molecular weight, balanced equation, and mole.

A. MOLECULAR FORMULAS

A molecular formula expresses the composition of a molecule. Subscripts indicate multiple atoms. Examples include

    Ar—argon; 1 atom per molecule

    H_2O—water; 3 atoms per molecule

    C_2H_5OH—ethanol; 9 atoms per molecule

In addition, chemical formulas are written for a wide number of compounds whose atoms form extended structures rather than individual molecules; the formula shows the simplest ratio of the atoms in the compound. Example:

    $MgCl_2$—magnesium chloride: extended structure, with 2 chloride ions for every 1 magnesium ion.

B. MOLECULAR WEIGHT

The molecular weight of a compound is calculated by adding the separate atomic weights of all of the atoms that constitute the compound. The units of atomic weight and molecular weight are u (atomic mass units). Molecular weight is computed using the molecular formula and a table of atomic weights. The formula weight of an ionic compound is calculated in a similar way.

EXAMPLE

Find the molecular weight of sucrose, $C_{12}H_{22}O_{11}$.

SOLUTION

A table gives the following atomic weights, in units of u.

    C 12.01;

    H 1.008

    O 16.00

    $\text{wt} = 12(12.01) + 22(1.008) + 11(16.00)$

        $= 342.3 \text{ u}$

C. EMPIRICAL FORMULA

Often an elemental analysis of a compound will enable an investigator to determine the **empirical formula** of a compound. This is the formula that expresses the *lowest whole-number ratio* of the atoms in the formula. For example, while the molecular formula of hydrogen peroxide is H_2O_2, the empirical formula is H_1O_1, or HO. (Examples of calculation of empirical formulas are given in section F.)

D. DESCRIPTION OF COMPOSITION USING PERCENT MASS

If H_2O_2 is analyzed, it is found to contain 5.9% hydrogen by weight and 94.1% oxygen by weight; this is a statement of its percent weight, or percent mass. We could predict these percentages by knowing the molecular (or empirical) formula, since each molecule of hydrogen peroxide must contain a fraction of hydrogen equal to:

$$\text{(at. wt. of 2 H's)}/\text{(at. wt. of 2 H's + at. wt. of 2 Os)} = (2.0)/(2.0 + 32.0)$$
$$= 0.059 \text{ (or 5.9%)}$$

A similar calculation for oxygen shows that water contains 94.1% oxygen.

E. METRIC UNITS

The units commonly employed in solving chemistry problems are metric units, or "SI" units. The principal units, with their common abbreviations, follow:

Length	meter (m)
Mass	kilogram (kg)
Time	second (s)
Temperature	Kelvin (K)
Current	ampere (A)
Quantity of substance	mole (mol)
Luminous intensity	candela (cd)

From these fundamental units several other very useful units can be derived:

Volume	liter (L)	0.001 m^3
Force	newton (N)	1 kg m/s^2
Energy	joule (J)	$1 \text{ kg m}^2/\text{s}^2$
Power	watt (W)	1 J/s
Pressure	pascal (Pa)	1 N/m^2
Electrical potential	volt (V)	1 W/A

The flexibility of SI units derives in large part from the prefixes that are used. For example, we may express a wavelength of 5.22×10^{-9} m in the more convenient form 522 nanometers (nm), where

$$1 \text{ nm} = 10^{-9} \text{ m}$$

We may also combine the prefix nano- with gram, second, liter, mole, or any other basic unit.

The following prefixes are most commonly used; here they are combined with gram:

megagram	(Mg)	10^6 gram
kilogram	(kg)	10^3 gram
decigram	(dg)	10^{-1} gram
centigram	(cg)	10^{-2} gram
milligram	(mg)	10^{-3} gram
microgram	(mg)	10^{-6} gram
nanogram	(ng)	10^{-9} gram
picogram	(pg)	10^{-12} gram

F. THE MOLE CONCEPT: AVOGADRO'S NUMBER

One **mole** of a substance is the amount equal to its molecular weight or formula weight expressed in units of grams. For example, since the atomic weight of iron is 55.85 amu, one mole of iron is a sample containing 55.85 g. Equivalently, we say that the **molar mass** of Fe = 55.85 g.

Each mole of any element or compound contains the same number of molecules. This number—quite a large one—is called Avogadro's number. Its value, expressed to four significant figures, is 6.022×10^{23}.

Here are a number of useful relationships involving mass of a compound, number of moles, and number of molecules:

1. number of moles $= \dfrac{\text{(mass in grams)}}{\text{(molar Mass)}}$

2. mass (g) = (number of moles) $\times$ (molar mass)

3. number of molecules = (Avogadro's number) $\times$ (number of moles)

These relationships are often expressed using "conversion factors," as in the examples that follow, which illustrate "modular" one-step calculations based on the above relationships.

1. "Grams → moles"
   Find the number of moles in 12.0 g of O_2
   12.0 g O_2 $\times$ (1 mol O_2/32.0 g O_2) = 0.375 mol O_2

2. "Moles → grams"
   Find the number of grams of H_2SO_4 in 0.100 mole of the compound.
   0.100 mol H_2SO_4 $\times$ (98.1 g/mol H_2SO_4) = 0.981 g

3. "Moles → number of molecules"
   How many molecules are represented by the 1.40 moles of H_2O produced above?
   1.40 mol $\times$ (6.022×10^{23} molecules/mol) = 8.43×10^{23} molecules

Here is an example that employs these relationships to calculate an empirical and a molecular formula.

EXAMPLE

A compound containing only carbon and hydrogen is found to have a composition that is 75.0% C and 25.0% H by weight. Its molar mass is determined to be 16.03 g/mol. Find its empirical and molecular formulas.

SOLUTION

1. Assume a given total mass of the compound, say 100 g.

2. From the percentages given, the sample must contain 75.0 g of C and 25.0 g of H.

3. moles C = 75.0 g/ (12.0 g/mol) = 6.25 mol
   moles H = 25.0 g/ (1.0 g/mole) = 25.0 mol

4. Ratio of moles H to moles C = 25.0/6.25 = 4.00

5. Round the result and determine that the empirical formula is CH_4.

6. Since the molar mass is known to be 16.03 g/mol, we can say that in this example, the molecular formula must also be CH_4. (This is not always the case; in general, the molecular formula is related to the empirical formula by whole number multiples.)

EXAMPLE

A sample of a hydrocarbon weighing 4.19 g is burned in oxygen to produce 12.5 g $CO_2(g)$ and 6.85 g $H_2O(l)$. Find the empirical formula of the sample.

SOLUTION

1. Moles of CO_2 = 12.5 g/ (44.0 g/mol) = 0.284 mol

2. Then moles C in original sample = 0.284 mol (since each original C leads to one CO_2 molecule)

3. Moles H_2O produced = 6.85 g/ (18.02 g/mol) = 0.380 mol

4. Then moles H in original sample = 2(0.380 mol) = 0.760 mol (since each H_2O resulted from 2 H's)

5. Calculate empirical formula using
   moles H/moles C = 0.760 mol/0.284 = 2.68 = 8/3
   empirical formula = C_3H_8

EXAMPLE

A sample of unknown metal "M" weighing 0.755 g reacts with oxygen to form 1.057 g of metal oxide MO. Find the molar mass of "M."

SOLUTION

1. The mass of oxygen that reacted was (1.057 − 0.755) g = 0.302 g

2. The moles of oxygen *atoms* that reacted was 0.302 g/(16.00 g/mol) = 0.0189 mol.

3. From the formula "MO," the moles of "M" must also be 0.0189 mol.

4. Then for "M,"
   molar mass = mass/# of moles = 0.755 g/(0.0189 mol) = 39.9 g/mol

In a later section, we will explain how the mole concept can be applied to a wide range of chemical problems.

G. DENSITY

The concept of **density** is defined as mass/volume. Densities of liquids and solids lie in the range of 0.5 to 23 g/cm^3, while densities of gases at 1 atm are typically on the order of 0.001 g/cm^3.

EXAMPLE

Find the density of a solid sample whose volume is 16.8 cm^3 and whose mass is 35.4 g.

SOLUTION

$$D = \frac{35.4 \text{ g}}{16.8 \text{ cm}^3} = 2.11 \text{ g/cm}^3$$

H. OXIDATION AND REDUCTION: OXIDATION NUMBERS

Oxidation is defined as the loss of electrons; **reduction** is the gain of electrons.

A redox reaction (or "oxidation-reduction reaction") is one in which oxidation and reduction take place.

When a neutral atom *loses* electrons, its **oxidation number** (or oxidation state) changes from 0 to a positive value, and it is said to be *oxidized*. When a neutral atom *gains* electrons, its oxidation number changes to a negative value and it is said to be *reduced*.

Rules for Assigning Oxidation Numbers

1. Neutral atoms have an oxidation number of 0.

2. In ions consisting of single atoms, the oxidation number is equal to the charge on the ion.

3. The H atom usually has an oxidation number of $+1$, except in H_2, where it is 0, and in hydride compounds such as CaH_2, where it is -1.

4. The oxidation number of O is usually -2; common exceptions are in O_2, where it is 0, and in H_2O_2, where it is -1.

5. The oxidation numbers of the atoms in a molecule or an ion must sum to the overall charge on that molecule or that ion.

Oxidizing and Reducing Agents

An oxidizing agent is reduced (its oxidation number is decreased) in the course of a reaction.

A reducing agent is oxidized (its oxidation number is increased) in the course of a reaction.

To avoid confusion, note what the term "agent" implies. A reducing agent causes another species to be reduced, while it is itself oxidized. The reverse is true for an oxidizing agent.

Reducing agents that are commonly used include:

$S_2O_3^{2-}$ (thiosulfate)
Cr^{2+}
Zn
HI
As_2O_3

Oxidizing agents commonly used include:

Ce^{4+}
I_2
$Cr_2O_7^{2-}$ (dichromate)
MnO_4^- (permanganate)

Oxidization-Reduction Titrations

An oxidizing agent or reducing agent of known concentration can be used to determine the amount of an unknown species in a solution. For example, the amount of Fe^{2+} in a solution can be determined by adding Ce^{4+} of known concentration. The titration reaction is

$$Ce^{4+}(aq) + Fe^{2+}(aq) \rightarrow Ce^{3+}(aq) + Fe^{3+}(aq)$$

During the reaction, the cerium ion (the oxidizing agent) oxidizes the ferrous ion from the +2 state to the +3 state. A chemical or electrochemical means is used to indicate the equivalence point. The balanced equation for the reaction is used to determine the amount of Fe^{2+} from the quantity of Ce^{4+} used.

I. CHEMICAL EQUATIONS: BALANCING

By use of formulas for molecules or salts, we can write equations that indicate entire chemical reactions. For example, when water is formed, the following **chemical equation** describes the reactants and product:

$$H_2 + O_2 \rightarrow H_2O$$

While the equation lists the participating species correctly, it fails to predict the proper weight relationship. The reaction needs to be **balanced**—to have coefficients added in front of the reactants and products that will cause the number of each atom on the left to equal that on the right.

The balanced equation is

$$2H_2 + O_2 \rightarrow 2H_2O$$

To confirm that the balancing is correct, we count total H atoms (4 on each side) and total O atoms (2 on each side). If the number of each atom is not the same on the left as on the right, we must have made an error.

Balancing can often be done by simple trial-and-error, but there are several rules that can be followed:

1. Isolate atoms that occur only once each on the right and left; balance for these atoms first.

2. If groups of atoms such as SO_4^{2-}, OH^-, etc., occur on the left and the right, it may be useful to balance these as groups rather than individual atoms.

3. Remember that you are not free to alter the subscripts; e.g., you can't change an H_2O to an H_3O as a means to balance hydrogen. Preserve the original molecular formulas.

4. Oxidation-reduction reactions have special procedures. To learn how to spot such reactions, and how to balance them, read the following section.

5. Always check the result by carefully counting atoms on each side. Be certain too that the total charge is the same on each side.

Balancing Oxidation-Reduction Reactions

The complexity of redox reactions requires a more systematic method than the one described above. The example below illustrates two general methods for balancing these reactions: (1) the "half reaction" method and (2) the "oxidation number" method.

EXAMPLE

Balance the following reaction, which occurs in acidic solution:

$$Ag + NO_3^- \rightarrow Ag^+ + NO$$

SOLUTION

Half-Reaction Method

Step 1

Separate the overall reaction into half reactions involving the species being oxidized and reduced:

(a) $Ag \rightarrow Ag^+$

(b) $NO_3^- \rightarrow NO$

Step 2

Balance the number of atoms in each half reaction:

(a) $Ag \rightarrow Ag^+$ No changes are needed here.

(b) $NO_3^- \rightarrow NO + 2H_2O$

In (b), we added O's to the right by adding H_2O's. Now we balance out the added H's on the left using H^+—acceptable since the solution is to be acidic (for basic solutions, see below):

(b) $NO_3^- + 4H^+ \rightarrow NO + 2H_2O$

Step 3

The atoms now balance in each half reaction but the charges don't, so add electrons as needed to the side that has the more positive total charge:

(a) $Ag \rightarrow Ag^+ + e^-$

(b) $NO_3^- + 4H^+ + 3e^- \rightarrow NO + 2H_2O$

As expected, this charge balance exercise confirms that (a) is an oxidation, (b) a reduction.

Step 4
Multiply (a) by 3 in order to have the same number of electrons in each half reaction:

(a) $3Ag \rightarrow 3Ag^+ + 3 e^-$

Step 5
Add the two half reactions together to get a result that contains no e^-'s, the same species as specified at the start, some H^+'s, and some H_2O's:

$$3Ag + NO_3^- + 4H^+ \rightarrow 3Ag^+ + NO + 2H_2O$$

Had the solution been specified as being alkaline rather than acidic, we could not have added H+ in Step 2. Methods for balancing reactions in basic solution are discussed at the end of this section.

Oxidation Number Method

Step 1
Identify the oxidation numbers of each reactant and product species that undergoes oxidation or reduction:

$$Ag(0) \rightarrow Ag(+1); \ N(+5) \rightarrow N(+2)$$

Step 2
Multiply the Ag or N species by coefficients; this will make the change in oxidation numbers the same for each atom (here, multiply each Ag species by 3):

$$3Ag + NO_3^- \rightarrow 3Ag^+ + NO$$

Step 3
Add H_2O and H^+ in order to balance H and O in the equation:

$$3Ag + NO_3^- + 4H^+ \rightarrow 3Ag^+ + NO + 2H_2O$$

EXAMPLE
Use the half reaction method to balance the following, which occurs in *basic* solution:

$$MnO_4^-(aq) + NH_3(aq) \rightarrow NO_3^-(aq) + MnO_2(s)$$

Method 1
Using OH^- to balance half-reactions.

Step 1
Separate the reaction into half-reactions:

(a) $MnO_4^- \rightarrow MnO_2$

(b) $NH_3 \rightarrow NO_3^-$

Step 2
Balance atoms. No changes needed here.

Step 3
Add OH^- and H_2O to balance O and H (this may take some time!)

    (a) $MnO_4^- + 2H_2O \rightarrow MnO_2 + 4OH^-$

    (b) $NH_3 + 9OH^- \rightarrow NO_3^- + 6H_2O$

Step 4
Add electrons to balance charge:

    (a) $MnO_4^- + 2H_2O + 3e^- \rightarrow MnO_2 + 4OH^-$

    (b) $NH_3 + 9OH^- \rightarrow NO_3^- + 6H_2O + 8e^-$

Step 5
Multiply the top reaction by 8 and the bottom reaction by 3, so that the electrons will cancel:

    (a) $8MnO_4^- + 16H_2O + 24\,e^- \rightarrow 8\,MnO_2 + 32\,OH^-$

    (b) $3NH_3 + 27OH^- \rightarrow 3NO_3^- + 18H_2O + 24e^-$

Step 6
Add the reactions, canceling electrons and combining H_2O's and OH^-'s:

$$8MnO_4^- + 3NH_3 \rightarrow 8MnO_2 + 3NO_3^- + 5OH^- + 2H_2O$$

Method 2
Using H^+ at the start, converting to OH^- at the end. (This method requires an extra step 2, but usually saves time in the half-reaction balancing process.) We'll use the same example as before.

Steps 1 and 2
Same as above.

Step 3
We balance half-reactions as if the reaction took place in acidic solution, adding H^+ and H_2O.

    (a) $MnO_4^- + 4H^+ \rightarrow MnO_2 + 2H_2O$

    (b) $NH_3 + 3H_2O \rightarrow NO_3^- + 9H^+$

Step 4
Add electrons to balance charge:

    (a) $MnO_4^- + 4H^+ + 3e^- \rightarrow MnO_2 + 2H_2O$

    (b) $NH_3 + 3H_2O \rightarrow NO_3^- + 9H^+ + 8\,e^-$

Step 5
Multiply the top reaction by 8 and the bottom by 3:

    (a) $8MnO_4^- + 32H^+ + 24e^- \rightarrow 8MnO_2 + 16H_2O$

    (b) $3NH_3 + 9H_2O \rightarrow 3NO_3^- + 27H^+ + 24e^-$

Step 6

Combine the 2 equations, canceling when possible:

$$8MnO_4^- + 3NH_3 + 5H^+ \rightarrow 8MnO_2 + 3NO_3^- + 7H_2O$$

Step 7

Now we must remove H^+ ions and insert OH^- ions, to reflect the reality that the reaction occurs in basic solution. To do this we add 5 OH^-'s to each side. On the left, these can be combined with the 5 H^+ ions, and the result will be 5 H_2O's. Those added to the right will remain unchanged:

$$8MnO_4^- + 3NH_3 + 5H_2O \rightarrow 8MnO_2 + 3NO_3^- + 7H_2O + 5OH^-$$

Step 8

Now cancel H_2O's;

$$8MnO_4^- + 3NH_3 \rightarrow 8MnO_2 + 3NO_3^- + 2H_2O + 5OH^-$$

The result is the same as that obtained by introducing hydroxide ion early in the process. Because the balancing in Step 3 is usually easier using H+ ions, the second method is generally faster.

We explore the implications of balanced reactions in the following examples.

J. APPLYING THE MOLE CONCEPT TO CALCULATIONS INVOLVING CHEMICAL REACTIONS

The Meaning of the Balanced Equation

Reconsider the equation—now balanced—for the formation of water:

$$2H_2 + O_2 \rightarrow 2H_2O$$

This equation can be used to make several meaningful statements about the proportions of reacting species:

There are 2 molecules of hydrogen gas that react with every 1 molecule of oxygen.

The number of water molecules produced equals the number of hydrogen molecules that react.

Twice as many water molecules are formed as there were oxygen molecules reacting.

1. "Grams → moles"

   Using the reaction $2NO + O_2 \rightarrow 2NO_2$, find the number of moles NO_2 produced by the complete reaction of 8.00 g of O_2.

   Plan: This problem requires two of the modular steps given earlier:

   $$g\ O_2 \rightarrow mol\ O_2 \rightarrow mol\ NO_2$$

   8.00 g O_2 × (1 mol O_2/32 g/mol O_2) × (2 mol NO_2/1 mol O_2) = 0.500 mol NO_2

2. "Grams → grams"

   Find the number of grams of NO that will react with 14.0 g of O_2 in the above reaction.

   Plan: $g\ O_2 \rightarrow mol\ O_2 \rightarrow mol\ NO \rightarrow g\ NO$

14.0 g O_2 $\times$ (1 mol O_2/32 g O_2/mol) $\times$ (2 mol NO/1 mol O_2) $\times$ (30.0 g NO/1 mol NO) = 26.2 g NO

3. Composition of a compound

5.00 g of a compound containing only C and H is burned in air, and 13.8 g of CO_2 is recovered. What was the mass composition of the original compound?

Plan: g CO_2 formed $\rightarrow$ mol CO_2 formed $\rightarrow$ mol C at outset $\rightarrow$ original g C $\rightarrow$ % of C

mol CO_2 = (13.8 g)/(44.0 g/mol) = 0.314 mol

original mol C = 0.314 mol as well

original g of C = 0.314 mol $\times$ 12.0 g/mol = 3.77 g C

% of C = (3.77/5.00) $\times$ 100% = 75.4%

% of H = (100% $-$ 75.4%) = 24.6%

Limiting Reactant Problems

In limiting reactant problems, there is always a mismatch between the relative amounts of two or more reactants, with the result that one, the limiting reactant ("LR"), is completely consumed, while some amount of the other remains. Here is an example:

EXAMPLE

2.0 moles each of H_2 and O_2 are reacted. How many moles of H_2O are formed?

SOLUTION 1

Recall that the balanced equation is $2H_2 + O_2 \rightarrow 2H_2O$.

If we needed equal numbers of moles of H_2 and O_2, we would have a simple problem—but instead we need twice as much H_2. Therefore, *all* the H_2 will be used up, and half the O_2 will remain. The 2.0 moles of hydrogen consumed will produce 2.0 moles of H_2O.

In the example above we could determine the "limiting reactant" by inspection. In a more general method, we assume that each reactant in turn is the limiting reactant and determine the amount of the second reactant that is needed. If there is a sufficient amount of the second reactant, then the first is the LR. Otherwise, the second reactant is the LR.

EXAMPLE

Consider the reaction

$2HCl(aq) + Na_2CO_3(s) \rightarrow 2NaCl(aq) + CO_2(g) + H_2O(l)$

If 0.126 moles of HCl(aq) are combined with 0.062 moles of $Na_2CO_3(s)$, find the moles of $CO_2(g)$ that will be produced.

SOLUTION

We solve the problem using the following chart:

	2HCl	+	Na$_2$CO$_3$	→	2NaCl	+	CO$_2$	+	H$_2$O
Initial	0.126		0.062(LR)		—		—		—
Change	2(−0.062)		−0.062		+0.124		+0.062	+	0.062
Final	0.002		—		0.124		0.062		0.062

Because the amount of HCl appears to be greater than twice the amount of Na$_2$CO$_3$, we assume that Na$_2$CO$_3$ is the LR. Had we guessed instead that HCl was the limiting reactant, we would have calculated that the amount of Na$_2$CO$_3$ needed was

$$(1/2)(0.126 \text{ moles}) = 0.063 \text{ moles},$$

which is more than we had available. The chart provides complete information about final quantities; in particular, there are 0.062 moles of CO$_2$ produced.

PRACTICE PROBLEMS

1. An unknown amount of C$_3$H$_8$ is burned completely to H$_2$O and CO$_2$, with 36 g of H$_2$O recovered. How many moles of the hydrocarbon were originally present?

   A. 0.25
   B. 0.50
   C. 2
   D. $\dfrac{36}{8}$

2. A compound having an empirical formula of SO$_3$ is found to have a molecular weight of 80. What is its molecular formula?

   A. SO$_3$
   B. S$_2$O$_6$
   C. S$_3$O$_9$
   D. SO$_4$

3. Consider the reaction

   2Mg + O$_2$ → 2MgO

   If 100 g of each reactant are present at the start, which of the following will still be present after the reaction has proceeded to the maximum extent?

   A. Mg
   B. O$_2$
   C. 2 Mg
   D. cannot be determined

4. What is the maximum weight of CO$_2$ that can be produced from 3.0 g each of carbon and O$_2$?

   A. 3.0 g
   B. 4.1g
   C. 6.0 g
   D. 11.0 g

5. Which of the following is (are) true of the reaction that follows? (Assume all reactants are lined up.)

   2MnO$_4^-$ + 5H$_2$O$_2$ + 6H$^+$ → 2Mn^{2+} + 5O$_2$ + 8H$_2$O

   I. The initial number of O atoms equals the final number of O atoms.
   II. The total number of moles are conserved during the reaction.
   III. The final number of moles of O$_2$ equal $\dfrac{6}{5}$ of the initial number of moles of H$^+$.

   A. I only
   B. II only
   C. III only
   D. I and III only

6. In the reaction in Question 5, which of the following quantities are equal?

    I.   initial moles MnO_4^- and final moles Mn^{2+}

    II.   initial grams H^+ and final grams H_2O

    III.   initial molecules H_2O_2 and final molecules H_2O

    A.   I only

    B.   II only

    C.   III only

    D.   I and II only

7. Using the reaction of Question 5, find the moles of oxygen gas that will be produced by the reaction of 0.335 moles MnO_4^-, 1.12 moles H^+, and excess H_2O_2.

    A.   0.335 mol

    B.   0.838 mol

    C.   0.933 mol

    D.   1.120 mol

8. Balance the following reaction.

$$S + O_2 \rightarrow SO_3$$

    A. $S + O_3 \rightarrow SO_3$

    B. $2S + 3O_2 \rightarrow 2SO_3$

    C. $\frac{1}{3}S + \frac{2}{3}O_2 \rightarrow \frac{1}{3}SO_3$

    D. $3S + 2O_2 \rightarrow 3SO_3$

9. What is the formula weight of $Al_2(SO_4)_3$?

    A.   123

    B.   150

    C.   315

    D.   342

10. In the reaction of C_2H_6 with O_2 to form H_2O and CO_2, how many grams of H_2O are produced by the complete reaction of 7.00 g of C_2H_6?

    A.   0.234 g

    B.   0.700 g

    C.   4.20 g

    D.   12.6 g

11. A sample of gaseous N_2 contains 0.10 moles and occupies a volume of 7.0 m^3. Find its density in g/cm^3.

    A. $0.40 \ g/cm^3$

    B. $4.0 \times 10^{-3} \ g/cm^3$

    C. $4.0 \times 10^{-5} \ g/cm^3$

    D. $4.0 \times 10^{-7} \ g/cm_3$

ANSWER KEY

1. B   2. A   3. B   4. B   5. A   6. A   7. B   8. B   9. D   10. D   11. D

ANSWERS AND EXPLANATIONS

1. **The correct answer is (B).** The 36 grams of water represented 2 moles. Since the original hydrocarbon contained 4 times as many H's per mole as did the water, there must have been $\frac{1}{4} \times 2$ moles, or 0.5 moles of original C_3H_8.

2. **The correct answer is (A).** We can simply use trial-and-error; and the first try, SO_3 itself, proves to have a molecular weight of 80.

3. **The correct answer is (B).** There are 4.12 mol Mg and 3.13 mol O_2. If all the Mg reacts, it will use one-half as much O_2, or 1.57 mol, leaving some O_2 left over.

4. **The correct answer is (B).** The balanced equation is $C + O_2 \rightarrow CO_2$, so equal numbers of moles of each reactant are needed. But the number of moles of C present are 3.0 g/ (12.0 g/mol) = 0.25 mol, while the number of moles of O_2 = 3.0 g/ (32.0 g/mol) = 0.094 mol. Thus, O_2 is the limiting reactant, and the number of moles of CO_2 produced will be equal to the number of moles of O_2, or 0.094 mol. Therefore the mass of the product equals (0.094 mol)(44.0 g/mol) = 4.1 g.

5. **The correct answer is (A).** In a balanced reaction, atoms are conserved, but moles may not be; in this case, every 13 moles of reactant yields 15 moles product. Choice III would be true if the fraction were $\frac{5}{6}$, but it is false as written because the H_2O_2 that reacts also contributes H's.

6. **The correct answer is (A).** For I, moles of reactant and product indicated are equal owing to the equality of their coefficients. II is false, since the final H_2O weighs more than the initial H^+. III is false, since the coefficients are different.

7. **The correct answer is (B).** If we assume that permanganate is the LR, then we calculate that 3 times as much H^+ will be needed, or 1.005 moles. Since more than this amount of H^+ is provided, our assumption is correct. (Had we guessed H^+ as the LR, we would have predicted that $\frac{1}{3}$ (1.12 mol) = 0.373 mol of permanganate was needed—more than we had available.)

   moles O_2 produced = (0.335 moles MnO_4^-)
   (5 moles O_2 / 2 moles MnO_4^-) = 0.838 mol O_2

8. **The correct answer is (B).** Note that in A some of the species have been altered. Fractions are allowable, but those in C do not give a balanced equation. D is correct for S but not O.

9. **The correct answer is (D).** Add up all the atomic weights, being careful of all subscripts.

10. **The correct answer is (D).** The balanced reaction is $2C_2H_6 + 7O_2 \rightarrow 4CO_2 + 6H_2O$

    $$7.00 \text{ g } C_2H_6 \times \left(\frac{1 \text{ mole } C_2H_6}{30.0 \text{ g } C_2H_6} \right) \times \left(\frac{6 \text{ mol } H_2O}{2 \text{ mol } C_2H_6} \right) \times \left(\frac{18.0 \text{ g } H_2O}{1 \text{ mol } H_2O} \right) = 12.6 \text{ g } H_2O$$

11. **The correct answer is (D).** Mass N_2 = (0.10 mol) (28.0 g/mol) = 2.8 g

    $$\text{density} = \frac{2.8 \text{ g}}{7.0 \text{ m}^3} \times \left(\frac{1m}{10^2 cm} \right)^3 = 4.0 \times 10^{-7} \text{ g/cm}^3$$

1.2 ELECTRONIC STRUCTURE AND THE PERIODIC TABLE

A. ATOMS

Atoms are the fundamental building blocks of matter. Most of an atom's mass is concentrated in its nucleus, which contains varying numbers of **protons** (of charge +1) and **neutrons** (uncharged), packed into a relatively small volume.

Surrounding the nucleus are **electrons** (charge −1), lighter particles that swarm around in a much greater total volume than the nucleus.

The masses of these three fundamental particles are often expressed in *atomic mass units* (u), where $1\ u = 1.6605 \times 10^{-27}$ kg:

Proton: charge = +1; mass = 1.00728 u

Neutron: charge = 0; mass = 1.00866 u

Electron: charge = −1; mass = 5.49×10^{-4} u

The number of protons in the nucleus of an atom is called its **atomic number**. An **element** is a substance made up exclusively of atoms of a given atomic number—e.g., the element hydrogen has atomic number 1.

The **mass number** is defined as the sum of the number of protons and neutrons.

Isotopes

The number of neutrons may vary for a given atomic number. As a result, there can be several **isotopes** of an element, each with a different number of neutrons and thus a distinct atomic mass number. For example, the element chlorine has an invariant atomic number of 17, but 75.5% of chlorine atoms have 18 neutrons, and the remainder have 20 neutrons.

The standard means of representing these isotopes is

$^{35}_{17}Cl$ and $^{37}_{17}Cl$

The lower number is the atomic number, while the upper is the mass number.

If an element has several isotopes, the observed atomic weight can be calculated in the following way, illustrated using chlorine: The observed **atomic weight** of naturally occurring chlorine is the weighted average of the two isotopes:

observed at. wt. = (0.755)(35.0) + (0.245)(37.0) = 35.5 u

Ions

In a neutral atom, the number of electrons equals the number of protons, which in turn equals the atomic number. Many atoms exist in stable forms where the number of electrons is greater or less than the atomic number; the resulting charged species is called an *ion*. For example, the commonly encountered "chloride" ion, Cl^-, has 18 electrons, one more than the neutral chlorine atom. The sodium ion, Na+, has 10 electrons, 1 less than the neutral sodium atom.

B. ENERGY OF THE HYDROGEN ATOM

To explain the spectrum of light emitted from heated objects ("blackbody radiation"), Max Planck proposed in 1901 that the energy gained or lost from matter was "quantized" in small units of energy that were a multiple of the quantity

$$\Delta E = h\nu$$

where ΔE is the change in energy of the system, h is **Planck's constant,** with a value of 6.626×10^{-34} J s, and ν is the frequency of the radiation that is emitted or absorbed.

In his work on the photoelectric effect, in which electrons are emitted from the surface of metals that are exposed to light of certain wavelengths, Einstein proposed that light itself is quantized. In other words, light, long thought of as a wave, also has particle qualities. Such particles came to be known as "photons."

As a consequence of the work of Planck and Einstein, the change in energy ΔE of an atom of molecule system owing to the absorption or emission of a photon of light whose frequency is ν and whose wavelength is λ is given by these expressions:

(a) Absorption of a photon: (Here ΔE is positive)

$$\Delta E = E_{\text{photon}}$$
$$= h\nu$$
$$= h(c/\lambda) \text{ since for light, } \nu = c/\lambda \text{ ,}$$

where c, the speed of light, $= 2.998 \times 10^8$ m/s

(b) Emission of a photon: (Here ΔE is negative)

$$-\Delta E = E_{\text{photon}}$$
$$= h\nu$$

In the expressions above, ΔE can either be positive (absorption of light by the atom) or negative (emission of light by the atom). In both cases, the energy, frequency, and wavelength of the photon are positive quantities.

EXAMPLE

Find the wavelength, in nanometers (nm), of light that is emitted when an atom loses an amount of energy equal to 5.00×10^{-19} J. (Note that 1 nm $= 10^{-9}$ m)

SOLUTION

$$\Delta E = E_{\text{photon}}$$
$$= h(c/\lambda)$$
$$\lambda = hc/\Delta E$$
$$= (6.626 \times 10^{-34} \text{ J s})(2.998 \times 10^8 \text{ m/s}) / (5.00 \times 10^{-19} \text{ J})$$
$$= 3.97 \times 10^{-7} \text{ m}$$
$$(3.97 \times 10^{-7} \text{ m}) \times (1 \text{ nm}/10^{-9} \text{ m}) = 397 \text{ nm}$$

The Bohr Atom and Hydrogen Energy Levels
In 1913, Neils Bohr published an explanation of the known absorption and emission spectra of the hydrogen atom. He assumed that the electron in hydrogen revolved around the proton in one of several circular orbits, so that the angular

momentum of the electron could only assume certain "quantized" values. As the electron absorbed more energy, it could move to orbits of greater diameter.

Bohr's theory was later shown to be incorrect; in particular, electrons do not move in simple orbits around the nucleus. But the theory correctly accounted for the energy levels of the hydrogen atom.

Energies of the Hydrogen Atom

The observed emissions from the hydrogen atom are explained by the following formulas, which describe different energy levels, each determined by a different value of "n," the principal **quantum number:**

$$E_n = \frac{-2.178 \times 10^{-18} \text{J/molec}}{n^2}$$

$$= \frac{-1312 \text{kj/mol}}{n^2}$$

$$n = 1, 2, 3, 4, \ldots$$

Note that the first expression gives the energy per atom, while the second expression gives the energy per mole of atoms.

When the hydrogen atom has its single electron in the "$n = 1$" level, it is most stable, with an energy of -1312 kJ/mol.

As the electron is placed in levels of higher n, its energy rises.

As n grows large, the associated energy approaches 0, which is the energy of a completely separated proton and electron.

Hydrogen Atom Energy Levels

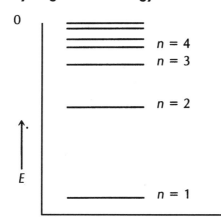

Energies of Hydrogen Transitions

The above formula can be applied to find the difference between a final level (of quantum number n_f) and an initial level (of quantum number n_i); the result is

$$\Delta E(\text{i} \rightarrow \text{f}) = (1312)(1/n_i^2 - 1/n_f^2)$$

in units of kJ/mol.

EXAMPLE

Find the energy (in kJ/mol) required to promote a hydrogen atom from the "ground state," where $n = 1$, to the particular excited state for which $n = 3$. What is the wavelength of the photon required?

SOLUTION

$$= \Delta E(1 \rightarrow 3) = (1312)\left(\frac{1}{1^2} - \frac{1}{3^2}\right)$$

$$= 1166 \text{ kJ/mol}$$

Because the answer is positive, the system must have a greater energy in the final state; i.e., its energy increases owing to absorption of a photon. To find the wavelength of this photon, we first convert energy in kJ/mol to J/photon:

$$(1166 \text{kJ/mol})(10^3 \text{ J/kJ})(1 \text{ mol}/6.022 \times 10^{23} \text{ photons})$$

$$= 1.936 \times 10^{-18} \text{ J/photon}$$

We now use the relationship between photon energy and wavelength, converting the final answer to nanometers (nm):

$$\lambda = hc/E_{\text{photon}}$$
$$= (6.626 \times 10^{-34} \text{ Js})(2.998 \times 10^8 \text{ m/s})(10^9 \text{ nm/m}) / (1.936 \times 10^{-18} \text{ J/photon})$$
$$= 102.6 \text{ nm}$$

Orbitals for the Hydrogen Atom

Electrons in the hydrogen atom occupy orbitals (or "wave functions") having the following properties:

- Each orbital corresponds to a definite energy determined by the principal quantum number of the orbital.

- The nature of the orbital determines the region of space in which the electron will be found. The probability that the electron will be found at a particular location is given by the square of the value of the wave function at that location.

- Each orbital in the hydrogen atom can hold up to 2 electrons.

- Each orbital is named by giving its principal quantum number and then a letter indicating its angular momentum quantum number, described below.

- A complete description of an orbital requires four different quantum numbers, also described below.

C. QUANTUM NUMBERS AND THEIR RELATIONSHIP TO HYDROGEN ORBITALS

n is the principal quantum number, which can equal 1, 2, 3 . . .

l is the angular momentum quantum number, which ranges from 0 to $n - 1$. The special names s, p, d, etc., refer to particular values of l:

if $l = 0$, the orbital is called "s"

if $l = 1$, the orbital is called "p"

if $l = 2$, the orbital is called "d"

if $l = 3$, the orbital is called "f"

m_l is the magnetic quantum number, which ranges from $-l$ to $+l$.

m_s is the electron spin quantum number, which can have values of $+\frac{1}{2}$ ("spin up") or $-\frac{1}{2}$ ("spin down").

Here are some examples of hydrogen atom states described by different values of the quantum numbers.

1. $n = 1$; $l = 0$; $m_l = 0$; $m_s = +\frac{1}{2}$: These values of the first three quantum numbers describe a 1s orbital (note that the "1" refers to the value of n and the "s" indicates that $l = 0$). The electron has a spin quantum number equal to $+\frac{1}{2}$.

2. $n = 2$, $l = 0$, $m_l = 0$, $m_s = -\frac{1}{2}$: The electron occupies a 2s orbital and has a spin quantum number equal to $-\frac{1}{2}$.

3. $n = 2$, $l = 1$, $m_l = 1$, $m_s = +\frac{1}{2}$: The electron occupies a 2p orbital and has a spin quantum number equal to $+\frac{1}{2}$.

4. $n = 3$, $l = 2$, $m_l = 2$, $m_s = -\frac{1}{2}$: The electron occupies a 3d orbital and has a spin quantum number equal to $-\frac{1}{2}$.

Figure 1 displays all the combinations that arise when $n \leq 4$. It also indicates two important consequences of the rules that define the quantum numbers:

1. For $n = 1$, the only orbital type possible is a 1s. For $n = 2$, a 2p orbital appears, and for $n = 3$, a 3d orbital is found. (At $n = 4$, a 4f orbital is found.)

2. For a given value of n, there will always be 1 orbital of "s" type. Where "p" orbitals are allowed, there will always be 3 of them, and where "d" orbitals are allowed, there will always be 5. (Similarly, where "f" orbitals are allowed, there will be 7.)

Figure 1
Allowed Quantum Numbers and Orbitals for the Hydrogen Atom (for $n = 1$ through $n = 4$)

n	l	m_l	m_s	orbital name	number of states per orbital	n	l	m_l	m_s	orbital name	number of states per orbital
1	0	0	$\pm\frac{1}{2}$	1s	2	4	0	0	$\pm\frac{1}{2}$	4s	2
2	0	0	$\pm\frac{1}{2}$	2s	2		1	−1	$\pm\frac{1}{2}$	4p	6
2	1	−1	$\pm\frac{1}{2}$	2p	6			0	$\pm\frac{1}{2}$		
		0	$\pm\frac{1}{2}$					+1	$\pm\frac{1}{2}$		
		+1	$\pm\frac{1}{2}$				2	−2	$\pm\frac{1}{2}$	4d	10
3	0	0	$\pm\frac{1}{2}$	3s	2			−1	$\pm\frac{1}{2}$		
3	1	−1	$\pm\frac{1}{2}$	3p	6			0	$\pm\frac{1}{2}$		
		0	$\pm\frac{1}{2}$					+1	$\pm\frac{1}{2}$		
		+1	$\pm\frac{1}{2}$					+2	$\pm\frac{1}{2}$		
3	2	−2	$\pm\frac{1}{2}$	3d	10		3	−3	$\pm\frac{1}{2}$	4f	14
		−1	$\pm\frac{1}{2}$					−2	$\pm\frac{1}{2}$		
		0	$\pm\frac{1}{2}$					−1	$\pm\frac{1}{2}$		
		+1	$\pm\frac{1}{2}$					0	$\pm\frac{1}{2}$		
		+2	$\pm\frac{1}{2}$					+1	$\pm\frac{1}{2}$		
								+2	$\pm\frac{1}{2}$		
								+3	$\pm\frac{1}{2}$		

Hydrogen states having the same value of n have the same energies regardless of the values of other quantum numbers—e.g., 2s has the same energy as 2p. (As we will see, for larger atoms, the energy of states such as 2s and 2p will *not* be equal.)

In its ground state, the hydrogen atom has one electron in the 1s orbital. Absorption of a photon can promote an electron to a higher state, if only for a short time.

Orbital Shapes

Many properties of atoms are explained by the shapes of atomic orbitals. Figure 2, on the following page shows the general shapes of the *s, p,* and *d* orbitals.

1. The probability of finding an electron in a small volume of space centered about a point is proportional to the square of the value of the wave function at that point in space.

2. The orbital diagrams are an attempt to show continuous distributions. The 1*s* orbital, for example, is not a sphere with a fixed radius, but rather a spherically symmetric function whose value falls off with increasing radius. (Figure 3 can help to clarify this.)

3. The orbitals can have positive or negative values, as well as "nodes" where the wave function equals 0. (The 2*s* orbital has a node that is evident in the radial electron density but not in the simple orbital drawing.) Note that a negative or positive value for the wave function (or orbital) has nothing to do with the sign of the electron's charge.

4. The *p* and *d* orbitals are "directional"—they point to a particular direction in space—while the *s* orbitals are not directional.

Electron Probability Density and Radial Distribution Functions

Figure 3 provides information about where the electron is likely to be found in a hydrogen atom. The "a" diagrams in the figure describe the ground state 1*s* orbital, while the "b" diagrams describe the 2*s* orbital, which the hydrogen electron might occupy in an excited state.

Figure 3

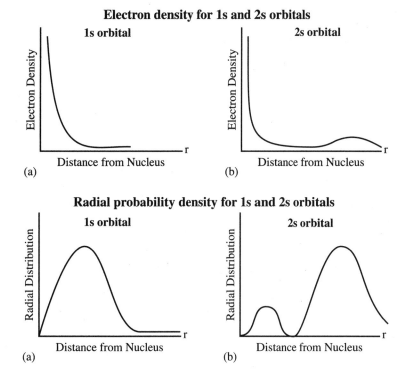

Electron density for 1s and 2s orbitals

Radial probability density for 1s and 2s orbitals

Figure 2

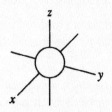

The 1*s* orbital

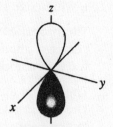

The 2p_z orbital

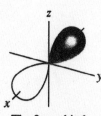

The 2p_x orbital

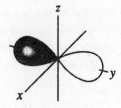

The 2p_y orbital

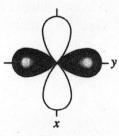

3$d_{x^2-y^2}$

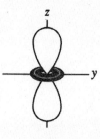

3d_{z^2}

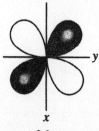

3d_{xy}

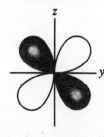

3d_{yz}

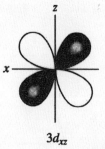

3d_{xz}

The 3*d* orbitals

The electron probability density function is the square of the wavefunction. It expresses the probability of finding the electron within a small volume element (e.g., in a cube that is 1 picometer on a side) at a given distance from the nucleus. For the 1s orbital, the function has its maximal value very close to the nucleus and falls off at greater distance. For the 2s orbital, the function is also highest near the nucleus, falls to zero (a "node"), then reaches a second maximum and again falls off far from the nucleus.

The radial distribution function provides different information. It indicates the likelihood that the electron will be found within a certain "shell" (e.g., in the region between 50 and 51 picometers from the nucleus). It is the function of choice to answer such questions as "What is the most likely distance of the electron from the nucleus?" By examining the radial distribution function for each type of orbital, we can conclude that a 2s electron is likely to be found at a greater distance from the nucleus than the 1s electron. We can also conclude from the radial distribution function that neither electron is likely to be found very close to the nucleus.

D. MANY-ELECTRON ATOMS

The energies and orbitals discussed so far apply only to the hydrogen atom, or with small modifications, to one-electron ions such as He^+. Other atoms are considered to have "hydrogen-like" orbitals that can be characterized by the same quantum numbers that are used to describe hydrogen.

The energies of the many-electron orbitals depend upon both n and l. For example, the 2p orbitals are slightly higher in energy than the 2s's, while the 3d's lie even higher than the 4s's. The general order of the energy levels of many-electron atoms is:

When studying this diagram, recall that the number of electrons that can occupy a set of orbitals depends upon the number of different sets of quantum numbers as described in section 3.2-C. (e.g., 2 electrons can occupy the 2s level, 6 can occupy the 3p level, and 10 can occupy the 3d level).

To help you remember the order of filling, you may want to use the following:

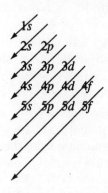

The Aufbau ("building-up") Principle

Hydrogen has a single electron in the 1s orbital; the next element, helium, has a second electron in the 1s orbital. Larger atoms must have electrons placed in higher orbitals. In placing electrons, we follow several rules:

1. Electrons are placed in the lowest energy orbital available.

2. **Pauli Exclusion Principle**
   No two electrons may have the same set of four quantum numbers. For example, the 1s orbital of He may hold two electrons, each with the same value of n, l, and m, provided that the electrons have different values of m_s ($\frac{1}{2}$ and $-\frac{1}{2}$).

3. **Hund's Rule**
   Orbitals having the same energy, such as the three 2p orbitals, are filled to maximize the number of unpaired electrons. Thus if 3 electrons are to be placed among the three 2p orbitals, one will enter each orbital. Only if four are to be placed will there be a need for two electrons to share an orbital.

Examples of configurations for various (elements exceptions to the usual order of filling are noted):

H $1s^1$ (i.e., there is 1 electron in a 1s orbital. In this notation the m_s quantum number is not specified.)

He $1s^2$

C $1s^2 2s^2 2p^2$

Ar $1s^2 2s^2 2p^6 3s^2 3p^6$ (Argon, a noble gas, has its uppermost "p" orbitals completely filled.)

K $1s^2 2s^2 2p^6 3s^2 3p^6 4s^1$ (Note that the last electron enters the 4s orbital, not the 3d.)

Sc $1s^2 2s^2 2p^6 3s^2 3p^6 4s^2 3d^1$

Ti $1s^2 2s^2 2p^6 3s^2 3p^6 4s^2 3d^2$

Cr $1s^2 2s^2 2p^6 3s^2 3p^6 4s^1 3d^5$ (We would expect the upper orbitals to be "$4s^2 3d^4$"—but this is not the case.)

Cu $1s^2 2s^2 2p^6 3s^2 3p^6 4s^1 3d^{10}$ (This is also an exception to the general order of filling.)

Br $1s^2 2s^2 2p^6 3s^2 3p^6 4s^1 3d^{10} 4p^5$

Pb $1s^2 2s^2 2p^6 3s^2 3p^6 4s^2 3d^{10} 4p^6\ 5s^2 4d^{10} 5p^6 6s^2 4f^{14} 5d^{10} 6p^2$

(Note the filled $4f$ level after the $6s$ levels.)

E. THE PERIODIC TABLE

Figure 4 shows the standard arrangement of elements into the **Periodic Table of Elements.** Note several general points concerning the table:

1. Elements with similar chemical properties occupy the same column, or *group*.

2. Two different sets of numbers are used to label the groups (columns). The representative elements, a subset of the total that excludes the transition metals, are labeled "1A, 2A . . . 8A." All of the columns are labeled with a newer designation, "1, 2, . . . 18."

3. Atomic weights of elements generally increase sequentially from left to right along a row, or *period*. Chemical properties are not consistent within a row, as will be shown below.

4. Movement from one square to the next along a row represents the addition of one proton and electron to form an atom of greater atomic number. Different electrons—*s, p, d,* or *f*—are added in different sections of the table.

5. In groups 1A through 8A, there is a range of properties as one moves along a given row. These elements differ from one another in the number of *s* and *p* electrons that each has in its outer ("valence") shell; there are no differences in the number of *d* or *f* electrons.

6. In general, metals occur on the left side of the table and nonmetals on the right. Note the zigzag line that divides metals from nonmetals.

7. Elements in Group 1A have a configuration of s^1, where the actual *s* orbital is $1s$ for H, $2s$ for Li, and so on. The lone valence *s* electron is readily given up, leading to a positively charged ion that readily forms metallic bonds.

8. Elements in Group 2A have a configuration s^2.

9. Elements in Group 3A have a configuration of $s^2 p^1$, those in Group 4A have $s^2 p^2$, and so on out to Group 7A with $s^2 p^5$ and Group 8A (the Noble Gases) with $s^2 p^6$.

Figure 4

PERIODIC TABLE OF ELEMENTS

1 1A Alkali metals	2 2A Alkaline earth metals		3	4	5	6	7 Transition Metals	8	9	10	11	12	13 3A	14 4A	15 5A	16 6A Halogens	17 7A	18 8A Noble gases
1 H 1.008																		2 He 4.003
3 Li 6.941	4 Be 9.012												5 B 10.81	6 C 12.01	7 N 14.01	8 O 16.00	9 F 19.00	10 Ne 20.18
11 Na 22.99	12 Mg 24.31												13 Al 26.98	14 Si 28.09	15 P 30.97	16 S 32.06	17 Cl 35.45	18 Ar 39.95
19 K 39.10	20 Ca 40.08		21 Sc 44.96	22 Ti 47.90	23 V 50.94	24 Cr 52.00	25 Mn 54.94	26 Fe 55.85	27 Co 58.93	28 Ni 58.70	29 Cu 63.55	30 Zn 65.38	31 Ga 69.72	32 Ge 72.59	33 As 74.92	34 Se 78.96	35 Br 79.90	36 Kr 83.80
37 Rb 85.47	38 Sr 87.62		39 Y 88.91	40 Zr 91.22	41 Nb 92.91	42 Mo 95.94	43 Tc (98)	44 Ru 101.1	45 Rh 102.9	46 Pd 106.4	47 Ag 107.9	48 Cd 112.4	49 In 114.8	50 Sn 118.7	51 Sb 121.8	52 Te 127.6	53 I 126.9	54 Xe 131.3
55 Cs 132.9	56 Ba 137.3		57 La* 138.9	72 Hf 178.5	73 Ta 180.9	74 W 183.9	75 Re 186.2	76 Os 190.2	77 Ir 192.2	78 Pt 195.1	79 Au 197.0	80 Hg 200.6	81 Tl 204.4	82 Pb 207.2	83 Bi 209.0	84 Po (209)	85 At (210)	86 Rn (222)
87 Fr (223)	88 Ra 226.0		89 Ac** (227)	104 Rf	105 Db	106 Sg	107 Bh	108 Hs	109 Mt	110 Uun	111 Uuu	112 Uub						

Nonmetals

Metals

*Lanthanides (Rare Earths)

58 Ce 140.1	59 Pr 140.9	60 Nd 144.2	61 Pm (145)	62 Sm 150.4	63 Eu 152.0	64 Gd 157.3	65 Tb 158.9	66 Dy 1.008	67 Ho 1.008	68 Er 1.008	69 Tm 1.008	70 Yb 1.008	71 Lu 1.008

**Actinides (Transuranium)

90 Th 232.0	91 Pa (231)	92 U 238.0	93 Np (237)	94 Pu (244)	95 Am (243)	96 Cm (247)	97 Bk (247)	98 Cf (251)	99 Es (252)	100 Fm (257)	101 Md (258)	102 No (259)	103 Lr (260)

10. Groups 1B through 8B (the *transition* elements) show some changes in properties from left to right along a row. These elements differ little in their arrangements of *s* and *p* electrons, but have more electrons in their outer *d* orbitals as one goes from left to right. Specifically, their configuration changes from d^1 for Group 3B to d^{10} for Group 2B.

11. The *inner transition* elements (the Lanthanides and Actinides, also called the *rare earth elements*) show little change in chemical properties from left to right along a row. These elements differ in the number of *f* electrons (either 4*f*, for the Lanthanides, or 5*f*, for the Actinides) added to their atomic configurations.

F. CHEMICAL PROPERTIES AND THE PERIODIC TABLE

General Principles

From top to bottom in a column (group) in the Periodic Table, outer electrons generally become *less* tightly bound.

From left to right across a row (period), outer electrons generally become *more* tightly bound.

Specific Consequences of These Principles

1. **Atomic Radius**

Atomic radius is one-half the average distance between centers of identical bonded atoms. It decreases from left to right across each row in the periodic table and increases from top to bottom down each column.

2. **Ionization Energy**

Ionization energy, or ionization potential, is the minimum energy required to remove one valence electron ("first" ionization energy) or two valence electrons ("second" ionization energy) from an atom to create a positive ion. For example, the first ionization energy for Na is the enthalpy change of the reaction

$$Na(g) \rightarrow Na+ (g) + e^- \qquad IE_1 = \Delta H = 496 \text{ kJ/mol}$$

Ionization energy increases *from left to right across a row* and *decreases from top to bottom down a column.*

3. **Electron Affinity**

Electron affinity is the energy change associated with the addition of an electron to a gaseous atom. Using fluorine as an example, the electron affinity is the enthalpy change for the following reaction:

$$F(g) + e^- \rightarrow F^-(g) \qquad EA = \Delta H = -328 \text{ kJ/mol}$$

Electron affinity does not vary as regularly as ionization energy, but *it is generally more negative for the nonmetals than for the metals,* with the halogens (Group 7A) displaying particularly large negative values.

4. **Electronegativity**

Electronegativity is the measure of the ability of an atom to attract shared electrons in a bond. Electronegativity increases from left to right across a row and decreases from top to bottom down a column. Electronegativities are commonly measured using Pauling's scale, which ranges from a minimum of 0.8 (Cs) to a high of 4.0 (F).

5. **Oxides**

Oxides are compounds formed by *reactions with oxygen*. The most stable oxides are those in which oxygen (in Group VIA) combines with an element far to the left of it in the Periodic Table of Elements. The acid-base properties of oxides depend on the position of the oxidized atom in the table: bases occur at the left of the table, acids at the right, with intermediate acid-base properties found in between.

PRACTICE PROBLEMS

1. Reading from top to bottom down a column of the Periodic Table of Elements, the atomic radius becomes:

   A. larger, owing to increased nuclear charge that is only partially shielded by additional valence electrons.
   B. smaller, owing to increased nuclear charge that is only partially shielded by additional valence electrons.
   C. smaller, owing to placement of additional electrons in orbitals that are farther from the nucleus.
   D. larger, owing to placement of additional electrons in orbitals that are farther from the nucleus.

2. Which of the following shows atoms in expected order of increasing ionization energy?

   I. Be, Mg, Ca
   II. B, C, N
   III. K, Na, Li

   A. I only
   B. II only
   C. III only
   D. II and III only

Questions 3–7 are based on the following chart showing some different possible combinations of quantum numbers describing electrons in a hydrogen atom. The values of m_s are not shown.

State	n	l	m
1	1	A	0
2	2	0	0
3	2	1	1
4	2	1	B
5	2	1	−1

3. What is the value marked A?

   A. 0
   B. 1
   C. −1
   D. −1, 0, or 1

4. Which of the states indicated have directional properties?

   A. 1
   B. 2
   C. 3 and 4
   D. 3, 4, and 5

5. What is the value marked B?

   A. 1
   B. 0
   C. −1
   D. 1, 0, or −1

6. Which state represents the hydrogen atom in its most stable configuration?

   A. 1
   B. 2
   C. 3
   D. 4

7. Now suppose that the chart represented a helium atom. How many of the states shown would have the same energy?

   A. 2
   B. 3
   C. 4
   D. 5

8. The $2p_z$ orbital is often written with a "+" and "−" sign in each part; this is not done for the $1s$ orbital. The explanation for the difference is:

   A. the $1s$ orbital can only hold 1 electron.
   B. the $2p$ electron is positively charged above the xy plane and negatively charged below.
   C. the sign of an orbital has no meaning.
   D. the value of the p_z wave function is positive above the xy plane and negative below it.

9. Ionization of the hydrogen atom could be caused by

   A. adding an electron of sufficient energy to promote a photon from a bound state so that it leaves the atom.
   B. adding a photon of sufficient energy to promote an electron from a bound state so that it leaves the atom.
   C. allowing a photon and an electron to be emitted from the atom.
   D. bringing a second hydrogen atom close enough to react to form H_2.

ANSWER KEY

1. D	2. D	3. A	4. D	5. B	6. A	7. B	8. D	9. B

ANSWERS AND EXPLANATIONS

1. **The correct answer is (D).** Choices "A" and "B" could be used to explain variation in radius across a row, but that is not asked for here. As one moves down a column, the highest-filled orbital becomes farther from the nucleus, causing the atomic radii to be greater; e.g., the radius of K, whose highest-filled orbital is $4s$, is greater than Na, whose highest-filled orbital is $3s$.

2. **The correct answer is (D).** I is in reverse order, since ionization requires less energy as valence electrons are placed in higher atomic orbitals.

3. **The correct answer is (A).** l ranges from $n - 1$ to 0; here, for $n = 1$, l must be 0 (we couldn't, for example, have a $1p$ orbital).

4. **The correct answer is (D).** 1 and 2 are s orbitals (since $l = 0$), but the others are p orbitals (since $l = 1$).

5. **The correct answer is (B).** *m* has values from $+l \ldots -l$. Because $l = 1$, *m* can have values of $+1$, 0, and -1. The $+1$ and -1 values are already listed in other states shown. Only $m = 0$ remains for a 2*p*.

6. **The correct answer is (A).** This is the 1*s* state, whose energy is lower than the 2*s* or 2*p* orbitals indicated in states 2 to 5. If a hydrogen electron were to occupy any of the last 4 states, the atom would be said to be in an "excited state."

7. **The correct answer is (B).** States 3, 4, and 5 involve the three 2*p* orbitals and are "degenerate." Because the atom is helium, which has more than one electron, the 2*s* orbital has a lower energy than the 2*p* orbitals. (Were the atom hydrogen, the correct answer would be "C.")

8. **The correct answer is (D).** The orbitals are functions with numeric values at each point in space. The $2p_z$ orbital has positive values above the *xy* plane and negative values below it.

9. **The correct answer is (B).** By providing energy in the form of a photon, an electron can be promoted beyond the bound states of the atom, so that it travels freely.

1.3 BONDING

A. THREE KINDS OF BONDING

Bonding is the attraction between different atoms in a molecule. There are three major types of bonding.

1. **Metallic Bonding**
   Metal atoms become positive ions by surrendering their outermost electrons to a sea of free electrons.

2. **Ionic Bonding**
   Electrons are transferred from one atom to another, resulting in a positive ion and a negative ion bound together by a strong electrostatic attraction.

3. **Covalent Bonding**
   Electron pairs are shared between two atoms and attracted by both nuclei.

B. IONIC BONDING IN CRYSTALS

Crystalline solids are extended arrays of positive and negative ions attracted by electrostatic interaction. The bonds in ionic crystals are much stronger than covalent bonds. The ions in the crystal are held in fairly tightly fixed positions by the electrostatic forces.

Ionic bonding is most likely to be found between elements on the far left and far right of the periodic table. Examples are sodium chloride (NaCl) and potassium bromide (KBr).

C. COVALENT BONDING

Covalent bonding involves the sharing of electrons between two nonmetallic atoms. The simplest descriptions of covalent bonding are **Lewis** or **electron-dot formulas,** which provide reasonable explanations of bonding for many compounds. In these formulas, dots are placed around each atom to symbolize the valence electrons (usually the outer s and p electrons), and the atoms are then combined so that each one is surrounded by a complete outer shell of eight electrons (an "octet"), including all electrons in any bond to that atom. (Hydrogen is an exception, since it has only two electrons around it.) Single bonds (one electron pair), double bonds (two pairs), and triple bonds (three pairs) are assigned as a consequence of the need to create octets.

For example, consider CH_3F, shown below. Here carbon forms four single covalent bonds, thus surrounding itself with the required eight electrons.

Four of these electrons came from carbon valence electrons, 3 came from the surrounding hydrogens, and 1 came from the fluorine, whose other electrons remain "unshared."

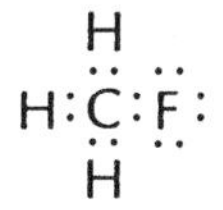

The oxygen molecule, O_2, requires a double bond:

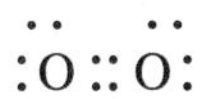

Here each oxygen contributes six valence electrons. Four of the total of 12 electrons form a double bond, leaving 2 unshared pairs on each oxygen.

D. RESONANCE STRUCTURES

For many compounds, several equivalent Lewis formulas can be written, as in the example below for ozone, O_3:

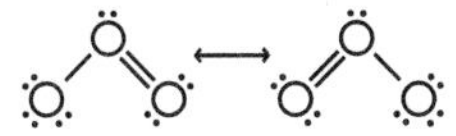

In such cases, no one diagram represents the actual molecule. The actual structure is somewhere in between and is called a resonance hybrid. This situation is indicated by drawing all the possible structures separated by a double-headed arrow.

EXAMPLE

Draw 2 resonance structures for the nitrite ion, NO_2^-.

SOLUTION

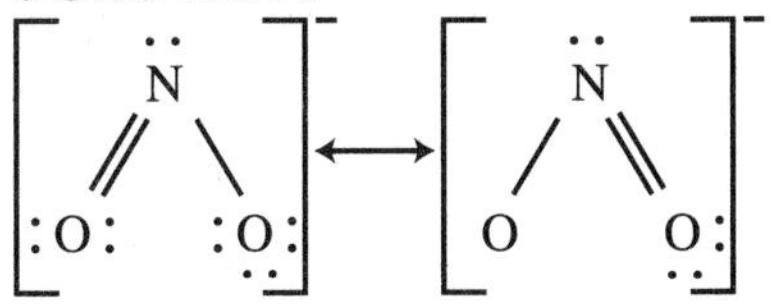

Note that we must indicate the overall charge of -1; a bracket is commonly used.

E. FORMAL CHARGE

When several valid Lewis structures are possible, the concept of "formal charge" on each atom helps to select the best structure.

Formal charge is defined as follows:

$$\text{Formal charge} = \left(\frac{\text{\# of}}{\text{valence } e\text{'s}}\right) - \frac{1}{2}\left(\frac{\text{\# of}}{\text{shared } e\text{'s}}\right) - \left(\frac{\text{\# of unshared}}{e\text{'s}}\right)$$

The most reasonable Lewis structure for a given compound will be the one that leaves the formal charge on each atom closest to zero. Further, any atom having a negative charge should have a high electronegativity value (see sec. J).

EXAMPLE

The molecule N_2O has several possible resonance structures. Use formal charge to determine which of the following is most favorable:

Structure 1: $\overset{..}{N} = N = \overset{..}{O}:$

Structure 2: $:N \equiv N - \overset{..}{\underset{..}{O}}:$

Structure 3: $:\underset{..}{N} - N \equiv O:$

By counting the electrons in each structure, we can construct the following table. ("Nitrogen #1" is on the left in the structure, and "nitrogen #2" is to the right of it.)

	Atom	# of valence e's	−	$\frac{1}{2}$ (# of shared e's)	−	# of unshared valence e's	=	Formal Charge
Structure 1	N#1	5	−	2	−	4	=	−1
	N#2	5	−	4	−	0	=	1
	O	6	−	2	−	4	=	0
Structure 2	N#1	5	−	3	−	2	=	0
	N#2	5	−	4	−	0	=	1
	O	6	−	1	−	6	=	−1
Structure 3	N#1	5	−	1	−	6	=	−2
	N#2	5	−	4	−	0	=	1
	O	6	−	3	−	2	=	1

Structure 1: $\overset{\ominus \,..}{} \overset{\oplus}{N} = N = \overset{..}{O}:$

Structure 2: $:N \equiv \overset{\oplus}{N} - \overset{..\ominus}{\underset{..}{O}}:$

Structure 3: $:\overset{\oslash..}{N} - \overset{\oplus}{N} \equiv \overset{\oplus}{O}:$

Structure 2 is the most reasonable, since it places the negative charge on the oxygen, which is more electronegative than nitrogen, and since it does not have large charge separations.

F. LEWIS ACIDS AND BASES

A **Lewis base** is a compound that donates an electron pair; a **Lewis acid** is a compound that accepts an electron pair. In the following example, the Lewis base is NH_3 and the Lewis acid is BF_3:

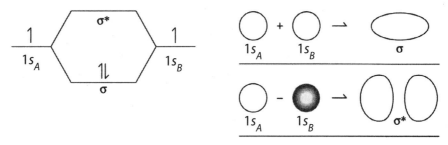

G. BONDING IN DIATOMIC MOLECULES

The lowest-energy orbitals in the H_2 molecule are two *linear combinations* of the $1s$ orbitals on each of the two atoms. If we designate these orbitals by "$1s_a$" and "$1s_b$," then the H_2 **molecular orbitals** can be written using the Greek letter σ (sigma),

$$\sigma = 1s_a + 1s_b \text{ (bonding)}$$
$$\sigma^* = 1s_a - 1s_b \text{ (anti-bonding)}$$

The figure below shows the shapes of the orbitals as well as the energies of the original atomic orbitals and the molecular orbitals. The **bonding orbital** is more stable because it places electrons between the nuclei most of the time, rather than concentrating them away from the region between the nuclei, as in the **anti-bonding orbital.**

Molecular Orbitals Arising From Two Hydrogen 1s Atomic Orbitals

The figure below shows electron configurations for the H_2^+ and H_2^- ions, which have one fewer and one more electron, respectively, than H_2. Each is predicted to exist, but with a bond roughly one-half the strength of that in H_2.

Bond strength can be assessed by the **bond order**, defined as

$$\text{bond order} = \frac{1}{2}(\text{\# of bonding } e^-\text{'s} - \text{\# of antibonding } e\text{'s})$$

When the bond order is 1.0, the bond is a single bond; when it is 2.0, a double bond, and when it is 3.0, a triple bond. "Half-bonds" are possible under this model, as in the following examples, each of which has a bond order of $\frac{1}{2}$.

It is not just the 1*s* atomic orbitals that may interact to form molecular orbitals. For example, in the C_2 molecule, where both the *2s* and *2p* orbitals are occupied, the molecular orbitals describing C_2 involve linear combinations of these higher atomic orbitals as well:

$$\sigma(2s) = 2s_a + 2s_b \text{ (bonding)}$$
$$\sigma(2s)^* = 2s_a - 2s_b \text{ (antibonding)}$$
$$\sigma(2p_z) = 2p_{z_a} + 2p_{z_b} \text{ (bonding)}$$
$$\sigma(2p_z)^* = 2p_{z_a} - 2p_{z_b} \text{ (antibonding)}$$

These examples show that σ-molecular orbitals are formed both from *2p* atomic orbitals and from $2p_z$ orbitals, where the *z*-direction is taken to be along the internuclear axis.

When we write similar expressions for the $2p_x$ and $2p_y$ orbitals on each carbon nucleus, we find that the orbitals lack the cylindrical symmetry of the sigma orbitals above. These orbitals, called **pi (π) orbitals,** are shown below.

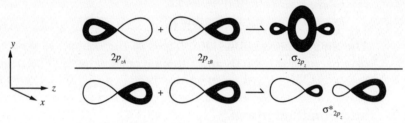

Formation of bonding (above) and antibonding (below) sigma orgitals from atomic *p* orbitals.

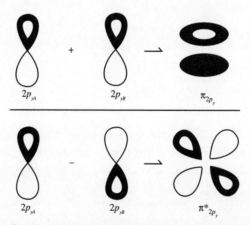

Formation of bonding (above) and antibonding (below) pi orbitals from atomic *p* orbitals.

Note: s atomic orbitals give rise to sigma molecular orbitals, but *p* orbitals can lead to either sigma or pi orbitals.

Order of Filling for $\sigma(2s, 2p)$ and $\pi(2p)$ Orbitals

The order of filling of these orbitals is shown below. One diagram is needed for Li_2 through N_2, and another for O_2 and F_2.

Similar π orbitals form from the $2p_x$ atomic orbitals.

(a) M.O.'s for O_2 through N_2

$$\underline{\quad} \; \sigma^*_{2p_z}$$

$$\pi^*_{2p_x} \; \underline{\quad} \qquad \underline{\quad} \; \pi^*_{2p_y}$$

$$\underline{\quad} \; \pi_{2p_z}$$

$$\pi_{2p_x} \; \underline{\quad} \qquad \underline{\quad} \; \pi_{2p_y}$$

$$\sigma^*_{2s} \; \underline{\quad}$$

$$\sigma_{2s} \; \underline{\quad}$$

(b) M.O.'s for O_2 and F_2

$$\sigma^*_{2p_z} \; \underline{\quad}$$

$$\pi^*_{2p_x} \; \underline{\quad} \qquad \underline{\quad} \; \pi^*_{2p_y}$$

$$\pi_{2p_x} \; \underline{\quad} \qquad \underline{\quad} \; \pi_{2p_y}$$

$$\sigma_{2p_z} \; \underline{\quad}$$

$$\sigma^*_{2s} \; \underline{\quad}$$

$$\sigma_{2s} \; \underline{\quad}$$

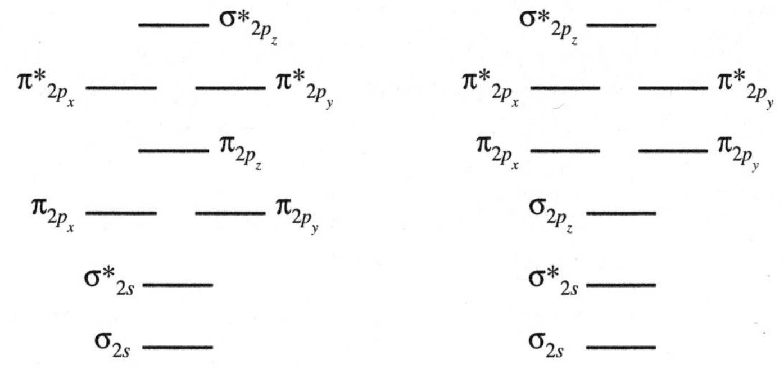

EXAMPLE

Using the appropriate molecular orbital diagram, predict the electron configuration and the bond order of the O_2^- ion.

SOLUTION

We will consider only valence electrons, e.g., those arising from the $2s$ and $2p$ atomic orbitals. This decision allows us to omit the σ_{1s} and σ^*_{1s}. Each neutral oxygen atom brings 6 electrons; there is also an additional electron owing to the net negative charge, for a total of 13 electrons. We use the chart that shows O_2 and F_2 orbitals, and fill it as below.

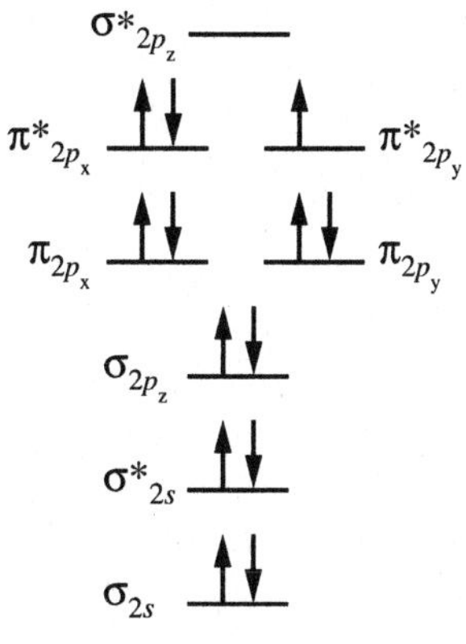

$$\sigma^*_{2p_z} \; \underline{\quad}$$

$$\pi^*_{2p_x} \; \underline{\uparrow\downarrow} \qquad \underline{\uparrow} \; \pi^*_{2p_y}$$

$$\pi_{2p_x} \; \underline{\uparrow\downarrow} \qquad \underline{\uparrow\downarrow} \; \pi_{2p_y}$$

$$\sigma_{2p_z} \; \underline{\uparrow\downarrow}$$

$$\sigma^*_{2s} \; \underline{\uparrow\downarrow}$$

$$\sigma_{2s} \; \underline{\uparrow\downarrow}$$

We now calculate

$$\text{bond order} = \frac{1}{2}(\text{bonding electrons} - \text{antibonding electrons})$$

$$= \frac{1}{2}(8-5)$$

$$= 1.5$$

H. VALENCE SHELL ELECTRON PAIR REPULSION (VSEPR)

Molecular orbital theory may be applied to molecules larger than diatomics, but at the price of great complexity. VSEPR provides a useful prediction of molecular geometry without detailed consideration of orbitals. It is frequently applied to compounds having a central atom surrounded by various other atoms or group of atoms.

The basic premise of VSEPR is that the most stable configuration of a molecule is the one that maximizes the distance between different pairs of electrons, either those in bonds or in nonbonding pairs.

To use VSEPR,

1. draw an electron-dot structure to determine the number of bonds and nonbonded electrons.

2. choose a structure that keeps the electron pairs farthest apart.

EXAMPLES

a) The BeH_2 molecule has two single bonds with no nonbonding pairs. A linear structure keeps the electrons in the bonds at greatest distance.

H—Be—H

b) The BF_3 molecule has three single bonds, also with no nonbonding pairs. Here the preferred structure is "trigonal planar," with bond angles of 120°. (Note that in this example, as in example a, the octet rule is violated.)

```
        F
        |
        B
       / \
      F   F
```

c) NH_3, ammonia, might be expected at first glance to resemble BF_3, but its electron-dot structure reveals a lone pair, which also needs to be kept away from the bonding pairs. The resulting structure is a pyramid with bond angles of 107.5°, somewhat less than the tetrahedral angle of 109.4° seen in CH_4 (next example). This distortion from ideal geometry is usually explained by stating that the repulsive force between electrons in a lone pair and those in a bonding pair is greater than the force between two pairs of bonding electrons. (Note that when characterizing the shape of a molecule, we don't include the lone pairs as part of the descriptive geometric shape.)

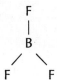

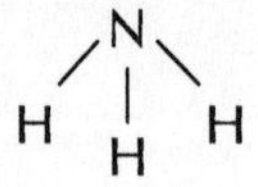

d) In CH_4 the bond angles are the tetrahedral angle of 109.5°.

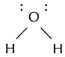

e) The water molecule is bent, with a bond angle 104.5°, somewhat less than the tetrahedral angle, owing to lone pair/bonding pair repulsions.

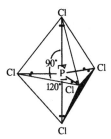

f) PCl_5 has a "trigonal bipyramid" shape, which best minimizes overlap among the five bonding electrons.

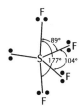

g) SF_4 has a shape that can be understood from that of PCl_5, in the same way NH_3 is related to CH_4: One of the bonding pairs in the PCl_5 is replaced by a lone pair, resulting in the "sawhorse" structure. Note the deviation from ideal geometry.

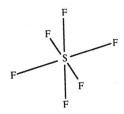

h) SF_6 has an "octahedral" (or "square bipyramidal") structure that best accommodates its 12 bonding pairs. There are no lone pairs, and 90° angles are expected.

I. HYBRID ORBITALS

The VSEPR theory does not address the issue of orbital types, focusing instead on a description of geometry. The **hybrid orbital** description relates particular molecular geometries, usually those predicted by VSEPR, to the original atomic orbitals on a central atom.

EXAMPLE

Describe the bonding in CH_4 in terms of hybrid orbitals.

1. First, determine the valence electron configuration of the central carbon: $2s^2 2p^2$. Electrons in the $2s$ orbitals would display no directional character, while those in two different p orbitals would show 90° bonding, in contrast to the 109.5° angles that are correctly predicted by VSEPR.

2. Next, imagine that energy is added to a $2s$ electron in order to promote it to the unoccupied $2p$ orbital.

3. Make linear combinations of the $2s$ orbital and each of the three p orbitals that point in four different directions, giving the shape needed for tetrahedral bonding. These four different orbital combinations are called "hybrids."

4. Form sigma bonds between each of the hybrids and a hydrogen $1s$ orbital.

Other Hybrids

sp	Linear molecules.
sp^2	Trigonal planar, or, if one of the hybrids is occupied by a lone pair, bent (e.g., SO_2).
sp^3	Tetrahedral, pyramidal (with lone pair), as above.
$sp^3 d$	Trigonal bipyramid, sawhorse (with lone pair).
$sp^3 d^2$	Octahedral, or with lone pairs, square pyramidal, square planar.

Illustrations of several hybrid orbitals are given in the Molecular Orbitals figure on page 45.

J. PARTIAL IONIC CHARACTER OF BONDS

It is not always possible to categorize a bond as purely ionic or purely covalent. In a bond between identical atoms, e.g., in H_2, the electrons in the bond are just as likely to be attracted to one hydrogen nucleus as another. In contrast, a bond between atoms that differ significantly in their electronegativity (e.g., in HF) will have the bonding **electrons** near the more electronegative fluorine atom most of the time.

We measure the degree to which electrons prefer one end of a molecule over another by the **dipole moment,** a vector whose direction indicates the separation of charge and whose magnitude is proportional to both the partial charge at each end of the molecule and the distance between the centers of the charges.

The dipole moment of any homonuclear diatomic molecule (H_2, N_2, etc.) is zero.

The dipole moment of a heteronuclear diatomic molecule whose atoms differ in their electronegativity is nonzero; the negative end of the dipole moment points to the more electronegative molecule.

The dipole moment of larger molecules is the vector sum of the bond dipole moments; totally symmetrical molecules such as linear CO_2 and tetrahedral CH_4 have zero dipole moments because the individual bond dipole moments cancel each other.

EXAMPLES

Predict whether each of the following molecules has a nonzero dipole moment:

1. HCl

2. H_2O

3. CCl_4

4. CCl_3F

5. NH_3

6.

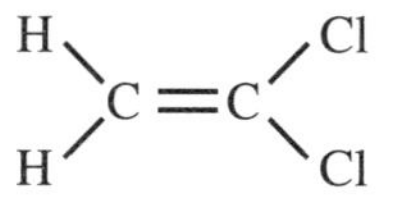

7.

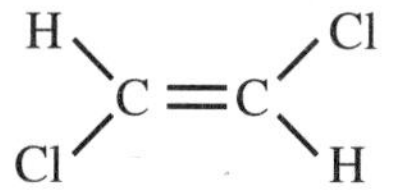

SOLUTIONS

1. Cl is more electronegative than H, so there will be a dipole moment, with the positive end at the hydrogen.

2. If water were a linear molecule, the 2 O-H bond dipoles would cancel. But since it is bent, there is a dipole moment, with its positive end toward the hydrogens.

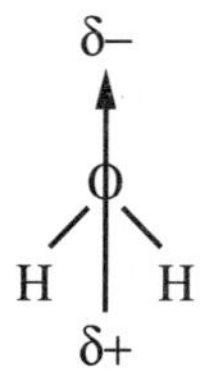

3. All 4 C-Cl bond dipoles cancel in this tetrahedrally symmetric molecule.

4. There will be a dipole moment here, since the C-F bond dipole is larger than the C-Cl bond dipoles.

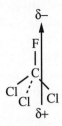

5. There will be a dipole moment here, because there is no fourth bond (as in CH_4) to cancel the other bond dipoles.

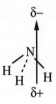

6. There will be a dipole moment, owing to the high electronegativity of Cl.

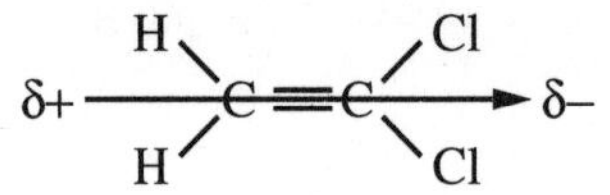

$$\delta+ \quad \begin{array}{c} H \\ \diagdown \\ \diagup \\ H \end{array} C \equiv C \begin{array}{c} \diagup Cl \\ \diagdown \\ Cl \end{array} \quad \delta-$$

7. Unlike 6, the C-Cl bond dipoles cancel, leaving a net dipole moment of zero.

PRACTICE PROBLEMS

1. Which of the following is a correct electron dot formula for acetylene, C_2H_2?

    A. H:C:C:H
    B. H:C::C:H
    C. H:C :::C:H
    D. H:C::C:H

2. The electronic configuration of N_2 (omitting orbitals arising from the $1s$ atomic orbitals) is

    $(\sigma2_s)^2(\sigma^*_2s)^2(\pi_{2p_x})^2(\pi_{2p_y})^2(\sigma_{2p_z})^2$

    What is its bond order?

    A. 0
    B. 1
    C. 2
    D. 3

3. Antibonding orbitals receive their name from the fact that

    A. they concentrate electrons between the nuclei, causing repulsion.
    B. they are lower in energy than the original atomic orbitals.
    C. they repel electrons in other molecules.
    D. they require the electrons to spend most of their time away from the region between the nuclei.

4. The configuration of F_2 is

$$(\sigma 2_s)^2(\sigma^*_2 s)^2(\sigma_{2p_z})^2(\pi_{2p_x})^2(\pi_{2p_y})^2(\sigma^*_{2p_x})^2(\pi^*_{2p_y})^2$$

The F_2^- ion is

A. expected to exist and be more strongly bonded than F_2.
B. expected to exist and be less strongly bonded than F_2.
C. expected to have the same bond strength as F_2.
D. expected not to exist, since its bond order would be 0.

5. The molecule CCl_2F_2 is expected to have what kind of geometry?

A. bent
B. trigonal planar
C. tetrahedral
D. sawhorse

6. The molecule NF_3 is expected to have what kind of geometry?

A. bent
B. trigonal planar
C. tetrahedral
D. pyramidal

7. The molecules CF_4 and XeF_4

A. have the same shape: tetrahedral.
B. have different shapes: CF_4 is square planar and XeF_4 is tetrahedral.
C. have different shapes: CF_4 is tetrahedral and XeF_4 is square planar.
D. have different shapes: CF_4 is tetrahedral and XeF_4 is pyramidal.

8. The molecules H_2O and H_2S

A. have the same geometry: linear.
B. have the same geometry: bent.
C. have different geometries: H_2O, bent; H_2S, linear.
D. have different geometries: H_2O, linear; H_2S, bent.

9. Two chemists argue about the geometry of the NH_3 molecule. Chemist A says that the molecule is trigonal planar, while Chemist B says it is pyramidal. Which of the following could help them decide their argument?

I. VSEPR reasoning
II. Careful molecular weight determination
III. Measurement of dipole moment

A. I only
B. II only
C. III only
D. I and III only

ANSWER KEY

1. C   2. D   3. D   4. B   5. C   6. D   7. C   8. B   9. D

ANSWERS AND EXPLANATIONS

1. **The correct answer is (C).** This is the only structure that gives each carbon an octet and also shows the correct number of electrons.

2. **The correct answer is (D).** Bond order = (8 bonding electrons − 2 antibonding electrons)/2 = 3. N_2 has a triple bond.

3. **The correct answer is (D).** Because antibonding electrons are not primarily in the internuclear region, they do not shield the positively charged nuclei from each other. Consequently, they do not support bonding.

4. **The correct answer is (B).** The extra electron must go into an antibonding orbital, making the overall bond order less than that of F_2.

5. **The correct answer is (C).** Analogous to CH_4. Note that choice D would be appropriate if the central atom were phosphorus.

6. **The correct answer is (D).** As in NH_3, the lone pair on the nitrogen prevents the molecule from taking on a planar configuration.

7. **The correct answer is (C).** Since there are no lone pairs on the carbon, CF_4 maximizes the distance between its bonding electrons by a tetrahedral arrangement. But the xenon atom has two unshared pairs that occupy opposite sites in an octahedral arrangement, leaving the 4 fluorines to occupy the 4 other sites and form a square complex.

8. **The correct answer is (B).** Both are bent. Each central atom has 2 unshared pairs, which occupy 2 corners of a tetrahedron; the other two corners contain bonding pairs.

9. **The correct answer is (D).** VSEPR predicts a pyramidal shape, and measurement of a nonzero dipole moment would confirm the prediction from theory. The molecular weight of each shape would, however, be the same.

1.4 PHASES AND PHASE EQUILIBRIUM

A. THE GAS PHASE

Gases are characterized by the following variables: pressure, volume, and temperature.

Pressure, P

Pressure is defined as force per unit area; in SI units, it is measured in Pascals (Pa), whose units are N/m^2.

Other units:

1 mm of Hg = 1 torr = 133.3 Pa

1 standard atmosphere (or atmosphere or atm) = 760 mm Hg

= 101,325 Pa

Temperature, T

Temperature is commonly expressed in absolute (or Kelvin) units (symbolized by K) for gas problems, and the relationships that follow assume this choice of units.
Temperatures in the Celsius scale can be converted using

$$T(\text{Kelvin}) = T(\text{Celsius}) + 273.15$$

Ideal Gas

An ideal gas is one in which both intermolecular forces and molecular volumes can be assumed to be negligible.

B. RELATIONSHIPS AMONG P, V, AND T FOR IDEAL GASES

Avogadro's Law

The number of moles of a gas is proportional to the volume of the gas, provided temperature and pressure are held constant. In particular, 22.4 L of an ideal gas at 1 atm and 273K contain one mole.

Boyle's Law

$$PV = \text{const.}$$

where moles and temperature are held constant. Also, $P_1V_1 = P_2V_2$, where the subscripts 1 and 2 denote different states.

Charles' Law

$$V = \text{const.} \times T$$

where volume and pressure are held constant. Also, $V_1/V_2 = T_1/T_2$.

Molar Volume at STP

At standard temperature and pressure ("STP"), i.e., at 1.00 atm and 273 C, one mole of any ideal gas occupies 22.4 L.

Ideal Gas Law

$$PV = nRT$$

where n is the number of moles, R is the gas constant $= 0.08206$ L atm/K mol. (R can also be expressed in other units, as discussed in the section on kinetic theory.)

EXAMPLE

A sample of an ideal gas occupies 0.142 L at a pressure of 0.862 atm. Find the volume to which the sample must be compressed to raise the pressure to 14.6 atm. (Assume constant temperature and a constant amount of gas.)

SOLUTION

$P_1 V_1 = P_2 V_2$

$V_2 = P_1 V_1 / P_2 = (0.862 \text{ atm})(0.142 \text{ L})/(14.6 \text{ atm})$

$= 8.38 \times 10^{-3}$

EXAMPLE

A sample of an ideal gas weighing 1.650 g occupies 653 mL at 29.0°C and 755 torr. Find its molar mass.

SOLUTION

Since we know the mass, we can find the molar mass by first solving for n:

$$n = \frac{PV}{RT} = \frac{(755 \text{ torr})(\text{atm}/760 \text{ torr})(0.653\text{L})}{(0.08206 \text{ L atm/K mol})(273.2 + 29.0)\text{K}}$$

$= 0.0262 \text{ mol}$

Now we use n to find the molar mass:

molar mass $= 1.650 \text{ g}/0.0262 \text{ mol}$

$= 63.0 \text{ g/mol}$

Dalton's Law of Partial Pressures

$$P_{\text{total}} = \Sigma p_i$$

The total pressure in a gas mixture equals the sum of the partial pressures of the component gases.

To determine the **partial pressure,** p_i, we use the mole fractions X_i to compute

$$p_i = X_i P_{\text{total}}$$

where $X_i = n_i/n_{\text{total}}$, n_i is the number of moles of the gas in question, and n_{total} is the total number of moles.

EXAMPLE

A gas mixture contains 0.850 mol of O_2, 0.465 mol of N_2, and 0.0250 moles of H_2, at a total pressure of 0.995 atm. Find the partial pressure of N_2 in the mixture.

SOLUTION

First, find the mole fraction of N_2:

$$X_{N_2} = \frac{n_{N_2}}{n_{total}} = \frac{(0.465 \text{ mol})}{(0.850 + 0.465 + 0.0250) \text{ mol}}$$

$$= 0.347$$

$$P_{N_2} = X_{N_2} P_{total}$$

$$= (0.347)(0.995 \text{ atm})$$

0.345 atm

Kinetic Theory of Gases

This theory, developed in the nineteenth century, assumes that molecules can be considered small, hard spheres that are constantly in motion and that collide elastically. The kinetic theory interprets pressure on the wall of a container as the result of collisions of the molecules with the wall.

Kinetic Energy of a Gas

The kinetic theory predicts that the **kinetic energy** of one mole of an ideal gas is equal to $\left(\frac{3}{2}\right)RT$. (Note that the atomic weight of the gaseous substance does not enter the equation.)

Molecular Speeds

The expression above for total kinetic energy can be used to show that the root-mean-square speed of the molecules in a gas (a quantity close to the average speed) is given by

$$v = \sqrt{\frac{3RT}{M}},$$ where M is the molecular weight expressed in kg/mol, and R, the gas constant, is 8.315 J/mol K.

Note that not all molecules have this speed; rather, speeds are distributed above and below this central value. Actual speeds will range as low as just above 0, with no absolute limit on the highest speed.

For many purposes, the expression above can be more usefully applied as a ratio of speeds of:

1. Two molecules of differing molecular weights:

$$\frac{v_1}{v_2} = \sqrt{\frac{M_2}{M_1}}$$

Note the inverse square-root relationship, which predicts that heavy molecules travel less rapidly than light ones if both are at the same temperature.

This expression describes **diffusion,** the spread of gases through space, as well as **effusion,** the special case of flow of gas molecules through a narrow opening.

2. The same molecule at two different temperatures:

$$\frac{v_1}{v_2} = \sqrt{\frac{T_1}{T_2}}$$

This expression implies that as temperature increases so does speed, although it requires, for example, a fourfold increase in absolute temperature in order to double the speed of a molecule.

EXAMPLE

Find v_{rms} for oxygen molecules at 60°C.

SOLUTION

$$v_{rms} = \sqrt{\frac{3RT}{M}}$$
$$= \sqrt{3(8.315\text{J/K mol})(273 + 60)\text{K}/(0.032 \text{ kg/mol})}$$
$$= 509 \text{ m/s}$$

Note that in order to use SI units throughout, we have expressed the molar mass in kg/mol. In order to combine J with the other units in the expression, we changed J to $kg\ m^2\ s^{-2}$.

C. NON-IDEAL GASES

Real gases (**non-ideal gases**) differ from the ideal gas described above in two important ways:

1. The molecules have some volume, even if it is small compared to the total gas volume. Thus, the volume available to molecules in a container is less than the overall measured volume.

2. The molecules attract one another. These attractions pull molecules from straight-line paths, increasing the time between wall collisions and lowering the pressure.

These properties of a real gas can be expressed by the **van der Waals equation,** which resembles the ideal gas law but contains additional terms:

$$(P + [n^2a/V^2])(V - nb) = RT$$

where P is the measured pressure, V is the measured volume, n is the number of moles of the gas, a is a constant related to the intermolecular attraction, and b is a volume somewhat larger than the molecular volume. The constants a and b depend on the particular gas molecule.

Note that as the gas is made less concentrated, the correction terms become less important, and the gas appears to behave more ideally. Gases behave ideally at low pressures and high temperatures.

D. CONDENSED PHASES

While intermolecular forces are often of secondary importance in the gas phase, where molecules are far apart, they are vital to the understanding of the "condensed phases," liquids and solids, where molecules approach within a few diameters of each other.

London Dispersion Forces

These forces cause molecules without permanent dipole moments to attract one another based on "instantaneous" dipole moments caused by the momentary concentration of electron density on one side of the molecule or another. These forces are strongest at short ranges, and are greatest in atoms of high atomic number or in large molecules.

An important consequence of London dispersion forces is that freezing and boiling temperatures will generally be higher in a series of compounds as molecular weight increases.

Dipole-Dipole Forces

If one of two nearby molecules in a liquid or solid has a dipole moment, then the attraction between those molecules is greater than the London dispersion forces described above. In a series of molecules, the interactive forces increase as the dipole moment increases.

Hydrogen Bonds

A hydrogen bond occurs between a hydrogen that is covalently bonded to a highly electronegative atom on one molecule and a highly electronegative atom on a nearby molecule. For example, a hydrogen bond may form between the hydrogen attached to oxygen in CH_3OH and the oxygen of a neighboring H_2O molecule. Hydrogen bonds can occur between different types of molecules or between molecules of the same substance, such as H_2O or NH_3.

One effect of hydrogen bonding is to raise melting and boiling points. For example, without the strong hydrogen bonding present in water, water would be expected to be gaseous at room temperature.

Note that the hydrogen bond is not a covalent bond between hydrogen and another atom in the same molecule, but is rather a weak bond between two molecules. The strength of a hydrogen bond between hydrogen and oxygen is about 20 kJ/mol, an order of magnitude weaker than a covalent bond.

E. PHASE EQUILIBRIA

Phase Changes

Melting

Melting is the endothermic (heat-absorbing) process by which a solid is transformed to a liquid. The positive enthalpy change in the process is called the heat of fusion, $\Delta H°_{fus}$.

In general, the volume increases slightly on melting (with accompanying drop in density), although water does not obey this trend; it contracts from 0° to 4°C, then begins to expand on further heating.

Evaporation

Evaporation is the process by which a liquid changes to a gas.

The positive enthalpy change in the process is called the heat of vaporization, $\Delta H°_{vap}$, which is generally greater than the heat of fusion for the same substance.

Evaporation is accompanied by a large increase in volume of the substance.

Note that the gaseous form of a substance coexists with the liquid form at temperatures below the boiling point, with the vapor pressure growing larger as the temperature is increased. At the boiling point, the vapor pressure is equal to the external pressure.

Sublimation

Sublimation is a process by which molecules of the solid convert directly to the gas, without passing into the liquid phase.

Critical Point

The temperature and pressure at the critical point, illustrated below, are called the critical temperature and critical pressure. At the critical point, the density of the gas phase becomes equal to the density of the liquid, so that the distinction between the two phases vanishes. The resulting substance is called a "supercritical fluid."

Phase Diagrams

The phase behavior of carbon dioxide is summarized on a traditional "phase diagram" below.

Phase Diagram For CO₂

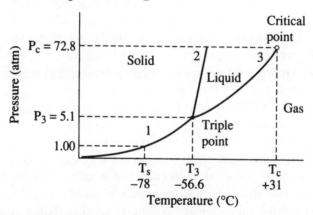

Note the following:

1. For values of *P* and *T* along line 1, a sublimation transition can occur; note in particular that at standard temperature and pressure, sublimation occurs rather than melting.

2. Along line 2, melting or freezing can occur. By choosing a given pressure, one can determine the freezing temperature.

3. Along line 3, evaporation or condensation can occur. By choosing a given pressure on that line, one can determine the boiling temperature.

4. Within the regions marked "Solid," "Liquid," and "Gas," only one phase occurs.

5. At the "Triple point" all three phases coexist; any change in P or T will cause at least one of the phases to disappear.

6. At the critical point, the liquid and gas phases disappear and the system becomes homogeneous.

F. COLLIGATIVE PROPERTIES

When a nonvolatile substance is dissolved in a liquid, it causes several **colligative**—i.e., collective—**effects.** These effects depend only on the number of particles of solute in the solution.

1. The Vapor Pressure of the Solvent Is Reduced (Raoult's Law)

This effect comes about owing to the decrease in the number of solvent molecules available to escape from the surface of the liquid. For "ideal solutions," Raoult's Law allows us to calculate the reduction in vapor pressure:

If a solution of nonvolatile solute with a mole fraction of X_1 is prepared using a solvent whose pure vapor pressure is P_2^0, then the vapor pressure of the solvent will be lowered by

$$\Delta P = X_1 P_2^0$$

EXAMPLE

At 25.0°C, the vapor pressure of pure water is 23.76 torr. Find the vapor pressure of a solution formed by dissolving 22.0 g of sucrose (molar mass = 342 g/mol) in 100.0 g of water. Sucrose may be considered to be nonvolatile (to have no appreciable vapor pressure) at 25°C.

SOLUTION

$$n_{sucrose} = \frac{22.0 \text{ g}}{342 \text{ g/mol}} = 0.0643 \text{ mol}$$

$$n_{H_2O} = \frac{100.0 \text{ g}}{18.0 \text{ g/mol}} = 5.56 \text{ mol}$$

$$X_1 = X_{sucrose} = \frac{0.0643 \text{ mol}}{(0.643 + 5.56) \text{ mol}}$$

$$= 0.0114$$

$$\Delta P = X_1 P_2^0 = (0.0114)(23.76 \text{ torr})$$

$$= 0.27 \text{ torr}$$

$$P_{vap} = P_{H_2O} - \Delta P = 23.49 \text{ torr}$$

2. The Boiling Point of the Solution Is Increased

If a solvent is diluted, it will no longer exhibit a vapor pressure of 1 atm at its normal boiling point, since somewhat fewer molecules will be available at the surface. Thus, the temperature must be raised to cause the solution to boil.

The elevation in the boiling point is found to be proportional to the "molality" (not the molarity) of the solute, where molality = m = (moles solute)/(kg solvent):

$$\Delta T_b = K_b m$$

where m is the molality calculated above, and K_b is the boiling point depression constant of the solvent. Values of K_b are tabulated for many solvents. For water, $K_b = 0.51°C$ kg/mol.

3. The Freezing Point of the Solution Is Decreased

If a solvent at its freezing temperature is diluted through the addition of a solute, then Le Chatelier's Principle predicts that the solid will melt in order to increase the concentration of the solvent in the liquid phase. Thus, the temperature must be lowered further in order to freeze the solution.

The expression for the freezing point lowering is

$$\Delta T_f = -K_f m$$

where K_f is the freezing point depression constant, tabulated for various solvents.

Molar Masses from Colligative Properties

The following example illustrates the use of a freezing point depression experiment to determine a molar mass.

EXAMPLE

A solution of 40.0 g of phosphoric acid in 2.00 kg water has a freezing point depression of 0.380° C. What is the molar mass of phosphoric acid? (K_f for water = 1.86°C kg H_2O/mol)

SOLUTION

First find the molality of the solution:

$$m = \frac{\Delta T}{K_f}$$

$$= \frac{0.380°C}{1.86°C \text{ kg } H_2O/\text{mol solute}}$$

$$= \frac{0.204 \text{ mol solute}}{\text{kg } H_2O}$$

We now have a ratio of moles of solute to kg of water, which can be used as a conversion factor to find the total moles of phosphoric acid solute present in 2.00 kg of water.

$$\text{moles solute} = (2.00 \text{ kg } H_2O)\left(\frac{0.204 \text{ mol solute}}{\text{kg } H_2O}\right)$$
$$= 0.408 \text{ mol solute}$$

Osmotic Pressure

If a solution containing a solute is separated from the pure solvent by a semipermeable membrane, one that allows solvent but not solute molecules to pass through, the solvent will diffuse from the dilute solution into the concentrated one.

The **osmotic pressure** of the solution is the external pressure that must be applied to the concentrated solution in order to stop the flow from the pure solvent.

The osmotic pressure is usually symbolized as π and can be related to other solution variables through the expression

$$\pi V = nRT \text{ or } \pi = MRT$$

where V is the volume of the solution, n is the number of moles of solute, M is the molarity, R is the gas constant, and T is the temperature. The equation, called the van't Hoff equation, resembles the Ideal Gas Law in its form.

PRACTICE PROBLEMS

1. A sample of H_2 gas occupies 0.30 L at 400°C and 760 torr pressure. To find the number of moles of gas in the sample, a student should calculate which of the following? (Units have been omitted.)

   A. (0.082)(400)/(760)(0.30)
   B. (0.082)(400)/(1.00)(0.30)
   C. (1.00)(0.30)/(0.082)(400)
   D. (1.00)(0.30)/(0.082)(673)

2. 4.0 moles of H_2O vapor at 0.20 atm and 298K are allowed to expand so that volume doubles. The temperature is unchanged. What is the new pressure (in atm)?

   A. 0.10
   B. 0.20
   C. 0.40
   D. 0.80

3. In Question 2, what is the final volume?

   A. 0.48 L
   B. 240 L
   C. 490 L
   D. 978 L

4. A sample of liquid weighing 0.15 g is heated to 100°C, a temperature high enough to change it to a vapor. The gas exerts a pressure of 1 atm when isolated in a 300-mL flask. Which of the expressions below could be used to determine the molecular weight of the gas?

   A. (0.15)(1.0)(273)/(0.082)(0.300)
   B. (0.15)(0.082)(273)/(1.00)(300)
   C. (0.15)(0.082)(373)/(1.00)(0.300)
   D. (0.300)(0.082)(373)/(1.00)(0.15)

5. In a mixture of H_2 and O_2, the ratio of speeds of the hydrogen to the oxygen molecules is

   A. 1:16
   B. 1:4
   C. 1:1
   D. 4:1

6. The molecules in a gas have a root-mean-square speed of 5.0×10^5 m/s at 300K. To what temperature will the gas have to be raised to have a root-mean-square speed of 1.5×10^6 m/s?

   A. 600K
   B. 900K
   C. 2100K
   D. 2700K

7. Hydrogen gas generated in a reaction is collected over water at 25°C and is found to have a pressure of 746 torr. (The vapor pressure of water at 25°C is 24 torr.) Which expression can be used to find the pressure of H_2, in atm?

   A. 24
   B. 746
   C. 746 + 24
   D. (746 − 24)/760

8. Which of the following are *not* characteristic of ideal gas behavior?

   I. Gas molecules move more rapidly at higher temperatures.
   II. It is difficult to compress gases beyond certain pressures, owing to intermolecular repulsions.
   III. Gases liquefy as they are cooled beyond a certain point.

   A. I only
   B. II only
   C. III only
   D. II and III only

9. In order to determine the partial pressure of O_2 in a mixture of several gases, a student should use

   A. Raoult's Law.
   B. Charles' Law.
   C. Boyle's Law.
   D. Dalton's Law.

10. In order to protect a car's engine from excessive cold, "antifreeze" added to the radiator water must

    A. depress the boiling point of the radiator water.
    B. increase the vapor pressure of the cooling liquid.
    C. elevate the freezing point of the radiator water.
    D. depress the freezing point of the radiator water.

11. Which of the following are arranged in order of increasing intermolecular forces? (Assume all are in the liquid phase, at the same temperature.)

    A. O_2, He, HCl
    B. HCl, O_2, He
    C. He, O_2, HCl
    D. O_2, HCl, He

12. What is the vapor pressure of H_2O at 100°C?

    A. 0.2 atm
    B. 0.5 atm
    C. 0.75 atm
    D. 1.0 atm

13. Which of the following statements about the Ideal Gas Law and the van der Waals equation are true?

 I. At low densities, a real gas behaves like an ideal gas.
 II. The "*b*" term in the van der Waals equation describes intermolecular forces.
 III. The product *PV* equals a constant (for constant *T*) for real and ideal gases alike.

 A. I only
 B. II only
 C. III only
 D. I and II only

14. Which of the following best anticipates the intermolecular attractive forces between molecules in H_2 and F_2, each in the same phase and at the same temperature?

 A. The forces will be stronger in H_2 owing to its greater speed.
 B. The forces will be stronger in F_2 owing to its greater dipole moment.
 C. The forces will be stronger in F_2 owing to its greater polarizability.
 D. The forces will be stronger in H_2 owing to its greater polarizability.

15. Which of the following best anticipates the relationship among the boiling points in argon, Cl_2, and FBr?

 A. $Ar < FBr < Cl_2$
 B. $FBr < Cl_2 < Ar$
 C. $Cl_2 < Ar < FBr$
 D. $Ar < Cl_2 < FBr$

ANSWER KEY

1. D	3. D	5. D	7. D	9. D	11. C	13. A	15. D
2. A	4. C	6. D	8. D	10. D	12. D	14. C	

ANSWERS AND EXPLANATIONS

1. **The correct answer is (D).** Use $n = PV/RT$

$$= \frac{(760 \text{ torr})(1 \text{ atm}/760 \text{ torr})(0.30 \text{ L})}{(0.082 \text{ L atm/K mol})(400 + 273) \text{ K}}$$

2. **The correct answer is (A).** You can use $P_1V_1 = P_2V_2$, since *T* is constant.

3. **The correct answer is (D).** One approach is to solve for the final *P* as in (2), then use the gas law to find *V*:

$$V = nRT/P = (4.0)(0.0821)(298)/(.1) = 979 \text{ L}$$

4. **The correct answer is (C).** Use $PV = nRT$ where $n = \text{grams}/MW$. Then solve for *MW*. Note *V* must be in liters, *T* in K.

5. **The correct answer is (D).** Use $v_1/v_2 = \left(\dfrac{m_2}{m_1}\right)^{\frac{1}{2}} = \left(\dfrac{32}{2}\right)^{\frac{1}{2}} = 4$. Check using physical intuition: H_2 is lighter, should move faster.

6. **The correct answer is (D).** Use $v_1/v_2 = \left(\dfrac{T_1}{T_2}\right)^{\frac{1}{2}}$

$$300/T_2 = \left[\dfrac{(5 \times 10^5)}{(1.5 \times 10^6)}\right]^2$$
$$T_2 = 2700K$$

As an alternate, more intuitive explanation, note that since the speed needs to be tripled, the temperature must be multiplied by 3^2, or 9.

7. **The correct answer is (D).** You must subtract the pressure of water vapor from the total pressure, and change torr to atm.

8. **The correct answer is (D).** While ideal gases move more rapidly at high temperature, they are "infinitely" compressible and they do not liquefy.

9. **The correct answer is (D).** Dalton's law of partial pressures states that the partial pressure of each is proportional to its mole fraction.

10. **The correct answer is (D).** Antifreeze is a solute that depresses the freezing temperature of the cooling water to a point below the outside temperature; solutes depress, rather than elevate, the freezing point.

11. **The correct answer is (C).** Forces between single atoms are lowest, then diatomic molecules with no dipole moment, then finally diatomics with dipole moments.

12. **The correct answer is (D).** We know that water boils at this temperature. "Boiling" means that the vapor pressure is equal to the external pressure.

13. **The correct answer is (A).** At low densities the correction terms to P and V become very small. Both correction terms, nb and an^2/V^2, depend on the number of gas molecules in a given volume, which is small at low densities. PV is not constant for the real gas as it is for an ideal gas.

14. **The correct answer is (C).** F_2 has more electrons, occupying a greater volume, than does H_2. Thus, it is more polarizable and will have stronger London forces.

15. **The correct answer is (D).** A low boiling point corresponds to weak intermolecular forces. Argon has the lowest of these: As a neutral atom, it is less polarizable than the larger Cl_2. The latter has no dipole moment, so exerts weaker forces than does FBr.

1.5 SOLUTION CHEMISTRY

A. IONS IN SOLUTION

Many of the compounds that dissolve, whether sparingly or completely, in aqueous solution, do so by dissociating into ions. These are called **cations** if positively charged, and **anions** if negatively charged. The ions may derive from single atoms (e.g., Na^+) or consist of several atoms (e.g., $Cr_2O_7^{2-}$).

B. CHARGES ON COMMONLY ENCOUNTERED IONS

In order to write chemical formulas easily for ionic compounds, it is useful to memorize the most common ions and their charges. The table below lists a number of these:

Cations			Anions		
+1	+2	+3	−1	−2	−3
Na^+	Mg^{2+}	Al^{3+}	F^-	O^{2-}	PO_4^{3-}
Cu^+	Ca^{2+}	Fe^{3+}	Cl^-	S^{2-}	
Ag^+	Ba^{2+}		Br^-	CO_3^{2-}	
K^+	Mn^{2+}		I^-	SO_4^{2-}	
NH_4^+	Fe^{2+}		OH^-	CrO_4^{2-}	
	Ni^{2+}		NO_3^-	$Cr_2O_7^{2-}$	
	Cu^{2+}		NO_2^-		
	Zn^{2+}		CN^-		
	Hg^{2+}		ClO_4^-		
	Sn^{2+}		MnO_4^-		
	Pb^{2+}		SCN^-		

C. SOLUBILITY

The **solubility** of a solute is usually specified as the number of moles of the solute that will dissolve in 1.00 liter of water. The dimensions of solubility are mol/L.

Salts that are highly soluble in water include those that contain Na^+, K^+, NH_4^+, and NO_3^-.

Fundamental Solubility Rules

Soluble

1. Most nitrate and acetate salts.

2. Most salts containing Na^+, K^+, and NH_4^+.

3. Most salts containing chloride. (Exceptions: $AgCl$, $PbCl_2$, and Hg_2Cl_2)

4. Most salts containing sulfate. (Exceptions: $PbSO_4$, $CaSO_4$, $SrSO_4$, $BaSO_4$, and Hg_2SO_4)

Insoluble
1. Most hydroxides and oxides. (Exceptions: compounds containing Group IA metals, Ca^{2+}, Sr^{2+}, and Ba^{2+}) Note that when oxides dissolve, they form hydroxide ions in water.

2. Most phosphates, carbonates, sulfites, and sulfides. (Exceptions: compounds containing Group IA metals or NH_4^+)

Example
Find the concentration (in units of *molarity*, abbreviated M) of a solution of Na_2SO_4 that is made by dissolving 0.345 g of the salt in 675 mL of water.

Solution
moles Na_2SO_4 = mass of salt / molar mass
$$= (0.345 \text{ g}) / (142 \text{ g/mol})$$
$$= 2.43 \times 10^{-3} \text{ mol}$$

concentration of Na_2SO_4 = (moles Na_2SO_4) / (L of solution)
$$= (2.43 \times 10^{-3} \text{ mol}) / (0.675 \text{ L})$$
$$= 3.60 \times 10^{-3} \text{ M}$$

Example
Find the number of moles of KBr in 15.5 mL of a 0.0788 M solution of KBr.

Solution
moles KBr = (vol of KBr)(concentration KBr)
$$= (0.0155 \text{ L})(0.0788 \text{ mol/L})$$
$$= 1.22 \times 10^{-3} \text{ moles KBr}$$

Example
Find the concentration of a solution that is 0.556 M in KNO_3 if 5.00 mL of the solution is diluted by the addition of 245 mL of water.

Solution
The key concept in this problem is that dilution does not change the moles of solute present.

moles solute = (concentration of solute)(volume of solution)

Thus, if the concentration and volume *before* the dilution are C_1 and V_1, and the concentration and volume *after* the dilution are C_2 and V_2, then

$$C_1V_1 = C_2V_2$$
$$C_2 = C_1V_1 / V_2$$
$$= (0.556 \text{ M})(5.00 \text{ mL}) / (5.00 + 245)\text{mL}$$
$$= 0.0111 \text{ M}$$

Note that in this problem, volumes did not have to be converted from mL to L, as they must in certain other problems. Note also that in this problem, the final volume is the sum of the original volume and the added volume of water.

D. SOLUBILITY PRODUCT

The solubility product is the equilibrium constant for a particular reaction, that of the dissociation of a sparingly soluble salt. Taking silver chloride as an example,

$$AgCl(s) \rightleftharpoons Ag^+(aq) + Cl^-(aq)$$
$$K_{sp} = [Ag^+(aq)][Cl^-(aq)]$$

Values of K_{sp} are given in tables. The use of K_{sp} is illustrated in the examples below. Note that the solubility product is not the same as the solubility.

Example 1

The solubility of AgCl in pure water is 1.26×10^{-5} M. Find K_{sp} in a solution of H_2O to which excess silver chloride has been added.

Solution

In 1.0 liter of H_2O, 1.34×10^{-5} moles of AgCl must have dissociated, producing a like amount of each ion.

$$K_{sp} = [Ag^+][Cl^-] = (1.26 \times 10^{-5})^2 = 1.59 \times 10^{-10}$$

Example 2

Find the concentration of Ni^{2+} and CO_3^{2-} in equilibrium with solid $NiCO_3$, whose K_{sp} is 1.4×10^{-7}.

Solution

We let x = the concentration of Ni^{2+} and CO_3^{2-}.

$$NiCO_3(s) \rightleftharpoons \underset{x}{Ni^{2+}} + \underset{x}{CO_3^{2-}}$$
$$x^2 = 1.4 \times 10^{-7}$$
$$x = (1.4 \times 10^{-7})^{\frac{1}{2}} = 3.7 \times 10^{-4}$$
$$[Ni^{2+}] = [CO_3^{2-}] = 3.7 \times 10^{-4} M$$

Because each mole of $NiCO_3$ that dissolves leads to one mole of Ni^{2+}, we can say that the solubility of $NiCO_3$ is 3.7×10^{-4}.

Example 3

Find the concentration of Ca^{2+} and F^- in a solution saturated with CaF_2 for which $K_{sp} = 3.9 \times 10^{-11}$.

Solution

$$CaF_2(s) \rightleftharpoons \underset{x}{Ca^{2+}} + \underset{2x}{2F^-}$$
$$x(2x)^2 = 4x^3 = 3.9 \times 10^{-11}$$
$$x = (9.8 \times 10^{-12})^{\frac{1}{3}} = 2.1 \times 10^{-4} M$$
$$[Ca^{2+}] = 2.1 \times 10^{-4} M$$
$$[F^-] = 2(2.1 \times 10^{-4}) = 4.2 \times 10^{-4} M$$

In this problem, the value of x that we have determined equals the solubility.

E. COMMON ION EFFECT

We found the solubility of AgCl in pure H_2O. Suppose AgCl were added to a solution of 0.10 M NaCl—recall that all salts containing Na^+ are soluble. As the AgCl dissociates, the Ag^+ ions liberated will encounter Cl^-'s from the NaCl solution and will precipitate as AgCl(s). Thus, the solubility of AgCl in NaCl is expected to be lower than in pure water.

To find the exact concentration, we use

$$AgCl(s) \rightleftharpoons Ag^+ + Cl^-$$
$$x(0.10 + x)$$
$$1.6 \times 10^{-10} = (x)(0.10 + x) = (x)(0.10)$$

Let us assume that x can be neglected in the second factor. Then,

$$1.6 \times 10^{-10} = x(0.10)$$
$$x = [Ag^+] = 1.6 \times 10^{-9}$$

Now we must justify neglecting x compared to 0.10, using the calculated value:

$$x = \frac{1.6 \times 10^{-9}}{0.10} = 1.6 \times 10^{-8}$$

Thus, the approximation was justified.

Note that:

1. $[Ag^+]$ is equal to the solubility in this solution, since each Ag^+ must have come from the dissociation of one AgCl.

2. The solubility is much less than the value found in pure water. This is consistent with what Le Chatelier's Principle would predict, since the presence of excess product—in this case, chloride ion—causes the equilibrium to shift to the left, diminishing the solubility of the solid AgCl.

F. SELECTIVE PRECIPITATION

We often wish to separate a mixture of ions. This can be accomplished if one of the ions in the mixture reacts with an added ion to form a solid while the remaining ions remain in solution. The following example shows how solubility calculations can lead to a successful separation.

Example

100 mL of a solution is 0.0100 M in both NaCl(aq) and NaBr(aq). If 0.100 M $AgNO_3$(aq) is added to the mixture, which salt will precipitate first—AgCl(s) or AgBr(s)? Give an estimate of the concentration of the first salt that will remain in solution when the second salt begins to precipitate. (K_{sp} for AgCl is 1.6×10^{-10}; K_{sp} for AgBr is 5.0×10^{-13})

Solution

Since AgCl and AgBr each contain two ions, we can predict that AgBr will precipitate first because its K_{sp} is lower. To verify this statement, we can calculate the concentration of Ag^+ needed to establish equilibrium with AgBr(s) when $[Br^-] = 0.0100$ M:

$$[Ag^+] = K_{sp}\,(AgBr)/[Br^-]$$
$$= (5.00 \times 10^{-13})/\,(0.0100)$$
$$= 5.00 \times 10^{-11}\text{ M}$$

Repeating this calculation with the equilibrium of Ag^+ and AgCl(s), we find

$$[Ag^+] = K_{sp}\,(AgCl)/[Cl^-]$$
$$= (1.6 \times 10^{-10})/\,(0.0100)$$
$$= 1.6 \times 10^{-8}\text{ M}$$

Since a smaller value of $[Ag^+]$ is needed to precipitate AgBr(s) than to precipitate AgCl(s), AgBr(s) will precipitate first. As the Br^- ion is depleted, the value of $[Ag^+]$ will rise above its initial value of 5.00×10^{-11} M; when it reaches 1.6×10^{-8} M, AgCl(s) will begin to appear. For effective separation, the addition of $AgNO_3$ should be stopped at this point. The concentration of Br^- remaining in solution can be calculated:

$$[Br^-] = K_{sp}(KBr)/[Ag^+]$$
$$= (5.0 \times 10^{-13})\,/\,(1.6 \times 10^{-8})$$
$$= 3.12 \times 10^{-5}\text{ M}$$

Thus, by precipitating AgBr(s) using $AgNO_3$(aq), we have reduced the amount of Br^- in the solution from its original value of 0.0100 M to 3.12×10^{-5} M, for a percentage reduction of

$$\frac{(0.0100\text{ M} - 3.12 \times 10^{-5})}{0.0100\text{ M}} \times 100\% = 99.7\%$$

PRACTICE PROBLEMS

1. Three solutions are prepared as follows:

   Solution I. Pure H_2O

   Solution II. 0.10 M KCl

   Solution III. 1 M $AgNO_3$

   A student places 2.0 g of solid AgCl in 100 mL of each solution. The solubility of the AgCl will be greatest in

   A. I
   B. II
   C. III
   D. I and II

2. K_{sp} for salt A is 2×10^{-10}; for salt B it is 2×10^{-14}. We can say that

   A. salt A is more soluble in plain water than salt B.
   B. salt B is more soluble in plain water than salt A.
   C. salt A is more soluble, provided it dissociates into the same number of ions as salt B.
   D. salt B is more soluble, provided it dissociates into the same number of ions as salt A.

3. The solubility of AgCl in pure water is approximately 10^{-5} M. Which expression gives the value of K_{sp}?

   A. $(10^{-5})^{\frac{1}{2}}$
   B. (10^{-5})
   C. $(10^{-5})^2$
   D. $(10^{-5})(2 \times 10^{-5})^2$

4. A solution of 0.10 M $AgNO_3$ is added to a second solution containing various halides, all of which precipitate with silver ion. The *last* anion to precipitate will be that with

   A. the greatest K_{sp} for the salt of Ag^+ with the halide.
   B. the smallest K_{sp} for the salt of Ag^+ with the halide.
   C. the greatest K_a.
   D. the smallest K_a.

5. Which of the following correctly expresses both a correct statement *and* a correct explanation for that statement?

   A. The solubility of $Fe(OH)_3$ is pH-dependent, owing to the half-cell potential of Fe^{3+}/Fe^{2+}.
   B. The solubility of $Fe(OH)_3$ is pH-dependent, owing to the presence of $[OH^-]$ in the solubility expression.
   C. The solubility product of $Fe(OH)_3$ is pH-dependent, owing to the presence of $[OH^-]$ in the solubility expression.
   D. The solubility product of $Fe(OH)_3$ is not pH-dependent, since $[H^+]$ does not appear in the solubility expression.

Questions 6–8 are based on the data in the chart below (the "halide" in the fourth column refers to the anion of the salt in that row):

Salt	K_{sp}	Solubility in Water	Solubility in 0.1 M halide
AgCl	1.8×10^{-10}	(1)	—
AgBr	(2)	7×10^{-7}	—
AgI	(3)	—	8.5×10^{-16}

6. What is the value of (1) in the table?

   A. 1.8×10^{-10}
   B. $(1.8 \times 10^{-10})^{\frac{1}{2}}$
   C. $(1.8 \times 10^{-10})^2$
   D. 0.1

7. What is the value of (2) in the table?

   A. 7×10^{-7}
   B. $(7 \times 10^{-7})^{\frac{1}{2}}$
   C. $(7 \times 10^{-7})^2$
   D. 0.1

8. What is the value of (3) in the table?

   A. 8.5×10^{-16}
   B. $(8.5 \times 10^{-16})^2$
   C. $(8.5 \times 10^{-16})^{\frac{1}{2}}$
   D. $(8.5 \times 10^{-16})(0.1)$

9. What happens if 0.1 mol $AgNO_3$ is added to 0.1 mol NaCl?

  A. No reaction occurs.
  B. There is slight formation of AgCl.
  C. Approximately 0.05 mol AgCl is formed.
  D. Approximately 0.10 mol of AgCl is formed.

10. If 100 mL of 0.1 M $AgNO_3$ is added to a solution containing both 0.1 M NaBr and 0.1 M NaCl, the result is

  A. no net reaction.
  B. precipitation of AgBr and AgCl.
  C. precipitation of mostly AgBr.
  D. precipitation of mostly AgCl.

11. The solubility products for $Mg(OH)_2$ and $Mn(OH)_2$ are 7.1×10^{-12} and 6×10^{-14}, respectively. If 50 mL each of 0.1 M $Mg(NO_3)_2$ and 0.1 M $Mn(NO_3)_2$ are mixed with 50 mL of 0.1 M NaOH, the predominant product will be solid _____.

  A. $Mg(OH)_2$
  B. $Mn(OH)_2$
  C. equal amounts of $Mg(OH)_2$ and $Mn(OH)_2$
  D. NaOH

ANSWER KEY

1. A   2. C   3. C   4. A   5. B   6. B   7. C   8. D   9. D   10. C   11. B

ANSWERS AND EXPLANATIONS

1. **The correct answer is (A).** Pure water. Solutions II and III have ions in common with the AgCl, and will inhibit dissociation.

2. **The correct answer is (C).** K_{sp} is not a reliable index of solubility for salts with different numbers of ions. As an example, consider the pure water solubility of a salt symbolized as AB, such as AgCl, whose K_{sp} is 1.8×10^{-10}.

sol. $= (K_{sp})^{\frac{1}{2}} = 1.3 \times 10^{-5}$ mol/L

Now consider salt CD_2 such as Ag_2CrO_4, whose K_{sp} is 1.2×10^{-12}.

sol. $= (K_{sp}/4)^{\frac{1}{3}} = 6.7 \times 10^{-5}$ mol/L

Even though the K_{sp} of AgCl is more than 100 times greater than the K_{sp} of Ag_2CrO_4, AgCl is less soluble.

3. **The correct answer is (C).** In pure water, sol. $= [Ag^+] = [Cl^-]$.

4. **The correct answer is (A).** Because each has the same number of ions, the salt with the *greatest* K_{sp} is the one most "willing" to dissociate, or, conversely, least "willing" to precipitate.

5. **The correct answer is (B).** Note solubility, not solubility *product*, is hydroxide-dependent. D is wrong because $[H^+]$ and $[OH^-]$ are related.

6. **The correct answer is (B).** In pure water, the solubility is $(K_{sp})^{\frac{1}{2}}$.

7. **The correct answer is (C).** This problem is the reverse of (6); K_{sp} is the square of the solubility.

8. **The correct answer is (D).** In the presence of 0.1 M of a common anion, the solubility $= [Ag^+]$, so

$K_{sp} = (0.1)(8.5 \times 10^{-16})$

9. **The correct answer is (D).** The reaction is essentially complete, since its K is $1/K_{sp}$.

10. **The correct answer is (C).** The salt with the smaller K_{sp} will precipitate when each has the same number of ions.

11. **The correct answer is (B).** The salt with the smaller K_{sp} precipitates first, and there is not enough NaOH to precipitate the second salt.

1.6   ACIDS AND BASES

A.   DEFINITIONS

Three definitions of acids and bases are in common use:

1. An **Arrhenius acid** donates H^+ ions (protons) in solution, while an **Arrhenius base** donates OH^- ions.

    ### Example
    HNO_3 is an Arrhenius acid; KOH is an Arrhenius base.

2. A **Brønsted-Lowry acid** donates H^+ while a **Brønsted-Lowry base** accepts H^+. This definition is the most useful one for acids and bases in aqueous solution.

    ### Example
    H_3O^+ is a Brønsted-Lowry acid, while OH^-, $HCOO^-$, etc., are Brønsted-Lowry bases.

3. A **Lewis acid** *accepts an electron pair*, while a **Lewis base** *donates* such a pair. Examples of acid and base under this definition are H^+ and OH^-, respectively, but also include such non-hydrogen compounds as BF_3 (Lewis acid) or Cl^- (Lewis base).

B.   IONIZATION OF WATER

The ionization of water, described by the following equilibrium reaction, is of fundamental importance to acid-base chemistry in aqueous solution:

$$H_2O \rightleftharpoons H^+ + OH^-$$

The extent of dissociation is indicated by the dissociation constant, K_w

$$K_w = 10^{-14} = [H^+][OH^-]$$

K_w varies slightly with temperature, but is usually assigned the value of 1.0×10^{-14}. It does not vary with concentration of any species dissolved in the water.

Note that if $[H^+]$ is known, then $[OH^-]$ can be determined, and vice versa.

Note also that although $[H^+]$ need not equal $[OH^-]$, if the two are equal ("neutral water"), each must equal 1.0×10^{-7}.

C. DEFINITION OF pH

The quantity **pH** is defined as follows:

$$pH = -\log_{10}[H^+]$$

Similarly,

$$pOH = -\log_{10}[OH^-]$$

Example

Find the pH of a solution if $[H^+] = 1.0 \times 10^{-9}$ M.

Solution

$$
\begin{aligned}
pH &= -\log [H^+] \\
&= -\log (1.0 \times 10^{-9}) \\
&= -(-9.00) \\
&= 9.00
\end{aligned}
$$

Note the rule for significant figures in logarithm calculations: Because $[H^+]$ is given to 2 significant figures, log $[H^+]$ must have 2 digits to the right of the decimal place.

Note also that while $[H^+]$ has units of M, pH is dimensionless.

Example

Find $[H^+]$ in a solution whose pH is 3.76.

Solution

Since $pH = -\log [H^+]$,

$$
\begin{aligned}
[H^+] &= 10^{-pH} \\
&= 10^{-3.76} \\
&= 1.7 \times 10^{-4} M
\end{aligned}
$$

(Two digits to the right of the decimal place in the value of pH requires 2 significant figures in the value of $[H^+]$.)

Comments on the pH scale

The pH scale is a way of taking very great differences in $[H^+]$ and reducing them to a shorthand scale of roughly 0 to 14.

Each change in pH of 1.0 represents a factor of 10 difference; e.g., if pH is 1.0 in one solution and 7.0 in another, the ratio of concentrations is 10^6.

pH values *can* be negative or greater than 14, representing very concentrated strong acids or bases, respectively.

pH can be quickly estimated as follows:

Find the pH if $[H^+] = 2.0 \times 10^{-3}$.

Because $[H^+] > 10^{-3}$, its logarithm is slightly *greater than* -3, so its pH is slightly less than $+3$. (A calculator gives a pH of 2.7.)

D. CONJUGATE ACIDS AND BASES

If a weak acid is symbolized by HA, then its conjugate base is formed by removing a hydrogen to form A^-. Together the two species are referred to as a conjugate acid-base pair. (Note that the acid species need not be neutral, as in the second example below.)

Examples of conjugate acid-base pairs:

1. Acetic acid/acetate: $C_2H_3O_2H/C_2H_3O_2^-$

2. Ammonium/ammonia: NH_4^+/NH_3

3. Amino acid: cationic form/neutral form (zwitterion):

    $$H_3N^+-CHR-COOH \ / \ H_3N^+-CHR-COO^-$$

    where "R" is a side group that differs with different amino acids. (An anionic form, in which one H^+ on the N is removed, also exists.)

4. An example using an amino acid. Amino acids have the general formula

where R is one of several different organic groups.

The structure is more accurately given using the zwitterion form, in which the ends of the molecule have opposite charges:

For the amino acid alanine, R is a $-CH_3$ group, so the structures of the conjugate acids and base are

Amino acids are discussed in more detail in the Organic Chemistry section.

E. STRONG ACIDS

A strong acid dissociates virtually completely. The most common strong acids are HCl, HNO_3, H_2SO_4 (first hydrogen ion), and $HClO_4$.

F. STRONG BASES

The common strong bases which, like strong acids, dissociate completely, are $NaOH$, KOH, and $Ba(OH)_2$.

G. STRENGTHS OF WEAK ACIDS AND BASES: K_A AND K_B

Weak Acids

The dissociation of a weak acid can be illustrated for hydrofluoric acid, HF:

$$HF \rightleftharpoons H^+ + F^-$$

The dissociation constant, K_a, is the equilibrium constant for this reaction:

$$K_a = [H^+][F^-]/[HF] = 3.5 \times 10^{-4}$$

The relatively small value of K_a confirms the fact that the equilibrium "lies to the left" and thus dissociation is not appreciable.

Weak Bases

The fluoride ion, F^-, which is the conjugate base of HF, reacts in plain water—no additional H^+ present—as follows:

$$F^- + H_2O \rightleftharpoons HF + OH^-$$

The equilibrium constant is given by

$$K_b = [HF][OH^-]/[F^-] = 2.9 \times 10^{-11}$$

The constants K_a and K_b are related by the expression

$$K_a K_b = 10^{-14}$$

Because of this relationship, an acid with a relatively large K_a will have a correspondingly low K_b.

The quantities pK_a and pK_b are also widely used:

$$pK_a = -\log K_a$$
$$pK_b = -\log K_b$$

H. CLASSIFICATION OF WEAK ACID-BASE PROBLEMS

1. Monoprotic Acids and Bases

Problems involving weak, monoprotic acids and bases are simplified by classifying them into three fundamental groups.

Case 1. Pure Weak Acid

Example

Find the pH of 0.10 M solution of acetic acid, "HOAc," for which $K_a = 1.8 \times 10^{-5}$.

$$HOA_C \rightleftharpoons H^+ \ OA_c^-$$
$$(.10 - x) \ x \ \ x$$
$$x^2/(0.10 - x) = 1.8 \times 10^{-5}$$

Neglect the x in the denominator (check validity of approximation afterward):

$$[H^+] = x = [(0.10)(1.8 \times 10^{-5})]^{\frac{1}{2}}$$
$$= 1.3 \times 10^{-3}$$
$$pH = -\log(1.3 \times 10^{-3})$$
$$= 2.89$$

We confirm the approximation made earlier, noting that $x/0.10 = 0.013$.

When an approximation similar to that above holds, for an acid of concentration C_a and dissociation constant K_a, we can write the following approximate formula:

$$[H^+] = (K_a C_a)^{\frac{1}{2}}$$

When the approximation that $x << C_a$ is *not* valid, we may use additional approximations (also referred to as *successive* approximations) that reinsert a result into the next calculation:

Example

Use a series of successive approximations to determine $[H^+]$ in a solution of 0.20 M HX for which $K_a = 3.0 \times 10^{-3}$. Compare the result with that given by the quadratic formula.

Solution

Because K_a is fairly high, we suspect that the usual approximation, which in this case becomes

$$x << 0.20 \text{ M,}$$

may not prove to be justified.

We set up the usual equation:

$$3.0 \times 10^{-3} = x^2/(0.20 - x)$$

As before, let us set $x = 0$ in the denominator. Then our first approximation for x is found to be

$$x = ((0.20)(3.0 \times 10^{-3}))^{\frac{1}{2}}$$
$$x = 0.013 \text{ M}$$

To check the approximation, we compute

$$x/(0.20 \text{ M}) = 0.065$$

It is common to accept an approximate answer if this ratio is 0.05 or less; here we evidently need to refine the result.

To achieve a second (and, presumably, more accurate) approximation, we again write the equation that needs to be solved:

$$3.0 \times 10^{-3} = x^2/(0.20 - x)$$

Now, rather than let $x = 0$ in the denominator, we set x equal to the previously determined approximate value, and solve for the remaining x in the numerator:

$$3.0 \times 10^{-3} = x^2/(0.20 - 0.013)$$
$$x^2 = (3.0 \times 10^{-3})(0.20 - 0.013)$$
$$x = 0.024 \text{ M}$$

This new, approximate value is considerably larger than the first one. If we repeat the process, inserting 0.024 M for the value of x in the denominator, we obtain 0.023 M.

We may use the quadratic formula to solve the equation exactly. We expand the original equation:

$$3.0 \times 10^{-3} = x^2/(0.20 - x)$$
$$x^2 + (3.0 \times 10^{-3})x - (6.0 \times 10^{-4}) = 0$$

Now we insert the three coefficients into the quadratic formula, choosing only the positive root:

$$x = \frac{-(3.0 \times 10^{-3}) + ((3.0 \times 10^{-3})^2 - 4(1)(-6.0 \times 10^{-4}))^{\frac{1}{2}}}{2(1)}$$
$$= 0.023 \text{ M}$$

The exact result is consistent with the result obtained using successive approximations. In general, approximate methods are faster for solving quadratic equations such as this one, and are essential for the higher-order equations that occur in other kinds of equilibrium problems.

Case 2. Pure Weak Base

Example
Find the pH of 0.20 M NH_3.

The value of K_b for NH_3 is 1.8×10^{-5}.

In water, NH_3 behaves as F^- did in the earlier example:

$$NH_3 + H_2O \rightleftharpoons NH_4 + OH^-$$
$$(0.20 - x) \qquad x \qquad x$$
$$x^2/(0.20 - x) = K_b = 1.8 \times 10^{-5}$$

Approximating as before:

$$x = [OH^-] = [(0.20)(1.8 \times 10^{-5})]^{\frac{1}{2}}$$
$$= 1.9 \times 10^{-3}$$
$$pOH = -\log(1.9 \times 10^{-3}) = 2.72; pH = 11.28$$

In general, when the above approximation is valid, we can write the following approximate formula:

$$[OH^-] = (C_b K_b)^{\frac{1}{2}}$$

Case 3. Buffer

A **buffer** is a mixture of a weak acid and its conjugate base or of a weak base and its conjugate acid; the mixture should have appreciable amounts of both; e.g., 1:1 or even 10:1 mixtures of each species may be buffers, but 1000:1 mixtures will not.

Example

0.50 mol of NaOH is added to 1.00 mol of formic acid (HCOOH) so that the total volume is 1.00 L. (K_a for formic acid is 1.9×10^{-4}.) Find the pH that results.

After the NaOH and the formic acid react, the resulting solution has approximately 0.50 mol each of HCOOH and HCOO$^-$. Rearranging the K_a expression:

$$[H^+] = K_a [HCOOH]/[HCOO^-]$$
$$= K_a (0.5 \text{ mol}/1.00 \text{ L})/(0.5 \text{ mol}/1.00 \text{ L})$$
$$= K_a = 1.9 \times 10^{-4}$$

The result is approximate, because we have neglected the slight dissociation of formic acid to formate, a process that will decrease the numerator and increase the denominator.

Several points are worth noting:

1. The result shows that for a buffer, $[H^+] = K_a$ multiplied by a simple ratio.

2. Because the solution volume is the same in numerator and denominator, the approximation can also be written

    $$[H^+] = K_a (\text{moles weak acid})/(\text{moles weak base})$$

3. If the concentrations of conjugate acid and base are equal, then

    $$[H^+] = K_a$$

4. The result can be used to predict how to make a buffer solution of a given $[H^+]$: Find a ratio of conjugate acid to conjugate base that leads to the desired value of $[H^+]$.

5. The result given can also be transformed into the Henderson-Hasselbalch equation for pH. If HA is a weak acid, then

    $$pH = pK_a + \log([A^-]/[HA])$$

2. Polyprotic Acids and Bases

Polyprotic acids are those that lose more than one hydrogen ion in solution.

The common acid sulfuric acid, H_2SO_4, has the unusual property that one of its hydrogens comes off completely, making it a strong acid:

$$H_2SO_4(aq) \rightarrow H^+(aq) + HSO_4^-(aq) \qquad \text{(reaction goes completion)}$$

The resulting hydrogen sulfate ion then dissociates slightly, exhibiting the characteristics of a weak acid:

$$HSO_4^-(aq) \leftrightarrow H^+(aq) + SO_4^{2-}(aq) \qquad {}^\Delta K_a = 1.2 \times 10^{-2}$$

Most diprotic acids are weak in each of their dissociations. An example is ascorbic acid (Vitamin C), whose formula is $H_2C_6H_6O_6$:

$$H_2C_6H_6O_6(aq) \leftrightarrow H^+(aq) + HC_6H_6O_6^-(aq) \qquad {}^\Delta K_1 = 7.9 \times 10^{-5}$$
$$HC_6H_6O_6^-(aq) \leftrightarrow H^+(aq) + C_6H_6O_6^{2-}(aq) \qquad {}^\Delta K_2 = 1.6 \times 10^{-12}$$

Note that K_2 is considerably smaller than K_1; often successive acid constants differ by factors of 10^3 or even more. When such large differences exist, calculations of pH and other quantities are facilitated, as we will see below.

Example
Find $[H^+]$ in a 0.10 M solution of $H_2C_6H_6O_6$.

Solution
Because $K_1 >> K_2$, we may assume that when starting with the fully protonated species, *only the first dissociation is important in producing hydrogen ion.* Therefore we may solve the problem as we did in Case 1 for a monoprotic acid, using K_1 as the acid dissociation constant. The approximate value of $[H^+]$ is given by

$$[H^+] = (K_1C_a)^{\frac{1}{2}}$$
$$= 2.8 \times 10^{-3} \text{ M}$$

Example
Find $[H^+]$ in a 0.10 M solution of $Na_2C_6H_6O_6$.

Solution
We have a sodium salt of the most basic of the three possible species, i.e., of the ascorbate ion, $C_6H_6O_6^{2-}$. This salt gives 0.10 M $C_6H_6O_6^{2-}(aq)$ in solution:

$$Na_2C_6H_6O_6(aq) \rightarrow 2Na^+(aq) + C_6H_6O_6^{2-}(aq)$$

The major pH-determining reaction will be the hydrolysis of ascorbate ion, which is analogous to the hydrolysis of ammonia in the previous monoprotic example. Here we find the hydrolysis constant using the relationship

$$K_{b_2} = (1 \times 10^{-14})/K_2$$
$$= 6.25 \times 10^{-3}$$

The approximate formula for $[OH^-]$ in a basic solution is

$$[OH^-] = (K_{b_2}C_b)^{\frac{1}{2}}$$
$$= 0.025 \text{ M}$$

but the approximation is not justified owing to the large value of the hydrolysis constant. The quadratic formula gives a value of 0.022 M.

Finally, we solve for $[H^+]$:

$$[H^+] = (1.00 \times 10^{-14})/(0.022)$$
$$= 4.5 \times 10^{-13} \text{ M}$$

The answer is reasonable: The small value of K_2 for ascorbic acid led us to predict that ascorbate, while a weak base, would still hydrolyze to a fair extent to produce a large number of OH^- ions, driving the pH well above 7.

Example

Find $[H^+]$ in a solution that is 0.12 M in $H_2C_6H_6O_6$ and 0.36 M in $NaHC_6H_6O_6$.

Solution

This is a buffer solution in which the conjugate acid is $H_2C_6H_6O_6$ and the conjugate base is $HC_6H_6O_6^-$. (The second dissociation of ascorbic acid may be neglected.) The relevant acid constant is K_1.

$$[H^+] = K_1[H_2C_6H_6O_6(aq)]/[HC_6H_6O_6(aq)]$$
$$= \frac{(7.9 \times 10^{-5})(0.12)}{(0.36)}$$
$$= 2.6 \times 10^{-5} \text{ M}$$

Example

Find $[H^+]$ in a solution that is 0.35 M in $NaHC_6H_6O_6$ and 0.28 M in $Na_2C_6H_6O_6$.

Solution

This is a buffer solution in which the conjugate acid is $HC_6H_6O_6^-$ and the conjugate base is $C_6H_6O_6^{2-}$. The relevant acid constant is K_2.

$$[H^+] = K_2[HC_6H_6O_6^-]/[C_6H_6O_6^{2-}]$$
$$= \frac{(1.6 \times 10^{-12})(0.35 \text{ M})}{(0.28 \text{ M})}$$
$$= 2.0 \times 10^{-12} \text{ M}$$

Example

Find $[H^+]$ in a solution of 0.10 M $NaHC_6H_6O_6$.

Solution

Unlike the previous two examples, this solution does not involve a mixture of $HC_6H_6O_6$ with another ascorbic acid species. And unlike the first two examples, $HC_6H_6O_6$ is neither fully protonated nor completely unprotonated; rather it has 1 acidic hydrogen ion. (Such a species, which can act as either a weak acid or weak base, is called an *ampholyte*.) This class of problem has a special approximate solution:

$$[H^+] = (K_1K_2)^{\frac{1}{2}}$$

or, equivalently,

$$pH = \frac{1}{2}(pK_1 + pK_2)$$

where $pK_1 = -\log K_1$ and $pK_2 = -\log K_2$

In this example,

$$[H^+] = ((7.9 \times 10^{-5})(1.6 \times 10^{-12}))^{\frac{1}{2}}$$
$$= 1.1 \times 10^{-8} \text{ M}$$

Note that when using the approximate formula, $[H^+]$ does not depend on the concentration of the weak acid species.

I. PROPERTIES OF BUFFER SOLUTIONS

Buffers receive their names because they lessen the effect that adding a strong acid or base has on the pH of a system. For example, if 0.010 mol of HNO_3 is added to 1.0 L of plain water, the pH will move from 7 to 2—a significant change.

Yet, suppose the same amount of strong acid is added to a buffer solution that is 0.10 M in both acetic acid (for which $pK_a = 4.75$) and acetate.

The Henderson-Hasselbalch equation gives the pH of the initial solution:

Initial pH $= 4.75 + \log(0.10 \text{ M}/0.10 \text{ M})$
$= 4.75$

The 1.0 L of solution originally contains 0.10 mol (or 100 mmol) of both acetate ion and acetic acid. The addition of H^+ from HNO_3 converts 0.010 mole (or 10 mmol) of $C_2H_3O_2{}^-$(aq) into $HC_2H_3O_2$(aq):

	H^+(aq)	+	$C_2H_3O_2{}^-$(aq)	→	$HC_2H_3O_2$(aq)
Init.	10 mmol		100		100
Reacts	−10		−10		+10
Final	—		90		110

Now we use the Henderson-Hasselbalch equation again, using mmol of each species inside the log term:

Final pH $= 4.75 + \log (90 \text{ mmol}/110 \text{ mmol})$
$= 4.66$

The buffer solution deserves its name, having allowed the pH to drop only 0.09 pH units.

J. TITRATION CURVES

A typical **titration curve** for a strong acid is shown below. In this case, sodium hydroxide is added to a solution of nitric acid.

Titration Curve for a Strong Acid

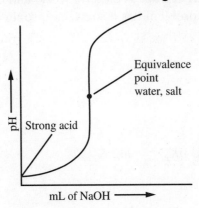

To find the volume of base needed to reach the **equivalence point,** we use the balanced equation for the titration reaction.

Example

Find the volume of 0.02200 M $Ba(OH)_2$ (a strong base) required to titrate 25.55 mL of 0.06680 M HCl to an equivalence point.

Solution

The balanced equation is $2HCl(aq) + Ba(OH)_2(aq) \rightarrow 2H_2O(l) + BaCl_2(aq)$

$$\text{mol HCl} = (0.02555 \text{ L})(0.06680 \text{ mol/L}) = 1.707 \times 10^{-3} \text{ mol}$$

$$\text{mol Ba(OH)}_2 = (1.707 \times 10^{-3} \text{ mol HCl})(1 \text{ mol Ba(OH)}_2 / 2 \text{ mol HCl})$$
$$= 8.535 \times 10^{-4} \text{ mol}$$

$$\text{L Ba(OH)}_2 = \frac{(8.535 \times 10^{-4} \text{ mol})}{(0.0220 \text{ mol/L})}$$
$$= 0.03880 \text{ L}$$
$$= 38.8 \text{ mL}$$

To find the pH during a titration (but before the equivalence point) of a strong acid with a strong base, we can use the relation

$$[H^+] = \frac{(\text{moles orig. } H^+) - (\text{moles added } OH^-)}{(\text{original volume} + \text{volume NaOH added})}$$

At the equivalence point, $[H^+] = [OH^-] = 1.00 \times 10^{-7}$.

The figure below shows the titration of a monoprotic weak acid, acetic acid, with NaOH.

Titration Curve for a Weak Acid

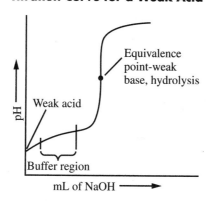

Note several points of interest in the above figure:

1. The increase in pH near the equivalence point is not as great as for a strong acid.

2. At the far left, the solution pH is that of the original weak acid, so $[H^+]$ is approximately $(C_a K_a)^{\frac{1}{2}}$.

3. Every mole of strong base that is subsequently added converts a mole of acetic acid to a mole of acetate; the mid-region of the curve is a buffer solution, and its pH increases only slowly with added strong base.

4. Finally, at the equivalence point the solution consists almost entirely of sodium acetate, and the pH is determined by the acetate's hydrolysis. (The pH will not, in general, be 7.0.) Here $[OH^-]$ is approximately $(C_b K_b)^{\frac{1}{2}}$.

For a weak acid titration where the acid is monoprotic and the strong base carries only one hydroxide, the endpoint volume of base is determined by the relation

$$C_a V_a = C_b V_b$$

Example

Propanoic acid, $HC_3H_5O_2$, is a monoprotic acid having $K_a = 1.3 \times 10^{-5}$. A sample of 25.0 mL of 0.100 M $HC_3H_5O_2$ is titrated with 0.100 M NaOH. Calculate the pH when the following volumes of base have been added:

    a) 0.00 mL

    b) 8.00 mL

    c) 22.0 mL

    d) 25.0 mL

Solution

It is useful to calculate the equivalence point at the outset. Because the acid and base react 1-to-1 and each is 0.100 M, the equivalence point will come at 25.0 mL. Therefore the first two additions of base will result in mixtures of the weak acid and its conjugate base, while the final addition will bring the titration exactly to its equivalence point.

a) The initial pH is determined by the approximate formula for a pure weak base:

$$[H^+] = (C_aK_a)^{\frac{1}{2}}$$
$$= ((0.100 \text{ M})(1.3 \times 10^{-5}))^{\frac{1}{2}}$$
$$= 1.1 \times 10^{-3} \text{ M}$$

(The assumption underlying the approximation, namely that $[H^+] << C_a$, can be verified.)

$$pH = -\log(1.1 \times 10^{-3})$$
$$= 2.96$$

b) We can determine the composition of the buffer solution using the following chart:

	$HC_3H_5O_2(aq)$	+	$OH^-(aq)$	$\rightarrow$	$C_3H_5O_2^-(aq)$
Init.	2.50 mmol		0.80		—
Reacts	−0.80		−0.80		+0.80
Final	1.70		—		0.80

$$[H^+] = K_a(HC_3H_5O_2(aq))/(C_3H_5O_2^-(aq))$$
$$= (1.3 \times 10^{-5})(1.70\text{mmol})/(0.80\text{mmol})$$
$$= 2.8 \times 10^{-5} \text{ M}$$
$$pH = -\log (2.8 \times 10^{-5})$$
$$= 4.55$$

Shortcut
An alternative way to calculate the ratio of

$$[HC_3H_5O_2(aq)]/[C_3H_5O_2^-(aq)]) = (1.70\text{mmol})/(0.80\text{mmol})$$
$$= 2.13$$

is to note that since added base converts weak acid to weak base, and since the equivalence point comes at 25.00 ml, at 8.00 mL the value of the ratio is simply

$$(25.00 \text{ mL} - 8.00 \text{ mL})/(8.00 \text{ mL}) \text{ mL} = 2.13$$

c) The procedure is similar to (b); our chart reveals a greater conversion of the weak acid to its conjugate base:

$HC_3H_5O_2$(aq)	+	OH^-(aq)	$\rightarrow$	$C_3H_5O_2^-$(aq)	+	H_2O

	$HC_3H_5O_2$(aq)	OH^-(aq)	$C_3H_5O_2^-$(aq)	H_2O
Init.	2.50 mmol	2.20	—	
Reacts	−2.20	−2.20	+2.20	
Final	0.30	—	2.20	

$$[H^+] = K_a(HC_3H_5O_2(aq))/(C_3H_5O_2^-(aq))$$
$$= (1.3 \times 10^{-5})(0.30 \text{ mmol})/(2.20 \text{ mmol}) = 1.8 \times 10^{-6} \text{ M}$$
$$pH = -\log(1.8 \times 10^{-6})$$
$$= 5.74$$

d) At 25.0 mL of added base, we have reached the equivalence point. The solution is equivalent to a solution of sodium propionate, $NaC_3H_5O_2$, whose concentration has been diluted from its original concentration by a factor of 2.00 (i.e, to a final value of 0.0500 M), since the volume in the titration flask has increased from 25.0 mL to 50 mL.

We recognize the equivalence point pH calculation as identical to the problem of finding the pH of a solution 0.0500 M $C_3H_5O_2^-$ that undergoes hydrolysis.

We first calculate the base constant for $C_3H_5O_2^-$:
$$K_b = (1.00 \times 10^{-14})/(1.3 \times 10^{-6})$$
$$= 7.7 \times 10^{-9}$$

$$[OH^-] = (C_bK_b)^{\frac{1}{2}}$$
$$= (0.050)(7.69 \times 10^{-9})^{\frac{1}{2}}$$
$$= 2.0 \times 10^{-5} \text{ M}$$

$$[H^+] = (1.00 \times 10^{-14})/(2.0 \times 10^{-5})$$
$$= 5.0 \times 10^{-10} \text{ M}$$

$$pH = -\log(5.0 \times 10^{-10})$$
$$= 9.30$$

The figure on page 85 shows the titration curve that results when a weak diprotic acid is titrated with a strong base. Many diprotic acids exhibit the general shape illustrated, which differs from the monoprotic case in having 2 distinct endpoints. The following example illustrates the calculation of pH values at several values of added base; as we will see, such calculations follow directly from the previous examples showing pH in different diprotic systems. (The concepts involved can be extended to acids with 3 or more hydrogens.)

Example

Oxalic acid, $H_2C_2O_4$, is a diprotic acid for which $K_1 = 5.9 \times 10^{-2}$ and $K_2 = 6.5 \times 10^{-5}$. A sample of 20.0 mL of 0.200 M $H_2C_2O_4$ is titrated with 0.200 M NaOH. Calculate the pH when the following volumes of base have been added:

a) 18.00 mL

b) 20.00 mL

c) 27.0 mL

d) 40.0 mL

Solution

First we establish the equivalence points. We note that the first equivalence point, corresponding to the completion of the reaction

$$H_2C_2O_4(aq) + OH^- \rightarrow H C_2O_4^-(aq) + H_2O$$

will come when

$$C_aV_a = C_bV_b$$

so

$$V_b = C_aV_a/C_b = (0.200 \text{ M})(20.00 \text{ mL})/(0.200 \text{ M})$$
$$= 20.00 \text{ mL}$$

Therefore, the second equivalence point, corresponding to the completion of the reaction

$$HC_2O_4^-(aq) + OH^- \rightarrow C_2O_4^{2-}(aq) + H_2O$$

will come at 40.00 mL, since each millimole of original oxalic acid leads to one millimole of $HC_2O_4^-(aq)$.

a) At 18.00 mL, we have not yet reached the first equivalence point, so the principal species are $H_2C_2O_4(aq)$ and $HC_2O_4^-$.

$$[H^+] = K_a[H_2C_2O_4(aq)]/[HC_2O_4^-]$$

Using the shortcut introduced in a previous example, we can write

$$[H^+] = (5.9 \times 10^{-2})(20.00 \text{ mL} - 18.00 \text{ mL})/(18.00 \text{ mL})$$
$$= 6.6 \times 10^{-3} \text{ M}$$
$$pH = 2.18$$

b) At 20.00 mL, the first equivalence point, we have only 1 major species, $HC_2O_4^-$. As we saw in the earlier discussion, the pH in this case can be calculated using

$$[H^+] = (K_1K_2)^{\frac{1}{2}}$$
$$= ((5.9 \times 10^{-2})(6.5 \times 10^{-5}))^{\frac{1}{2}}$$
$$= 2.0 \times 10^{-3} \text{ M}$$
$$pH = 2.7$$

c) At 27.00 mL we have passed the first equivalence point by 7.00 mL and are on our way to the second equivalence point at 40.00 mL, 20.00 mL past the first equivalence point. The principal species are $HC_2O_4{}^-$ and $C_2O_4{}^{2-}$. The shortcut expression, using K_2, gives

$$[H^+] = (6.5 \times 10^{-5})(20.00 \text{ mL} - 7.00 \text{ mL})/(7.00 \text{ mL})$$
$$= 1.2 \times 10^{-4} \text{ M}$$
$$\text{pH} = 3.92$$

d) At 40.00 mL, the second equivalence point, we have only $C_2O_4{}^{2-}$(aq) as the principal species. The hydrolysis of this weak base leads to the following pH calculation, as in an earlier example for sodium propionate.

First we find K_b, using K_2 for oxalic acid:

$$K_b = (1.00 \times 10^{-14})/(6.5 \times 10^{-5})$$
$$= 1.5 \times 10^{-10}$$

Next we use the approximate result derived earlier for hydrolysis, noting that

$$C_b = 0.200 \text{ M}(20 \text{ mL}/40 \text{ mL}) = 0.10 \text{ M}$$

owing to the dilution of the original solution during the titration.

$$[OH^-] = (C_b K_b)^{\frac{1}{2}}$$
$$= ((0.10 \text{ M})(1.5 \times 10^{-10}))^{\frac{1}{2}}$$
$$= 3.9 \times 10^{-6} \text{ M}$$

$$[H^+] = (1.00 \times 10^{-14})/(3.9 \times 10^{-6})$$
$$= 2.6 \times 10^{-9} \text{ M}$$

$$\text{pH} = 8.6$$

An *indicator* can be used to determine the *equivalence point* of a titration, i.e., the exact volume of NaOH at which the moles of strong base added equal the original moles of acid. Different indicators, which are themselves weak acids or bases, are chosen for different titrations; what is important is that the indicator change color at a pH near that of the equivalence point.

As an example, the well-known indicator phenolphthalein has a range of pH 8.2–10. This is acceptable for titrations of many weak acids with strong bases, where the equivalence point is somewhat basic owing to hydrolysis of the conjugate base. (See previous examples.) Phenolphthalein is also a satisfactory indicator for a strong acid/strong base titration, whose equivalence point is expected to come at 7.0; the change in pH near the equivalence point is so steep that any "overshoot" is negligible.

On the other hand, a titration of a weak base with a strong acid will result in an acidic equivalence point pH and a curve less steep than that for a strong acid/strong base titration. In that case, an indicator suitable for an acidic range is required.

Example

A 10.00-mL sample of 0.150 M ammonia, NH_3(aq), is titrated with HCl until the equivalence point is reached at 12.50 mL of acid. Which of the following indicators would be suitable? (K_b for ammonia = 1.8×10^{-5})

Methyl orange	3.2–4.4
Ethyl red	4.0–5.8
Bromcresol purple	5.3–6.8
Phenolphthalein	8.2–10

Solution

At the equivalence point, the principal species is ammonium ion, NH_4^+(aq), which is the conjugate acid of NH_3. To find [H^+] in the solution, we use the approximate formula for a weak acid in water:

$$[H^+] = (C_a K_a)^{\frac{1}{2}}$$

To determine C_a, we adjust the original concentration of NH_3 by the appropriate dilution factor, noting that the sample volume increases from 10 mL to 17 mL in the course of the titration:

$$C_a = (0.150 \text{ M})(10.00 \text{ mL} / 17.00 \text{ mL})$$
$$= 0.0882 \text{ M}$$

We find K_a for ammonium ion from the given value of K_b for NH_3:

$$K_a = (1.00 \times 10^{-14})/K_b = (1.00 \times 10^{-14})/(1.8 \times 10^{-5})$$
$$= 5.6 \times 10^{-10}$$

Now we can solve for [H^+]:

$$[H^+] = (C_a K_a)^{\frac{1}{2}}$$
$$= ((0.0882)(5.6 \times 10^{-10}))^{\frac{1}{2}}$$
$$= 7.0 \times 10^{-6} \text{ M}$$
$$pH = 5.15$$

The chart shows that ethyl red has a color change in this range.

PRACTICE PROBLEMS

1. The pH of a 0.10 M solution of acetic acid ($K_a = 1.8 \times 10^{-5}$) is closest to which of the following?

   A. 0.1
   B. 3
   C. 7
   D. 0

2. Which of the following has (have) buffer properties?

   I. 50 mL of 0.1 M HCl
   II. 100 mL of 0.1 M acetic acid
   III. 50 mL of 0.1 M NaOH

   A. I only
   B. II only
   C. III only
   D. the solution resulting when II and III are mixed

3. The endpoint of a titration of 50 mL of 0.2 M HCl with 0.1 M $Ba(OH)_2$ will come after the addition of how many mL of the base?

   A. 25 mL
   B. 50 mL
   C. 100 mL
   D. 200 mL

4. If 25 mL of 0.1 M HNO_2 ($K_a = 6.0 \times 10^{-4}$) is titrated with 0.1 M NaOH, what will happen to the pH of the solution?

   A. It will fall gradually, until 25.0 mL of base is added, then drop sharply.
   B. It will rise gradually, until 25.0 mL of base is added, then rise sharply.
   C. It will reach the value of pK_a at 25 mL of base.
   D. It will remain constant.

5. The relationship among the species in a buffer solution (where the weak acid is HA) may be expressed by the *Henderson-Hasselbalch* equation, $pH = pK_a + \log [A^-]/[HA]$.

   According to this equation,

   I. $[H^+]$ increases as $[A^-]$ increases.
   II. a good buffer is one with a pK_a close to the pH desired.
   III. it is the ratio of the conjugate base to acid, not the actual amounts, that determine the pH of a buffer.

   A. I only
   B. II only
   C. III only
   D. II and III only

6. The equilibrium constants K_a and K_b for a conjugate acid-base pair are related by $K_a K_b = 1 \times 10^{-14}$. This relation implies which of the following?

   A. Strong acids have strong conjugate bases.
   B. Weak acids have weak conjugate bases.
   C. The stronger the base, the weaker its conjugate acid.
   D. The extent of dissociation of a weak base is almost always greater than that of a weak acid.

7. A student is asked to calculate the volume of 0.10 M NaOH that must be added to 60 mL of 0.20 M acetic acid ($K_a = 1.8 \times 10^{-5}$) in order to produce a solution for which $[H^+] = 9.0 \times 10^{-6}$ M. Which of the following volumes is closest to that which she will need?

   A. 30 mL
   B. 60 mL
   C. 80 mL
   D. 120 mL

Questions 8–11 are based on the following chart, which describes the composition of various buffer solutions made from several conjugate acid/base pairs.

Acid/base	K_a	pK_a	[acid]	[base]	[H$^+$]	pH
acetic/acetate	1.8×10^{-5}	—	0.1	0.1	1.8×10^{-5}	**(1)**
acetic/acetate	1.8×10^{-5}	—	0.2	0.1	**(2)**	—
ammonium/ammonia	5.6×10^{-10}	9.3	**(3)**	0.1	2.8×10^{-10}	—
ammonium/ammonia	5.6×10^{-10}	9.3	0.1	0.01	**(4)**	—

8. The value indicated by (1) is closest to which of the following?

    A. −5
    B. 1.8
    C. 4
    D. 5

9. The value indicated by (2) is closest to which of the following?

    A. 1.8×10^{-5}
    B. 9×10^{-6}
    C. 3.6×10^{-5}
    D. −5

10. The value indicated by (3) is closest to which of the following?

    A. 0.025
    B. 0.05
    C. 0.10
    D. 0.20

11. The value indicated by (4) is closest to which of the following?

    A. 5.6×10^{-11}
    B. 5.6×10^{-10}
    C. 5.6×10^{-9}
    D. 9.3

Questions 12–14 refer to a 0.10 M solution of acid HA, whose $K_a = 1.0 \times 10^{-5}$. The diagram shows a titration curve of this acid with 0.10 M NaOH.

a) Titration of HA with 0.10 M NaOH

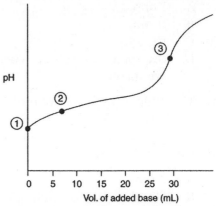

b) Titration of B with 0.10 M HNO$_3$

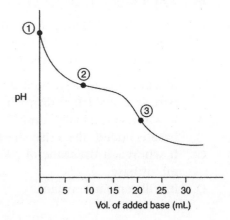

12. Which of the following is closest to the pH at point 1?

    A. 1
    B. 2
    C. 6
    D. 8

13. Which of the following is closest to the pH at point 2?

A. 2
B. 4
C. 7
D. 9

14. Which of the following is closest to the pH at point 3?

A. 2
B. 4
C. 7
D. 9

15. Diagram b) shows a titration curve for a weak base, *B*, whose conjugate acid is BH^+. K_b for the base is 1×10^{-7}. For which of the labeled points is the pH closest to 7?

A. 1
B. 2
C. 3

16. You are given a diprotic acid H_2A having $K_1 = 10^{-6}$ and $K_2 = 10^{-12}$. You are also given a large supply of 0.100 M NaOH. Which of the following buffer solutions would you be *unable* to prepare?

A. A buffer of pH 5
B. A buffer of pH 6
C. A buffer of pH 9
D. A buffer of pH 12

ANSWER KEY

1. B	3. B	5. D	7. C	9. C	11. C	13. B	15. B
2. D	4. B	6. C	8. D	10. B	12. B	14. D	16. C

ANSWERS AND EXPLANATIONS

1. **The correct answer is (B).** For a weak acid in water, you can often use the approximation that

   $$[H^+] = (C_a K_a)^{\frac{1}{2}} = 1.3 \times 10^{-3}; \ pH = 2.88$$

2. **The correct answer is (D).** By mixing a weak acid with NaOH, we convert some of the acetic acid to acetate. The resulting mixture of the acid and its conjugate base is a buffer, and $[H^+]$ will be within an order of magnitude of K_a.

3. **The correct answer is (B).** Moles $[H^+]$ at the start = moles OH^- to reach endpoint:

   $$(0.2)(.050) = 2(0.1)V$$

   where *V* is the volume of base to be added, and the factor of 2 on the right expresses the fact that the concentration of OH^- ions is twice the concentration of the $Ba(OH)_2$ solution.

4. **The correct answer is (B).** The pH curve is the familiar one for a weak acid titrated with a strong base; as base is added, the pH rises gradually through the buffer region, then slopes steeply upward at the endpoint. Choice C would be correct at the "halfway" point, or 12.5 mL.

5.   **The correct answer is (D).** Note that A would be true if it said that "pH increases
     . . ." (II) is true because when pK_a is close to pH, the ratio of acid to salt is close to
     1, with the result that both acid and salt can have reasonably large concentrations.
     This property allows the buffer to resist pH changes resulting from appreciable
     quantities of strong acid or base that are added.

6.   **The correct answer is (C).** For a conjugate pair, strength of acid and base are
     inversely related. Note that neither can be said to be "strong," however.

7.   **The correct answer is (C).** In a buffer, we know that to be a good approximation,

$$[H^+] = K_a \frac{[HA]}{[A^-]}$$

Since we know $[H^+]$ and K_a, we can find the ratio of acid to conjugate base:

$$\begin{aligned}
[HA]/[A^-] &= [H^+]/K_a \\
&= (9.0 \times 10^{-6})[1/8] \times 10^{-5} \\
&= 0.50
\end{aligned}$$

The starting amount of HA is 0.012 mol (12 mmol). To create the 1:2 ratio of HA to
A^- that is required, we must add 0.008 mol (8 mmol) of strong base, since we will
then have 4 mmol of HA remaining, with 8 mmol of A^- created. We can accomplish
this by adding 80 mL (0.080 L) of NaOH, since (0.08L)(0.10 mol/L) = 0.0080 mol.

8.   **The correct answer is (D).** pH = $-\log (1.8 \times 10^{-5})$ = 4.74

9.   **The correct answer is (C).** $[H^+] = K_a /[A^-] = K_a(.2/.1)$

10. **The correct answer is (B).** See answer 9; solve for [HA].

11. **The correct answer is (C).** Refer to answer 9; solve for $[H^+]$.

12. **The correct answer is (B).** We calculate $[H^+]$ using the approximate expression
     for a solution of a pure weak acid:

$$\begin{aligned}
[H^+] &= (C_a K_a)^{\frac{1}{2}} \\
&= [(0.10)(1.0 \times 10^{-5})]^{\frac{1}{2}} \\
&= 1.0 \times 10^{-3} \, M
\end{aligned}$$

   pH = 3

13. **The correct answer is (B).** We can estimate that 8 mL of base have been added, so
     27% of the original HA has been converted to A^-, leaving 73%. Thus (moles HA) /

   $(\text{moles } A^-) = \dfrac{0.73}{0.27} = 2.7$

$$\begin{aligned}
[H^+] &= K^a \text{ moles HA / (moles } A^-) \\
&= (1.0 \times 10^{-5})(2.7) \\
&= 2.7 \times 10^{-5}
\end{aligned}$$

   pH = 4.57

14. **The correct answer is (D).** At the equivalence point, we have a solution of NaA whose concentration is half of that of the original acid owing to dilution during the titration. We find $[OH^-]$ by the approximate expression for hydrolysis of a weak base (in this case, A^-).

$$K_b = (1.00 \times 10^{-14}) / (1.0 \times 10^{-5}) = 1.0 \times 10^{-9}$$
$$[OH^-] = (C_b K_b)^{\frac{1}{2}}$$
$$= [(0.05)(1.0 \times 10^{-9})]^{\frac{1}{2}}$$
$$= 7.1 \times 10^{-6}\ M$$
$$[H^+] = (1.00 \times 10^{-14}) / (7.1 \times 10^{-6}) = 1.4 \times 10^{-9}$$
$$pH = 8.95$$

15. **The correct answer is (B).** We may calculate pH in a base titration by using the buffer formula for a weak acid:

$$K^a = (1.00 \times 10^{-14}) / K^b = 1.0 \times 10^{-7}$$
$$[H^+] = K_a [HB^+]/ [B]$$
$$1.0 \times 10^{-7}\ M = (1.0 \times 10^{-7}\ M)\ [HB^+]/[B]$$
$$[HB^+] / [B] = 1.0$$

But if the ratio of conjugate acid to conjugate base equals 1.0, we must be at the midpoint of the titration.

Note that answer C is attractive because we are used to neutral equivalence points in *strong acid/strong base* titrations. But here the base is weak, so the equivalence point pH is less than 7.0; similarly, the earlier discussion showed that when the acid is weak and the base is strong, the equivalence point pH is greater than 7.0.

16. **The correct answer is (C).** Recall that the expression for finding $[H^+]$ in a buffer solution is

$$[H^+] = K_a\ [\text{weak acid}]/[\text{weak base}]$$

As we have seen, a diprotic acid has two sets of weak acid/weak base pairs, so it can be used to make buffers in 2 regions, one centered around pK_1 and one around pK_2.

In this case, a pH-6 buffer can be made by adding NaOH to the solution of H_2A until we have made a mixture of equal parts H_2A and HA^-. To make a pH-5 buffer, the ratio of acid to base needs to be 10:1.

For the pH 12 buffer, we add more NaOH, past the first equivalence point, until the ratio of HA^- to A^{2-} is 1:1.

The problem with making a pH 9 buffer here is twofold. First, the ratio of H_2A and HA^- would need to be 1:1000, but ratios much past 1:10 make poor buffers. Further, this pH is just that expected at the first equivalence point, for which we have seen that we can make the approximation

$$[H^+] = (K_1 K_2)^{\frac{1}{2}}$$
$$= [(1.0 \times 10^{-6})(1.0 \times 10^{-12})]^{\frac{1}{2}}$$
$$= 1.0 \times 10^{-9}\ M$$

At this equivalence point, the pH changes rapidly with added base or acid: not a good property for a buffer.

1.7 THERMODYNAMICS

A. THERMOCHEMISTRY

Systems and State Functions

A thermodynamic **system** is a portion of the universe that we choose to identify in solving a problem; it might be an open container of gas, a closed vessel in which a reaction takes place, etc.

Everything outside the system is referred to as the **surroundings.**

State functions are properties of systems that have definite values for each state of the system, values that do not depend on the way in which the system reaches a given state. In most instances, knowledge of some of the state functions leads to knowledge of all the others.

The important state functions are

P (pressure)	V (volume)
T (temperature)	E (internal energy)
H (enthalpy)	S (entropy)
G (free energy)	

Note that the symbols for state functions are written as capital letters.

Pressure-Volume Work

In many chemical processes, the type of work that must be considered involves expansion or compression of a gas against an external pressure. The work is given by

$$w = -\int_{V_1}^{V_2} P_{ext} \, dV$$

where w is negative when work is done by the system on its surroundings.

If the external pressure is constant, this expression reduces to $w = -P_{ext} \, \Delta V$.

Note that we use lowercase w for work, and that we write simply w, not Δw. These rules are followed because work is *not* a state function.

B. TEMPERATURE SCALES

The fundamental SI temperature scale is the Kelvin scale, which varies from 0K upward; the freezing and boiling points of water in this scale are 273.15K and 373.15K, respectively. The Celsius (formerly called Centigrade) scale is a commonly used scale, having the advantage that common temperatures on the Earth's surface are generally in the range 0–30°C. The relation between the two is

$$T(K) = T(°C) + 273.15$$

Fahrenheit temperature is little-used in scientific work; the conversion from Celsius to Fahrenheit is

$$T(°F) = \frac{9}{5} \times T(°C) + 32$$

Heat

When a temperature difference exists between a system and its surroundings, heat, symbolized by q, can flow toward the cooler region. Note that q is not a state function.

C. FIRST LAW OF THERMODYNAMICS

If heat is added to a system, or if the surroundings do work on the system, then E, the **internal energy** of the system, will increase. This statement leads to the First Law

$$\Delta E = q + w$$

where ΔE is the change in the internal energy of the system. The units of ΔE are J or J/mol.

Note that heat *added to* the system is positive, and *work done* on the system is positive as well.

D. THE EQUIVALENCE OF DIFFERENT FORMS OF ENERGY

Energy may take different forms; e.g., the First Law indicates that the mechanical work represented by PV expansion or compression of a gas may be converted to heat. Similarly, energy generated in chemical reactions may be converted to other energy forms. In chemical problems, all forms of energy are typically given in units of kJ/mol.

Constant Volume Processes

If the volume is held constant, no PV work is done, and $\Delta E = q$.

Ideal Gas at Constant Temperature

If T is constant, then E is constant ($\Delta E = 0$) for an ideal gas, and $q = -w$.

Constant Pressure Processes

The heat in a constant pressure process can be symbolized by q_p. In such a process, heat is a state function.

$$q_p = \Delta H = \Delta E + \Delta(PV)$$

where H is the **enthalpy** defined as

$$H = E + PV$$

If $\Delta H < 0$, the reaction is "exothermic."

If $\Delta H > 0$, the reaction is "endothermic."

Standard Enthalpy Change

The standard enthalpy change, $\Delta H°$, is the enthalpy of a given reaction when products and reactants are at their standard states, i.e., in the most stable form, at 1 atm pressure for gases and 1.0 M concentration for solutions. There is no single standard temperature, although 298°C is often chosen.

Hess's Law

Since ΔH is a state function, two different paths leading from the specified reactants to the desired products should yield the same value for ΔH.

In practice, Hess's Law amounts to a statement that if two or more reactions can be added or subtracted in order to give a desired reaction, then ΔH for that reaction can be found by combining the enthalpy changes for the individual reactions in a similar way.

Example

Find $\Delta H°$ for the conversion of solid ethanol, C_2H_5OH, directly to its vapor (sublimation), using the $\Delta H°$ values for the two reactions that follow:

ethanol (*s*) → ethanol (*l*)	4.8 kJ
ethanol (*l*) → ethanol (*g*)	39.3 kJ

Solution

By adding the two reactions and canceling the term "ethanol (*l*)" on each side, we obtain the reaction that is wanted. Its enthalpy is the sum of the two enthalpies:

ethanol(s) → ethanol(l)	4.8 kJ
ethanol(l) → ethanol(s)	39.3 kJ
ethanol(s) → ethanol(g)	44.1 kJ

Example

Using the following reactions and enthalpies,

(1) $\frac{1}{2} N_2$ (g) + O_2 (g) → NO_2(g)   33.8 kJ

(2) N_2 (g) + O_2 (g) → 2NO(g)   180.7 kJ

Find the enthalpy for the reaction

(3) 2NO(g) + O_2 (g) → 2 NO_2(g) ΔH = ?

Solution

We need to find a way to combine equations (1) and (2) so that they will add to equation (3). As we do so, we manipulate the ΔH value associated with each in these ways:

1. If a reaction is multiplied by a constant, then ΔH is multiplied by the same constant.

2. If a reaction is reversed, then the sign of ΔH is reversed.

By inspecting the products and reactants that occur in equation (3), we conclude that we must double equation (1), then subtract equation (2) (i.e., reverse the equation, then add it):

$2 \times$ eq. (1):	$N_2(g) + 2O_2(g) \rightarrow 2NO_2(g)$ $2x(33.8 \text{ kJ}) =$	67.6 kJ
$-$ eq. (2):	$2NO(g) \rightarrow N_2(g) + O_2(g)$	$= -180.7$ kJ

$2 \times$ eq.(1) $-$ eq.(2):

$$2NO(g) + O_2(g) \rightarrow 2NO_2(g) \qquad \Delta H = \quad 67.6 \text{ kJ}$$
$$-180.7 \text{ kj}$$
$$= -113.1 \text{ kJ}$$

Standard Heats of Formation

The most common application of Hess's Law is through standard heats of formation, $\Delta H°_f$, which are tabulated for numerous compounds. $\Delta H°_f$ is the enthalpy change, at standard conditions, when *1 mole of a substance is created from its constituent elements in their most stable state.*

As an example, $\Delta H°_f$ for CaO is the enthalpy change for the reaction

$$Ca + \tfrac{1}{2}O_2 \rightarrow CaO \qquad \Delta H°_f = -636 \text{ kJ/mol}$$

From this definition, we see that $\Delta H°_f$ for an element already in its standard state is zero.

To find $\Delta H°$ for a particular reaction, use the relation

$$\Delta H° = \Sigma \Delta H°_f \text{ (products)} - \Sigma \Delta H°_f \text{ (reactants)}$$

where coefficients (denoted by n in the formula) in the reaction are treated as in the example below:

Example

Find $\Delta H°$ for the reaction

$$C_2H_6 + \left(\tfrac{7}{2}\right) O_2 \rightarrow 2CO_2 + 3H_2O$$

using the table below:

Substance	$\Delta H°_f$ (kJ/mol)
C_2H_6	-84
CO_2	-394
O_2	0
H_2O	-242

Solution

$$\Delta H° = 2\Delta H°_f (CO_2) + 3\Delta H°_f (H_2O) - \Delta H°_f(C_2H_6) - (7/2) \Delta H°_f (O_2)$$
$$= 2(-394) + 3(-242) - (-84) - \left(\frac{7}{2}\right)(0)$$
$$= -1430 \text{ kJ/mol}$$

E. BOND DISSOCIATION ENERGY

The bond dissociation energy is actually an *enthalpy* and is defined in one of two ways:

1. ΔH for a reaction in which a diatomic molecule separates into two atoms in the gas phase, e.g.,

$$Br_2 \rightarrow 2\ Br \qquad \Delta H = D_{Br-Br} = 193\ kJ/mol$$

2. An average ΔH for the breaking of a bond between two atoms within a larger molecule. In practice, the ΔH for a given bond depends somewhat on the surrounding atoms and bonds, but by averaging enthalpy data from a large number of molecules, it is possible to derive the following table:

Bond	Bond Dissociation Energy (kJ/mol)
C—C	348
C=C	615
C—H	413
C=O	728
N—H	391
C—N	292
H—H	432

As an example of the application of bond energies, let us calculate the enthalpy of the reaction $2H_2(g) + C(g) \rightarrow CH_4(g)$.

We make use of the principle that ΔH = (sum of bonds broken) − (sum of bonds formed)

$$= 2D_{H-H} - 4D_{C-H}$$
$$= 2(432) - 4(413)$$
$$= -788\ kJ/mol$$

Now let us calculate ΔH for this reaction using heat of formation data. (Note that $\Delta H°_f$ for *gas-phase* carbon is not zero.)

$$\Delta H = \Delta H°_f\,(CH_f(g)) - 2\Delta H°_f\,(H_2\,(g)) - \Delta H°_f\,(C(g))$$
$$= (-75 - 2(0) - 717)\ kJ/mol$$
$$= -792\ kJ/mol$$

The two methods agree surprisingly well, considering that the bond dissociation energies used in the first method were average values taken from many molecules.

F. MEASUREMENT OF HEAT CHANGES

Heat Capacity

The heat capacity is the amount of energy needed to raise the temperature of a body by one Kelvin degree. When applied to a mole of substance, it is commonly signified by C_p (constant pressure) or C_v (constant volume). The heat transferred to a body at constant pressure, when no phase changes occur, is given by

$$q = nC_p(\Delta T)$$

where q is the heat, n is the number of moles, C_p is the molar heat capacity (approximated as a constant over the temperature interval under consideration), and ΔT is the change in temperature.

Under conditions of constant volume, C_p is replaced by C_v; for gases, these quantities are quite different, whereas for liquids and solids they are almost identical.

For an ideal monatomic gas,

$$C_v = (3/2)RT$$

$$C_p = (5/2)RT$$

where $R = 8.315$ J/mol K.

Specific Heat

The specific heat is the heat capacity per unit mass. Thus the specific heat c at constant pressure is given by

$$c = C_p/(\text{molar mass})$$

The heat transferred to a body of mass m to raise the temperature ΔT is given by

$$q = m(\text{spec. heat})\Delta T$$

The specific heat of water has the value 4.18 J/gK (or 1.00 cal/°Cg) over the temperature range 0° to 100° C.

Example

Find the heat, in J, needed to raise the temperature of 22.5 g of water from 12.4°C to 88.4°C.

Solution

$q = m(\text{spec. heat}) \Delta T$

$\quad = (22.5 \text{ g})(4.18 \text{ g J/ g°C})(88.4°C - 12.4°C)$

$\quad = 7.15 \times 10^3 \text{ J}$

G. ENTROPY

The state function entropy, S, measures the disorder of a system. When a gas expands or a bond breaks, ΔS usually increases. Entropy is low for ordered crystalline solids, higher for liquids, and higher still for gases.

The function ΔS can be expected to be positive for reactions that result in more gaseous products than were present at the start, and for phase changes that go from solid to liquid or from liquid to gas.

At constant T,

$$\Delta S = q_{rev}/T$$

where q_{rev} is the heat released or absorbed during a reversible process. Note that the units of ΔS are J/mol K (different from those of enthalpy).

Absolute entropies ($S°$) are tabulated in texts and reference books, most commonly for 273K. $\Delta S°$ for a given reaction can be calculated from the formula

$$\Delta S° = \Sigma S° \text{ (products)} - \Sigma S° \text{ (reactants)}$$

Example

Do you expect ΔS to be greater or less than zero for each of the following reactions?

a)	CH_3OH (l)	$\rightarrow$	CH_3OH (g)
b)	NaCl (s)	$\rightarrow$	NaCl (aq, 1 M)
c)	HCl (g)	$\rightarrow$	HCl (aq, 1 M)
d)	C (graphite)	$\rightarrow$	C (diamond)
e)	$3 H_2$ (g) + N_2 (g)	$\rightarrow$	$2NH_3$ (g)

Solution

a) Since the gas phase is more disordered than the liquid, we expect that ΔS will be positive.

b) Since the solution of the salt in water will be more disordered than the solid, we expect that ΔS will be positive.

c) The gaseous form of HCl is expected to become more ordered in the solution, so we expect that ΔS will be negative.

d) Both of these phases are solid, but graphite, with its weak bonds between planes, is expected to be less well ordered. We expect that ΔS will be negative.

e) Since every 5 molecules that react turn into only 2 product molecules, the system becomes more ordered, and we expect that ΔS will be negative.

H. SPONTANEITY—THE INTERPLAY OF ΔH AND ΔS

From the standpoint of entropy, the criterion for a **spontaneous reaction** is that $\Delta S > 0$—disorder should increase. But a consideration of enthalpy provides a different criterion, namely that $\Delta H < 0$ for a reaction to be spontaneous. We assess the contribution of both entropy and enthalpy by using the last major state function, the **free energy** G, defined as

$$G = H - TS$$

For a process where the temperature is unchanged,

$$\Delta G = \Delta H - T\Delta S$$

The general criterion for spontaneity can now be written

$$\Delta G < 0 \text{ for a spontaneous reaction}$$

As a reaction proceeds spontaneously, its free energy decreases until equilibrium is reached, and no further change in the free energy results.

The maximum amount of work, other than pressure-volume work, that a system can theoretically perform during a chemical reaction is equal to $-\Delta G$.

Calculation of ΔG

The free energy can be calculated when ΔH, ΔS, and T are known. Alternatively, $\Delta G°$, the standard free energy, can be calculated from tables of $\Delta G°_f$. (Note that $\Delta G° = 0$ for an element in its standard state.)

$$\Delta G° = \Sigma \Delta G°_f \text{ (products)} - \Sigma \Delta G°_f \text{ (reactants)}$$

Example

Determine $\Delta G°$ at 298 K for the reaction in the last example, using the value of -46 kJ/mol for $\Delta H_f°(NH_3(g))$ and the value -196J/mk for $\Delta S°$ the reaction.

Solution

$\Delta H° = 2\Delta H_f°(NH_3(g)) - 3\Delta H_f° (H_2(g)) - \Delta H_f°(N_2(g))$

$\quad = 2(-46\text{kJ/mol}) - 3(0) - (0) = -92 \text{ kJ/mol}$

$\Delta G° = \Delta H° - T\Delta S°$

We change the units of $\Delta S°$ to kJ/mol:

$\Delta G° = (-92 \text{ kJ/mol}) - (298)(-0.196 \text{ kJ mol})$

$\quad\quad = -34 \text{ kJ/mol}$

I. HEAT TRANSFER

Conduction

In heat transfer owing to conduction, molecules at the high temperature end of a solid body, or of a container holding liquid or gas, pass along some of their energy to adjacent molecules by vibrations or collisions. Although the molecules themselves do not move appreciably from their starting point, heat is transferred over long distances. The rate of transfer depends on the material, on the cross-sectional area, and on the temperature gradient ($\Delta T/\Delta x$) along the substance.

Convection

Heat transfer by convection involves the actual movement of molecules in a gas or liquid. For example, warm air from a heating duct may physically move into a room, displacing cooler air; warm ocean currents have a similar effect. An insulator such as the down in a sleeping bag minimizes heat transfer from the inside of the bag to the outer air by trapping air in small cells, preventing convection currents.

Radiation

Heat transfer by radiation of electromagnetic waves, such as solar energy, does not require any conducting or convecting medium. The energy radiated has a broad spectrum of wavelengths. The intensity of the radiant energy is proportional to the surface area of the energy source and to the fourth power of the temperature of the source.

J. COEFFICIENT OF EXPANSION

Most substances expand when heated. (A notable exception is water, which contracts when heated between 0° and 4° C.) The change in length that an object undergoes during a temperature change is given by

$$\Delta \ell = \alpha \ell_0 \Delta T$$

where $\Delta \ell$ is the change in length, ΔT is the temperature change, ℓ_0 is the original length, and α is the "coefficient of linear expansion."

K. HEATS OF FUSION AND VAPORIZATION

The heat of fusion of a substance is the change in enthalpy at the point that it goes from solid to liquid at a constant temperature. Similarly, the *heat of vaporization* is the enthalpy change on going from liquid to vapor. Both of these quantities are positive.

They may be expressed either as *molar* heat of fusion and vaporization (with units of kJ/mol), or as *specific* heat of fusion and vaporization (with units of J/g).

As an example, the molar heat of fusion of water at 0°C is defined as the enthalpy change for the reaction

$$H_2O(s) \rightarrow H_2O(l) \qquad \Delta H_{fus} = 6.02 \text{ kJ/mol}$$

In a similar way, we define the molar heat of vaporization of hexane, C_6H_{14}, as

$$C_6H_{14}(l) \rightarrow C_6H_{14}(g) \qquad \Delta H_{vap} = 30.1 \text{ kJ/mol}$$

The example below shows some applications of these enthalpies.

Example

Find the mass of ice that can be melted by 625 J of heat at 0°C.

Solution

The specific heat of fusion is the heat required to melt 1 g of substance at its melting point. We compute it as

specific heat of fusion = (molar heat of fusion) / (molar mass)

For water,

$$\text{specific heat of fusion} = (6.02 \times 10^3 \text{ J/mol}) / 18.0 \text{ g/mole}$$
$$= 334 \text{ J/g}$$

To solve for the total heat, we substitute into the following relation:

$$q = (\text{mass of sample})(\text{specific heat of fusion})$$

So (mass of sample) = q / (specific heat of fusion)

$$= (625 \text{ J}) / (334 \text{ J/g})$$

$$= 1.87 \text{ g}$$

Notice that there is no ΔT term in the equation, since the melting process occurs entirely at 0°C. If the sample is to be warmed further, we would add an additional term using the specific heat formula introduced earlier.

Suppose we now ask how much heat will be released if the 1.87 g of water at 0°C is to be frozen again. Since this process is the reverse of the first, the answer will be that $q = -625$ J, where the negative sign indicates that heat leaves the system.

Example

A student finds that 260 J of heat are released when 0.115 g of steam at 100°C condenses to liquid at the same temperature. Use her results to calculate the specific heat of vaporization for water at 100°C.

Solution

The problem tells us about the heat that is *released* when steam changes to liquid. In order to better fit the definition of specific heat of vaporization given above, we could rephrase it, saying that 260 J must be added to vaporize 0.115 g of liquid water. Then

heat needed = (mass of sample)(specific heat of vaporization)

(specific heat of vaporization) = (heat needed) / (mass of sample)

$$= (260 \text{ J}) / (0.115 \text{ g})$$

$$= 2{,}260 \text{ J} / \text{g}$$

PRACTICE PROBLEMS

1. Consider the data for the reactions below whose equilibrium constants are given at the right:

    $BaCO_3 \rightleftharpoons Ba^{2+} + CO_3^{2-}$ K_1
    $HCO_3 \rightleftharpoons H^+ + CO_3^{2-}$ K_2
    $BaCO_3 + H^+ \rightleftharpoons Ba^{2+} + HCO_3^-$ K_3

    Which of the following expressions can be used to calculate K_3?

    A. $K_1 K_2$
    B. $K_1 - K_2$
    C. K_1/K_2
    D. K_2/K_1

2. In using a table of standard enthalpies of formation to calculate $\Delta H°$ for the reaction

    $4NH_3(g) + 5O_2(g) \rightarrow 4NO(g) + 6H_2O(g)$

    how many nonzero enthalpies must be looked up?

    A. 1
    B. 2
    C. 3
    D. 4

3. A student wishes to use bond energies to calculate the enthalpy change for the reaction

    $(CH_3)_3CCl + (CH_3)_2NH \rightarrow$
    $(CH_3)_3CN(CH_3)_2 + HCl$

    Which of the following shows the most efficient means of doing the calculation would be to compute energies of bonds broken and formed using which of the following inventories?

    A. bonds broken: 15 C—H, 3 C—C, 2 C—N, 1 C—Cl, 1 N—H; bonds formed: 15 C—H, 3 C—C, 2 C—N
    B. bonds broken: 1 C—Cl, 1 N—H; bonds formed: 1 C—N, 1 H—Cl
    C. bonds broken: 14 C—H, 3 C—C, 2 C—N; bonds formed: 14 C—H, 3 C—C, 2 C—N, 1 C—Cl, 1 N—H
    D. bonds broken: 1 C—N, 1 H—Cl; bonds formed: 1 C—Cl, 1 N—H

4. Use the following reactions and enthalpies

    (1) $C_8H_{18}(l) + (17/2)O_2(g) \rightarrow 8CO(g) + 9H_2O(l)$ ($\Delta H_1 = -3.21$ kJ)

    (2) $2CO_2(g) \rightarrow 2CO(g) + O_2(g)$ ($\Delta H_2 = 0.57$ kJ)

    to find the enthalpy for the reaction:

    (3) $2C_8H_{18}(l) + 25O_2(g) \rightarrow 16CO_2(g) + 18H_2O(l)$

    A. -10.98 kJ
    B. -9.62 kJ
    C. -2.64 kJ
    D. 10.98 kJ

5. What does the standard free energy of a reaction measure?

    A. Its tendency to react at equilibrium
    B. Its tendency to react at standard concentrations
    C. Its tendency to react at standard temperature
    D. The heat that will be given off as it reacts

For questions 6–8, consider reactions I–VI, whose molar enthalpy changes are symbolized as ΔH_1 to ΔH_6.

   I. $CO_2(s)$ (195K) $\rightarrow CO_2(g)$ (195K) ΔH_1

  II. $CO_2(g)$ (273K) $\rightarrow CO_2(g)$ (373K) ΔH_2

 III. $C(s) + O_2(g)$ (273K) $\rightarrow CO_2(g)$ (273K) ΔH_3

 IV. $C(s)$ (200K) $\rightarrow C(s)$ (273K) ΔH_4

  V. $O_2(g)$ (200K) $\rightarrow O_2(g)$ (273K) ΔH_5

 VI. $CO_2(g)$ (200K) $\rightarrow CO_2(g)$ (273K) ΔH_6

Express the enthalpy change of each process described in terms of the ΔH's given. Assume 1 mole of each substance.

6. CO_2 vapor condenses directly to CO_2 ("dry ice") at 195K.

   A. ΔH_1
   B. $-\Delta H_1$
   C. ΔH_3
   D. $-\Delta H_3$

7. Carbon and $O_2(g)$ at 200K are heated to 273K, reacted completely to form CO_2, and heated to 373K.

   A. $\Delta H_3 - \Delta H_4 - \Delta H_5$
   B. $\Delta H_2 + \Delta H_3 + \Delta H_4 + \Delta H_5$
   C. $-\Delta H_3 + \Delta H_4 + \Delta H_5$
   D. $\Delta H_1 + \Delta H_4 + \Delta H_5$

8. Carbon and O_2 at 200K react to form gaseous CO_2 at 200K.

   A. ΔH_3
   B. $-\Delta H_3$
   C. $\Delta H_3 + \Delta H_4$
   D. $\Delta H_3 + \Delta H_4 + \Delta H_5 - \Delta H_6$

ANSWER KEY

1. C   2. C   3. B   4. A   5. B   6. B   7. B   8. D

ANSWERS AND EXPLANATIONS

1. **The correct answer is (C).** To obtain the reaction described by K_3, you can reverse the second reaction and add it to the first. The equilibrium constant for the resulting reaction is then K for the first times, the reciprocal of K for the second.

2. **The correct answer is (C).** All but $O_2(g)$, which is an element in its standard state, having a value of 0 for $\Delta H°_f$.

3. **The correct answer is (B).** Answer A is also correct but is not as efficient since it requires extraneous calculation; try to write down only bonds that change from reactants to products.

4. **The correct answer is (A).** To combine the 2 reactions given into the final reaction, we use

   $2 \times$ eq.(1) $- 8 \times$ eq.(2)

   So $\Delta H_3 = \Delta H_1 - 8\Delta H_2 = -10.98$ kJ

5. **The correct answer is (B).** $\Delta G°$ gives ΔG for 1 M concentrations of solutions and 1 atm pressures of gases; only by accident will these be equilibrium conditions. Heat released is measured by ΔH at constant pressure, and contributes to ΔG but is not equal to it.

6. **The correct answer is (B).** The reaction is the reverse of the sublimation described by Reaction I.

7. **The correct answer is (B).** The four processes to be carried out are specified as written in Reactions IV, V, III, and II.

8. **The correct answer is (D).** Heat the reactants: Reactions IV and V; react at 273K: Reaction III; cool product to 200K: Reaction VI (in reverse).

1.8 KINETICS AND EQUILIBRIUM

Chemical kinetics is concerned with the **rates of chemical reactions.** To explain how rate is defined, let us consider the reaction

$$2NO(g) + Br_2(g) \rightarrow 2NOBr(g)$$

The rate of this reaction can be measured in three ways:

1. The rate of disappearance of NO, measured in units of mol $L^{-1}s^{-1}$.

2. The rate of disappearance of Br_2, which will be half the value measured in (1).

3. The rate of appearance of NOBr, whose observed value will be the same in absolute value as that measured in (1).

For example, using (2) as the definition of the rate, we can relate it to the changes in the other species as follows:

$$\text{rate} = \frac{-d[B_2]}{dt} = \left(-\frac{1}{2}\right)\frac{d[NO]}{dt} = \left(\frac{1}{2}\right)\frac{d[NOBr]}{dt}$$

A. RATE LAW

One goal of many kinetics investigations is to find the **rate law** for the reaction. It is often possible to write the law in terms of reactant concentrations as follows:

$$\text{rate} = k[A]^a[B]^b \ldots$$

where A, B. . . . are the reactants, the quantity k is the **rate constant,** and the letters a, b . . . . are usually integers or half-integers, sometimes having negative values (e.g., 0, -1, $+1$, $+\frac{1}{2}$, $-\frac{1}{2}$, etc., are possible values).

B. DETERMINATION OF RATE LAWS FROM RATE/CONCENTRATION DATA

Consider the data below, showing the rate of the reaction

$$2A + B \rightarrow C$$

(in units of mol L^{-1} s^{-1}) for various initial concentrations of A and B:

Trial	Init.[A]	Init.[B]	Init. rate
1	0.30	0.10	6.0×10^{-4}
2	0.60	0.10	1.2×10^{-3}
3	0.30	0.20	2.4×10^{-3}

The above data may be used to determine the rate law:

1. Trials 1 and 2 show that if [A] is doubled while [B] is held constant, the rate doubles. Therefore the rate is proportional to [A].

2. Trials 1 and 3 show that when [B] is doubled while [A] is held constant, the rate quadruples. Therefore the rate is proportional to $[B]^2$.

3. We now know that the rate law has the form

$$\text{rate} = k[A][B]^2$$

4. Data from any row can be used to determine k once the rate law is known; e.g., from the first trial,

$$k = 6 \times 10^{-4}/(0.30)(0.10)^2 = 0.20 \ M/s$$

C. RELATION OF REACTION COEFFICIENTS TO EXPONENTS IN THE RATE LAW

Note that in the previous example, the coefficient in front of A and B in the balanced reaction did not correspond to the exponents in the final rate law. However, if we can be certain that a reaction occurs *in only one step* (often called an *elementary step*), then we can predict the exponents from the coefficients. For example, if

$$X + 2Y \rightarrow \text{products}$$

is known to occur in only one step, then the rate law must be

$$\text{rate} = k[X][Y]^2$$

D. INTEGRATED RATE LAWS

The previous equations show rates of change of concentration; in simple cases, they can lead to **integrated rate laws** that show the behavior of reactant or product concentrations as a function of time. These laws can be described by different types of reactions, categorized as **orders of reactions.**

1. **"Zero-th order" reactions.** Some reactions of the form

$$A \rightarrow B + C$$

follow the rate law

$$-d[A]/dt = k[A]^0 = k$$

This leads to the following integrated rate law:

$$[A(t)] = A_0 - kt$$

where A_0 is the initial concentration of A. Thus, a plot of concentration of A against time *gives a straight line*.

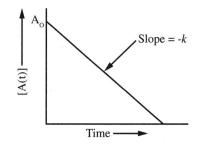

2. **"First-order" reaction.** In this case, $-d[A]/dt = k[A]$. Then $[A(t)] = [A]_0 e^{-kt}$ where A_0 is the initial concentration of A; the concentration of A *decreases exponentially*. Also,

$$\ln[A] = -kt + \ln[A_o]$$

This relationship implies that a plot of $\ln[A]$ against t should give a straight line.

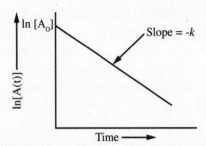

A first-order reaction has the useful property that its "half-life"—the time required for the concentration of reactants to fall to one-half their original value—is independent of what that original value is.

The half-life $t_{1/2}$ is related inversely to the rate constant k by the following expression:

$$t_{1/2} = \frac{0.693}{k}$$

3. **"Second-order" reaction.** For this reaction type,

$$-d[A]/dt = k[A]^2$$

The resulting integrated rate law is

$$\frac{1}{[A(t)]} - \frac{1}{[A]_O} = kt$$

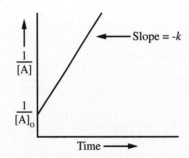

The figure above illustrates this relationship—note that the reciprocal of the concentration is plotted on the *y*-axis.

Example

The following data are obtained in a kinetics study in which the concentration of reactant X is measured at 5-minute intervals. Using appropriate plots, determine (a) the order of the reaction and (b) the rate constant.

T(min)	[A]	T(min)	[A]
0	0.280	40	0.097
5	0.245	45	0.085
10	0.215	50	0.075
15	0.188	55	0.065
20	0.165	60	0.057
25	0.145	65	0.050
30	0.127	70	0.044
35	0.111		

Solution

Our plan is to test the data by graphing according to the three models we have just seen.

The figure below shows a simple plot of [A] versus time. This would be linear if the kinetics were 0th-order; instead, the graph seems to display exponential decay.

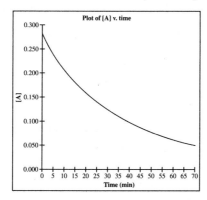

We then plot ln[A] v. time.

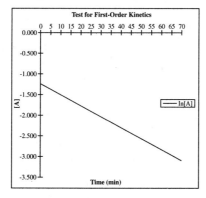

We do indeed find a straight line here, whose slope is equal to -0.0264 s^{-1}. Thus,

$$k = 0.0264$$

and

$$t_{1/2} = \frac{0.693}{0.0264\text{s}^{-1}} = 26.3 \text{ s}$$

For completeness, we can test the data for 2nd-order behavior as well, as shown in the plot of 1/[A] v. time in the figure below.

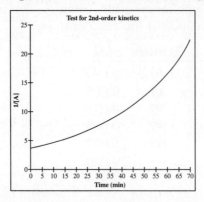

The result is not a straight line, and we conclude that the data represents first-order kinetics.

E. ACTIVATION ENERGY AND TEMPERATURE-DEPENDENCE OF RATE CONSTANTS

Molecules must collide to react, yet not every collision results in a reaction. In order to react, a pair of reactants must possess between them *enough kinetic energy to overcome a large potential energy "barrier"* whose height is referred to as the **activation energy, E_a**.

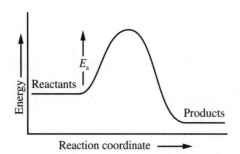

If E_a is large, relatively few reactions will occur, and k will be small. Increasing the temperature increases the kinetic energy of the reactants, with a consequent increase in k. The specific dependence of k on E_a and T is

$$k = Ae^{-(Ea/RT)}$$

where the factor A is approximately temperature-independent. This expression leads to an equation that relates E_a to the values of the rate constant at two different temperatures:

$$\ln\left(\frac{k_2}{k_1}\right) = -\frac{E_a}{R}\left(\frac{1}{T_2} - \frac{1}{T_1}\right)$$

F. MULTISTEP REACTIONS

Many reactions take place in multiple steps, each with its own activation energy. When we list these steps in their correct order, we are said to be stating the "reaction mechanism." In many cases, the activation energy barrier for one of these steps considerably exceeds all the others, with the result that this step is by far the slowest. Such a reaction step is called **rate-determining.**

Example

The overall reaction for "nucleophilic addition" of t-butyl bromide with OH^- ion can be written as follows:

$$(CH_3)_3CH\ _2Br + OH^- \rightarrow (CH_3)_3CH_2OH + Br^-$$

It is proposed that the reaction actually occurs through a mechanism involving the following two steps:

Step 1: $(CH_3)_3CH_2Br \rightarrow (CH_3)_3CH_2^+ + Br^-$ (slow)
Step 2: $(CH_3)_3CH_2^+ + OH^- \rightarrow (CH_3)_3CH_2OH$ (fast)

The "slow," or "rate-determining," step involves the dissociation of the t-butyl bromide. Since this is an elementary (i.e., 1-step) reaction, then according to Sec. C we can write the rate for this step as

$$-\frac{d[CH_3)_3CH_2Br}{dt} = k(CH_3)_3CH_2Br$$

After a molecule undergoes this slow reaction, it quickly adds a hydroxide ion in Step 2. Thus, the rate law for the overall reaction is that of the slow reaction only: It is first-order in $(CH_3)_3CH_2Br$ and does not depend at all on the concentration of OH^-.

Example

The experimental rate law for the reaction

$$H_2(g) + I_2(g) \rightarrow 2\ HI(g)$$

is found to be

$$-\frac{d[H_2(g)]}{dt} = k[H_2(g)]I_2(g)$$

Propose a 2-step mechanism that is consistent with this rate law.

Solution

We should note that the rate law for this reaction involves both reactants, unlike the rate law in the previous problem. We might also note that the rate law is simply that which would be found if the reaction occurred in one step only. We must, however, find a 2-step reaction mechanism, so we try the following:

Step 1: $I_2(g) \underset{k_{-1}}{\overset{k_1}{\rightleftharpoons}} 2I(g)$ (fast equilibrium)

Step 2: $H_2(g) + 2\ I(g) \rightarrow 2\ HI(g)$ (slow)

Because the second step is the rate-determining one, we can write the following, using k' as a rate constant that is different from the k used originally.

$$\frac{d[H_2(g)]}{dt} = k'\,[H_2(g)][I(g)]^2$$

The right-hand side of the reaction involves the concentration of the intermediate species, $I(g)$. We can re-express this more conveniently using the following reasoning, which is further explained in Section 1.8 I.

Because Step 1 represents a rapid equilibrium, the forward rate (with rate constant k_1) equals the reverse rate (with rate constant k_{-1}). Therefore

$$k_1[I_2(g)] = k_{-1}[I(g)]^2$$
$$[I(g)]^2 = k_1[I^2(g)]\,/\,k_{-1}$$

Now we can substitute into the rate law proposed above:

$$\frac{d[H_2(g)]}{dt} = k'\,[H_2(g)][I(g)]^2$$
$$= k'\,(k_1/k_{-1})[H_2(g)][I_2(g)]$$

This result is what was proposed initially, namely a rate law that is first-order in both $[H_2(g)]$ and $[I_2(g)]$.

G. KINETIC V. THERMODYNAMIC CONTROL OF REACTIONS

Many reactions are capable of following multiple paths, yielding different products. The path that is chosen may depend upon temperature or other variables.

The reaction is said to be "under **kinetic control**" if the activation energy is large enough to prevent a large fraction of molecules from overcoming it. Thus E_a determines the path rather than ΔG.

Conversely, if the activation energy is low enough that at the temperature in question many molecules can overcome the activation barrier (and in particular if equilibrium can be established), then the reaction is said to be "under **thermodynamic control**," and the products with the most favorable (more negative) ΔG will be formed.

Example

The following diagram shows the reaction coordinates for 2 reactions, #1 and #2. (Both are drawn on the same scale for easier comparison.) Both reactions involve identical reactants. When one of the reactions dominates, the overall process is said to be under "kinetic control," while when the other is dominant, the process is said to be under "thermodynamic control." Explain the circumstances that lead to each type of control in this example.

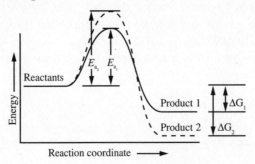

Solution

The reaction leading to Product 1 (solid line) has a lower activation energy than the other reaction; therefore the reaction leading to Product 1 will have a faster rate and the process is said to be under "kinetic control." Product 1 is expected to be the dominant product at low temperatures and within a short time of the start of the reaction.

Yet Product 2 has a significant advantage over Product 1 when the free energies of the final states are compared: Product 2 is more stable. At temperatures high enough that a large fraction of reactants can surmount the large E_a leading to Product 2, and at moderate to long reaction times, Product 2 may be expected to be the dominant product. In this case, the process is said to be under "thermodynamic control."

H. CATALYSTS

A catalyst is most frequently used to raise a reaction rate when the K_{eq} for a reaction is large, favoring its completion, but the E_a is substantial, leading to a slow rate. Catalysts are substances that differ from the original reactants and products, and they generally are not consumed in the reaction.

They open new reaction pathways that decrease the activation energy and thus raise the rate of the reaction.

In *homogeneous catalysis*, both reactants and catalyst are in the same phase; e.g., in solution.

In *heterogeneous catalysis*, the reaction is catalyzed by a new phase, as in the case of a solid boundary acting as a catalyst for a gas-phase reaction. For example, when $H_2(g)$ is mixed with an alkene, the addition of hydrogen to the double-bonded carbons is extremely slow unless a metallic surface such as platinum is present. Evidently the H_2 molecules dissociate to hydrogen atoms at the surface of the metal and then add more effectively to the double bond than they would in the absence of platinum.

Enzyme Catalysis

Enzymes are large protein molecules that catalyze reactions of biological molecules in highly specific ways. The general form of an enzyme-catalyzed reaction is

$$E + S \underset{k_{-1}}{\overset{k_1}{\rightleftharpoons}} ES \qquad ES \overset{k_2}{\rightarrow} E + P$$

where E is the enzyme, S is the "substrate," i.e., the molecule with which the enzyme reacts, ES is the "enzyme-substrate complex," and P is the product into which S is changed by the reaction.

Analysis of this system gives the following expression for the rate or velocity, v:

$$v = \frac{dP}{dt} = \frac{k_2[E_0][S]}{K_m + S}$$

where

$$K_m = \frac{k_{-1} + k_2}{k_1}$$

This expression, the Michaelis-Menten equation, leads to two types of behavior in the cases where substrate concentration is either very small or very large.

1. When the initial concentration of substrate is very low, the rate is found to be first-order with respect to both the enzyme and the substrate.

   i.e., when $[S] << K_m$,
   $V = k_2[E_o][S] / K_m$

2. In contrast, when the substrate concentration is quite high, the rate is first-order with respect to the enzyme concentration but zero-th-order with respect to the concentration of substrate.

   i.e., when $[S] >> K_m$,
   $V = k_2[E_o]$

This is the maximum reaction rate; at high substrate concentration, all of the active sites on the enzyme are occupied, so any further increase in [S] will fail to increase the rate of the reaction.

I. RELATION OF REACTION RATES TO EQUILIBRIUM CONSTANTS

A reaction that reaches **equilibrium** does so because of a balance of one or more subreactions that propel it forward, and another set of reactions that cause it to move backward. Let us consider a simple equilibrium,

$A \rightleftharpoons B$

which proceeds in the forward direction by

$A \rightarrow B$ (k_f)

and in the reverse direction by

$B \rightarrow A$ (k_r)

Equilibrium occurs when the forward rate is equal to the reverse rate; when this is true we have

forward rate $= k_f[A]$; reverse rate $= k_r[B]$;
$k_f[A] = k_r[B]$
$[B]/[A] = k_f/k_r$
$= K_{eq}$

The result shows that an **equilibrium constant** is a ratio of forward and backward rate constants; for example, a reaction whose equilibrium lies far to the right has a much greater rate constant for its forward reaction than the reaction that drives it back toward reactants. For such a reaction, $K_{eq} > 1$. Conversely, for an equilibrium that favors the reactants, $K_{eq} < 1$.

The **Law of Mass Action** extends the argument above to multistep reactions for which equilibrium is reached. If the balanced equation for an overall reaction is

$aA + bB \rightleftharpoons cC + dD$

where the lowercase letters represent coefficients and the uppercase letters represent chemical species, then according to the Law of Mass Action, the equilibrium constant K_{eq} is given by

$$K_{eq} = [C]^c[D]^d/[A]^a[B]^b$$

Here, the brackets represent concentrations in mol/L for solutions, or partial pressures in atto for gases. When one of the species is a solid or pure liquid, its concentration is written by convention as 1.0; similarly, the concentration of the solvent is also written as 1.0.

J. THE RELATIONSHIP OF ΔG TO K_{EQ}

We have just seen that $K_{eq} > 1$ for a spontaneous reaction, while we learned earlier that $\Delta G° < 0$ for such a reaction. We might suppose that K_{eq} is related to $\Delta G°$, and this is in fact the case:

$$\Delta G° = -RT \ln K_{eq}$$

or

$$K_{eq} = e^{(-\Delta G°/RT)}$$

PRACTICE PROBLEMS

1. In the reaction A + 3B → 2C, the concentration of C is found to build from 0 to .002 M in 20 s. What is the rate of appearance of C in M/s?

    A. 1×10^{-4}
    B. 2×10^{-4}
    C. 2×10^{-3}
    D. 6×10^{-3}

2. In the reaction in Problem 1, the rate of disappearance of A is how many times the rate of appearance of C?

    A. $\dfrac{1}{2}$

    B. $-\dfrac{1}{2}$

    C. 1

    D. $\dfrac{1}{3}$

3. For the reaction in Question 1, the rate is expected to be given by which of the following?

    A. $k[A]^2[B]$
    B. $k[A][B]^2$
    C. $k[A][B]^2/[C]^3$
    D. cannot be determined

4. The reaction A → 3C is found to have a rate law of

    $$-d[A]/dt = k[A]^2$$

    If the initial concentration of A is 0.02 M and $k = 1.5 \times 10^{-3}$, what is the initial rate?

    A. 3×10^{-7}
    B. -6×10^{-7}
    C. 6×10^{-7}
    D. 3×10^{-5}

Questions 5–7 are based on the following graph, which shows the kinetics of two reactions:

A → products   Rxn A
B → products   Rxn B

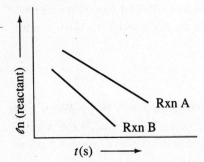

5. What is the order of each reaction with respect to the reactants?

   A. 0th order
   B. 1st order
   C. 2nd order
   D. 3rd order

6. The slopes of the lines

   I.   can be used to calculate rate constants.
   II. indicate that reactant concentrations decrease with time.
   III. indicate the nature of the transition state.

   A. I only
   B. II only
   C. III only
   D. I and II only

7. The rate constants for the two reactions can be determined as

   A. greater for A than B.
   B. greater for B than A.
   C. equal for A and B.
   D. cannot be determined.

Questions 8–12 are based on the following figure, which shows the energy change during the chemical reaction A + B → C.

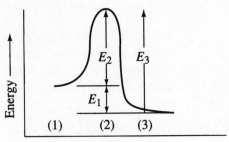

Extent of reaction ⟶

8. The activated complex is formed at which point(s) on the horizontal axis?

   A. 1
   B. 2
   C. 3
   D. 1 and 2

9. The energy required to cause the reaction A + B → C to proceed is given by which of the following?

   A. E_1
   B. E_2
   C. E_3
   D. $E_1 + E_2$

10. The equilibrium constant for the reaction is most closely related to which of the following?

   A. E_1
   B. E_2
   C. E_3
   D. $E_1 + E_2$

11. The energy needed to form the activated complex for the reaction C → A + B is which of the following?

   A. E_1
   B. E_2
   C. E_3
   D. $E_3 - E_1$

12. Raising the temperature at which the reaction takes place will

    I. increase the rate of the reaction.
    II. increase E_1.
    III. increase E_2.

    A. I only
    B. II only
    C. III only
    D. I and II only

13. The decomposition reaction $A_2 \rightarrow 2A$ is found to have zero-th-order kinetics. In 40 s, the concentration of A increases from 0.0960 M to 0.0980 M. What is the rate constant?

    A. 5.0×10^{-6} M/s
    B. 2.5×10^{-5} M/s
    C. 5.0×10^{-4} M/s
    D. 2×10^4 s/M

14. The concentration of a reactant in a first-order decomposition reaction is decreased to $\dfrac{1}{16}$ of its original value in 160 s. What is the half-life of the reactant?

    A. 10 s
    B. 20 s
    C. 40 s
    D. 80 s

15. A chemist measures the rate of the reaction $D \rightarrow E + F$ as a function of time, and finds that a plot of ln[D] against time gives a straight line. What is the order of the reaction with respect to D?

    A. 0
    B. 1
    C. 2
    D. 3

16. What is the slope of the line in Question 15?

    A. 0
    B. negative
    C. positive
    D. positive, turning to 0

17. A gas Y_2Z dissociates as follows:

    $$Y_2Z(g) \rightleftharpoons 2Y(g) + Z(g) \qquad K_{eq} = 35$$

    If 0.5 atm of Y_2Z is placed in an empty container, which of the following expressions can be used to determine the equilibrium concentrations of the species?

    A. $35 = (0.5)^2(0.5)/(0.5)$
    B. $35 = (x)(x)/(0.5)$
    C. $35 = (2x)(x)/(0.5 - x)$
    D. $35 = (2x)^2(x)/(0.5 - x)$

18. If the gas-phase reaction in Problem 17 is carried out in a closed container, what will be the effect of decreasing the total volume available?

    A. Shift the equilibrium to the right
    B. Shift the equilibrium to the left
    C. Leave the equilibrium unchanged
    D. Shift the equilibrium in such a way as to leave the total pressure unchanged

19. For the endothermic reaction

    $$2NH_3 \rightleftharpoons N_2(g) + 3H_2(g)$$

    raising the temperature will have what effect?

    A. It will shift the equilibrium to the right.
    B. It will shift the equilibrium to the left.
    C. It will leave the equilibrium unchanged.
    D. Its effect will vary depending upon the initial temperature.

ANSWER KEY

1. A	3. D	5. B	7. B	9. B	11. C	13. B	15. B	17. D	19. A
2. A	4. C	6. D	8. B	10. A	12. A	14. C	16. B	18. B	

ANSWERS AND EXPLANATIONS

1. **The correct answer is (A).** Rate = $\Delta[C]/\Delta t = (2 \times 10^{-3}M)/(2 \times 10^1 \text{ s}) = 1 \times 10^{-4}$ M/s

2. **The correct answer is (A).** The factor of $\frac{1}{2}$ of comes from the reaction coefficients; the minus sign comes from the fact that we are comparing products and reactants; one disappears as the other appears.

3. **The correct answer is (D).** If we knew that the reaction occurred in a single step, then the answer would be B. But we don't know this, and we have no experimental data to help us infer the rate law.

4. **The correct answer is (C).** Rate = $k[A]^2 = (1.5 \times 10^{-3})(2 \times 10^{-2})^2 = 6 \times 10^{-7}$

5. **The correct answer is (B).** First-order reactions show a linear plot of log(concentration) v. time.

6. **The correct answer is (D).** The negative slope shows that the reactant concentration decreases over time, and the magnitude of the slope gives $(-k)$. Knowing two slopes at different temperatures could tell us what E_a is; but we have no T-dependent data.

7. **The correct answer is (B).** The slope of the line equals $(-k)$; thus, k for reaction B is positive and larger than that for reaction A.

8. **The correct answer is (B).** The activated complex requires energy for its formation, and point 2 represents the place along the reaction coordinate where the energy of the system is a maximum.

9. **The correct answer is (B).** The activation energy is the energy barrier that the system faces as it travels from left to right along the reaction coordinate.

10. **The correct answer is (A).** K_{eq} can be derived from ΔG, the difference in free energy between the initial and final states. Assuming the "energy" measured in the diagram is the free energy—textbooks often are not specific on this point—then E_1 can be used to calculate K_{eq}. The activation energy E_2 is *not* related to K_{eq}.

11. **The correct answer is (C).** Starting at the right and moving left, the system sees a potential barrier whose height is E_3. This is the activation energy that must be overcome for the reverse reaction.

12. **The correct answer is (A).** The barrier heights are temperature-independent, but the ability of reacting species to cross the barrier depends very much on temperature, with greater T leading to higher reaction rates.

13. **The correct answer is (B).** For a zero-th-order reaction,

$$rate = k = \frac{-d}{dt}[A_2] = \frac{1}{2}\frac{d[A]}{dt}$$

$$= \frac{1}{2}\frac{(0.098 - 0.096)\,M}{40s}$$

$$= 2.5 \times 10^{-5}\,M/s$$

14. **The correct answer is (C).** In a first-order reaction, the concentration requires four half-lives to drop to $\frac{1}{16}$ of its initial value.

15. **The correct answer is (B).** First-order reactions decay exponentially, so a plot of the natural log of the reactant against time will be linear.

16. **The correct answer is (B).** Since [D] declines, so does ln[D].

17. **The correct answer is (D).** We've substituted as shown below:

$$Y_2Z \;\rightleftharpoons\; 2Y \;+\; Z$$
$$0.5 - x \qquad 2x \qquad\qquad x$$
$$K_{eq} = (2x)^2(x)/(0.5 - x)$$

Note that $2x$ has to be squared, following the rule for writing equilibrium expressions.

18. **The correct answer is (B).** By decreasing the volume, we've increased the total pressure. The system can react to relieve this "stress" in part by shifting to the left, thus decreasing the total moles and hence the total pressure. The total pressure will not, in general, remain constant, as choice D claims.

19. **The correct answer is (A).** The intuitive way to respond to the question is the following:

In an endothermic reaction, heat is a reactant in the reaction, just as NH_3 is. Then from LeChatelier's Principle, raising the temperature, which can be thought of (very loosely!) as providing more heat to the system, causes the equilibrium to shift from left to right.

More rigorously,

$$\ln K = -\Delta G/nRT = -\Delta H/nRT + \Delta S/nR$$

Only the first term involves T; since ΔH is positive, then increasing T increases $\ln K$ (and also K), shifting the equilibrium to the right.

1.9 ELECTROCHEMISTRY

A. ELECTROLYTIC CELL

The **electrochemical cell** shown in the figure below employs an external **voltage** to force electrons to flow through the wire in order to cause a redox reaction to occur, even though it would not do so spontaneously. Such a cell is called an **electrolytic cell.**

The cell contains a solution of $CuSO_4$(aq). Electrons flow toward the right-hand electrode and reduce Cu^{2+}(aq) ions from the solution, plating out metal on the electrode, which is called the **cathode** (a name consistently applied to an electrode where reduction takes place).

Simultaneously, Cu metal is oxidized at the left-hand electrode, renewing the supply of Cu^{2+}(aq) in solution. Because oxidation takes place at this electrode, it is called the **anode.** Although SO_4^{2-}(aq) ions are neither oxidized nor reduced, their diffusion through the solution is important in transferring charge between the two electrodes.

B. FARADAY'S LAW

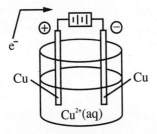

Electrolytic cell

Left-hand electrode (anode):

$$Cu(s) \rightarrow Cu^{2+}(aq) + 2e^- \text{ (oxidation)}$$

Right-hand electrode (cathode):

$$Cu^{2+}(aq) + 2e^- \rightarrow Cu(s) \text{ (reduction)}$$

The previous example of an **electrolytic cell** leads to an important question: How many moles of a substance will be oxidized or reduced in a given time? Suppose that a redox reaction results in the transfer of n moles of electrons for every mole of substance oxidized or reduced, with a constant **current** I, of i amperes (A), in t seconds.

The charge, q, in Coulombs (C) is given by

$$q = it$$

The moles of electrons transferred are then found by

$$\text{moles } e^- = \frac{q}{\mathscr{F}}$$

where $\mathscr{F}$ is **Faraday's Constant**, 96,485 C/mol.

Example

In the previous cell, suppose that a current of 0.400 A runs for 25.0 min. Find the mass of copper metal that will be deposited at the cathode.

Solution

We first calculate q, the total charge transferred (note that the unit *Coulomb* is equivalent to *amp* $\times$ *second*):

$$q = it = (0.400 \text{ A}) (25.0 \text{ min} \times 60 \text{ s/min})$$
$$= 6.00 \times 10^2 \text{ C}$$

Next, we calculate the moles of electrons used:

$$\text{mol } e^- = q/F = \frac{6.00 \times 10°\text{C}}{96,485\text{C/mol}}$$
$$= 6.22 \times 10^{-3} \text{ mol}$$

Finally, we convert to moles of copper, then mass of copper:

$$\text{mass Cu} = (6.22 \times 10^{-5} \text{ mol}_{e^-})(1 \text{ mol Cu/2 mol}_{e^-})(63.55 \text{ g/mol Cu})$$

C. GALVANIC CELL

A **galvanic cell,** which produces a spontaneous voltage (i.e., no external battery needs to be applied), is shown below.

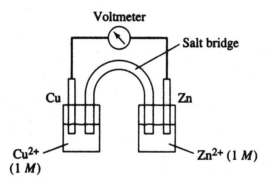

In galvanic cells, the species being oxidized is in one part of the cell; that being reduced is in the other.

A barrier, e.g., a **salt bridge** or porous wall, prevents the redox species from direct mixing but allows other ions (e.g., Na^+ and NO_3^-) to pass back and forth in order to balance the charge.

As in the case of the electrolytic cell, the side where oxidation takes place has an electrode called the anode; the side where reduction takes place has an electrode called the cathode. A wire connects the electrodes, with a voltmeter in between.

When this cell is connected, copper is plated out on the left-hand electrode, while zinc is dissolved from the right-hand electrode. The results observed in the galvanic cell imply that the following reaction occurs spontaneously:

$$Zn + Cu^{2+} \rightarrow Zn^{2+} + Cu$$

This is a redox reaction, since two electrons are transferred from zinc to copper as the reaction proceeds. We can artificially separate the reactions into two "half-reactions":

$$Cu^{2+} + 2e^- \rightarrow Cu \qquad E^\circ{}_{Cu}{}^{2+} = .34 \text{ V}$$
$$Zn^{2+} + 2e^- \rightarrow Zn \qquad E^\circ{}_{Zn}{}^{2+} = -.76 \text{ V}$$

The quantities labeled "E°" to the right of each half-reaction represent the standard **reduction potential** of each half-reaction. In combining the two half-reactions, we find the half-reaction with the greater value of E°, then reverse the other half-reaction, change the sign of its E°, and add both the reactions and the **potentials.**

In this example, the result is

$$Zn + Cu^{2+} \rightarrow Zn^{2+} + Cu \qquad E^\circ{}_{cell} = .34 + (.76) = 1.10 \text{ V}$$

Here, $E^\circ{}_{cell}$ is the *standard cell potential:* It is used when all of the reactants and products are at 1 M concentrations. (For other concentrations, a correction must be made using the Nernst Equation, which we will not cover here.)

Facts to Note about This Galvanic Cell

- In this cell, as we have seen above, Cu^{2+} ion must be reduced and Zn metal must be oxidized.
- The above redox reactions will both occur if electrons flow through the voltmeter from the Zn electrode toward the Cu electrode.
- Thus the Cu electrode is the cathode and the Zn electrode is the anode.
- Because electrons flow toward the Cu electrode, it must be positive. The Zn electrode is thus negative.

Example
Predict the anode and cathode if a cell similar to the one above is constructed using Pb^{2+}/Pb ($E^\circ = -0.13$ v) on the left and Fe^{2+}/Fe ($E^\circ = -0.41$ v) on the right. Write the overall reaction that the cell illustrates.

Solution
Reduction will occur on the left, since the reduction potential is higher for the lead half-cell. Thus, the cathode is on the left, the anode on the right. The overall reaction is

$$Pb^{2+} + Fe \rightarrow Pb + Fe^{2+}$$

D. CONCENTRATION CELL

The figure below shows a cell with the same half-reaction occurring on each side.

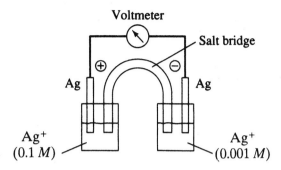

Will the meter register a nonzero voltage? Yes; although $E° = 0$, the system is not at equilibrium, the electrons will flow in such a way as to achieve equal concentrations of silver on each side, just as if the solutions were allowed to mix. Thus, reduction will occur at the electrode that is immersed in the most concentrated solution, which must be the positive electrode since electrons flow toward it in order to reduce Ag^+ to neutral silver.

PRACTICE PROBLEMS

1. In the reaction below,

   $$H_2S + 2NO_3^- + 2H^+ \rightarrow S + 2NO_2 + 2H_2O$$

   How many moles of electrons are transferred for each mole of H_2S that reacts?

   A. 1
   B. 2
   C. 3
   D. 6.02×10^{23}

2. Three electrolytic cells are constructed, each with a different composition:

   Cell 1: Ag electrodes, 0.1M Ag^+ solution

   Cell 2: Zn electrodes, 0.1M Zn^{2+} solution

   Cell 3: Al electrodes, 0.1M Al^{3+} solution

   If a current of 0.250 amp is passed through each cell for 1.00 min, which cell will have the greatest number of moles of solid metal deposited at the cathode?

   A. Cell 1
   B. Cell 2
   C. Cell 3
   D. All will have the same amount

3. The values of $E°$ for two half-reactions are given below:

$$Cl_2 + 2e^- \rightarrow 2\,Cl^- \qquad 1.36\ V$$
$$Br_2(l) + 2e^- \rightarrow Br^- \qquad 1.09\ V$$

Now consider the overall reaction:

$$Br_2(l) + 2Cl^- \rightarrow Cl_2 + 2\,Br^-$$

This reaction can be described as

A. spontaneous, with $E°_{cell} = .27\ V$.
B. spontaneous, with $E°_{cell} = 2.45\ V$.
C. not spontaneous, with $E°_{cell} = -.27\ V$.
D. not spontaneous, with $E°_{cell} = -2.45\ V$.

4. To obtain an overall spontaneous reaction from the two half-reactions

$$2Pb^{2+} + 2e^- \rightarrow Pb \qquad E° = -.13\ V$$
$$\text{and}$$
$$Ag^+ + e^- \rightarrow Ag \qquad E° = .80\ V$$

a student should calculate which of the following expressions for $E°_{cell}$?

A. $E° = .80 - (-.13)$
B. $E° = 2(.80) - (.13)$
C. $E° = 2(.80) - 2(-.13)$
D. $E° = .80 - 2\,(.13)$

5. In the cell shown below, which of the following is (are) true? (Note that no $E°$ values are needed.)

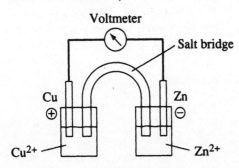

I. Electrons flow through the meter from left to right.
II. Cu is the anode.
III. The spontaneous reaction is

$$Cu^{2+} + Zn \rightarrow Cu + Zn^{2+}$$

A. I only
B. II only
C. III only
D. I and II

6. Referring to the diagram of the previous problem, suppose that the voltmeter reads 1.10 v. (Assume that the concentration of each solution is 1.00 M.) When the copper electrode and solution on the left are replaced with a silver electrode immersed in 1.00 M $AgNO_3$, the voltmeter reading changes to 1.56 v. Which of the following is a correct conclusion?

A. $E°(Ag^+/Ag) = 0.46\ v$
B. $E°(Ag^+/Ag) = 1.56\ v$
C. $E°(Ag^+/Ag) - E°(Cu^{+2}/Cu) = 0.46\ v$
D. $E°(Ag^+/Ag) - E°(Cu^{+2}/Cu) = 1.56\ v$

7. Which of the following is (are) true of the cell shown?

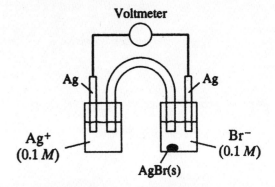

I. The cathode is on the left.
II. The anode is on the left.
III. The Ag electrode on the left is positive.

A. I only
B. II only
C. III only
D. I and III only

ANSWER KEY

| 1. B | 2. A | 3. C | 4. A | 5. C | 6. C | 7. D |

ANSWERS AND EXPLANATIONS

1. **The correct answer is (B).** Each sulfur atom is oxidized from the (-2) state to the (0) state, requiring 2 electrons per atom, or 2 moles of electrons per mole of H_2S.

2. **The correct answer is (A).** The same number of moles of electrons flows through each cell. But since Cell 1 contains Ag^+, which requires 1 mole of electrons to reduce 1 mole of silver ions, it will have the greatest number of moles of solid deposited. Cu^{2+} and Al^{3+} require 2 moles and 3 moles, respectively, of electrons to deposit one mole of solid.

3. **The correct answer is (C).** Add the reverse of the first reaction to the second to get the reaction desired:

   $E° = -.27$ V

4. **The correct answer is (A).** Note you have to subtract a *negative* number, and that there is *no need* to double $E°$, even though the half-reaction had to be multiplied by two.

5. **The correct answer is (C).** III only. First notice that copper is positive; this implies that electrons flow toward it through the meter. There reduction takes place (making it the cathode). Reaction III shows Cu^{2+} being reduced.

6. **The correct answer is (C).** The increase in overall cell voltage reflects the increase in reduction potential of the silver half-cell relative to the copper half cell that it replaced.

7. **The correct answer is (D).** To solve this problem, it is necessary to interpret the cell as a silver ion concentration cell. A small amount of Ag^+ can dissociate from the solid AgBr, so that the right side has diluted Ag^+ and the left side has concentrated Ag^+. Therefore electrons will flow through the wire from right to left in order to electrically reduce Ag^+ on the left and thus lower the concentration of Ag^+ ions on that side. Since electrons flow spontaneously toward the left electrode, the left side must be positive.

CHAPTER 2

Physics

2.1 UNITS

Physical quantity is a value used to numerically describe or define a physical phenomenon. This is done by first establishing a standard value and assigning it a unit or dimension. For example, the physical quantity of **length** can be defined (i.e., measured) in terms of the standard unit of the meter. A **numerical quantity** can be completely described by a pure number without any units: for example, 63.5. A dimensional quantity requires a numerical component and a unit component: for example, 63.5 inches. A measured dimensional quantity has different numerical values in different unit systems. Thus, 63.5 inches equals 1.61 meters. **Units** are the standard definitions against which physical quantities are measured.

A. COMMON UNIT SYSTEMS

There are three common unit systems encountered in physics problems—the SI, cgs, and British systems.

The **SI system** is the abbreviation for Système International d'Unités. It is a metric system, also referred to as the **mks system** because the basic units of **length, mass,** and **time** are the meter, kilogram, and second, respectively. This is the most common system used in physics.

The **cgs system** is an older metric system that was replaced by the SI system. It uses the centimeter, gram, and second as its basic units of length, mass, and time.

The **British system,** also called the **English** or the **Engineering system,** is a nonmetric system. Its basic units of length, mass, and time are the foot, slug, and second, respectively.

The conversions for length and for mass among the three systems are listed below.

Length and Mass Conversions

SI	cgs	British
1 m =	100 cm =	3.28 ft
10^{-2} m =	1 cm =	3.28×10^{-2} ft
0.305 m =	30.5 cm =	1 ft
1 kg =	10^{3} g =	6.85×10^{-2} slug
10^{-3} kg =	1 g =	6.85×10^{-5} slug
14.6 kg =	1.46×10^{4} g =	1 slug

B. BASIC UNITS

There are seven basic physical quantities, each with an assigned unit that defines the property. The values of these units are established by international treaty. All other physical quantities are measured using units that are derived from some combination of the basic seven.

The seven basic physical quantities with their symbols and the corresponding SI units with their symbols are as follows:

Physical Property	SI Unit
length, d	meter, m
mass, m	kilogram, kg
time, t	second, s
electrical charge, q	coulomb, C
temperature, T	degree kelvin, K
amount of material, n	mole, mol
luminous intensity, I	candela, cd

C. DERIVED UNITS

All other units are defined in terms of the basic units. For example, velocity is length per unit time.

$$\text{velocity} = \frac{\text{length}}{\text{time}}$$

Some **derived units** are given an alternative equivalent unit name and symbol. For example, the derived SI unit that measures the physical quantity force is the kilogram meter per square second, $kg\ m/s^2$, which is also called the **newton**, N.

Commonly encountered physical quantities and their derived SI units are as follows:

Physical Quantity	Derived Unit	Equivalent Unit
acceleration, a	m/s^2	
area, A	m^2	
capacitance, c	$C^2 s^2/kg\ m^2$	farad, f
electric current, I	C/s	ampere, a
electric resistance, R	$kg\ m^2/C^2\ s$	ohm, Ω
electromotive force, emf	$kg\ m^2/C\ s^2$	volt, V
energy, E	$kg\ m^2/s^2$	joule, J
force, F	$kg\ m/s^2$	newton, N
frequency, v	s^{-1}	hertz, Hz
potential difference, V	$kg\ m^2/C\ s^2$	volt, V
power, P	$kg\ m^2/s^3$	watt, W
velocity, v	m/s	
volume, V	m^3	
work, W	$kg\ m^2/s^2$	newton meter

Notice that the derived units for energy and work are the same. The derived units for *emf* and potential difference are also identical.

D. UNIT CONVERSION

Unit conversion is a procedure used to convert one unit into an equivalent unit.

Step 1

Start with a definition. A definition is a mathematical equation that relates two equivalent quantities such as:

$$A = B$$

EXAMPLE

$$1 \text{ inch} = 2.54 \times 10^{-2} \text{ m}$$

The definition can relate equivalent units of the same unit system or equivalent units in different unit systems.

Step 2

Rewrite each definition into two **conversion factors,** CF. A CF is the ratio of the two terms, A and B, in the definition:

$$\frac{A}{B} \text{ and } \frac{B}{A}$$

such as:

$$\frac{1 \text{ in}}{2.54 \times 10^{-2} \text{m}} \text{ and } \frac{2.54 \times 10^{-2} \text{m}}{1 \text{ in}}$$

Step 3

Use the appropriate CF to convert from one unit into the other:

$$\text{Convert from } A \text{ to } B: A\left(\frac{B}{A}\right) = \frac{AB}{A} = B$$

The like terms A in the numerator and denominator cancel to leave only the B term. Similarly:

$$\text{Convert from } B \text{ to } A: B\left(\frac{A}{B}\right) = \frac{BA}{B} = A$$

such as:

$$(63.5 \text{ in.})\frac{2.54 \times 10^{-2} \text{ m}}{1 \text{ in}} = 1.61 \text{ m}$$

and

$$1.61 \, m\frac{1\text{n}}{2.54 \times 10^{-2} \text{ m}} = 63.5 \text{ in.}$$

Part of the strength of unit conversion is that you don't need to intimately understand the units of the second system as long as you have a definition that relates them to the unit system you do understand. A conversion factor has two component parts:

1. The numerical component is the pure number part of the quantity. Such components are arithmetically manipulated.

2. The unit component is the nonnumerical part of the term (inches, meters, etc.). Such components are manipulated algebraically.

   a) Like terms multiplied together give the term raised to the appropriate power:
   $$m \times m \times m = m^3$$

   b) Like terms divided into each other cancel:
   $$\frac{m^3}{m} = m^2$$

E. DIMENSIONAL ANALYSIS

Dimensional analysis is a powerful tool for checking the validity of equations and results. In an exam situation, dimensional analysis can often be used to eliminate one or more of the possible answers because the units are incorrect. In dimensional analysis, an expression is evaluated in terms of the units of the variables rather than by their numerical values.

To perform dimensional analysis, proceed as follows:

1. Rewrite the equation in terms of the units of the variables. Ignore the numerical factors.

2. Reduce the equation algebraically to a simple form.

3. Compare each additive term and the result for consistency. Make sure you're not adding apples and oranges.

For example, we can check the validity of the range equation,

$$x = x_0 + v_0 t + \frac{1}{2} a_0 t^2$$

where x_0 is in mi, v_0 is in mi/hr, a_0 is in mi/hr^2, and t is in hr.

We begin by rewriting the equation:

$$\text{mi} = \text{mi} + (\text{mi/hr})(\text{hr}) + (\text{mi/hr}^2)(\text{hr}^2)$$

Canceling factors like (hr/hr), we find that all terms reduce to mi and conclude that the units are consistent.

Dimensional analysis can also be useful for determining the units of unknown quantities. For example, suppose we want to know the units for the gravitational constant, G, knowing only the gravitational force equation:

$$F = \frac{GMm}{r^2}$$

We write

$$G = \frac{Fr^2}{Mm} = \frac{Nm^2}{kg \cdot kg} = \frac{\left(kg\frac{m}{s^2}\right)m^2}{kg \cdot kg} = \frac{m^3}{kg\,s^2}$$

PRACTICE PROBLEMS

1. Kinetic energy is given by the formula $E_k = \dfrac{mv^2}{2}$, where m is the mass and v is the velocity. The derived SI unit of energy is the joule, J, which is equivalent to which combination of basic units?

   A. $kg\ m^2/s^2$
   B. $g\ cm^2/s^2$
   C. $g\ m^2/s^2$
   D. $kg\ m/s^2$

2. If 1 inch is equal to 2.5 cm, approximately how many inches are in 1000 kilometers?

   A. 2.5×10^4 in.
   B. 4×10^4 in.
   C. 2.5×10^9 in.
   D. 4×10^7 in.

3. A marathon race is about 26 miles long. What is the length in kilometers? (1 km = 0.623 mi)

   A. 0.024 km
   B. 16 km
   C. 42 km
   D. 52 km

4. If a man is 6 ft. 4 in. tall, what is his approximate height in centimeters? (1 in. = 2.54 cm)

   A. 230 cm
   B. 190 cm
   C. 150 cm
   D. 120 cm

5. The equation for the velocity of a falling drop of water is

   $$v = (2/9\pi)(r^2 g\rho/\eta)$$

   where v is the velocity in m/s; r is the radius of the drop in m; g is the acceleration due to gravity in m/s^2; ρ is the density of the drop in kg/m^3. What must be the units of η, the coefficient of viscosity?

   A. $kg\ m/s$
   B. $m\ s/kg$
   C. $kg\ s^2/m$
   D. $kg/m\ s$

ANSWER KEY

1. A	2. D	3. C	4. B	5. D

ANSWERS AND EXPLANATIONS

1. **The correct answer is (A).** In the SI system, the units of mass, length, and time are kg, m, and s. This eliminates choices B and C immediately. Velocity is length over time, which is m/s in the SI system. The square of the velocity, v^2, must have the units m^2/s^2 so that $mv^2 = kg\ m^2/s^2$, which is choice A.

2. **The correct answer is (D).** This is a unit conversion problem:

   10^3 km $(10^3\ m/1\ km)(10^2\ cm/1\ m)(1\ in./2.54\ cm) = (1 \times 10^8/2.5)$ in. $= 4 \times 10^7$ in.

3. **The correct answer is (C).** One kilometer is less than 1 mile, so the length measured in km is larger than the value measured in mi. This eliminates A and B. Choice D is eliminated because it would require 1 km to equal 1/2 mi so that each mi gave 2 km.

   26 mi (1 km/0.623 mi) = 42 km

4. **The correct answer is (B).** 2.54 cm lies between 2 cm and 3 cm. Since 1 in. = 2.54 cm. you expect the height in cm to be more than twice but less than three times the corresponding value in inches:

76 in (2 cm/1 in.) = 152 cm

and

76 in. (3 cm/1 in.) = 228 cm

The actual value is:

76 in. (2.54 cm/1 in.) = 193 cm ≈ 190 cm

5. **The correct answer is (D).** This is a dimensional analysis problem. Rearrange the equation so that η is alone on one side of the equal sign. Since pure numbers like 2, 9, and π have no units, they can be ignored in this problem.

$$\eta = r^2 \, g\rho/v = m^2(m/s^2)(kg/m^3)/(m/s) = kg/m \, s$$

2.2 VECTORS

A scalar quantity is a physical quantity that has only magnitude (size). It is completely described by a single number or numbers plus appropriate unit(s). **Scalar** calculations involve only ordinary arithmetic operations.

A vector quantity is a physical quantity that has both magnitude and direction. **Vector** quantities are printed in boldface (**F** = force). The magnitude of a vector is a scalar quantity (F = magnitude of force). Calculations involving vectors require vector mathematical methods.

A. PROPERTIES OF VECTORS

- A vector can be moved anywhere in the plane that contains it, as long as the magnitude and direction of the vector are not changed in the process.
- Two vectors are identical (equal) if they have the same magnitude and direction.
- The negative of a vector is a vector with the same magnitude but opposite direction.
- A vector multiplied by a positive scalar quantity produces a vector with a different magnitude but the same direction.
- A vector multiplied by a negative scalar quantity produces a vector with a changed magnitude and an exactly reversed direction.
- Two or more vectors can be added together to give a vector sum called a resultant. The **resultant** is a single vector that can replace the other vectors acting on a body to produce the same effect as the set of vectors.
- Vector subtraction is the same as vector addition except that the negative of the vector is added.

B. GRAPHICAL ANALYSIS

Graphically, vector addition is accomplished by moving the vectors so that the tail of each successive vector in the addition is connected to the head of the next vector in the addition. The resultant vector **R** is the vector that connects the remaining free tail to the free head.

The order in which the vectors are added doesn't matter. All combinations must give a resultant vector of the same magnitude and direction.

If only two vectors are being added, they can be placed so that their tails are at the same origin point:

- The two vectors form the adjacent legs of a parallelogram with their resultant vector as its diagonal.

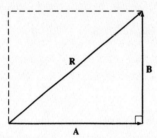

- The two vectors and their resultant also form the sides of a triangle with an area equal to half the area of the parallelogram.

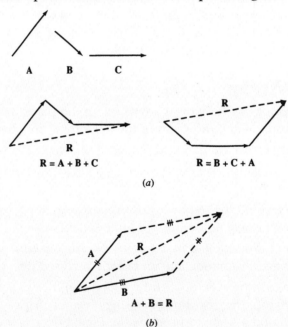

(a) The resultant of the addition of a set of vectors is independent of the order in which they are added.

(b) The resultant of the addition of two vectors is the diagonal of the parallelogram for which the two vectors are legs.

- If the two vectors are mutually perpendicular, the parallelogram formed is a rectangle and the two vectors and their resultant form a right triangle.

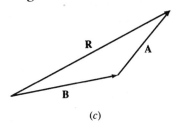

(c)

(c) The two vectors and their resultant from the sides of a triangle.

C. TRIGONOMETRIC ANALYSIS

Every vector can be resolved into two mutually perpendicular components. The components represent the projection of the vector onto the axes of a Cartesian coordinate axis system. Each axis of the coordinate system, x, y, or z is itself a vector. The direction of the component is specified by the axis onto which it is projected, and the component can then be given as the scalar multiplier of the unit vector for the axis.

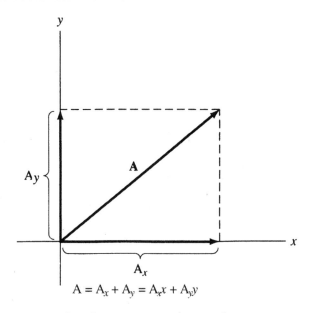

$$A = A_x + A_y = A_x x + A_y y$$

The magnitude of a projection ranges from a minimum value of zero to a maximum value equal to that of the vector. The minimum occurs if the vector is perpendicular to the axis; the maximum occurs if the vector is collinear to an axis. Collinear vectors can either be parallel, both pointed in the same direction, or antiparallel, pointed in opposite directions. A vector and its components form the hypotenuse and legs of a right triangle; therefore, the vector can be analyzed using the trigonometric relationships of a right triangle.

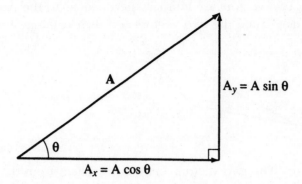

Letting theta, θ, be the angle between the vector and the x-axis, the magnitude of the components of the vector can be found using the following relationships:

$$\sin \theta = \text{opposite leg/hypotenuse} = A_y/A$$

therefore,

$$A_y = A \sin \theta$$

$$\cos \theta = \text{adjacent leg/hypotenuse} = A_x/A$$

therefore,

$$A_x = A \cos \theta$$

Applying the Pythagorean theorem, the magnitude of the vector is found by taking the square root of the sum of the squares of the components:

$$A = (A_x{}^2 + A_x{}^2)^{1/2}$$

The angle θ can be found from any of the following relations:

$$\sin \theta = \text{opposite leg/hypotenuse} = A_y/A$$

$$\theta = \text{arc sin } A_y/A$$

$$\cos \theta = \text{adjacent leg/hypotenuse} = A_x/A$$

$$\theta = \text{arc cos } A_x/A$$

$$\tan \theta = \text{opposite leg/adjacent leg} = A_y/A_x$$

$$\theta = \text{arc tan } A_y/A_x$$

D. VECTOR MULTIPLICATION

There are two forms of vector multiplication. One produces a scalar quantity and the other produces another vector quantity.

Dot Product

The result of this process is a scalar quantity, not a vector:

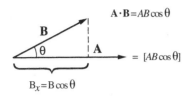

The magnitude of the projection of B onto A is given as $B_x = B \cos \theta$.

1. $\mathbf{A} \cdot \mathbf{B} = 0$ if the two vectors are perpendicular because $\theta = 90°$ and cos 90° = 0.

2. $\mathbf{A} \cdot \mathbf{B} = AB$, the maximum value possible, if the two vectors are parallel because $\theta = 0$ and cos 0° = 1.

Cross Product

The result of this process is a vector quantity, C, that is perpendicular to the plane that contained the two original vectors, A and B.

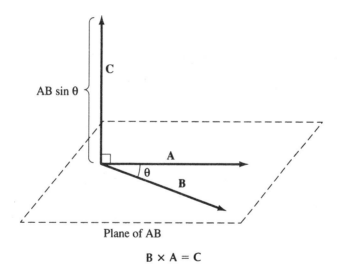

$$\mathbf{B} \times \mathbf{A} = \mathbf{C}$$

The magnitude of the resultant vector **C** is always a positive number given by

$$\mathbf{C} = \mathbf{AB} \sin \theta$$

If **A** and **B** are parallel or antiparallel, then the angle θ between them is 0° or 180°, respectively. The sin 0° = sin 180° = 0, and the vector product is zero.

Right Hand Rule

There are always two directions that are perpendicular to a given plane. The direction of the vector product is determined by applying the right hand rule. Imagine an axis perpendicular to the plane of the two interacting vectors **A** and **B**. Let's imagine vector B being projected onto vector **A**. Wrap your right hand around this axis so that the fingers curl in the direction vector **B** would have to move to become collinear with **A**. Your thumb will point in the direction of the resultant vector **C**.

The "Right-Hand Rule"

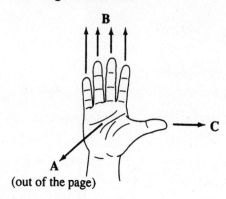

(out of the page)

PRACTICE PROBLEMS

1. A car travels due east for a distance of 3 miles and then due north for an additional 4 miles before stopping. What is the shortest straight line distance between the starting and ending points of this trip?

    A. 3 mi
    B. 4 mi
    C. 5 mi
    D. 7 mi

2. In the previous example, what is the angle a of the shortest path relative to due north?

    A. $\alpha = \text{arc cos } 3/5$
    B. $\alpha = \text{arc sin } 5/3$
    C. $\alpha = \text{arc sin } 4/3$
    D. $\alpha = \text{arc tan } 3/4$

3. A vector **A** makes an angle of 60° with the x-axis of a Cartesian coordinate system. Which of the following statements is true of the indicated magnitudes?

    A. A_x is greater than A_y.
    B. A_y is greater than A_x.
    C. A_y is greater than A.
    D. A_x is greater than A.

4. Force is a vector quantity measured in units of newtons, N. What must be the angle between two concurrently acting forces of 5 N and 3 N, respectively, if the resultant vector is 8 N?

    A. 0°
    B. 45°
    C. 90°
    D. 180°

5. Two forces, **A** and **B**, act concurrently on a point C. Both vectors have the same magnitude of 10 N and act at right angles to each other. What is the closest estimate of their resultant?

    A. 0 N
    B. 14 N
    C. 20 N
    D. 100 N

ANSWER KEY

1. C	2. D	3. B	4. A	5. B

ANSWERS AND EXPLANATIONS

1. **The correct answer is (C).** The two legs of the trip are perpendicular, therefore the shortest distance is given by the hypotenuse of the corresponding 3-4-5 right triangle. The value can be confirmed using the Pythagorean theorem:

    $$R = (3^2 + 4^2)^{\frac{1}{2}} = 5 \text{ mi}$$

2. **The correct answer is (D).** The angle α that gives the direction of the hypotenuse relative to the y-axis is given by:

    $\tan \alpha = $ opposite leg/adjacent leg $= 3/4$

    $\alpha = $ arc tan 3/4

    Similarly, it can be given as:

    $\alpha = $ arc cos 4/5 and $\alpha = $ arc sin 3/5

3. **The correct answer is (B).** Choices C and D can be eliminated immediately because the projection of a vector can never be greater than the vector itself. As the angle between the vector and the axis increases towards 90°, the magnitude of the projection decreases toward zero. The angle between the vector and the x-axis is 60°, which means the angle between the vector and the y-axis must be 30°. Therefore, the projection onto the y-axis, A_y, must be greater than the projection onto the x-axis, A_x.

4. **The correct answer is (A).** The only way the vector sum of a 3 N and a 5 N force can equal 8 N is if both forces act in the same direction. Therefore, the angle between them must be zero degrees.

    $5 \text{ N} + 3 \text{ N} = 8 \text{ N}$

5. **The correct answer is (B).** The two vectors form the legs of a right triangle. The resultant vector is the hypotenuse. A and C are eliminated immediately because they require that the two forces be antiparallel or parallel respectively. Choice D can also be eliminated since it is too large to be the hypotenuse. The magnitude of the resultant is confirmed by using the Pythagorean theorem:

    $$R = (10^2 + 10^2)^{1/2} = (200)^{1/2} = 10(2)^{1/2} = 10(1.41) \approx 14 \text{ N}$$

2.3 MOTION: DEFINITION OF TERMS

A. MECHANICS

Mechanics is the study of the relationships among matter, force, and motion. It is divided into the two broad categories of statics and dynamics.

- **Statics**

  Statics covers the conditions under which a body at rest remains at rest. The position of the body does not change with time.

- **Dynamics**

  Dynamics, or kinematics, studies the laws that govern the motion of a body. The position of the body does change with time.

B. POSITION

Position gives the coordinate(s) for the location of a body with respect to the origin of some frame of reference. Position is a vector quantity having both magnitude and direction measured from the origin. Position is given in units of length.

- **Frame of Reference**

  Frame of reference is any coordinate axis system that establishes a location called the origin. Changes in the position of a body—and, therefore, in the motion of the body—are measured with respect to this origin.

- **Cartesian Coordinate Axis System**

  The Cartesian coordinate axis system is a three-dimensional system with three mutually perpendicular axes labeled x, y, and z. This system is used to define the position, or change in position, of a body.

If the position of a body must be specified within a volume of space, then all three coordinate values are required to locate it. Each coordinate gives the body's position with respect to one of the three axes.

If the position or motion of a body is confined to an area of space, only two axes are required (usually x and y, by convention) to locate the body within the area. This applies to motion in a plane.

If the position of a body is further restricted to motion along a straight line, only one axis is required to locate the body. Linear motion is called translational motion. By convention, horizontal motion is along the x-axis and vertical motion is along the y-axis.

Relativity of Position and Motion

The values for the position and motion of a body depend on the frame of reference selected. Once the frame of reference has been defined, motion is the change in position with reference to the coordinates of the chosen frame. Generally, questions concerning position, speed, velocity, and acceleration use the Earth as the frame of reference.

Since position is relative, motion (which is a change in position) must also be relative. Therefore, the perception of motion also depends on the frame of reference. If two bodies appear to be approaching each other, then without an external reference point it is impossible to determine if:

- both bodies are moving toward each other from opposite directions

- one body is stationary and the other is moving toward the first

- both bodies are moving in the same direction, but one is moving faster and is therefore overtaking the other body

Optional Aside

If you are sitting down reading this text, how fast are you moving? This answer is not as obvious as you might expect. The Earth circles the sun with an average speed of 19 miles per second, so that if your frame of reference has its origin at the sun, your speed as you sit and read is a staggering 19 mi/s. If, however, the frame of reference is centered on the Earth, then although both you and the planet are still revolving around the sun at 19 mi/s, relative to each other neither you nor the Earth is moving. You are stationary as you sit and read.

C. MOTION

Motion is the change in position of a body. It is the displacement of a body with respect to bodies that are at rest (stationary) or to a fixed point (origin).

Displacement, d

Displacement, d, is a vector quantity that gives the direction and magnitude of the change in the position of a body. The vector is given by the difference between the coordinates of the initial and final positions.

For linear motion (along the x axis):

$$d = \Delta x = x_{\text{final position}} - x_{\text{initial position}}$$

Distance, *d*

Distance, *d*, gives the magnitude of the change in the position of a body. It is always a positive scalar quantity. The unit of distance and displacement is length.

$$d = |\Delta x|$$

Velocity, v

Velocity, v, is a vector quantity that gives the change in position as a function of time. It tells how fast the position of a body is changing in a given direction. It is the ratio of displacement to the time interval Δt during which the displacement occurs.

$$v = d/\Delta t$$

For linear motion, this is given by:

$$v = d/\Delta t = \Delta x/\Delta t = (x_2 - x_1)/(t_2 - t_1)$$

The units of velocity and speed are m/s, cm/s, and ft/s in the SI, cgs, and British systems, respectively.

Velocity is the slope of the curve that results from plotting the change in position vs. time.

Uniform Velocity

For uniform velocity, the ratio of displacement to time is constant. The graph for uniform velocity gives a straight line. For linear motion:

$$v = d/\Delta t = \Delta x/\Delta t = (x_2 - x_1)/(t_2 - t_1)$$

A net force must act on a body to change either its speed or its velocity. The result of this force is acceleration, a. The requisite for uniform linear motion is that there is no net acceleration; a = 0.

Nonuniform Velocity

Nonuniform velocity is the rate at which the body changes its position. It is not constant. For this to occur, the body must experience a net acceleration; a ≠ 0.

There are two broad categories for nonuniform velocity:

1. **uniform acceleration** (the velocity of the body changes at a steady rate)

2. **nonuniform acceleration** (the velocity of the body does not change uniformly)

Average Velocity, v_{av}

The average velocity is the ratio of the total displacement over the total time. The total displacement is the difference between the final position and the initial position and is independent of the actual path.

For a body with constant velocity (zero acceleration), the velocity of the body and its average velocity are identical:

$$v_{av} = v = d/\Delta t = \Delta x/\Delta t = d/t \; ; a = 0$$

For a body with nonuniform velocity (nonzero acceleration), the total displacement vector is not necessarily the same as the vector sum for the displacement vectors of all points along the path. The average velocity over a given time interval is the numerical average of the initial and final velocity for the time interval:

$$v_{av} = 1/2 \, (v_{final} + v_{initial})$$

Instantaneous Velocity, v_{inst}

If the velocity is nonuniform, the graph of velocity vs. time will be a curve. The velocity at any point is the instantaneous velocity at that point. Graphically, it is given by the slope of a tangent to the curve at that point.

For nonuniform velocity, the value of the average velocity approaches that of the instantaneous velocity as the time interval decreases:

$$\lim_{\Delta t \to 0} \frac{\Delta x}{\Delta t} = \lim_{\Delta t \to 0} v_{av} = v_{inst}$$

For uniform velocity, the average and instantaneous velocities are identical.

Speed, v

v is a scalar quantity that gives the rate at which motion is occurring, which is the magnitude of the velocity of the body. It is the ratio of distance traveled to the time involved in traveling that distance.

$$v = d/\Delta t$$

Graphically, speed is the slope to the curve of distance vs. time.

Average Speed, v_{av}

v_{av} equals the total path length divided by the total elapsed time. Your speed at any point along the path may be different from this average value.

Instantaneous Speed, v_{inst}

v_{inst} is the speed at a given moment or point along the path traveled. It is defined as the slope of the line tangent to the curve at that point.

When the speed of a body is constant (uniform), the ratio of distance to time is constant and

$$v_{inst} = v_{av} = v = d/\Delta t$$

When the rate at which a body changes position is not constant, then its speed is nonuniform and generally, $v_{inst} \neq v_{av}$.

Acceleration, a

Acceleration, a, is the vector quantity that gives the rate of change of the velocity:

$$a = \Delta v/\Delta t = (v_f - v_i)/(t_f - t_i) = (v_f - v_i)/t$$

Therefore,

$$v_f = v_i + at$$

and

$$x_f = x_i + v_i t + \frac{1}{2} at^2$$

The units of acceleration are the units of velocity divided by the unit of time. In the SI system, the unit is m/s². In the cgs and British systems, the units are cm/s² and ft/s², respectively.

The acceleration vector can change the magnitude and/or the direction of the velocity vector. A body undergoing acceleration has a nonlinear change in position with time because the distance covered in any time interval will be changed by the acceleration.

The acceleration vector can either increase or decrease the velocity vector depending on its direction with respect to the velocity vector.

Graphically, acceleration is the slope of the curve of velocity vs. time. For uniform acceleration, the graph of velocity vs. time is linear. For nonuniform acceleration, the graph is a curve and the acceleration at a given point is the tangent to the curve at that point.

Average and Instantaneous Accelerations

Like velocity, acceleration can be expressed as an average value, a_{av}, or as an instantaneous value, a_{inst}. For uniform acceleration, the acceleration, average acceleration, and instantaneous accelerations are numerically identical since the graph of velocity vs. time is a straight line:

$$a_{av} = a_{inst} = \Delta v/\Delta t = (v_{final} - v_{initial})/(t_{final} - t_{initial})$$

D. GRAPHS OF POSITION, VELOCITY, AND ACCELERATION WITH RESPECT TO TIME

Linear displacement is the change in the position of a body along a straight line (axis), Δx. Plots giving position, velocity, and acceleration as functions of time are given on the following pages for four cases of motion.

Case 1: Body at rest; therefore velocity and acceleration are zero.

Case 2: Body moves with uniform velocity; therefore zero acceleration.

Case 3: Body moves with nonuniform velocity and with uniform nonzero acceleration.

Case 4: Body moves with nonuniform velocity and nonuniform acceleration.

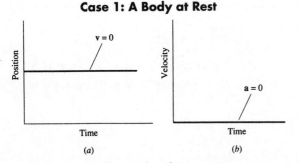

Case 1: A Body at Rest

For a body at rest, the graphs of (a) position vs. time and (b) velocity vs. time are all straight lines of constant zero slope. There is no acceleration.

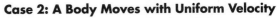
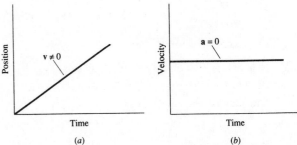

Case 2: A Body Moves with Uniform Velocity

For a body experiencing uniform velocity, (a) the graph of position vs. time gives a straight line with nonzero slope. The slope gives the velocity. (b) The graph of velocity vs. time gives a straight line with a zero slope. This slope is the acceleration experienced by the body. There is no acceleration.

Case 3: A Body Moves with Nonuniform Velocity and with Uniform Nonzero Acceleration

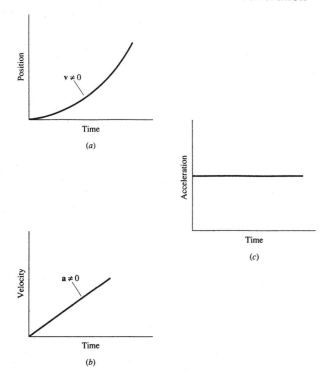

(a)

(c)

(b)

For a body that moves with nonuniform velocity and with uniform nonzero acceleration, the graphs of (a) position vs. time, (b) velocity vs. time, and (c) acceleration vs. time are all straight lines of constant zero slope.

Case 4: A Body Moves with Nonuniform Velocity and Nonuniform Acceleration

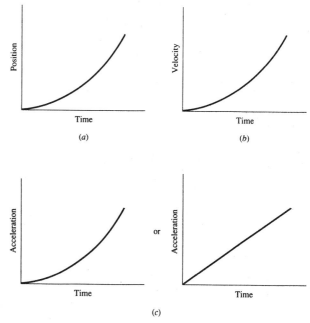

(a)

(b)

or

(c)

For a body that moves with nonuniform velocity and nonuniform acceleration, the graph of (a) the plot of position vs. time is a curve. The instant velocity at a given point is the slope of a tangent at that point. (b) The graph of velocity vs. time is also a curve. The instant acceleration at a given point is the slope of a tangent at that point. (c) The graph of acceleration vs. time can either be a curve or a straight line with a nonzero slope.

PRACTICE PROBLEMS

A bird flies 4.0 meters due north in 2.0 seconds and then flies 2.0 meters due west in 1.0 seconds. What is the bird's average speed?

A. 2.0 m/s
B. 4.0 m/s
C. 8.0 m/s
D. $2/3 \sqrt{5}$ m/s

2. If a car is traveling due south with a decreasing speed, then the direction of the car's acceleration is

A. due east.
B. due west.
C. due north.
D. due south.

3. A hiker travels 60 meters north and then 120 meters south. What is her resultant displacement?

A. 20 m north
B. 60 m south
C. 120 m north
D. 180 m south

4. If the average velocity of a plane is 500 km per hour, how long will it take to fly 125 km?

A. 4.00 h
B. 2.00 h
C. 0.50 h
D. 0.25 h

5. Applying the brakes to a car traveling at 45 km/h provides an acceleration of 5.0 m/s^2 in the opposite direction. How long will it take the car to stop?

 A. 0.40 s
 B. 2.5 s
 C. 5.0 s
 D. 9.0 s

6. An airplane is flying in the presence of a 100 km/h wind directed due north. What must be the velocity and heading of the plane if it is to maintain a velocity of 500 km/h due east with respect to the ground?

 A. 510 km/h E
 B. 300 km/h SE
 C. 510 km/h SE
 D. 600 km/h E

7. A ball rolls down a frictionless inclined plane with a uniform acceleration of 1.0 m/s^2. If its velocity at some instant of time is 10 m/s, what will be its velocity 5.0 seconds later?

 A. 5 m/s
 B. 10 m/s
 C. 15 m/s
 D. 16 m/s

8. A ball rolls down a frictionless inclined plane with a uniform acceleration of 1.0 m/s^2. If its initial velocity is 1.00 m/s, how far will it travel in 10 s?

 A. 10 m
 B. 12 m
 C. 60 m
 D. 100 m

9. Displacement is to distance as

 A. position is to change in position.
 B. velocity is to speed.
 C. acceleration is to velocity.
 D. speed is to velocity.

10. A body with an initial speed of 25 m/s accelerates uniformly for 10 seconds to a final speed of 75 m/s. What is the acceleration?

 A. 3 m/s^2
 B. 5 m/s^2
 C. 25 m/s^2
 D. 50 m/s^2

11. A body initially at rest is accelerated at 5 m/s^2 for 10 seconds. What is its final velocity?

 A. 0.50 m/s
 B. 2.0 m/s
 C. 5 m/s
 D. 50 m/s

12. Which graph represents the motion of a body accelerating uniformly from rest?

 A.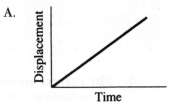

 B.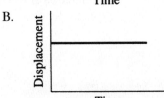

 C.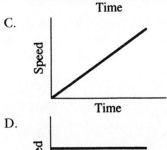

 D.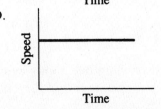

13. The speeds of a body at the ends of five successive seconds are: 180, 360, 540, 720, 900 m/h. What is the acceleration of the body?

 A. 0.05 m/s^2
 B. 20 m/s^2
 C. 180 m/s^2
 D. 180 m/h^2

ANSWER KEY

1. A	3. B	5. B	7. C	9. B	11. D	13. A
2. C	4. D	6. C	8. C	10. B	12. C	

ANSWERS AND EXPLANATIONS

1. **The correct answer is (A).** The average speed is the ratio of the distance traveled per unit time.

   v = 6.0 m/3.0 s = 2.0 m/s

2. **The correct answer is (C).** In order to change the magnitude but not the direction of the car's velocity, the acceleration vector must point in the opposite direction.

3. **The correct answer is (B).** Displacement is the vector that represents change in position of a body. The resultant vector is the vector sum of 60 m north and 120 m south to give 120 m south − 60 m north to give 60 m south.

4. **The correct answer is (D).** The average speed is distance traveled per time required:

   $t = d/v_{av}$ = 125 km/500 km/h = 0.25 h

   Since the plane travels 500 kilometers in one hour, it should take less than one hour to fly 125 kilometers. This eliminates A and B.

5. **The correct answer is (B).** $t = (v_f - v_i)/a$. The final velocity is 0 km/h and the acceleration is −5.0 m/s². (The negative sign appears because the acceleration is antiparallel to the velocity.) Remember to convert from kilometers to meters and from hours to seconds. Find t as follows:

$$[(0 - 45 \text{ km/h})/(-5 \text{ m/s}^2)](10^3 \text{m/km})(1 \text{ h}/3600 \text{ s}) = (45 \times 10^3/5 \times 3600) \text{ s}$$
$$= (9 \times 10^3/36 \times 10^2) \text{ s}$$
$$= 2.5 \text{ seconds}$$

6. **The correct answer is (C).** The desired velocity of the plane must have both an eastward component (direction of travel) and a southward component to overcome the northward force of the wind. This eliminates choices A and D. The vector due east is the projection of the plane's velocity vector on the east axis. Since a projection cannot be greater than the vector producing it, 500 km/h is the minimum velocity the plane could have. This eliminates choice C.

   This can be confirmed by applying the Pythagorean theorem:

   $\{(100 \text{ km/h})^2 + (500 \text{ km/h})^2\}1/2 = 510 \text{ km/h SE}$

7. **The correct answer is (C).** $v_f = v_i + at$ = 10 m/s + (1.0 m/s²)(5.0 s) = 15 m/s

8. **The correct answer is (C).**
   d = $v_i t$ + 1/2 at^2
   = (1.0 m/s)(10 s) + 1/2 (1.0 m/s₂)(10 s)₂
   = 10 + 50 = 60 m

9. **The correct answer is (B).** Distance is the scalar equivalent of the displacement vector and speed is the scalar equivalent of the velocity vector. A and C are eliminated because all the terms are vectors. D is eliminated because the ratio is vector to scalar instead of scalar to vector.

10. **The correct answer is (B).** $a = \Delta v / \Delta 3t = (75 \text{ m/s} - 25 \text{ m/s})/10 \text{ s} = 5 \text{ m/s}^2$

11. **The correct answer is (D).** $v_f = v_i + at = 0 + (5 \text{ m/s}^2)10 \text{ s} = 50 \text{ m/s}$

12. **The correct answer is (C).** Acceleration is the rate of change in velocity or speed of a body. A and B are eliminated because they are not velocity or speed vs. time graphs. D is eliminated because the zero slope means zero acceleration.

13. **The correct answer is (A).**

    $a = \Delta v / \Delta t$

    $= (180 \text{ m/h})(1\text{h}/3600 \text{ s})/1 \text{ s} = 0.05 \text{ m/s}_2$.

    Remember to convert from hours to seconds.

2.4 MOTION: TRANSLATIONAL AND IN A PLANE

A. TRANSLATIONAL MOTION WITH UNIFORM ACCELERATION

This kind of motion is the simplest type of accelerated motion. The body moves in a straight line with constant acceleration, which means the velocity of the body is changing at a uniform rate.

Uniform acceleration can be completely described by these four variables:

1. The position, x, or its change, $\Delta x = x - x_0$

2. The velocity, v, or its change, $\Delta v = v - v_0$

3. The time, t, or its change, $\Delta t = t - t_0$

4. The acceleration, a

Where x_0, v_0, and t_0 are the initial position, velocity, and time; x, v, and t are the values at some other time; a is the acceleration.

Questions involving uniform acceleration can be solved using the following set of six interrelated equations. The appropriate equation depends on which of the four variables are known. The pertinent missing variable(s) is listed next to the equation.

Equation	Missing Variables
1. $v = v_0 + at$	$\Delta x = x - x_0$
2. $v_{av} = \frac{1}{2}(v + v_0) = (v_0 + \left(\frac{1}{2}\right) at)$	$\Delta x = x - x_0$
3. $\Delta x = x - x_0 = v_0 t + 1/2 \, at^2$	v
4. $\Delta x = x - x_0 = vt - 1/2 \, at^2$	v_0
5. $\Delta x = x - x_0 = 1/2 \, (v + v_0)t$	a
6. $v^2 - v_0^2 = 2a(x - x_0) = 2a\Delta x$	t

Acceleration Due to Gravity, g

Acceleration due to gravity, g, is a vector quantity that is always directed towards the center of the earth. The magnitude of gravity, g, for the Earth in each of the three unit systems is:

SI:	$g = 9.8 \text{ m/s}^2$
cgs:	$g = 980 \text{ cm/s}^2$
British:	$g = 32 \text{ ft/s}^2$

In a vacuum, the acceleration due to gravity is the same for all falling bodies regardless of their size or composition. This may seem counterintuitive to everyday observations until you remember that in a vacuum, g supplies the only force acting on the body, and other forces—such as air resistance and buoyancy—are absent. For most real (nonvacuum) conditions, the effects of these other forces, while present, are assumed to be negligible.

The value of g is constant and doesn't change as the body falls.

Optional Aside

Actually, the effect of gravity on a body decreases as the distance between the body and the Earth's center of gravity increases. However, if the distance the body falls is small compared to the radius of the Earth, the variation in gravity is negligible. This is ensured by restricting free fall to points near the surface of the Earth. The value of gravity also varies slightly with latitude and with the rotation of the Earth, but these perturbations are negligible.

The force of gravity depends on the body producing the force, called the gravitating body. All the remarks about the acceleration of gravity due to the Earth apply to the gravity due to any other body. The only difference will be the magnitude of g. The acceleration due to gravity near the surface of the moon is 1.67 m/s^2, while that near the surface of the sun is 274 m/s^2.

Free-Falling Body

Free fall is an example of translational motion with uniform acceleration. The acceleration is supplied by gravity. Free fall describes the motion of bodies rising and/or falling on or near the surface of the Earth.

The equations that describe free fall are identical to those for any translational motion with uniform acceleration. The vector for gravitational acceleration, g, replaces the acceleration vector a. Since vertical motion is, by convention, associated with the y-axis of a coordinate system, the gravitational vector is parallel to the y-axis. The vector carries a negative sign because it is always directed downward toward the negative y leg of the y-axis:

$$-g = a_y = \text{constant}$$

Velocity in Free-Fall Calculations

The velocity is given by the equation $v = v_0 + at$ where the acceleration is due to gravity:

$$v = v_0 - gt$$

The velocity at any time during free fall is the vector sum of any initial velocity, v_0, and the change to that initial velocity due to the acceleration of gravity, g. This change depends on how long the acceleration has been acting on the body, t.

Position in Free-Fall Calculations

The position of a free-falling body is given by the equation $\Delta x = x - x_0 = v_0 t + 1/2\, at^2$ with the horizontal axis, x, replaced by the vertical axis, y, and the acceleration due to gravity, g:

$$y = v_0 t - 1/2\, gt^2$$

Free-Falling Body Problems

The three common free-falling body problems that involve pure translational motion are outlined below.

1. **A Body Dropped from a Height**

   This is the simplest free-falling body problem. The body starts from rest so $v_0 = 0$ and the equations for velocity and position reduce to:

   $$v = -gt \text{ and } y = -1/2\, gt^2$$

2. **A Body Thrown Vertically Down from a Height**

   Here the body starts with an initial velocity directed in the same direction as the acceleration. Velocity and position are given by the equations $v = v_0 - gt$ and $y = v_0 t - 1/2gt^2$, respectively.

3. **A Body Thrown Vertically Up**

   This problem can be divided into three distinct regions of motion:

   a) The body moves vertically upward. The velocity and position are given by the equations $v = v_0 - gt$ and $y = v_0 t - 1/2gt^2$. The initial velocity and the force of gravity vectors are antiparallel so that the velocity of the upward motion decreases with time and eventually becomes zero. The maximum height reached depends on the amount of time the body rises, which in turn depends on the magnitude of the initial velocity. The greater the v_0, the longer it takes for g to cancel it.

   b) Eventually the effect of the gravitational acceleration cancels (overcomes) the effect of the initial upward velocity. At this point, called the zenith, the velocity becomes zero and the body stops rising.

   $$v_0 = gt_{maximum}, v = 0$$

   Once the time ($t_{maximum}$) has been determined, the maximum height can be found:

   $$y_{maximum} = v_0 t_{maximum} - 1/2\, gt^2_{maximum}$$

   c) At the zenith the initial velocity is zero and the only force acting on the body is the force of gravity, which starts accelerating the body toward the Earth. A description of this part of the motion is identical to the case above in which a body is dropped from a height.

B. MOTION IN A PLANE WITH UNIFORM ACCELERATION

A body following a curved path requires two axes to define its position at any time. By convention, we use the x- and y-axes and the motion is said to occur in the xy plane.

Projectile Motion

A body following a curvilinear path is called a projectile and the path is called its trajectory. The **range** is the horizontal distance traveled by the projectile along the x-axis.

If a free-falling body has a horizontal velocity component, instead of moving only along a single vertical line it will follow the curved path of a parabola. Any vector associated with the body can be resolved into two mutually perpendicular components that are parallel to the x- and y-axes.

Components of the Velocity Vector

The initial velocity v_0 can be resolved into two components:

$$v_{0x} = v_0 \cos \theta_0 \text{ and } v_{0y} = v_0 \sin \theta_0$$

where θ_0 is the initial angle between the velocity vector and the horizontal axis.

If the only nonnegligible force acting on the projectile is gravity, the velocity component along the x-axis is constant; its value at any point will be the same as its initial value:

$$v_x = v_{0x}$$

The velocity component along the y-axis feels the acceleration due to gravity. The effect of this acceleration depends on how long it has been acting on the body. Therefore, the magnitude of the component, v_y, at any time is the vector sum of its initial component and the effect of the gravitational acceleration:

$$v_y = v_{0y} - gt$$

Components of the Acceleration Vector

The only source of acceleration is gravity, which is directed down along the y-axis. The component along the x-axis is zero.

$$a_y = a_{0y} = -g$$
$$a_x = a_{0x} = 0$$

Components of the Position

1. The distance or position along the x-axis at any point must be the initial value plus the horizontal distance moved. The latter is the product of the horizontal velocity component and the time since the motion started.

$$x = x_0 + v_{0x}t$$

2. The height or position along the y-axis has an additional term due to the acceleration of gravity:

$$y = y_0 + v_{0y}t - 1/2\, gt^2$$

Range, *R*, and Time of Flight, *T*

The range, R, is the horizontal distance between the starting and ending points of the projectile's path. The time of flight, T, is the total time the projectile spends in flight. It is twice the time required for the projectile to reach its maximum height.

$$T = 2 v_{0y}/g = 2 v_0 \sin \theta/g$$

$$R = (v_0 \cos \theta)T = (v_{02}/g) \sin 2\theta$$

Both calculations assume air resistance is negligible.

The maximum range occurs for $\theta_0 = 45°$, because $\sin 2 \times 45° = \sin 90° = 1.00$ and $R_{max} = v_0^2/g$. For every range other than R_{max} there will be two angles that give the same range. This diagram shows range and the two equal range values produced by θ_1 and θ_2.

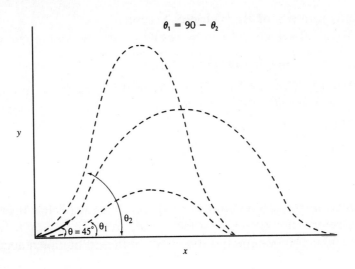

Summary of Position and Velocity

Equations

The initial value conditions can be modified to give values for v_x, v_y, x, and y at any point along the path by placing the origin at the starting point of the motion so that $x_0 = y_0 = 0$.

$$x = v_{0x}t = (v_0 \cos \theta_0)t$$
$$y = v_{0y}t - 1/2\, gt^2 = (v_0 \sin \theta_0)t - 1/2\, gt^2$$
$$v_x = v_0 \cos \theta_0$$
$$v_y = v_0 \sin \theta_0 - gt$$

General Trajectory Path

1. While the projectile is rising, v_y is antiparallel to gravity so its value decreases with time.

2. At the zenith, which is the maximum height reached by the projectile, $v_y = 0$.

3. On the descent, v_y and g are parallel so the vertical velocity increases.

4. The magnitude of the velocity (the instantaneous speed) of the projectile at any point is:

$$v = (v_x{}^2 + v_y{}^2)^{1/2}$$

5. The direction of the velocity at any point is:

$$\tan \theta = v_y/v_x$$

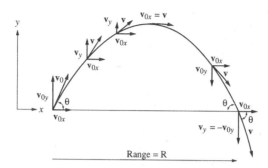

Diagram of the parabolic trajectory of a projectile launched with an initial velocity v_0. The velocity at any point is along the tangent at that point and can be resolved into components parallel to the x- and y-axes.

Uniform Circular Motion

In **uniform circular motion,** the speed of a body moving in a circular path is constant. However, since the direction of the body's motion is constantly changing, its velocity must be constantly changing. Furthermore, since the speed is constant, the magnitude of the velocity must be constant and it is the direction of the velocity vector that changes.

The **period,** T, is the time required to complete one revolution. If the radius of the path is R, the constant speed equals the ratio of the circumference to the period:

constant speed $= v = 2\pi R/T$

In projectile motion, the acceleration is constant in both magnitude and direction. In uniform circular motion, the acceleration is constant only in magnitude but not in direction. The acceleration is:

$$a = \Delta v/\Delta t = v^2/R = \text{speed}^2/\text{radius}$$

Circular Components of Acceleration

The acceleration vector can be resolved into two mutually perpendicular components with respect to the curve of the path rather than the coordinate axis system with its origin at the center of the circle.

The tangential or parallel component, $a_{\parallel}$, at any point on the curve is coincident with a line tangent to the curve at that point. This component changes the magnitude of the velocity vector but not its direction.

The normal or perpendicular component, $a_{\perp}$, is also called the centripetal or radial acceleration. At any point on the curve, it is perpendicular to the tangent at that point and directed along a radius toward the center of the circle. This component changes the direction of the velocity vector but not its magnitude. This component must have a nonzero value if the body is to remain moving in a circular path.

A body in uniform circular motion, therefore, must have a **tangential acceleration** of zero and a normal or centripetal acceleration that is constant. This means that the body is continually "falling" (accelerating) toward the center.

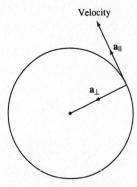

Components of acceleration for uniform circular motion. $a_{\parallel}$ is collinear with the velocity vector. For uniform circular motion, its magnitude is zero so it has no effect on the velocity. $a_{\perp}$ changes the direction of the velocity. It is radially directed.

PRACTICE PROBLEMS

1. A rock is dropped from a height of 19.6 meters above the ground. How long does it take the rock to hit the ground?

   A. 2 s
   B. 4 s
   C. 4.9 s
   D. 9.8 s

2. A spacecraft exploring a distant planet releases a probe to explore the planet's surface. The probe falls freely a distance of 40 meters during the first 4.0 seconds after its release. What is the acceleration due to gravity on this planet?

   A. 4.0 m/s^2
   B. 5.0 m/s^2
   C. 10 m/s^2
   D. 16 m/s^2

3. Which property is constant for a body in free fall?

   A. acceleration
   B. displacement
   C. velocity
   D. speed

4. Which graph represents the relationship between speed (v) and time (t) for a body falling near the surface of a planet?

   A.
   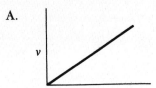

   B.
   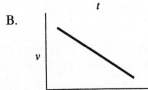

   C.
   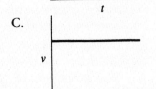

   D.
   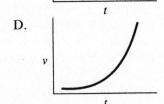

5. A ball is dropped from the roof of a very tall building. What is its velocity after falling for 5.00 seconds?

   A. 1.96 m/s
   B. 9.80 m/s
   C. 49.0 m/s
   D. 98.0 m/s

6. A quarterback throws a football with a velocity of 7 m/s and an angle of 15° with the horizontal. How far away should the designated receiver be?

   A. 1.25 m
   B. 2.50 m
   C. 5.00 m
   D. 6.25 m

7. What must be the minimum velocity of a missile if it is to strike a target 100 meters away?

   A. 19.6 m/s
   B. 31.3 m/s
   C. 98.0 m/s
   D. 980 m/s

8. An arrow is shot at an angle of 30° to the horizontal and with a velocity of 29.4 m/s. How long will it take for the arrow to strike the ground?

   A. 1 s
   B. 2 s
   C. 3 s
   D. 4 s

9. At what angle should a projectile be fired in order for its range to be at maximum?

   A. 30°
   B. 45°
   C. 60°
   D. 120°

10. A bomber is traveling due east with a velocity of 300 m/s when it releases a bomb. If the bomb takes 2.00 seconds to strike the ground, what was the range (horizontal distance) of the bomb's path?

    A. 100 m
    B. 150 m
    C. 300 m
    D. 600 m

11. A bomber is flying with a velocity of 500 m/h at an altitude of 1960 meters when it drops a bomb. How long does it take for the bomb to hit the ground?

    A. 0.50 s
    B. 20 s
    C. 50 s
    D. 200 s

12. A ball is thrown with a horizontal velocity of 6.0 m/s. What is its velocity after 3.0 seconds of flight?

    A. 30 m/s
    B. 15.8 m/s
    C. 18 m/s
    D. 4.9 m/s

13. What is the speed of a body moving in a horizontal circle of radius 5.00 m at a rate of 2.00 revolutions per second?

    A. 7.85 m/s
    B. 15.7 m/s
    C. 31.4 m/s
    D. 62.8 m/s

14. A 0.2-kilogram ball is tied to the end of a string and rotated in a horizontal circular path of radius 25 cm. If the speed is 10πcm/s, what is the centripetal acceleration?

    A. $2.5\ \pi$ cm/s^2
    B. $4.0\ \pi^2$ cm/s^2
    C. $0.40\ \pi$ cm/s^2
    D. $25\ \pi$ cm/s^2

15. A 70-kilogram woman standing at the equator rotates with the Earth around its axis at a speed of about 500 m/s. If the radius of the Earth is approximately 6×10^6 m, which is the best estimate of the centripetal acceleration experienced by the woman?

    A. 4×10^{-2} m/s^2
    B. 4 m/s^2
    C. 10^{-4} m/s^2
    D. 24 m/s^2

16. A missile is fired at an angle with the horizontal. The air resistance is negligible. The initial horizontal velocity component is twice that of the initial vertical velocity component. The trajectory of the missile is best described as

    A. semicircular.
    B. translational.
    C. parabolic.
    D. hyperbolic.

17. Which trajectory best describes a ball rolling down a curved ramp that ends at point P?

    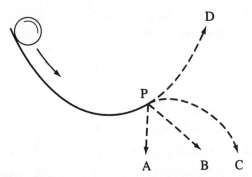

    A. A
    B. B
    C. C
    D. D

18. A cannon is placed on a flatcar of a train. The train is moving at a uniform speed 5.0 m/s when the cannon fires a ball vertically up at 10 m/s. Which vector best represents the resultant velocity of the cannonball?

    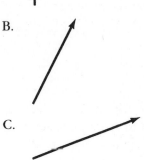

19. A bullet is fired from a gun with a muzzle velocity of 300 m/s and at an angle of 30° above the horizontal. What is the magnitude of the vertical component of the muzzle velocity?

    A. 0 m/s
    B   9.8 m/s
    C. 150 m/s
    D. 300 m/s

20. What is the centripetal acceleration of a 20.0 kilogram body traveling at a uniform speed of 40.0 m/s around a circular path of radius 10.0 m?

    A. 320 m/s^2
    B. 160 m/s^2
    C. 80 m/s^2
    D. 20 m/s^2

21. Car A has a mass twice that of car B. Both are traveling with the same uniform speed around a circular racetrack. The centripetal acceleration of car A is

A. twice that of car B.
B. half that of car B.
C. is the same as that of car B.
D. four times that of car B.

22. A ball rolls with uniform speed around a frictionless flat horizontal circular track. If the velocity of the ball is doubled, the centripetal acceleration is

A. quadrupled.
B. doubled.
C. halved.
D. unchanged.

23. The centripetal acceleration of a car traveling at constant speed around a frictionless circular racetrack

A. is zero.
B. has constant magnitude but varying direction.
C. has constant direction but varying magnitude.
D. has varying magnitude and direction.

ANSWER KEY

1. A	4. A	7. B	10. D	13. D	16. C	19. C	22. A
2. B	5. C	8. C	11. B	14. B	17. C	20. B	23. B
3. A	6. B	9. B	12. A	15. A	18. B	21. C	

ANSWERS AND EXPLANATIONS

1. **The correct answer is (A).** This is free fall with zero initial velocity and initial height of $y_0 = 19.6$ m. The position equation: $-y = v_0 t - 1/2\ gt^2$ becomes $y = 1/2\ gt^2$. Solving for time gives:

$$t = (2y_0/g)^{1/2}$$
$$= (2 \times 19.6\ m/9.8\ m/s^2)^{1/2}$$
$$= (4\ s^2)^{1/2} = 2\ s$$

2. **The correct answer is (B).** This is a free-fall problem. The object starts from rest, $v_0 = 0$. Rearrange the position equation to solve for the acceleration of gravity:

$$g = 2y/t^2 = 2(40\ m)/16\ s^2 = 5.0\ m/s^2$$

3. **The correct answer is (A).** By definition, a free-falling body experiences a constant acceleration due to gravity.

4. **The correct answer is (A).** A free-falling body feels a constant acceleration due to gravity. Therefore, its speed increases uniformly (linearly) as it falls. Choice B is eliminated because the speed is decreasing linearly, which is opposite to the effect expected for the fall. Choice C indicates constant speed, which means there is zero acceleration. Choice D is a curve. This indicates a nonlinear acceleration that causes the speed to increase in a nonlinear manner.

5. **The correct answer is (C).** The free-fall velocity starting with an initial velocity of zero is:

$$v = -gt = -(9.8\ m/s^2)5.00\ s = -49\ m/s$$

The velocity is 49 m/s downward (negative sign).

6. **The correct answer is (B).**

   Range, R = (v_0^2/g) sin 2q

   $$= \{(7 \text{ m/s})^2/(9.8 \text{ m/s}^2)\}(0.500)$$

   $$= 2.5 \text{ m}.$$

7. **The correct answer is (B).** Assume the range desired is the maximum range. It is achieved when $\theta = 45°$ so that sin 2θ = sin 90° = 1. $R_{max} = v_0^2/g$ therefore:

   $v_0 = (gR_{max})^{1/2}$

   $$= \{(9.8 \text{ m/s}^2)(100 \text{ m})\}^{1/2}$$

   $$= (980 \text{ m}^2/\text{s}^2)^{1/2}$$

   $$= 31.3 \text{ m/s}$$

8. **The correct answer is (C).** The time of flight is:

   $T = (2 \ v_0 \sin \theta)/g$

   $$= 2(29.4 \text{ m/s})(0.500)/9.8 \text{ m/s}^2$$

   $$= 3 \text{ s}$$

9. **The correct answer is (B).** By definition, R_{max} occurs when $\theta = 45°$.

10. **The correct answer is (D).** The horizontal and vertical components of velocity are independent of each other. The initial horizontal velocity of the bomb is the same as that of the plane. The range is the horizontal distance covered, which is the product of the horizontal velocity and the time in flight:

    $x = v_0 t = (300 \text{ m/s})(2.00 \text{ s}) = 600 \text{ m}$

11. **The correct answer is (B).** The horizontal and the vertical components of velocity are independent. The vertical component is due only to the acceleration of gravity:

    $y = 1/2 \ gt^2$

    rearranges to:

    $t = (2y/g)^{1/2}$

    $$= \{2(1960 \text{ m})/(9.8 \text{ m/s}^2)\}^{1/2}$$

    $$= (400 \text{ s}^2)^{1/2}$$

    $$= 20 \text{ s}$$

12. **The correct answer is (A).** The horizontal component of velocity is v_x = 6.0 m/s, and the vertical component is $v_y = gt = (9.8 \text{ m/s}^2)(3.0 \text{ s}) = 29.4$ m/s, and v = $(v_x^2 + v_y^2)^{1/2} = \{(6.0 \text{ m/s})^2 + (29.4 \text{ m/s})^2\}^{1/2} = (900 \text{ m}^2/\text{s}^2)^{1/2} = 30$ m/s.

13. **The correct answer is (D).** For a circular path, speed is $v = 2\pi R/T$. The distance covered by the body is one circumference per revolution. If the body completes 2 revolutions per second, its period (the time required to complete one revolution) must be 0.5 second.

    $v = 2\pi R/T$

    $$= (2\pi)(5.0 \text{ m})/(0.5 \text{ s})$$

    $$= 20\pi \text{ m/s}$$

    $$= 62.8 \text{ m/s}$$

14. **The correct answer is (B).** The mass of the ball is not needed to find the centripetal acceleration.

$$a_c = a_\perp = v^2/R = (10\pi \text{ cm/s})^2/25 \text{ cm} = 4\pi^2 \text{cm/s}^2$$

15. **The correct answer is (A).** The woman is moving in a circle whose radius is that of the Earth, and moving with a constant speed equal to the rotation of the Earth on its axis. The centripetal acceleration is:

$$a_c = v^2/R$$
$$= (500 \text{ m/s})^2/6 \times 10^6 \text{ m}$$
$$= (25 \times 10^4 \text{ m}^2/\text{s}^2)/6 \times 10^6 \text{ m}$$
$$a_c = 4.2 \times 10^{-2} \text{ m/s}^2 \sim 4 \times 10^{-2} \text{ m/s}^2$$

16. **The correct answer is (C).** If air resistance is neglected, the trajectories of all projectiles fired near the surface of the Earth follow a parabolic path because the horizontal velocity is constant while the vertical acceleration is also constant.

17. **The correct answer is (C).** The ball leaves the ramp with a horizontal component to its velocity and acquires a vertical acceleration due to gravity. The path is a typical parabolic trajectory.

18. **The correct answer is (B).** The cannon gives the ball vertical velocity while the train gives it horizontal velocity so the resultant cannot be purely vertical or purely horizontal. This eliminates choices A and D. Since the vertical component is greater than the horizontal component, the resultant should make an angle greater than 45° with the horizontal. Choice B is the better description.

19. **The correct answer is (C).** The velocity has two perpendicular components, one vertically oriented and the other, horizontal.

$$v_{0y} = v_0 \sin 30°$$
$$= (300 \text{ m/s})(0.500)$$
$$= 150 \text{ m/s}$$

The triangle formed is a 30°-60°-90° right triangle; therefore, the side opposite the 30° angle is half the length of the hypotenuse (300 m/s).

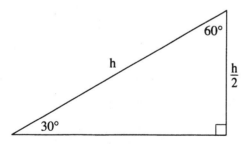

20. **The correct answer is (B).** The centripetal acceleration is the ratio of the square of the speed to the radius of the circle:

$$a_c = v^2/R$$
$$= (40 \text{ m/s})^2/10 \text{ m}$$
$$= 160 \text{ m/s}^2$$

21. **The correct answer is (C).** $a_c = v^2/R$. Since the speed v is the same for both cars and the radius of the track is the same, the centripetal acceleration is the same. The centripetal force on each car is different, however, because of the difference in mass.

22. **The correct answer is (A).** $a_c = v^2/R$. The acceleration and the square of the velocity are directly proportional. If you double the velocity, you quadruple the square of the velocity. Therefore, you quadruple the acceleration.

23. **The correct answer is (B).** Acceleration is always in the direction of the force producing the acceleration. In a circular path, the direction of the force is continuously changing. The magnitude of the acceleration remains the same because the magnitude of the force is constant.

2.5 FORCE AND NEWTON'S LAWS

A. FORCE

Force is a vector quantity that measures the interaction between two or more bodies. A force provides an acceleration; therefore, it changes the motion of a body.

The unit of force is a derived unit that defines the amount of acceleration (m/s^2), acting to move a mass (kg) some distance (m). The resulting units are summarized below:

System	Derived Unit	Basic Units
SI	newton, N	$1 \text{ N} = 1 \text{ kg m}^2 \text{ s}^{-2}$
cgs	dyne, dyn	$1 \text{ dyn} = 1 \text{ g cm}^2 \text{ s}^{-2}$
British	pound, lb	$1 \text{ lb} = 1 \text{ slug ft}^2 \text{ s}^{-2}$

All forces fall into four fundamental types:

Two long-range types:

    1. Gravitational force

    2. Electromagnetic force

Two short-range types (which are actually forms of electromagnetic forces):

    3. The strong force, which holds protons and neutrons together in the nucleus

    4. The weak force, which is involved in radioactive emissions

Contact Forces

Contact forces require that the interacting bodies be in physical contact with each other. Friction is a typical contact force.

Noncontact Forces

Noncontact forces can act through empty space without any physical contact between the interacting bodies. The force influences the motion of a body by producing a field that interacts with that body. Gravitational, electric, and magnetic forces produce fields and are typical noncontact forces.

Concurrent Forces

Concurrent forces are two or more forces that have lines of action that pass through some common point in the body. A set of concurrent forces can always be resolved into a single resultant force that produces the same effect on the body as the concurrent set. The resultant tends to produce translational motion.

Nonconcurrent Forces

Nonconcurrent forces are forces that act on the same body but do not act along the same line and do not all intersect at same common point. These forces tend to cause the body to rotate.

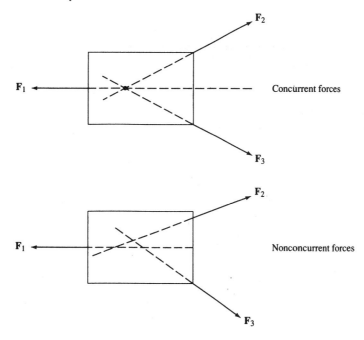

Parallel Forces

Parallel forces are a special case of nonconcurrent forces whose lines of action never intersect. However, they can be resolved into a single resultant force that is the algebraic sum of the parallel forces. Parallel forces tend to cause the body to rotate.

B. NEWTON'S FIRST LAW OF MOTION

A body remains in a state of rest or of uniform motion (traveling along a straight line with constant speed) unless it is acted on by a net applied force. This first law is also called the law of inertia or the law of equilibrium.

- **Inertia**
  Inertia is the tendency of a body to resist a change in its motion. That is, a body will not change its motion spontaneously; some outside force must act on it.

- **Equilibrium**
  Equilibrium describes the condition where there is no net change in the motion of a system or body. A body can have forces acting on it and still be in equilibrium, provided the vector sum of the forces is zero.

C. NEWTON'S SECOND LAW

A net force acting on a body will cause an acceleration of the body. The acceleration vector is directly proportional to the force vector and occurs in the same direction. The proportionality constant is the **mass** of the body:

$$\mathbf{F} = m\mathbf{a} = m\mathbf{v}/t = m\mathbf{d}/t^2$$

1. The greater the force acting on a body, the greater the acceleration it experiences.

2. If equal forces are applied to bodies of different masses, the more massive body will experience the smaller acceleration because mass and acceleration are inversely proportional.

3. If no net force is applied to a body, the acceleration is zero and the second law gives rise to the first law.

    *   A body at rest has zero velocity. Since the acceleration is also zero, the body remains at rest.

    *   A body in uniform motion has a constant velocity. Since the acceleration is zero, the velocity remains unchanged.

4. If a sufficient net force is applied to a body that is initially at rest, the body will start to move in the same direction as the applied force. The longer the force is applied, the faster the body moves.

5. If a force is applied to a body with uniform motion, the following changes are possible:

    *   If the force is in the same direction as the motion, the body will increase its speed. The angle between **F** and **v** is 0°.

    *   If the force is in the opposite direction to the motion, the body will decrease its speed. The angle between **F** and **v** is 180°.

    *   If the force is applied at some angle other than 0° or 180° to the direction of the motion, the body will acquire nonlinear motion. That is, the direction as well as the magnitude of its motion will change.

    *   **Weight,** w, is the effect of the acceleration due to gravity, g, on the mass of a body. Therefore, weight is equal to the force of gravity on a body. It is a vector quantity that is always directed toward the center of the Earth.

        $$\mathbf{w} = \mathbf{F}_{grav} = m\mathbf{g}$$

        Two bodies of equal mass will have different weights on different planets because the acceleration due to gravity on the two planets will be different.

Note: A common source of error in calculations occurs when the SI and cgs units for mass are incorrectly used to denote weight:

	SI	cgs	British
mass	kg	g	slug
weight	N	dyn	lb

D.   NEWTON'S THIRD LAW

For every action there is an equal and opposite reaction. If a body exerts a force on a second body, that second body must exert an equal counterforce on the first. The two forces form an **action-reaction pair.**

The forces of the action-reaction pair cannot act on the same body. This distinguishes them from forces that are not action-reaction pairs, but are rather pairs that happen to operate in opposite directions at some common point.

Consider a system composed of a block being pulled along a frictionless horizontal surface by a rope (see figure below). Assume the rope is massless and the box sits on a frictionless surface.

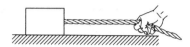

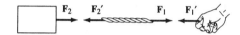

Forces acting on a rope and box system.

The following forces act on the system:

- The hand on the rope produces force F_1 that is equal and opposite to the force F'_1 exerted by the rope on the hand.

- At the other end of the diagram, the force F_2 exerted by the rope on the box is equal and opposite to the force F'_2 exerted by the box on the rope.

- F_1 and F'_1 form one action-reaction pair, while F_2 and F'_2 form the other.

Note: Although F_1 and F'_2 are equal and opposite to each other, they do not form an action-reaction pair because they both operate on the same body, the rope.

E.   NEWTON'S LAW OF UNIVERSAL GRAVITATION

Every body in the universe attracts every other body with a force that is directly proportional to the product of the masses of the two bodies and inversely proportional to the square of the distance separating the two bodies. The proportionality constant is the gravitational constant, G.

$$F_{gravity} = G \frac{m_1 m_2}{r^2}$$

where m_1 and m_2 are the masses of body 1 and body 2, r is the distance between them, and $G = 6.67 \times 10^{-11}$ N m^2/kg^2.

The force of gravity is the gravitational attraction a body feels near the surface of a celestial body, such as the Earth. The gravitational forces are directed along the line that connects the centers of gravity of the two interacting bodies. For a body on or near the surface of the Earth, it is reasonable to assume that:

1. The height of the body above the surface is negligible compared to the radius of the Earth, so $r^2 \approx r^2_{Earth}$.

2. $\mathbf{g} = \mathbf{F}/m = G m_{Earth}/r^2_{Earth}$, which means g depends only on the distance of the body from the center of the Earth.

F. FRICTIONAL FORCE

The force of friction, F_f, is a nonconservative contact force that resists the motion of one surface sliding across another.

1. Friction acts parallel to the surfaces that are in contact.

2. Friction acts in the direction opposite to that of the net force that acts to move the body along the surface.

3. Friction depends on the identities of the materials in contact and on the conditions of their surfaces (wet, dry, oiled, rough, smooth).

Optional Aside

The two main sources of friction are:

Mechanical Interactions
Imperfections in the surfaces of the two bodies tend to interlock them together, making it more difficult for one to slide over the other.

No surface can be made perfectly smooth, and even if it could, polishing surfaces only reduces friction to some limiting value. Polishing beyond this point actually increases the amount of friction observed.

Electrical Interactions
The same interatomic and intermolecular forces that hold atoms and molecules together in solids can act between the atoms or molecules of the two sliding surfaces.

4. The frictional force is directly proportional to the force pressing the two surfaces together. This force is the normal force, F_N. The normal force simply equals the component of the weight of the body that is perpendicular to the surface with which it is in contact unless some other force acting on the body also has a component perpendicular to the contact surfaces. As the angle of inclination of the surface increases, the value of F_N decreases and the frictional force decreases, making it easier for the body to slide as the incline becomes steeper.

5. The dimensionless proportionality constant for the ratio of the frictional force to the normal force is called the coefficient of friction, μ. The value of the coefficient depends not only on the identities of the two surfaces, but also on whether the body is in motion or not. For example, for two steel surfaces, the static coefficient is 0.5 and the dynamic coefficient is 0.4.

- **Static Coefficient of Friction, μ_s**
  Static coefficient of friction, μ_s, is the unitless coefficient prior to the onset of motion and describes the static frictional force that helps prevent motion:

  $$\mu_s = F_f/F_N$$

  The static frictional force has a maximum value given by:

  $$F_{f\,max} = \mu_s F_N$$

  If the applied force exceeds this maximum static frictional force, motion will begin.

- **Dynamic Coefficient of Friction, μ_d**

  Dynamic coefficient of friction, μ_d, is the coefficient once motion starts and describes the sliding frictional force that resists that motion. It is also called the *kinetic coefficient of friction:*

  $$\mu_d = F_f/F_N$$

  The sliding frictional force of a body is approximately independent of the body's speed or change in speed.

6. For any given body on a surface, the frictional force is greater when the body is stationary than when it is in motion. This means it takes a greater force to put a body at rest into motion than to maintain the motion of a body that is already moving.

   For a given pair of surfaces, the static coefficient is greater than the dynamic coefficient:

   $$\mu_s > \mu_d$$

7. The frictional force is approximately independent of the size of the contact area between the two interacting surfaces. This is not a contradiction of item 5 above. The weight of the body doesn't change, so if the area supporting the weight decreases, the pressure per unit area will increase, so:

   $$F_f = \mu_s F_N = \mu_s PA \sim \text{constant}$$

Friction on a Horizontal Plane

On a horizontal surface, the normal force is exactly equal and opposite to the weight of the body, so they cancel out. The only opposition to motion is the frictional force.

To initiate motion, the net component of the applied force that is parallel to the surface, $F_{\parallel}$, must exceed the opposing static frictional force:

$$F_{\parallel} > F_f = \mu_s F_N$$

Once motion has been started, the value of the frictional force drops because the coefficient changes from its static value to its corresponding, lower, dynamic value.

To maintain uniform motion, the net component of the applied force that is parallel to the surface, $F_{\parallel}$, must equal the opposing sliding frictional force:

$$F_{\parallel} = F_f = \mu_d F_N$$

Friction on an Inclined Plane

For a horizontal surface, the normal force of a given body is constant. In an incline, the normal force is not equal to the weight of the body, but only to the component of the weight force that is perpendicular to the surface of the incline. The second component is parallel to the surface of the incline and pointed downward. The frictional force opposes this component.

If the angle of inclination is changed, the value of F_N will likewise change. The minimum angle required to produce uniform speed can be determined from the fact that uniform speed means zero acceleration. Therefore, the net force in the direction of the motion must be zero. This occurs when the parallel force exactly equals the frictional force:

$$F_{\parallel}/F_N = \mu = \tan \theta$$

where θ gives the angle where the block should slide uniformly.

For a given incline, the value of the frictional force, F_f, determines the motion of the body on the incline:

1. If the net applied parallel force is less than the frictional force, the body remains at rest on the incline.

2. If the parallel force exactly equals the frictional force, the body slides down the incline with a constant speed.

3. If the parallel force exceeds the frictional force, the body will accelerate as it slides down the incline.

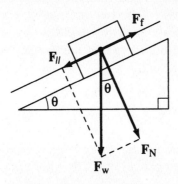

Forces acting on the surface of an inclined plane when friction is present. The two components are the legs of a right triangle with F_w as the hypotenuse. $F_{\parallel} = F_w \sin \theta$, *and* $F_N = F_w \cos \theta$.

PRACTICE PROBLEMS

1. A net resultant force acting on a body will have which effect?

   A. The velocity of the body will remain constant.
   B. The velocity of the body remains constant, but the direction in which the body moves will change.
   C. The velocity of the body will change.
   D. None of the above.

2. A box rests on a level table. Which of the following is an action-reaction pair of forces?

   A. The weight of the box and the upward force of the table on the box
   B. The weight of the table and the upward force of the Earth on any of the legs of the table
   C. Both A and B
   D. None of the above.

3. Body A has a mass that is twice as great as that of body B. If a force acting on body A is half the value of a force acting on body B, which statement is true?

   A. The acceleration of A will be twice that of B.
   B. The acceleration of A will be half that of B.
   C. The acceleration of A will be equal to that of B.
   D. The acceleration of A will be one fourth that of B.

4. What is the force required to impart an acceleration of 10 m/s^2 to a body with a mass of 2.0 kg?

   A. 0.2 N
   B. 5 N
   C. 12 N
   D. 20 N

5. The force of gravity between two bodies is

   A. inversely proportional to the distance between them.
   B. directly proportional to the distance between them.
   C. inversely proportional to the square of the distance between them.
   D. directly proportional to the square of the distance between them.

6. Newton's second law can be stated as which of the following?

   A. For every action there is an equal and opposite reaction.
   B. Force and the acceleration it produces are directly proportional.
   C. A body at rest tends to remain at rest unless acted upon by a force.
   D. None of the above.

7. If two forces act concurrently on a body, the resultant force will be greatest when the angle between them is

   A. 0°
   B. 45°
   C. 90°
   D. 180°

8. A force acting on a box can have one of the four orientations, A, B, C, or D, indicated below.

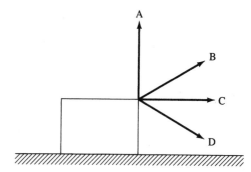

   In which orientation will the force have the smallest vertical component?

   A. A
   B. B
   C. C
   D. D

9. As the vector sum of the forces acting on a body increases, the acceleration of the body must

   A. increase.
   B. remain the same.
   C. decrease.
   D. either increase or decrease depending on the direction of the resultant.

10. After a rocket is launched, its engines are shut off. The rocket continues to move in a straight line at constant speed. This is an example of

    A. acceleration.
    B. inertia.
    C. gravitation.
    D. action-reaction.

11. For a body experiencing zero acceleration, which statement is *most* true?

    A. The body must be at rest.
    B. The body may be at rest.
    C. The body must slow down.
    D. The body may speed up.

12. What is the weight of a 2.0-kg body on or near the surface of the Earth?

    A. 4.9 N
    B. 16 lbs
    C. 19.6 N
    D. 64 kg m s^{-2}

13. A body accelerates at 2.5 m/s^2 when acted on by a net force of 5.0 N. The mass of the body is

    A. 0.5 kg
    B. 2.0 kg
    C. 12.5 kg
    D. 25 kg

14. Two bodies of equal mass are separated by a distance of 2 meters. If the mass of one body is doubled, the force of gravity between the two bodies will

    A. be half as great.
    B. be twice as great.
    C. be one fourth as great.
    D. be four times as great.

15. If the mass of a moving body is doubled, the inertia of the body will be

    A. half as great as its original value.
    B. twice as great as its original value.
    C. four times as great as its original value.
    D. unchanged from its original value.

16. On a large asteroid, the force of gravity on a 10 kg body is 20 N. What is the acceleration due to gravity on the asteroid?

    A. 0.5 m/s^2
    B. 2.0 m/s^2
    C. 9.8 m/s^2
    D. 98 m/s^2

17. The distance between a spaceship and the center of the Earth increases from one Earth radius to three Earth radii. What happens to the force of gravity acting on the spaceship?

    A. It becomes 1/9 as great.
    B. It becomes 9 times as great.
    C. It becomes 1/3 as great.
    D. It becomes 3 times as great.

18. A 100-kg astronaut lands on a planet with a radius three times that of Earth and a mass nine times that of Earth. The acceleration due to gravity, **g**, experienced by the astronaut will be

    A. nine times the value of **g** on Earth.
    B. three times the value of **g** on Earth.
    C. the same value of **g** as on Earth.
    D. one third the value of g on Earth.

19. For the system of a man in an elevator, his weight will appear to be greatest when

    A. the elevator rises at a constant velocity.
    B. the elevator is accelerated upward.
    C. the elevator falls at a constant velocity.
    D. None of the above, because weight is constant.

20. Which graph best represents the relation between the force of gravity and the mass of a free-falling body?

A.

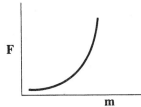

B.

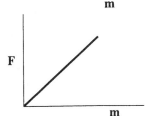

C.

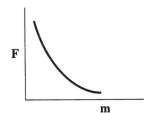

D.

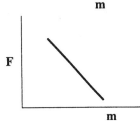

ANSWER KEY

1. C	3. D	5. C	7. A	9. A	11. B	13. B	15. B	17. A	19. B
2. A	4. D	6. B	8. C	10. B	12. C	14. B	16. B	18. C	20. B

ANSWERS AND EXPLANATIONS

1. **The correct answer is (C).** Force produces acceleration, which by definition is a change in velocity.

2. **The correct answer is (A).** The forces in an action-reaction pair must be equal and opposite and operate on two different bodies at a point of interaction. Choice C is eliminated because weight is always directed toward the center of the Earth so that both forces are in the same direction. Choice B is incorrect because the force on any one leg is only equal to 1/4 the total weight of the table.

3. **The correct answer is (D).** Get the ratio of the acceleration from Newton's Second Law, $\mathbf{F} = \mathbf{ma}$.

    $a_A/a_B = (\mathbf{F}_A m_B/\mathbf{F}_B m_A)$
    $\qquad\quad = (\mathbf{F}_B/2)(m_B/1)(1/2m_B)(1/\mathbf{F}_B)$
    $\qquad\quad = 1/4$

4. **The correct answer is (D).** Second law. $\mathbf{F} = ma = (2\text{ kg})(10\text{ m/s}^2) = 20\text{ N}$

5. **The correct answer is (C).** Law of universal gravitation.

6. **The correct answer is (B).** Second Law.

7. **The correct answer is (A).** Resultant of two forces is greatest when they are parallel and least when they are antiparallel.

8. **The correct answer is (C).** The force is along the horizontal. It has no vertical component.

9. **The correct answer is (A).** Second law. Force and acceleration are directly proportional.

10. **The correct answer is (B).** First law. Inertia is the tendency of a body to resist a change in its motion.

11. **The correct answer is (B).** Choices C and D are eliminated immediately because you cannot change speed or velocity without applying a force to supply the acceleration. Choice A is eliminated because the first law applies to both bodies at rest and those with uniform velocity.

12. **The correct answer is (C).** Second law.

    $$w = F = mg = (2.0 \text{ kg})(9.8 \text{ m/s}^2) = 19.6 \text{ N}$$

13. **The correct answer is (B).** Second law.

    $$m = F/a = (5.0 \text{ kg m s}^{-2})/(2.5 \text{ m s}^{-2}) = 2.0 \text{ kg}$$

14. **The correct answer is (B).** Law of universal gravitation. Force is directly proportional to the product of the masses. Doubling one of the masses doubles their product and therefore doubles the force.

15. **The correct answer is (B).** Inertia.

16. **The correct answer is (B).** Second law. $g = F/m = (20 \text{ kg m s}^{-2})/10 \text{ kg} = 2 \text{ m/s}^2$

17. **The correct answer is (A).** Choices B and D can be eliminated because the force of gravitational attraction doesn't increase with distance.

    $$\mathbf{F_G} = G\, m_1 m_2/r^2$$

    so $\mathbf{F_G}$ varies inversely with the square of the distance between the two bodies.

18. **The correct answer is (C).** $\mathbf{F}_{G \text{ earth}} = G\, m_{\text{earth}} m_{\text{body}}/r^2_{\text{ earth}}$

    On the planet we get:

    $$\mathbf{F}_{G \text{ planet}} = G\, (9\, m_{\text{earth}})(m_{\text{body}})/(3 r_{\text{earth}})^2 = \mathbf{F}_{G \text{ earth}}$$

    Since the force of gravity and the mass of the astronaut remain the same on both the planet and on Earth, the acceleration due to gravity must also be the same, $F/m = \mathbf{g}$ = constant.

19. **The correct answer is (B).** Weight is mass times the acceleration due to gravity. At uniform velocity there is no acceleration, so weight must remain constant. This eliminates A and C. It also eliminates D since it includes A.

20. **The correct answer is (B).** From Newton's Second Law, $F/m = \mathbf{g}$. This gives the graph of a straight line with a positive slope (equal to $\mathbf{g}$).

2.6 EQUILIBRIUM AND MOMENTUM

A. EQUILIBRIUM

Equilibrium describes the condition of a body experiencing no net acceleration. In order to obtain equilibrium, a body cannot experience any unbalanced or net forces.

Concurrent forces act at the same point; they supply a push or a pull to the body that can produce translational motion. Parallel forces are forces that do not act at the same point; they supply a twist or rotation to the body that can produce rotational motion.

1. In dynamic equilibrium, the magnitude and direction of the velocity are constant. The body has uniform linear motion.

2. In static equilibrium, the velocity is zero. A body at rest remains at rest.

3. A rigid body is one that cannot be replaced by a particle. Because an ideal particle is a point, only translational motion is possible. For a real, rigid body, rotational as well as translational motion is possible.

4. For equilibrium to occur, the body must have both translational and rotational equilibrium.

- *Translational Equilibrium*
  Translational equilibrium occurs when the resultant of all forces acting on a body is zero. If the resultant force is zero, its perpendicular components must also be zero.

  Newton's second law is:

  $$\text{net } F = \Sigma F = ma$$

  For equilibrium, $a = 0$ and we get the mathematical statement of Newton's first law: If no net force acts on a body, the motion of the body will continue unchanged.

  $$\Sigma F = 0 \text{ which means } \Sigma F_x = 0 \text{ and } \Sigma F_y = 0$$

  This is the condition for translational equilibrium and it is called the first condition of equilibrium.

Vector Analysis of Force

1. A force F can be resolved into two mutually perpendicular components, F_x and F_y. The force is the resultant of the vector sum of its components.

2. Any force can be replaced by its components acting at the same point on the body.

3. If several forces act simultaneously on a body, they can be replaced by a single equivalent force called the resultant, R, or by the components of the resultant:

   $$R = \Sigma F \quad R_x = \Sigma F_x \quad R_y = \Sigma F_y$$

- *Rotation Equilibrium*

  Parallel forces tend to cause the rotation of a body in a plane. The point around which the body rotates is called its axis of rotation. In order to determine the effects of parallel forces on the motion of a body in a given plane, a reference point called a pivot or fulcrum is selected.

  Torque, τ, is the moment of force, given by the product of the magnitude of the force producing the rotation and the torque arm:

  > torque = force × torque arm
  >
  > $\tau = Fr$

  The **torque arm** or lever, r, is the perpendicular distance between the line of action of the force and the axis of rotation.

  The torque depends on the magnitude of the force, the point of application of the force, and the direction of the force.

  The SI unit of torque is the newton-meter, $N\,m = kg\,m^2/s^2$.

  Rotational equilibrium occurs when the resultant torque on a body is zero.

  > net $\tau = \Sigma\tau = 0$

  which means that the sum of the clockwise torques is equal to the sum of the counterclockwise torques about some pivot point.

  Torques Acting on a Body

  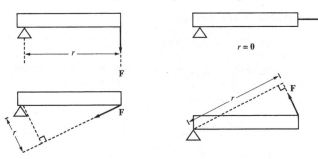

- **Center of Mass and Center of Gravity**

  A body is generally extended in space. That is, it occupies volume. However, for many calculations an extended body can be treated as if it were a particle, with no volume and all of its mass concentrated at a single point. The **center of mass** of a body is that point at which all of its mass can be considered to be concentrated. Similarly, the **center of gravity** of a body is that point at which all of its weight can be considered to be concentrated. In a uniform gravitational field, the centers of mass and gravity coincide.

Optional Aside

In almost all real situations, the center of gravity is slightly displaced from the center of mass, although the displacement is generally negligible. A solid cube of uniform composition rests on a table. If the mass of the cube is uniformly distributed, its center of mass is located at its geometric center. Its weight, however, is not uniformly distributed because the effect of gravity depends on the distance of the body from the center of the Earth. Since the bottom half of the cube is closer to the center of the Earth than the top, the bottom half weighs slightly more than the upper half. Therefore, its center of gravity lies slightly below its center of mass.

B. MOMENTUM

Momentum, p, is a vector quantity given by the mass of a body times its velocity. If the velocity is linear, the momentum of the body is linear. (Rotating bodies have rotational momenta.) Momentum is a product of a mass and a velocity:

$$\text{p} = m\text{v}$$

If two bodies have the same velocity, the body with the greater mass will have the greater momentum. If a small car and a big truck have the same speed, the truck will be harder to stop.

If two bodies have the same mass, the one with the greater speed will have the greater momentum. A bullet shot from a gun can do more damage to a target than a bullet thrown by hand.

- **Impulse** is the product of a force and the time interval over which it acts. This is equal to the change in the momentum that the force brings about on the body:

$$\text{F}\Delta t = \Delta\text{p} = m\Delta\text{v}$$

- **Conservation of linear momentum:** If no outside forces act on a system of bodies, the total momentum of the system remains constant. For example, if two bodies collide, their total momentum is conserved. Therefore, if one of the bodies slows down as a result of the interaction, the other must speed up:

$$m_A\text{v}_{A\text{ initial}} + m_B\text{v}_{B\text{ initial}} = m_A\text{v}_{A\text{ final}} + m_B\text{v}_{B\text{ final}}$$

$$m_A(v_{A\text{ initial}} - v_{A\text{ final}}) + m_B(\text{v}_{B\text{ initial}} - \text{v}_{B\text{ final}}) = 0$$

where A and B are two bodies that undergo a change in velocity and therefore in momentum.

Newton's Third Law of Motion is a special case of the law of conservation of momentum that covers contact forces. The law of conservation of momentum also covers noncontact forces such as gravitational and electromagnetic forces.

The conservation of momentum is used to study the motions of colliding bodies.

- In **elastic collisions,** two colliding bodies rebound without loss of kinetic energy. The sum of the kinetic energy of the bodies before the collision is equal to the sum of the kinetic energies after the collision. Perfectly elastic collisions only occur with atomic and subatomic particles.

- In **inelastic collisions,** two colliding bodies become joined or coupled together with a resultant loss of kinetic energy. Most real collisions are partly elastic and partly inelastic.

Kinetic energy is conserved only in perfectly elastic collisions. Momentum, however, is always conserved, whether the collision is elastic or inelastic.

PRACTICE PROBLEMS

1. A 5.00-meter steel beam of uniform cross section and composition weighs 100 N. What is the minimum force required to lift one end of the beam?

   A. 25 N
   B. 50 N
   C. 250 N
   D. 500 N

2. A nonuniform bar 8.0 meters long is placed on a pivot 2.0 meters from the lighter end of the bar. The center of gravity of the bar is located 2.0 meters from the heavier end. If a 500 N weight on the light end balances the bar, what must be the weight of the bar?

   A. 125 N
   B. 250 N
   C. 500 N
   D. 1000 N

3. A car with a mass of 800 kg is stalled on a road. A truck with a mass of 1200 kg comes around the curve at 20 m/s and hits the car. The two vehicles remain locked together after the collision. What is their combined velocity after the impact?

   A. 3 m/s
   B. 6 m/s
   C. 12 m/s
   D. 24 m/s

4. A 1000-kg car traveling at 5.0 m/s overtakes and collides with a 3000-kg truck traveling in the same direction at 1.0 m/s. During the collision, the two vehicles couple together and continue to move as one unit. What is the speed of the coupled vehicles?

   A. 2.0 m/s
   B. 4.0 m/s
   C. 5.0 m/s
   D. 6.0 m/s

5. A rifle with a mass of 0.20 kg fires a 0.50-gram bullet with an initial velocity of 100 m/s. What is the recoil velocity of the rifle?

   A. 0.25 m/s
   B. 0.50 m/s
   C. 1.0 m/s
   D. 10 m/s

6. A 0.2-kg ball is bounced against a wall. It hits the wall with a speed of 20 m/s and rebounds elastically. What is the magnitude of the total change in momentum of the ball?

   A. 0 kg m/s
   B. 4 kg m/s
   C. 8 kg m/s
   D. 10 kg m/s

7. A tennis ball is hit with a tennis racket and the change in the momentum of the ball is 4 kg m/s. If the collision time of the ball and racket is 0.01 second, what is the magnitude of the force exerted by the ball on the racket?

   A. 2.5×10^{-3} N
   B. 4×10^{-2} N
   C. 3.99 N
   D. 400 N

8. A 160-pound jogger runs at a constant speed. What is his momentum if he covers 100 yards in 10 seconds?

   A. 6 ft lb /s
   B. 16 slug ft /s
   C. 100 ft lb /s
   D. 150 slug ft /s

9. How fast must a 2000-kg body travel in order to have the same momentum as a 200-g body traveling at 200 m/s?

   A. 0.02 m/s
   B. 0.05 m/s
   C. 5.0 m/s
   D. 20 m/s

10. A spacecraft with a total mass of 10,000 kg lifts off from the Kennedy Space Center in Florida. Its rockets burn for 15 seconds and produce a thrust of 3.0×10^5 N. Assuming that the net mass of the spaceship does not change as the rocket fuel is consumed, what is the final velocity of the spaceship?

    A. 2.0×10^2 m/s
    B. 4.5×10^2 m/s
    C. 3.0×10^2 m/s
    D. 5.0×10^2 m/s

11. Gas is burned in a combustion engine. The resulting explosion produces a force that drives the pistons in the engine. The force of the explosion on the piston is due to the change in momentum of the gas molecules. A 0.4-g sample of gas produces a force of 2400 N in an explosion that lasts 10^{-3} seconds. What must be the speed of the gas molecules?

    A. 6×10^3 m/s
    B. 6 m/s
    C. 3×10^3 m/s
    D. 3 m/s

12. A 30-kg cart traveling due north at 5 m/s collides with a 50-kg cart that had been traveling due south. Both carts immediately come to rest after the collision. What must have been the speed of the southbound cart?

    A. 3 m/s
    B. 5 m/s
    C. 6 m/s
    D. 10 m/s

13. A rod of negligible mass is 10 m in length. If a 30-kg weight is suspended from one end of the rod and a 20-kg weight from the other, where must the pivot point be placed to ensure equilibrium?

    A. 4 m from the 30-kg weight
    B. 4 m from the 20-kg weight
    C. 6 m from the 30-kg weight
    D. 5 m from the 20-kg weight

ANSWER KEY

1. B   3. C   5. A   7. D   8. D   9. A   10. B   11. C   12. A   13. A
2. B   4. A   6. C

ANSWERS AND EXPLANATIONS

1. **The correct answer is (B).** This is a torque arm problem. Since the beam is uniform, its center of gravity is at the midpoint of the beam, 2.50 m from either end. The weight acts at the center of gravity. Because we are lifting one end of the rod, the pivot point must be at the opposite end. The system can be pictured as:

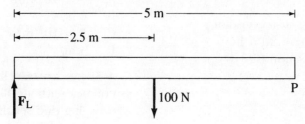

F_L is the lifting force required and it acts through a length of 5.00 m from the pivot point, P. It must counter the force of the weight acting through the length 2.50 m. At equilibrium:

$(5.00 \text{ m})F_L = (2.50 \text{ m})(100 \text{ N})$

The minimum force to lift the beam must be half the weight of the beam:

$F_L = (2.50 \text{ m}/5.00 \text{ M})(100 \text{ N}) = 50 \text{N}$

2. **The correct answer is (B).** The center of gravity occurs 4.0 m from the pivot point. At equilibrium:

$(2.0 \text{ m})(500 \text{ N}) = (4.0 \text{ m})(w)$

$w = 1/2 (500 \text{ N}) = 250 \text{ N}$

3. **The correct answer is (C).** Conservation of momentum ensures that the total momentum after the collision must equal the total momentum before the collision. If A is the 800-kg car and B is the 1200-kg truck, then:

(initial sum) $m_A v_A + m_B v_B = m_A v_A + m_B v_B$ (final sum)

Since the car is stalled, its initial velocity is zero and $m_A v_A$ initial is zero. After collision the vehicles are joined and $v_A = v_B = v_{final}$. The equation becomes:

$m_B v_B = (m_A + m_B)v_{final}$

The final velocity is $(1200 \text{ kg})(20 \text{ m/s})/(1200 \text{ kg} + 800 \text{ kg}) = 12 \text{ m/s}$.

4. **The correct answer is (A).** Conservation of momentum gives:

$P_{before\ collision} = P_{after\ collision}$

The total momentum prior to the collision is the sum of momenta for the two vehicles. After the collision, p is the momentum associated with their coupled masses:

$(1000 \text{ kg})(5.0 \text{ m/s}) + (3000 \text{ kg})(1.0 \text{ m/s}) = (4000 \text{ kg})v_{final}$

$v_{final} = (5000 + 3000)(\text{kg m /s})/4000 \text{ kg} = 2.0 \text{ m/s}$

5. **The correct answer is (A).** The momentum is conserved because there are no external forces acting on the rifle-bullet system during the firing. The initial momentum, however, is zero. The final momentum is the sum of the momentum of the bullet and the recoil momentum of the rifle:

    $$P_{before} = P_{after}$$
    $$0 = m_{rifle}v_{rifle} + m_{bullet}v_{bullet}$$
    $$v_{rifle} = -(0.5 \text{ g})(100 \text{ m/s})/0.2 \times 10^3 \text{ g} = 0.25 \text{ m/s}$$

    In order to be consistent, the mass of the rifle was converted into grams. The negative sign for v_{rifle} occurs because the recoil velocity of the rifle is in the opposite direction to the velocity of the bullet.

6. **The correct answer is (C).** The change in momentum is given by:

    $$\Delta p = mv_r - mv_0$$

    where v_0 is the initial velocity and v_r is the rebound velocity. Since the collision is elastic, the ball rebounds in the opposite direction but with the same speed with which it hit the wall. Therefore, $v_r = -v_0$, and the change in momentum is:

    $$\Delta p = m(-v_0) - mv_0 = -2mv_0$$
    $$= -2(0.2 \text{ kg})(20 \text{ m/s})$$
    $$= -8 \text{ kg m/s}$$

    The magnitude of a number is its absolute value:

    $$|-8 \text{ kg m/s}| = 8 \text{ kg m/s}$$

7. **The correct answer is (D).** Force is related to momentum by the impulse-momentum equation:

    $$Ft = \Delta p$$

    Therefore,

    $$F = \Delta p/t = (4 \text{ kg m/s})/0.01 \text{ s}$$
    $$= 400 \text{ kg m/s}^2 = 400 \text{ N}$$

8. **The correct answer is (D).** To be consistent with the British units, the distance must be converted from yards to feet and the weight in pounds into the corresponding mass in slugs.

    The units immediately eliminate A and C as possible answers.

    $$m = w/g = 160 \text{ lb}/ 32 \text{ ft/s}^2 = 5 \text{ slugs } 100 \text{ yds}(3 \text{ ft/yd}) = 300 \text{ ft}$$

    $$p = mv = (5 \text{ slugs})(300 \text{ ft}/ 10 \text{ s}) = 150 \text{ slug ft/s}$$

9. **The correct answer is (A).** $P_{body\ 1} = P_{body\ 2}$, therefore,

    $$v_1 = m_2v_2/m_1$$
    $$= (200 \times 10^{-3} \text{ kg})(200 \text{ m/s})/2000 \text{ kg}$$
    $$= 0.02 \text{ m/s}$$

    In order to be consistent, the masses of the two bodies must be in the same units, either both in grams or both in kilograms.

10. **The correct answer is (B).** From the impulse-momentum equation, $Ft = mv$ or $F\Delta t = m\Delta v$:

$F\Delta t/m = \Delta v = v_{final} - v_{initial} = v_{final}$

Since the spacecraft started from rest, $v_{initial} = 0$. Substitution gives:

$v_{final} = (3.0 \times 10^5 \text{ kg m/s}^2)(15 \text{ s})/10^4 \text{ kg} = 450 \text{ m/s}$

11. **The correct answer is (C).** The impulse-momentum equation rearranges to:

$\Delta v = F_{net}\Delta t/m$

There are two points to consider in solving the problem.

First is the application of dimensional analysis. Do the units agree?

$F\Delta t/m = \text{N s/g} = (\text{kg m/s}^2)\text{s/g}$

It is necessary to change grams into kilograms (or vice versa) in order to end up in the desired units of speed, meters/second. This eliminates choices B and D.

Second is the value of the change in velocity. Since the collisions are perfectly elastic, the gas molecules leave with the same speed they hit with. The only difference is that their direction has been reversed. Each molecule goes from a velocity of +v to one of −v so that $\Delta v = +v - (-v) = 2v$. Solving the equation gives C.

12. **The correct answer is (A).** Momentum is conserved. Since both carts come to rest, the total momentum after the collision must be zero, which means the total momentum prior to the collision was also zero. If the two carts are labeled A and B, then:

$m_A v_A = m_B v_B$

$v_B = (30 \text{ kg})(5 \text{ m/s})/50 \text{ kg} = 3 \text{ m/s}$

13. **The correct answer is (A).** Choices B and C can be eliminated because the position of the pivot is identical for both. D can also be eliminated because it puts the pivot at the center of the rod, which would only give equilibrium if the two weights were identical. The choice must be A.

This can be confirmed as follows. For equilibrium, $\Sigma\tau = 0$ which means

$\Sigma\tau_{clockwise} = \Sigma\tau_{counterclockwise} = 0$

The two weights cause rotation in opposite directions; therefore, if x is the distance of the pivot from the 30-kg weight, then $10 - x$ is the distance from the pivot to the 20-kg weight, and:

$(30 \text{ kg})(x \text{ m}) = (20 \text{ kg})(10 - x \text{ m})$

$50x = 200, x = 4 \text{ m}$

2.7 WORK AND ENERGY

A. WORK AND ENERGY

Work and energy are equivalent terms. **Energy** is the ability of a system or body to perform work. Work is the ability of a system or body to transfer energy usefully from one point to another.

- **Energy**
  The two broad categories of energy are **kinetic energy,** which depends on the motion of the body, and **potential energy,** which depends on its position.

    Energy comes in a variety of forms, such as mechanical, thermal, electrical, etc. Energy can be converted from one form into another and into work.

    In an ideal system, all of the energy transferred or converted can be used to do work.

    In a real system, only part of the total energy transferred may actually be available to do work, part being lost as thermal motion (heat) of the body.

- **The Law of Conservation of Energy**
  The law of **conservation of energy** states that energy cannot be created or destroyed. It can only be transferred from point to point or converted into some other form of energy. Energy is usually reported as a scalar quantity because we are generally interested only in the amount of energy involved.

- **Work**
  Work is the ability of a system to transfer energy usefully from one form to another or from one point to another. Work is the transference of energy, not the creation or destruction of energy.

    In an ideal system, all of the energy transferred can be used to do work.

    In a real system, only part of the energy transferred may actually be available to do work.

Work is described as the effect of a force acting to move a body through some distance. It is given by the dot product of a force and a displacement vector. The force can be a single force or the resultant of several forces:

$$W = \text{F} \cdot \text{d} = Fd \cos \theta$$

where F and d are the magnitudes of the two vectors and θ is the angle between them.

The physical significance of the dot product is that the amount of work a force can produce depends on the magnitude of its component in the direction of the displacement.

The maximum amount of positive work—that is, work done by the system—occurs when the force is parallel to the displacement. Then $\theta = 0°$ and $\cos 0° = +1$ so that $W = Fd = F\Delta d$ where Δd is the change in displacement.

The maximum amount of negative work—that is, work done on the system—occurs when the force is antiparallel to the displacement. Then $\theta = 180°$ and $\cos 180° = -1$ so that $W = -Fd$.

If F and d are perpendicular to each other, no work is done either by or on the system because $\theta = 90°$ and $\cos 90° = 0$, so that $W = 0$.

Optional Aside

This observation has an interesting, but, for many students, a counterintuitive, consequence: In lifting and carrying a suitcase, you supply a counterforce to gravity. This force is along the vertical axis.

When you lift a suitcase, you do work on it because the force (your counterbalance to gravity) is parallel to the displacement.

If you hold the suitcase, no work is done because there is no longer any displacement.

If you carry it on level ground, no work is done on or by the suitcase because F_g is perpendicular to the horizontal direction of the displacement.

Change of Volume Work

A common form of work is that done by an expanding or contracting gas against a constant external pressure.

$$W = P_{ext}\Delta V = P_{ext}(V_{final} - V_{initial}) = (F/d^2)d^3 = Fd$$

where d is length, d^2 is area, d^3 is volume, and the external pressure, P_{ext}, is the force per unit area.

- If the gas expands, the change in volume is positive so the work is positive, which means the gas does work on the surroundings.

- If the gas contracts, the change in volume is negative, so the work is negative, which means the surroundings do work on the gas.

Motion of a Spring

When a spring is stretched or compressed and then released, a restoring force tends to return it to its equilibrium (rest) position after it oscillates about this equilibrium position. Work can be done by an oscillating spring:

$$W = 1/2\ kx^2$$

where k is the spring constant that measures how difficult it is to compress or stretch a particular spring, and x gives the displacement from the equilibrium position.

- Units of energy and work are identical. However, for convenience or for historical reasons, units for the two quantities are sometimes reported in different but equivalent units.

  In the SI system, the derived unit of energy is the joule, J. The equivalent unit of work is the newton-meter, N m. These are related to the basic units by:

  $$1\,J = 1\,N\,m = 1\,kg\,m^2\,s^{-2}$$

- In the cgs system, the derived unit of energy is the erg. The equivalent unit of work is the dyne-centimeter, dyn cm. These are related to the basic unit by:

$$1 \text{ erg} = 1 \text{ dyn cm} = 1 \text{ g cm}^2 \text{ s}^{-2}$$

- In the British system, the unit of energy and work is the foot-pound, ft-lb.

- Two other commonly encountered energy/work units are the calorie, cal, frequently used to measure thermal energy, and the electron volt, eV, used to measure electronic energy.

- The energy units have the following conversion relationships:

$$1 \text{ J} = 10^7 \text{ erg} = 0.738 \text{ ft-lb}$$
$$1 \text{ cal} = 4.186 \text{ J}$$
$$1 \text{ eV} = 1.60 \times 10^{-19} \text{ J}$$

B. KINETIC ENERGY

Kinetic energy, E_k, is the energy associated with the motion of a body or the particles (atoms and molecules) composing the body. For translational motion, kinetic energy is:

$$E_k = 1/2 \ mv^2$$

where m is the mass and v is the speed (scalar) of the body or particle.

Macroscopic systems are those that are large enough that they obey classical or Newtonian physics. At the macroscopic level, E_k is the translational motion of the body as a whole.

Microscopic systems are those that are too small to follow classical laws and are described in terms of quantum mechanics. At the microscopic level, E_k is the change in the motion of the particles and is observed as a change in the thermal motion or temperature of the body.

Changes in kinetic energy can change the thermal motion of the particles without changing the translational motion of the body as a whole. Thus, changes in the E_k of a system are not always obvious at a macroscopic level.

Work-Energy Theorem

Work can be performed by changing a system's potential energy, kinetic energy, or both. The work-energy theorem applies only to systems where the energy changes are restricted to kinetic energy. The amount of work done by the system is equal to the change in its kinetic energy.

$$W = \Delta E_k = E_{k \text{ final state}} - E_{k \text{ initial state}}$$
$$= 1/2 \ mv^2_{\text{final state}} - 1/2 mv^2_{\text{initial state}} = 1/2 m \Delta(v^2)$$

If $E_{k \text{ final state}} > E_{k \text{ initial state}}$, the system has gained energy and ΔE_k is positive. Therefore, work is positive. This means work is done on the system and F and d have parallel components.

If $E_{k \text{ final state}} < E_{k \text{ initial state}}$, the system has lost energy and ΔE_k is negative. Therefore, work is negative. This means work is done by the system and F and d have antiparallel components.

Optional Aside

Interesting consequences of the work-energy theorem include:

Free Fall
A body drops under acceleration of gravity; that is, the force comes from mg, the weight of the body. The force acts in the same direction as the motion (downward). Therefore, work is positive and E_k increases as the body falls.

Vertical Projectile
For a body moving vertically upward the force acting on it is still mg, but it is opposite to the direction of the motion. Work is negative and E_k decreases.

Terminal Velocity
As a body falls in the atmosphere, it eventually reaches a terminal velocity where the force of mg pulling the body down equals the frictional drag of the air on the body. Since F_{grav} and F_{fric} are equal and opposite, there is no net force acting on the body once it reaches terminal velocity. No work is done and E_k remains constant.

Uniform Circular Motion
The speed is constant; therefore, E_k is constant and no work is done on the body by the force vector. F points toward the center of the circle and is therefore perpendicular to the velocity. Since force and direction of motion are 90° apart, $W = 0$.

C. POTENTIAL ENERGY

Potential energy, E_p, is the energy associated with the position of a body. It is the energy "stored" or contained in a system. The most common form of potential energy is gravitational:

$$E_p = mgh$$

where m is the mass of the body, g is the acceleration due to gravity, and h is the height of the body above the ground. **Gravitational potential energy** is the ability of the force of gravity to do work on a body.

Potential energy, like kinetic energy, is the ability of a body to do work. The work associated with a change in the gravitational potential energy of a body is called the gravitational work, W_{grav}:

$$W_{grav} = \Delta E_p = (E_{p\text{ final state}} - E_{p\text{ initial state}}) = mg\Delta h$$

A body can perform work by changing its position with respect to the surface of the planet. The acceleration due to gravity, g, is directed vertically down.

A decrease in the vertical height of the body means the displacement and the acceleration are parallel. The gravitational force does work as the potential energy of the body decreases. Work is done by the system.

An increase in the vertical height of the body means the displacement and the acceleration are antiparallel. The body is working against the gravitational force. The vertical force does work on the system, and the potential energy of the body increases.

D. THE LAW OF CONSERVATION OF MECHANICAL ENERGY

This law states that the total mechanical energy, which is the sum of the kinetic and potential energy of a system, remains constant. This means that all of the energy must remain in the system, changing only in how it is distributed between the kinetic and the potential forms.

$$E_{tot} = E_k + E_p$$

In order for conservation of energy to be valid, the system must be isolated from the rest of the universe. That is, the system cannot exchange either matter or energy with the outside world. Only ideal systems are truly isolated. Real systems show deviations from conservation.

Conservative Forces

Conservative forces are forces that conform to the conservation of energy law. These are forces that have a potential energy associated with them. The change in potential energy is equal and opposite to the work done by the conservative force:

$$\Delta E_p = -W_{con}$$

Gravitational and spring forces are examples of conservative forces.

For a force to be conservative, it must have one of the following three properties. Since these properties are equivalent, compliance with any one ensures that the force complies with all three.

1. A force is conservative if it does no work in a closed cycle. The work for the round trip is zero.

    If W is the work involved in going from A to B, then $-W$ must be the work involved in going from B back to A via the same path. Therefore, the total work for the round trip is zero.

2. A force is conservative if the amount of work depends only on the initial and final positions of the body and is independent of the path taken.

3. The change in kinetic energy, ΔE_k, for the round trip is zero.

Nonconservative Forces

Nonconservative forces are forces that produce deviations from the law of conservation of energy. If a force doesn't have a potential energy associated with it, then it is a nonconservative force or dissipative force. Friction is an example of a nonconservative force.

Nonconservative forces produce nonmechanical forms of energy, such as heat which is not included in the sum. The total of mechanical and nonmechanical energy is always conserved:

$$E_{tot} = E_{mech} + E_{nonmech}$$

E. POWER

Power is a scalar that gives the rate of doing work or transferring energy into or out of a system.

If the power is constant, it is equal to the ratio of the work to the time:

$$P = W/\Delta t$$

Therefore, the product of power and time gives the amount of energy used (work done).

If the power is variable, it is given as the instantaneous power, P_{inst}, which is the dot product of the force and the velocity:

$$P = F \cdot v = Fv \cos \theta$$

If the force and velocity are parallel, then $P = Fv$.

The SI unit of power is J/s. Another SI unit for power is the **kilowatt,** kW. Be careful not to confuse this with kilowatt hour, kW h, which is a unit of energy.

PRACTICE PROBLEMS

1. If the speed at which a car is traveling is tripled, by what factor does its kinetic energy increase?

    A. $3^{1/2}$
    B. 3
    C. 6
    D. 9

2. Work is measured in the same units as

    A. force.
    B. energy.
    C. momentum.
    D. power.

3. What is the magnitude of the force exerted by air on a plane if 500 kilowatts of power are needed to maintain a constant speed of 100 meters per second?

    A. 5 N
    B. 50 N
    C. 500 N
    D. 5000 N

4. What happens to the speed of a body if its kinetic energy is doubled?

    A. It is multiplied by $2^{1/2}$.
    B. It is doubled.
    C. It is halved.
    D. It is multiplied by 4.

5. What is the total amount of work done when a 100 N force pushes a box to the top of an incline that is 5.0 m long, and then a 50 N force pushes the box another 5.0 m along a horizontal surface?

    A. 5.0×10^2 J
    B. 7.5×10^2 J
    C. 1.0×10^3 J
    D. 1.5×10^3 J

6. A ball with a mass of 1.0 kg sits at the top of a 30° incline plane that is 20.0 meters long. If the potential energy of the ball is 98 J at the top of the incline, what is its potential energy once it rolls halfway down the incline?

    A. 0 J
    B. 49 J
    C. 98 J
    D. 196 J

7. The rate of change of work with time is

A. energy.
B. power.
C. momentum.
D. force.

8. In the diagram, a box slides down an incline. Toward which point is the force of friction directed?

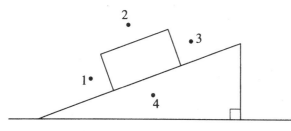

A. 1
B. 2
C. 3
D. 4

9. If the velocity of a body is doubled, its kinetic energy

A. decreases to half its original value.
B. increases to two times its original value.
C. decreases to one fourth its original value.
D. increases to four times its original value.

10. What is the velocity of a car if its engine is rated at 100 kW and provides a constant force of 5.0×10^3 N?

A. 0.05 m/s
B. 0.02 m/s
C. 20 m/s
D. 50 m/s

11. The total energy of a body free falling in a vacuum

A. increases.
B. decreases.
C. remains the same.
D. depends on the shape of the body.

12. How much work is done when a 0.50-kg mass is pushed by a 20-N force over a distance of 10.0 meters?

A. 5 J
B. 10 J
C. 49 J
D. 200 J

13. A body located 10.0 meters above the surface of the Earth has a gravitational potential energy of 490 J. What is the new gravitational potential energy if the body drops to a height of 7.00 meters above the Earth?

A. 70 J
B. 147 J
C. 280 J
D. 343 J

14. What is the power output by a weight lifter lifting a 10^3-N weight a vertical distance of 0.5 meters in 0.1 s?

A. 50 W
B. 500 W
C. 5000 W
D. 50,000 W

15. Cart A has a mass of 1 kg and a constant velocity of 3 m/s. Cart B has a mass of 1.5 kg and a constant velocity of 2 m/s. Which of the following statements is true?

A. Cart A has the greater kinetic energy.
B. Cart B has the greater kinetic energy.
C. Cart A has the greater acceleration.
D. Cart B has the greater acceleration.

16. What is the kinetic energy of a 10.0-kg mass with a velocity of 2.00 m/s?

A. 20 J
B. 10 J
C. 5 J
D. 2.5 J

17. The derived unit for energy and work is called the joule, J. It is equivalent to which combination of SI units?

A. $kg\ m^2$
B. N/m^2
C. $kg\ m^2/s^2$
D. W/N

18. Two carts A and B have equal masses. Cart A travels up a frictionless incline with a uniform velocity that is twice that of Cart B. Which statement is most accurate?

A. The power developed by A is the same as that of B.
B. The power developed by A is half that of B.
C. The power developed by A is twice that of B.
D. The power developed by A is 4 times that of B.

19. The work done in raising a body must

A. increase the kinetic energy of the body.
B. decrease the total mechanical energy of the body.
C. decrease the internal energy of the body.
D. increase the gravitational potential energy.

20. A frictionless incline has a ramp length of 5.0 meters and rises to a height of 4.0 meters. How much work must be done to move a 50-N box from the bottom to the top of the incline?

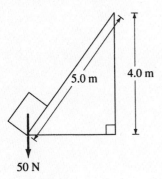

5.0 m   4.0 m

50 N

A. 100 J
B. 150 J
C. 200 J
D. 250 J

21. Work is done when a force

I. acts vertically on a box moving along a horizontal surface.
II. exerted on one end of a box is equal and opposite to a force exerted on the other end of the box.
III. pushes a box up a frictionless incline.
IV. of gravitational attraction acts between a box and the surface of the Earth.

A. I and III only
B. II and IV only
C. I only
D. III only

22. A 100-kilogram box is pulled 10 meters across a frictionless horizontal surface by a 50-N force. What is the change in the potential energy of the box?

A. 0 J
B. 2 J
C. 20 J
D. 50 J

23. What is the average power output of a 50-kg boy who climbs a 2.0-m step ladder in 10 seconds?

A. 10 W
B. 49 W
C. 98 W
D. 250 W

24. How much work must be done to raise a 5.0-kg block of steel from the ground to a height of 2.0 m?

A. 2.5 N
B. 10 N
C. 49 N
D. 98 N

ANSWER KEY

1. D	3. D	5. B	7. B	9. D	11. C	13. D	15. A	17. C	19. D	21. D	23. C
2. B	4. A	6. B	8. C	10. C	12. D	14. C	16. A	18. C	20. C	22. A	24. D

ANSWERS AND EXPLANATIONS

1. **The correct answer is (D).** The kinetic energy is directly proportional to the square of the velocity. If the velocity is tripled, then its square becomes $(3v)^2 = 9v^2$; and E_k must increase by the same ninefold amount.

2. **The correct answer is (B).** By definition, energy is the ability to do work and shares the same units (joules).

3. **The correct answer is (D).** The average power is the product of the force acting on the plane and the speed, $P = Fv$. Solving for the required force gives:

   $F = P/v = 500 \times 10^3$ W$/(100$ m/s$) = 5 \times 10^3$ N

   Watch the units: W $=$ J/s, J $=$ Nm, N $=$ kg m^2/s^2

4. **The correct answer is (A).** E_k and v^2 are directly proportional. If E_k is doubled, then v^2 is doubled and the square root of v^2 gives $2^{1/2}$. The velocity, v, must increase to $2^{1/2}$ its original value.

5. **The correct answer is (B).** The total work done on the body is the sum of the products of the applied force and the distance moved:

   Work $= (100$ N$)(5$ m$) + (50$ N$)(5$ m$) = 750$ N m $= 750$ J

6. **The correct answer is (B).** Since the height is decreasing, the E_p is decreasing and must have a value less than its initial reading of 98 J. Choice D is eliminated because its value is higher than the initial E_p value. Choice C is eliminated because its value is the same as the initial value of the E_p. Choice A is eliminated because the only way to have zero E_p is if the body is at ground level. That leaves B as the only option.

   Confirm by:

   $E_p = mgh = (1.0$ kg$)(9.8$ m/s$^2)(5.0$ m$) = 49$ J

   The 5.0 m height comes from treating the incline as a right triangle. Since sin 30° $=$ 0.500, the length of the side opposite the 30° angle is half the length of the hypotenuse. When the ball has rolled halfway down the ramp, the hypotenuse is 10.0 m long.

7. **The correct answer is (B).** Power is the rate of doing work and is given by the ratio of the work done over the time required to do the work.

8. **The correct answer is (C).** Friction acts in the direction opposite to the motion. The force moving the box is directed toward point 1, so the resulting frictional force must be toward point 3. Point 2 is the direction of the normal; point 4 is the direction of the weight.

9. **The correct answer is (D).** Doubling v means quadrupling v^2; therefore, E_k must increase to 4 times its original value.

10. **The correct answer is (C).** Power is force times speed, $P = Fv$, so

    $v = P/F = 100 \times 10^3$ W$/5 \times 10^3$ N $= 20$ m/s

11. **The correct answer is (C).** Apply the law of conservation of energy. As the body falls, its E_p decreases. However, the body's E_k increases because the velocity at which it is falling increases. Therefore, the sum of the energies remains the same.

12. **The correct answer is (D).** Since you are not given information to the contrary, assume that the force acts in the same direction as the motion. Then:

$W = Fd = (20\ N)(10.0\ m/s) = 200\ J$

13. **The correct answer is (D).** The gravitational potential energy and the height of the body above the ground are directly proportional. Since the weight of the body (wgt $= mg$) remains constant, reducing the height to 7/10 of its value must reduce $E_{p\ grav}$ by the same proportion. We can eliminate choices A and B because both are less than half the original E_p requiring that the body drop to less than half its original height. By inspection, choice C is only a little more than 1/2 and choice D is almost 3/4 the original value of E_p, making D the likely answer.

Confirm this by:

$E_{p\ new} = E_{p\ old}\ (h_{new}/h_{old}) = (490\ J)(7/10) = 343\ J$

14. **The correct answer is (C).** Power = rate of doing work, $P = W/t = Fd/t$:

$P = (10^3\ N)(0.5\ m)/0.1\ s = 5 \times 10^3\ W$

15. **The correct answer is (A).** Since the velocity is constant, the acceleration must be zero and we can eliminate choices C and D. Solving $E_k = 1/2\ mv^2$ for the two carts gives:

$E_{kA} = (1\ kg)(9) = 9\ J$
$E_{kB} = (1.5)(4) = 6\ J$

16. **The correct answer is (A).** $E_k = 1/2\ mv^2 = (1/2)(10.0\ kg)(2.00\ m/s)^2 = 20\ J$

17. **The correct answer is (C).** Work is the product of force ($N = kg\ m/s^2$) and distance (m).

$W = Fd = kg\ m^2/s^2$

18. **The correct answer is (C).** Since each cart has a constant velocity, the acceleration on each must be zero. Thus, the only force acting on a cart must be the force that counters the cart's weight. Both carts have the same mass, so both are subject to the same force. Power is the product of force and velocity, so:

$P_A/v_A = P_B/v_B = F = $ constant

Power and velocity are directly proportional. Cart A travels at twice the velocity and must develop twice the power.

19. **The correct answer is (D).** By definition, $E_{p\ grav}$ changes with the height of a body above the ground.

20. **The correct answer is (C).** Because the incline is frictionless, the work done is that associated with the change in vertical distance, 4 m. The work is that done against gravity and equals the weight of the box, $F = $ wgt $= mg$.

$W = Fd = (50\ N)(4\ m) = 200\ J$

21. **The correct answer is (D).** $W = Fd$, so we can eliminate II and IV because no motion (change in distance) occurs. The force described in I is perpendicular to the direction of the motion so I is also eliminated. Only III fits the definition of work.

22. **The correct answer is (A).** $\Delta E_p = mg\Delta h$. The height of the box doesn't change, so its potential energy doesn't change.

23. **The correct answer is (C).** $P = W/t$. Work is force times distance and force is mass times acceleration. The acceleration here is that of gravity. So:

$$P = (m \times a \times d)/t$$
$$= (50 \text{ kg})(9.8 \text{ m/s}^2)(2.0 \text{ m})/10 \text{ s}$$
$$= 98 \text{ W}$$

24. **The correct answer is (D).** The work done is against the force of gravity. The force of gravity is the weight of the block:

$$W = Fd = mgh = (5.0 \text{ kg})(9.8 \text{ m/s}^2)(2.0 \text{ m}) = 98 \text{ N}$$

2.8 SOLIDS AND FLUIDS

A. PHASES OF MATTER

Matter exists in three phases or states: solid, liquid, and gas, distinguished by the strength of the intermolecular forces holding the component molecules together.

Note: All remarks about molecular interactions also apply to substances where the component particles are atoms instead of molecules; their interactions are due to analogous interatomic forces.

Solids

In solids, the particles are held in a fixed pattern by strong intermolecular forces, and each molecule oscillates around its fixed or equilibrium position. It is the fixed position of the constituent molecules that gives solids their rigidity. A sample of a solid has a definite volume and a definite shape that it maintains regardless of the shape of the vessel in which it is placed. There are well-defined boundaries or interfaces between the surface of the solid and the surrounding environment.

Crystalline solids are solids in which the fixed arrangement of the molecules forms a regular and repeating pattern. This three-dimensional pattern is called the crystal lattice of the solid. Salts and minerals are examples of crystalline solids. A crystalline solid is characterized by a sharp, well-defined melting point, which is the temperature at which the substance makes the transition between its solid and liquid phases.

In **amorphous solids,** the positions of the molecules are fixed, but the pattern of their arrangement is random. Glass is an example of an amorphous solid. An amorphous solid will not have a well-defined melting point.

Fluids and Gases

Fluids are liquids and gases are nonrigid substances in which the molecules are essentially free to move about or flow.

In liquids the intermolecular forces are weaker than in solids and the molecules are farther apart. A liquid has a definite volume but not a definite shape. It assumes the shape of the vessel containing it. There is usually a single interface between the upper surface of the liquid and the environment (usually air) above it.

In a gas the molecules ideally do not interact with each other. A gas has neither a definite volume nor a definite shape, but will expand to completely fill any closed vessel containing it. There is no interface between the gas sample and the surrounding environment, just the walls of the vessel.

Molecular Motion

Molecular motion is described by the kinetic theory of matter, which states that molecules of all substances are in constant motion. The square of the velocity of the particles is directly proportional to the kinetic energy, E_k, of the substance, which in turn is directly proportional to its temperature.

In changes of phase, the substance is transformed from one physical state into another. Phase changes are equilibrium phenomena, and therefore occur at a constant temperature that depends on the identity of the substance, the transition occurring, and the pressure.

Melting is the transition between the solid and liquid phases of a substance. Its reverse, from liquid to solid, is called freezing or solidification.

Boiling or vaporization is the transition from liquid to gas. The reverse transition is called condensation.

Sublimation is the change from solid to gas.

Each of these processes is reversible. If the molecular motion is great enough to overcome the attractive intermolecular forces holding the particles together, the transition will be to a less structured phase (such as solid to liquid). If the intermolecular forces overcome the molecular motion, the transition will be to a more structured phase (such as liquid to solid).

Cohesion is the attractive force between molecules of the same substance. This is the force that holds like molecules together and opposes the dissolving of one substance in some other substance.

Adhesion is the attractive force between molecules of different substances. This is the force that allows one substance to become dissolved in another.

Diffusion is the penetration of molecules of one substance into a sample consisting of a second substance. It can occur among all three phases but is most common in fluids.

Pressure

Pressure is a physical quantity that gives the ratio of the magnitude of a force, F, perpendicular to a given surface area, A:

$$P = F/A$$

Pressure is an example of a physical quantity called stress.

Units of Pressure

The SI system has three equivalent units of pressure, the Pascal, Pa; the Newton per square meter, N/m^2; and the kilogram per meter per square second, $kg/m\ s^2$:

$$1\ Pa = 1\ N/m^2 = 1\ kg/ms^2$$

Some conversions between different units of pressure are:

$$1 \text{ atm} = 760 \text{ mm Hg} = 760 \text{ torr} = 1.01 \times 10^5 \text{ Pa} = 14.7 \text{ lb/in}^2$$

Density

Density, ρ, is the ratio of the mass to volume of a substance:

$\rho = m/V$

An SI unit of density is kg/m^3. Other units include kg/L where one liter is the volume of a perfect cube with sides of length 0.1 meters:

$1 \text{ L} = 10^{-3} \text{ m}^3$

For most substances, the density of the liquid is less than that of the solid so that most solids sink in liquids of the same substance. A notable exception to this observation is water, where the solid form is less dense than the liquid. This is why ice floats.

The density of water, ρ_{H_2O}, is 1 g/cm^3 in the cgs system and 1000 kg/m^3 in the SI system.

For solids and liquids, the volume of a given sample at a given temperature is constant, making the density an intensive property, which means it is independent of the size of the sample. The value of the density depends on the identity of the solid or liquid substance and the temperature at which the measurements are made.

Optional Aside

The density of a solid or liquid is an intensive property of the substance that is given by the ratio of the two extensive properties: mass and volume. Intensive properties do depend on the physical size of the sample. However, the greater the mass of the sample, the greater the volume that mass tends to occupy, so that the ratio remains constant.

Increasing the temperature of a substance increases the thermal motion of the molecules so that they tend to move farther away from each other. Therefore, the volume occupied by a solid or liquid in most cases will increase slightly with increasing temperature. Since density and volume are inversely proportional, increasing the volume occupied by a given mass will decrease its density.

Specific gravity, s.g., is also called relative density. It is the ratio of the density of a given substance to the density of water at the same temperature. Since density is the ratio of mass to volume, the specific gravity also gives the ratio of the mass of a given volume of a substance to the mass of an equal volume of water. The specific gravity is a dimensionless physical property:

s.g. $= \rho_{body}/\rho_{H_2}O$

Gases

Since gases expand to fill the available volume, the density of a given sample will change as you change the volume of the vessel.

For gases, density changes significantly with changes in T and P and is more correctly described as the concentration of the gas. The mass of the gas is thus uniformly distributed throughout the vessel.

B. SOLIDS

Deformation

Deformation is the change in dimension or shape of a body due to the application of an external force.

Elasticity is the ability of a deformed body to return to its original dimensions once the external force causing the deformation is removed.

The **elastic limit** is the minimum stress that produces an irreversible deformation of the solid. Each sample of a substance has a maximum amount of deformation that it can undergo. If it is deformed beyond this point, called the elastic limit, the sample remains deformed even after the external deforming force is removed.

Tensile strength is the force required to actually break a rod with unit cross-sectional area of the substance.

Stress

Stress is the force acting on a solid divided by the area over which the force acts. It therefore has units of N/m^2 in the SI system. It is a physical quantity that is analogous to and has the same units as pressure. The difference is that stress gives the ratio of the internal force produced when the body is deformed to the area of the body that the force affects. There are three main types of stress. Two of them, **tension** and **compression,** are called **normal stresses** because the force is perpendicular to the area it affects.

normal stress $= F_\perp/A$

In contrast, a **shear stress** is a **tangential stress** because the force is coplanar with (parallel to) the area it affects.

Optional Aside

Deforming a substance usually changes the distance between its component molecules, which in turn changes the magnitude and/or direction of the intermolecular forces of the substance. When the external deforming force is removed, the intermolecular forces act as a restoring force, returning the molecules to their original equilibrium positions. This restoring force is the internal force used in the stress equation.

Tension or tensile stress is the effect of two external antiparallel forces with the same line of action pulling on opposite ends of a body. The two forces oppose each other and tension tends to elongate the body, increasing its length from ℓ to $\ell + \Delta\ell$ where $\Delta\ell$ is the change in length produced by the tension. Each force is normal to the area it acts on. The line of action of the forces corresponds to the axis of elongation.

Compression is the reverse of tension. It is due to the effect of two antiparallel collinear external forces pushing on opposite sides of the same body. The two forces again oppose each other but the net effect is to compress the body, decreasing its length by $\Delta\ell$ from ℓ to $\ell - \Delta\ell$. Each force is again perpendicular to the area on which it acts.

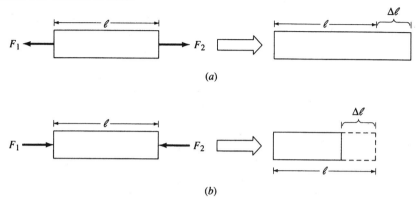

(a) Elongation and (b) compression of a rod under stress.

Note: For some substances, the tensile and compression stresses are equal in magnitude for a given force. In other substances, they may be quite different. For instance, concrete can generally withstand a larger compression force than tensile force before it breaks.

In shear stress, the two antiparallel forces do not have the same line of action. The net effect is that the forces act along opposite areas instead of perpendicular to them. One surface area is displaced a horizontal distance Δx with respect to the opposite surface. Shear stress is also called tangential stress.

shear stress $= F_{\parallel}/A$

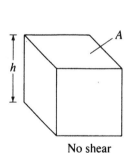

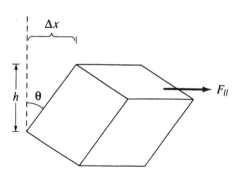

No shear

The shear force, $F_{\parallel}$, is parallel to the surface area, A, causing the surface to slip through an angle θ *or* $\dfrac{\Delta x}{h}$ for small angles.

Force F produces both normal force, $F_{\perp}$, and shear force, $F_{\parallel}$.

Strain

Strain is the deformation of a body that results from the application of stress. In other words, stress deforms a body and the actual deformation is called strain. Strain is the ratio of the change produced by the stress to the original length or volume. Therefore, strain is always dimensionless.

Elongation strain is associated with both tension and compression stresses. Both are the fractional change in length produced by the stress and given by the ratio of the change in length to the original length. Elongation strain is dimensionless:

elong. strain $= \Delta\ell/\ell$

Volume strain is the fractional change in volume produced by a stress. It is given by the ratio of the change in volume to the original volume:

volume strain $= \Delta V/V$

Note: The volume strain is also called the hydraulic strain. Tensile, compression, and shear stresses apply only to solids. The required restoring force is supplied by the fixed molecular structure of the solid. Fluids, however, cannot undergo these stresses, especially shear stress, because there is no fixed internal structure to supply the restoring force.

The only stress a fluid can undergo is called hydraulic stress. This kind of stress occurs when an external pressure is applied perpendicularly to the surface of the fluid.

Solids can also experience hydraulic stress as well as tensile, compression, and shear stresses.

Shear strain is the ratio of the parallel displacement, Δx, to the length of the distorted side, h.

shear strain $= \Delta x/h$

Elastic Moduli

Stress and strain are directly proportional. The proportionality constant is called a modulus of elasticity:

stress $=$ modulus $\times$ strain

There are three main elastic moduli. All of them have the units of pressure, N/m^2.
Moduli are always reported as positive numbers.

Young's modulus, Y, is the ratio of the tensile or compression stress to the corresponding strain:

$Y = (F/A)/(\Delta\ell/\ell) = (F\ell)/(A\Delta\ell)$

This can be rearranged to solve for the force, F:

$F = (YA)(\Delta\ell/\ell) = k\Delta\ell$

This equation has the form of Hooke's Law where k, called the force constant or the spring constant, is a constant for a given body. k is inversely proportional to the length, ℓ, of the body and directly proportional to the product, YA:

$k = YA/\ell$

Y depends on the temperature as well as the identity of the substance. Most values of Y are on the order of 10^{10} N/m^2.

Shear modulus, S, is also called the rigidity modulus. It is the ratio of the shear stress, $F_\parallel/A$, to the shear strain, $\Delta x/h$:

$$S = (F_\parallel/A)/(\Delta x/h) = Fh/A\Delta x$$

which is exactly analogous to the Young's modulus equation.

The greater the value of S, the more the substance resists shear stress.

Bulk modulus, B, gives the ratio of stress to hydraulic strain. The stress is the pressure applied to the solid or fluid; the strain is the fractional change in volume:

$$B = -P/(\Delta V/V) = -PV/\Delta V$$

The units of B are units of pressure, N/m^2. Since increasing the pressure always decreases the volume of the fluid or solid, the equation carries a negative sign to ensure that B is always a positive number.

B reflects how difficult it is to compress a substance. The more easily a substance is compressed, the smaller its value of B. For example:

$$B_{steel} = 16 \times 10^{10}\ N/m^2$$
$$B_{air} = 1.01 \times 10^5\ N/m^2$$

The values of B are usually measured at an external pressure of one atmosphere.

B for most gases is constant at $1.01 \times 10^5\ N/m^2$. Solids with large Young's moduli also tend to have large bulk moduli. The bulk moduli for liquids are not much lower than those of solids. Both generally have magnitudes of $\sim 10^{10}\ N/m^2$. This suggests that liquids are not very compressible.

The **compressibility constant,** K, is the reciprocal of the bulk modulus and gives the fractional decrease in volume produced by a small increase in pressure:

$$K = 1/B$$

The units of K are square meters per newton, m^2/N.

Summary of Stress and Strain

Type of Stress	Stress	Strain	Elastic Modulus
Tension or Compression	$F_\perp/A$	$\Delta \ell/\ell_0$	$Y = (F_\perp/A)/(\Delta \ell/\ell_0)$
Hydrostatic Pressure	$P = F_\perp/A$	$\Delta V/V_0$	$B = -P/(\Delta V/V_0)$
Shear	$F_\parallel/A$	$\tan \theta$	$S = (F_\parallel/A)/\theta$

Shear strain $= \Delta x/h = \tan \theta \sim \theta$ if $\Delta x \ll h$. Although the angle is measured in radians, shear strain has no units because it is the ratio of two distances, x and h. Modulus = stress/strain.

C. HYDROSTATICS

Hydrostatics is the study of fluids at rest.

Any force acting on (or produced by) a static fluid must be perpendicular to the surface of the fluid component it acts on because any force parallel to the fluid surface will cause the fluid to flow. This changes the fluid from a hydrostatic to a hydrodynamic system.

Note: The surface of a fluid component need not occur at an interface between the fluid and some other substance. It includes the internal surfaces of any arbitrary volume element within the sample of fluid.

Static fluids cannot have parallel force components.

Since the frictional forces are always parallel to a surface involved, a static fluid has no static coefficient of friction.

Optional Aside

Fluid lubricants are placed between two surfaces. Since the lubricant is at rest, there is no frictional force between it and either surface, which in turn reduces the friction between the two surfaces.

Pascal's Principle

Pascal's Principle states that any pressure or change in pressure applied to an enclosed fluid at rest is transmitted uniformly and without any loss to all parts of the fluid and to the walls of the vessel containing the fluid. The pressure, as usual, acts perpendicularly to the surface of the fluid.

The pressure in a static fluid can be described either under the condition of negligible gravity or the condition where the effect of gravity cannot be neglected. Pascal's Principle generally refers to the former condition and can be restated as follows: If the effect of gravity is negligible, then the weight of the fluid is negligible, and the pressure of the static fluid will be the same at all points in the fluid. This means that the pressure at the bottom of a tank of any fluid is the same as the atmospheric pressure applied at the top of the fluid.

The law of hydrostatic pressure is the application of Pascal's Principle to systems where the effect of gravity cannot be neglected. It states that the **hydrostatic pressure** of a fluid, P_h, at any given point is the sum of any external pressure, P_0, plus the weight of the fluid above that point:

$$P_h = F_{total}/A = (F_0 + F_g)/A = P_0 + F_g/A$$

where F_0 is the external force producing the external pressure, and F_g is the force due to gravity.

Since density, ρ, is mass over volume, m/v, and volume is area times height, Ah, then:

$$F_g = mg = \text{wgt} = \rho Ahg$$

where g is the acceleration due to gravity and wgt is the resulting weight. The contribution of the fluid to the hydrostatic pressure is the product of the density of the fluid, the height (or depth) at which the pressure is being evaluated, and g:

$$P = F_g/A = \rho hg$$

Since the external or atmospheric pressure is constant for a given sample, the change in pressure for any two points, A and B, in the sample depends only on their depths:

$$\Delta P = P_A - P_B = \rho g(h_A - h_B) = \rho g \Delta h$$

This means:

1. The pressure at the bottom of a tank of fluid must be greater than the pressure at the top.

2. Pressure depends only on the depth and is independent of the horizontal dimensions (area) of the surface. The pressure at any point in a static fluid is given by:

$$P = P_{\text{external}} + \rho g h$$

Therefore, if two surfaces are at the same depth in a fluid, they will both experience the same pressure regardless of their areas. (The pressure on a square-inch sample of a given fluid is the same as the pressure on a square-mile sample of the fluid, provided both samples are at the same depth.)

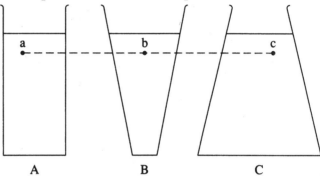

Three vessels with different shapes are filled with fluid to the same height. Points at the same height in the vessel will have the same pressure, $P_a = P_b = P_c$. Therefore, the pressure is the same at the bottom of the vessels despite their different shapes. However, the force exerted at levels of equal height in the different vessels will not be the same since the surface areas for the planes containing the points are different; $F_a \neq F_b \neq F_c$. The force exerted on the bottom of each vessel is different. Since force and area are directly proportional, the force is greatest for C and least for B.

Optional Aside

The atmosphere is a fluid that exerts a force on the surface of the Earth. It produces atmospheric pressure that decreases with increasing altitude, just as the pressure in a tank of water decreases from the bottom to the top.

There are several instruments that are used to measure the pressure in a static fluid. The two most common are the barometer and the manometer.

The **barometer** is an evacuated closed-end cylinder that is completely filled with a fluid such as mercury and inverted with its open end under the surface of a reservoir of the same fluid. If the pressure due to the weight of the fluid, $\rho g h$, is less than the external pressure, P_0, of the atmosphere acting on the surface of the fluid in the reservoir, fluid will flow out of the cylinder and into the reservoir until $\rho g h = P_0$. The temperature at which the observations occur must be noted because density is temperature dependent.

A **manometer** can be used as a gauge to measure the pressure of a system. It consists of a U-shaped tube that is partially filled with a liquid of known density, often mercury or water. One end is attached to the system to be monitored, and the other is either left open to the atmosphere or closed and evacuated. In an open-end manometer, the level of the fluid in each arm of the U tube adjusts itself so that the sum of the pressure of the system, P_{sys}, and the fluid in one arm, $\rho g h_1$, equals the sum of the pressure of the atmosphere, P_0, and the fluid in the other arm, $\rho g h_2$. Thus, the pressure of the system is:

$$P_{sys} = \rho g(h_2 - h_1) + P_0$$

In a closed-end manometer, $P_0 = 0$ because that side of the arm was evacuated. Therefore:

$$P_{sys} = \rho g(h_2 - h_1)$$

and depends only on the difference between the fluid levels in the two arms.

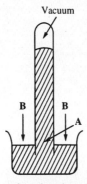

Vacuum

Illustration of a closed-end manometer.

The fluid in a barometer rises under a vacuum until the pressure in the cylinder, A, equals the atmospheric pressure on the reservoir, B.

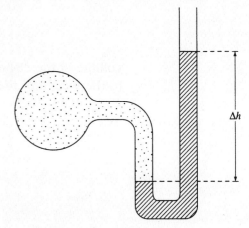

Illustration of an open-end manometer.

A hydraulic lever or lift is an example of the direct application of Pascal's Principle. A **hydraulic lift** consists of two pistons, one with a small surface area called the input piston, and the other with a larger area called the output piston, connected by an enclosed fluid.

For a given pressure or change in pressure, the larger the area subjected to that pressure, the greater the force produced:

$$P = F_{small}/A_{small} = F_{large}/A_{large}$$

A small force is applied to the piston with the smaller area. The resulting pressure is transmitted uniformly and undiminished throughout the fluid to the larger area piston where it exerts a proportionately larger force. The work done on the small piston must equal the work done by the large piston:

$$W = F_{input}d_{input} = F_{output}d_{output}$$

Since $F_{input} < F_{output}$, then $d_{input} > d_{output}$. The smaller piston moved a greater distance than the larger piston.

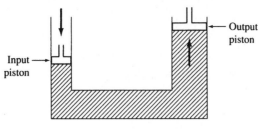

Hydraulic lift.

Archimedes' Principle

Archimedes' Principle states that a floating body is in static equilibrium and the upward or buoyant force, F_B, exerted by the fluid on a floating or on a submerged body equals the weight of the fluid displaced by the body. The body will sink until the weight of the fluid it displaces is equal to its own weight:

$$F_B = \rho v g = (m/v)(vg) = mg = \text{weight}$$

The volume of the object that is below the surface of the fluid is equal to the volume of the displaced fluid, and the density is that of the fluid. Thus, F_B is equal to the weight of the displaced fluid. Be careful: In order to float, the body must displace its own weight, not its own volume in fluid.

As a result of Archimedes' Principle:

1. If the density of the body is greater than the density of the fluid, $\rho_{body} > \rho_{fluid}$, then $\text{weight}_{body} > F_B$ and the body will sink in the fluid (be completely submerged).

2. If the density of the body is less than the density of the fluid, $\rho_{body} < \rho_{fluid}$, then $\text{weight}_{body} < F_B$ and the body will float on the surface of the fluid (be only partly submerged).

3. A body floating in a fluid appears to weigh less than it does in air because the buoyant force and the weight are antiparallel vectors. The weight apparently lost is equal to the weight of the fluid displaced by the body.

4. Since two masses cannot occupy the same space at the same time, the volume of a submerged body must equal the volume of the fluid it displaces.

The **center of buoyancy** is the point in a submerged or floating body where the total upward buoyant force can be considered to act. Since pressure increases with depth, the pressure at the top of a body is less than the pressure at the bottom of the body. Therefore, the center of buoyancy is not necessarily coincident with the center of mass (or gravity) for the body.

Surface Tension

Surface tension, γ, is the force per unit length perpendicular to the line of action of the force:

$$\gamma = F_\perp / L$$

The SI units are newtons per meter, N/m.

Liquid molecules are attracted to each other by cohesive forces and to molecules of other substances by adhesive forces.

The cohesive forces are great enough to produce definite surfaces or interfaces, but not so great that the liquid is rigid.

Internal molecules, those in the bulk of the liquid, are uniformly attracted in all directions by cohesive forces, and therefore feel no net force.

Molecules at interfaces are subject to both cohesive and adhesive forces, which do not cancel. Therefore, surface molecules experience a net force or surface tension. This net force means that work must be done in forming the surface; therefore, the surface molecules have a potential energy that is directly related to the surface area.

At the Air Interface

Adhesive forces between the liquid and a gas (such as air) act upward away from the bulk liquid and tend to be much weaker than the liquid's cohesive forces, which act downward, toward the bulk liquid. The resulting net force causes the liquid to behave as if it had formed a surface membrane or skin.

In a Vacuum

A volume of liquid falling in a vacuum forms a sphere because this shape provides the minimum surface area, and therefore the minimum potential energy, E_p, for the surface of a given volume. Liquid samples falling outside of a vacuum are distorted into nonspherical drops by gravity and air resistance.

At the Glass Interface

Adhesive forces between a liquid and a solid (such as the glass walls of a container) are usually greater than cohesive forces of the liquid-gas interactions and produce an effect known as capillary action.

Capillary Action

A capillary or capillary tube is a thin-walled narrow diameter tube, usually but not necessarily made of glass. When it is partially inserted vertically into a reservoir of liquid, the liquid will rise in the tube because of the adhesive forces. In the capillary, the surface molecules are subject to three forces:

1. The cohesive forces acting downward into the bulk of the liquid

2. The adhesive forces with the atmosphere, which are antiparallel with the cohesive force (since this force is almost always much less than the cohesive force, it can be neglected or added to give a slightly smaller cohesive force)

3. The liquid-glass adhesive forces act toward the wall of the tube

If the capillary is narrow, the liquid will form a hemispherically curved surface called the meniscus.

For most liquids, including water, the adhesive force exceeds the cohesive force and the meniscus curves upward forming a concave surface. Liquid rises in the capillary to a level greater than that of the reservoir liquid. This process is called *wetting*.

A small number of liquids, most notably mercury, are nonwetting. Here the cohesive forces are greater than the adhesive forces. The meniscus curves down at the edges forming a convex outer surface. The liquid in the capillary is usually depressed below that of the reservoir.

The height to which the liquid is elevated by capillary action is inversely proportional to the diameter of the capillary and to the density of the liquid, and directly proportional to the surface tension.

For two samples of the same liquid (therefore, γ and ρ are constant) the smaller the radius of the capillary tube, the greater the elevation.

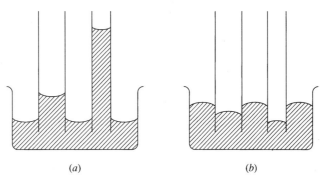

(a)   (b)

Meniscus for (a) a fluid where $F_{adhesive}$ is greater than $F_{cohesive}$ and (b) a fluid where $F_{adhesive}$ is less than $F_{cohesive}$.

Optional Aside

The upward force on the edges of the meniscus is the surface tension acting on the perimeter of the surface (where the liquid contacts the capillary wall):

$$F_{up} = \gamma \, (2\pi r)$$

The downward force is the weight of the liquid expressed as its volume $\pi r^2 h$ times its weight per unit volume, ρg:

$$F_{down} = (\pi r^2 h)(\rho g)$$

At equilibrium, $F_{up} = F_{down}$, and solving for the elevation, h, gives:

$$h = (2\gamma)/\rho g r$$

D. HYDRODYNAMICS

Hydrodynamics is the study of fluids in motion. It covers two broad categories of fluids, ideal fluids and real fluids.

Ideal Fluids

An ideal fluid is one that flows steadily around a body but exerts no force on the body. It is defined by four criteria:

1. It is nonviscous. There is no internal frictional resistance to its flow.
2. The density is constant; therefore, the fluid is incompressible.
3. Its flow is a steady-state flow. The magnitude and direction of the velocity at any given point is constant with respect to time.
4. The flow is irrotational. This means that the fluid will not cause a test body placed in it to rotate about an axis through the body's center of mass. However, the body can move in a circular path within the fluid.

Streamlines

Streamlines are fixed paths that fluids appear to flow along. The molecules of the fluid move without rotational motion or turbulence. The direction of the velocity of the fluid at a given point is the tangent to the streamline at that point.

1. The velocity at a given point in a streamline is constant.
2. The velocity at different points in a streamline can be different.
3. Streamlines can never cross. Since the velocity vector is tangent to the streamline, if two streamlines crossed it would imply that the fluid had two different velocities at that point.
4. The magnitude of the velocity at a given point is proportional to the density of the streamlines per unit of cross-sectional area at that point. Decreasing the diameter of a tube increases the velocity of the incompressible fluid. This is represented by compressing the spacing between streamlines.

In **laminar flow,** the fluid moves in layers between two surfaces in such a way that the resulting streamlines are parallel to the surfaces and to each other. These layers slide smoothly by each other. A layer is defined as the maximum thickness of a fluid where all parts have the same average velocity.

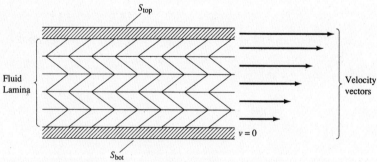

The top surface, S_{top}, is moving with a velocity, v. The bottom surface, S_{bot}, is stationary. The fluid moves in layers between the two surfaces. The layer closest to S_{top} moves with a velocity approximately equal to that of the surface. Each successive layer moves with a diminishing velocity. The layer closest to S_{bot} has a velocity close to zero.

Optional Aside

Different layers of a fluid with laminar flow tend to have different average velocities. The layer of fluid adjacent to a surface adheres to it and tends to move with the same speed as the surface. This layer of fluid tends to drag the next layer along with it, and so on. The net result is that the velocity of subsequent layers decreases as you move away from a moving surface or toward a stationary surface.

Volume Flow Rate, Q

The volume, V, of fluid flowing past a given area is the product of the cross-sectional area A, the velocity of the fluid v, and the time interval the flow is measured over, t:

$$V = Avt$$

The rate of flow Q is the volume per unit of time passing a given area and is given by the product of the velocity and the area crossed:

$$Q = V/t = Av$$

An SI unit of the volume rate is cubic meters per second, m^3/s.

The **equation of continuity** states that for an incompressible fluid flowing through an enclosed tube, the volume flow rate Q is constant. For two points along the tube, $A_1 V_1 = A_2 V_2 = $ constant. Since the cross-sectional area of the tube and the velocity of the fluid are inversely proportional, increasing the diameter of a tube decreases the velocity of the fluid and vice versa.

Bernoulli's equation states that for an incompressible fluid with negligible viscosity moving with streamline flow, velocity and pressure are inversely related so that any increase in velocity of the fluid will produce a decrease in the associated pressure. It is an application of the Laws of Conservation of Energy and Mass; specifically, it is the Work-Energy Theorem of moving fluids. It is used to describe the pressure associated with moving fluids when the viscosity is negligible, so that there is no loss of kinetic energy as thermal energy:

$$P + \rho gh + 1/2\ \rho v^2 = \text{constant}$$

Bernoulli's equation states that the sum of the three terms on the right-hand side is the same at every point in the fluid. Therefore, for any two arbitrary points:

$$P_1 + \rho gh_1 + 1/2\ \rho v^2_1 = P_2 + \rho gh_2 + 1/2\ \rho v^2_2 = \text{constant}$$

where P is the pressure; ρgh is the potential energy per unit volume, E_p/V; $1/2\ \rho v^2$ is the kinetic energy per unit volume, E_k/V. All three unit terms have units of pressure.

Case 1. Constant Height

For horizontal flow, $h_1 = h_2$ and the equation reduces to:

$$P_1 + 1/2\ \rho v^2_1 = P_2 + 1/2\ \rho v^2_2$$

Pressure is greatest when the velocity (and thus the second term on each side) is least. The kinetic energy term can only be changed if work is done; therefore, there must be a net force acting on the fluid.

Case 2. Constant Velocity

Here the equation reduces to:

$$P_1 + \rho g h_1 = P_2 + \rho g h_2$$

This is a manifestation of Pascal's Principle as observed in the operation of barometers and manometers.

Case 3. Constant Pressure

The equation becomes:

$$\rho g h_1 + 1/2\,\rho v^2_1 = \rho g h_2 + 1/2\,\rho v^2_2$$

If two leaks are created at different heights in a water tank, the liquid exiting from the lower leak must have the greater velocity (bigger $1/2\,\rho v^2$ term) since it will have the smaller height ($\rho g h$ term).

Real Fluids

Real fluids are all fluids that do not meet the four criteria of ideal fluids. A real fluid does exert a force on any body moving through it. This frictional force arises from intermolecular interactions; the viscosity of the fluid produces a resisting force that is parallel to the surface of the body. This in turn causes the conversion and loss of some of the kinetic energy of the fluid motion as thermal energy. Thus, fluid near a body (surface) tends to move more slowly, forming a boundary layer. The flow and the loss of kinetic energy are directly proportional; if the flow is slow, the frictional loss of energy will be low.

Viscous Force, F_v

A fluid flowing past a surface exerts a force, $F_{\parallel}$, that is parallel to the surface and in the same direction as the flow. In reaction, the surface exerts a force on the fluid called the viscous force, F_v, which is opposite to the direction of the flow. F_v represents the internal friction or internal inertia of a fluid that causes it to resist flowing. It is directly proportional to the velocity of the fluid, v, and to the area of the surface the fluid flows over, A, and inversely proportional to the distance between the fluid element and the surface, d. The proportionality constant is called the viscosity, η:

$$-F_{\parallel} = F_v = \eta A v/d$$

Note: In laminar flow, this internal friction produces a shear stress between adjacent layers.

Viscosity is the resistance of a fluid to flow. The greater the viscosity, the more difficult it is to get fluid motion. The difficulty with which a fluid flows is measured by the viscosity coefficient, η, which is temperature dependent and characteristic of the fluid. The SI unit of viscosity is the newton second per square meter, N s/m^2, which is also called the poiseuille, Pl. In the cgs system, the unit is the poise, P:

$$1 \text{ Ns/m}^2 = 1 \text{ Pl} = 10 \text{ P}$$

In laminar flow of fluids through pipes and tubes, the layers are arranged as concentric cylinders. The fluid velocity is greatest, V_{max}, for the central cylinder and is slowest for the outermost cylinder which is immediately adjacent to the walls of the pipe. The average velocity of different layers depends on the radial distance of the layer from the center of the pipe.

In turbulent flow, there is no steady-state streamline flow; the velocity at any given point is not constant but tends to change rapidly with time. Turbulence is the result of four factors: the density of the fluid, ρ; its average forward velocity, v; its viscosity, η; and the diameter of the pipe carrying the fluid, d.

The **Reynolds number,** $\mathcal{R}$, is a dimensionless quantity derived from the combination of the four factors above and used to predict the conditions of turbulent flow for a fluid system:

$$\mathcal{R} = \rho v d / \eta$$

1. If $\mathcal{R} < 2000$, the flow will be laminar.

2. If $\mathcal{R} > 3000$, the flow will be turbulent.

3. $\mathcal{R}$ values between 2000 and 3000 represent a transition region between laminar and turbulent flow patterns.

4. $\mathcal{R}$ is directly proportional to the density, velocity, and tube diameter, and inversely proportional to the viscosity. Changing any combination of these appropriately can drive a system from laminar to turbulent flow or vice versa.

PRACTICE PROBLEMS

1. A diver is swimming 10 meters below the surface of the water in a reservoir. There is no current, the air has a pressure of 1 atmosphere, and the density of the water is 1000 kilograms per cubic meter. What is the pressure experienced by the diver?

   A. 1.1 atm
   B. 1.99×10^5 Pa
   C. 11 atm
   D. 1.01×10^5 Pa

2. The Young's modulus for steel is 2.0×10^{11}N/m^2. What is the stress experienced by a steel rod that is 100 centimeters long and 20 millimeters in diameter when it is stretched by a force of 6.3×10^3 N?

   A. 2.00×10^8 N/m^2
   B. 12.6×10^{12} N/m^2
   C. 3.15×10^8 N/m^2
   D. 4.0×10^{11} N/m^2

3. A 100-centimeter-long steel rod experiences a stress of 4.0×10^8 N/m^2 when it is stretched by a force of 10 N. The Young's modulus of steel is 2.0×10^{11} N/m^2. What is the strain on the rod?

   A. 5.0×10^3 m
   B. 5.0×10^3
   C. 2.0×10^{-3} m
   D. 2.0×10^{-3}

4. The aorta of a 70-kilogram man has a cross-sectional area of 3.0 square centimeters and carries blood with a velocity of 30 centimeters per second. What is the average volume flow rate?

   A. 10 cm/s
   B. 33 cm^3/s
   C. 10 cm^2/s
   D. 90 cm^3/s

5. A closed-end tube is evacuated and placed with its open end beneath the surface of a reservoir of mercury. The mercury rises to a height of 93 cm. If the density of mercury is 1.36×10^4 kg/m^3, what is the pressure at the bottom of the column of mercury?

A. 1.24×10^5 Pa
B. 1.24×10^5 atm
C. 1.26×10^4 Pa
D. 1.26×10^4 atm

6. At 20°C the density of water is 1 g/cm^3. What is the density of a body that has a mass of 100 grams in air and 25 grams in water?

A. 0.25 g/cm^3
B. 0.75 g/cm^3
C. 1.3 g/cm^3
D. 4.0 g/cm^3

7. Brass has a density of 8.9 g/cm^3. A sample of brass is shaped into a perfect cube that has a mass of 71.2 grams. What is the length of each side of the cube?

A. 2.0 cm
B. 4.0 cm
C. 8.0 cm
D. 9.0 cm

8. What is the specific gravity of a bar of iron that has a mass of 192 grams and the dimensions 12 cm $\times$ 2 cm $\times$ 1 cm?

A. 8.0 g/cm^3
B. 8.0
C. 24 g/cm^3
D. 24

9. Two insoluble bodies, A and B, appear to lose the same amount of weight when submerged in alcohol. Which statement is most applicable?

A. Both bodies have the same mass in air.
B. Both bodies have the same volume.
C. Both bodies have the same density.
D. Both bodies have the same weight in air.

10. The bottom of each foot of an 80-kg man has an area of about 400 cm^2. What is the effect of his wearing snowshoes with an area of about 0.400 m^2?

A. The pressure exerted on the snow becomes 10 times as great.
B. The pressure exerted on the snow becomes 1/10 as great.
C. The pressure exerted on the snow remains the same.
D. The force exerted on the snow is 1/10 as great.

11. Two rectangular water tanks are filled to the same depth with water. Tank A has a bottom surface area of 2 m^2 and tank B has a bottom area of 4 m^2. Which statement about the forces and pressures at the bottom of the tanks is correct?

A. Since F_A is less than F_B, P_A is less than P_B.
B. Since F_A is equal to F_B, P_A is less than P_B.
C. Since F_A is less than F_B, P_A is equal to P_B.
D. Since F_A is equal to F_B, P_A is equal to P_B.

12. In a hydraulic lift, the surface of the input piston is 10 cm^2 and that of the output piston is 3000 cm^2. What is the work done if a 100 N force applied to the input piston raises the output piston by 2.0 meters?

A. 20 kJ
B. 30 kJ
C. 40 kJ
D. 60 kJ

ANSWER KEY

1. B	3. D	5. A	6. C	7. A	8. B	9. B	10. B	11. C	12. D
2. A	4. D								

ANSWERS AND EXPLANATIONS

1. **The correct answer is (B).** The fluid is at rest (no currents) so this is a hydrostatic pressure calculation. In SI units 1 atm = 1.01×10^5 Pa. Choice D can be eliminated because the pressure below the water must be greater than the pressure at the surface.

    $P_{diver} = P_{atm} + \rho gh$

    $= (1.01 \times 10^5 \text{ Pa}) + (10^3 \text{ kg/m}^3)(9.8 \text{ m/s}^2)(10 \text{ m})$

    $P_{diver} = 1.99 \times 10^5$ Pa

    This problem is easily solved by estimating the answer: $9.8 \sim 10$; $1.01 \times 10^5 \sim 10^5$, therefore:

    $P_{diver} \sim (10^5 \text{ Pa}) + (10^3 \text{ kg/m}^3)(10 \text{ m/s}^2)(10 \text{ m}) \sim 2 \times 10^5$ Pa which is closest to choice B.

2. **The correct answer is (A).** Stress is force per unit area, so neither the Young's modulus nor the length of the rod are needed to solve the problem. The area of the rod is $\pi r^2 = (3.15)(10 \times 10^{-3} \text{ m})^2 = 3.15 \times 10^{-5} \text{ m}^2$

    Stress $= F/A$
    $= (6.30 \times 10^3 \text{ N})/(3.15 \times 10^{-5} \text{ m}^2)$
    $= 2.00 \times 10^8 \text{ N/m}^2$

3. **The correct answer is (D).** Strain is the ratio of change in length to the original length. Therefore, start by finding the change in length:

    $\Delta \ell = (\text{Stress}/Y)$
    $= (1.00 \text{ m})(4.0 \times 10^8 \text{ N/m}^2)/(2.0 \times 10^{11} \text{ N/m}^2)$
    $= 2 \times 10^{-3} \text{ m}$

    Strain is dimensionless; therefore, choices A and C can be eliminated immediately.

    Strain $= \Delta \ell / \ell = (F/A)/Y = \text{Stress}/Y$
    $= (4 \times 10^8 \text{ N/m}^2)/(2 \times 10^{11} \text{ N/m}^2)$
    $= 2 \times 10^{-3} \text{ (no units)}$

4. **The correct answer is (D).** $Q = Av = (3.0 \text{ cm}^2)(30 \text{ cm/s}) = 90 \text{ cm}^3/\text{s}$.

5. **The correct answer is (A).** The pressure at the bottom of the column is due only to the weight of the mercury in the tube (because it was evacuated).

    $P = \rho gh$
    $= (1.36 \times 10^4 \text{ kg/m}^3)(9.8 \text{ m/s}^2)(93 \times 10^{-2}\text{m})$

    These values readily round off to:

    $P = (1.4 \times 10^4 \text{ kg/m}^3)(10 \text{ m/s}^2)(1 \text{ m}) \sim 1.4 \times 10^5$ Pa

    Since all the terms were rounded off, the actual answer will be a little smaller than the estimate. Choice A is the numerical closest match that also has the correct units.

6. **The correct answer is (C).** Archimedes' Principle. The apparent loss of weight (or mass) of a submerged body equals the weight (or mass) of the fluid displaced.

    1. The mass of the displaced water is: $100g - 25g = 75g$
    2. The volume occupied by this mass of water is: $75 \text{ g}/(1 \text{ g/cm}^3) = 75 \text{ cm}^3$
    3. The volume of the body must equal the volume of the water displaced.
    4. The density of the body is: $\rho = m/V = 100 \text{ g}/75 \text{ cm}^3 = 1.3 \text{ g/cm}^3$

7. **The correct answer is (A).** Volume $= m/\rho$, and $\text{side}_{cube} = V^{1/3}$

    This problem lends itself well to quick estimation; $8.9 \text{ g/cm}^3 \sim 9 \text{ g/cm}^3$; 71.2 g can be replaced by 72 which is the closest integer multiple of 9:

    $$\text{side} = (m/\rho)^{1/3} \sim (72 \text{ g}/9 \text{ g cm}^{-3})^{1/3}$$
    $$= (8 \text{ cm}^3)^{1/3}$$
    $$= 2 \text{ cm}$$

    Note: 2 cm is also the value of the length of the side calculated when the exact values are used.

8. **The correct answer is (B).** Specific gravity of solids is the ratio of the density of the solid to the density of water, 1.0 g/cm^3. Since it is a ratio of identical units, the specific gravity is dimensionless:

    $$\rho = m/V = 192 \text{ g}/24 \text{ cm}^3 = 8.0 \text{ g/cm}^3$$

    Therefore the specific gravity is simply 8.0.

9. **The correct answer is (B).** Archimedes' Principle. The weight lost is equal to the weight of the displaced fluid; therefore, both must have the same volume because the volume of the fluid equals the volume of the body.

10. **The correct answer is (B).** The force exerted by the man is his weight and it is assumed to be constant. This eliminates choice D. For a constant force, pressure and area are inversely proportional. The area of the snowshoes is ten times the area of the foot so that the pressure associated with the snowshoes is the inverse of 10 or 1/10 the pressure exerted by the foot.

11. **The correct answer is (C).** Hydrostatic pressure depends only on depth. Since both tanks are filled to the same depth, $P_A = P_B$. Since $P = F/A = $ constant, the tank with the larger bottom area will experience the greater force, $F_B > F_A$.

12. **The correct answer is (D).** The pressure produced by the input piston is:

    $$P = F/A = 100 \text{ N}/0.001 \text{ m}^2$$
    $$= 1.00 \times 10^5 \text{ N/m}^2$$

    Pascal's Principle insures that this pressure is transmitted uniformly and undiminished throughout the fluid. This pressure produces a larger force at the larger area output piston:

    $$F_{out} = PA = (1.00 \times 10^5 \text{ N/m}^2)(0.300 \text{ m}^2)$$
    $$= 3.00 \times 10^4 \text{ N}$$

    The work done is:

    $$W = Fd = (3.00 \times 10^4 \text{ N})(2 \text{ m})$$
    $$= 6.0 \times 10^4 \text{ N m}$$
    $$= 6.0 \times 10^4 \text{ J} = 60 \text{ kJ}$$

2.9 GENERAL WAVE CHARACTERISTICS AND PERIODIC MOTION

A. WAVES: GENERAL DESCRIPTION

A wave is a general disturbance that is propagated (moves) through matter and/or space. This disturbance can:

1. change its magnitude from point to point along the line of propagation, and/or

2. change its magnitude at a given point with respect to time.

The common defining property of all waves is that wave motion is a mechanism that transfers energy from one point to another.

If the wave propagates through matter, this transfer of energy occurs without any net transfer of matter.

Waves carry energy and momentum obtained from the source of the wave. Intensity, I, is the power transported across a unit cross-sectional area; it is directly proportional to the square of the amplitude, $I \propto A^2$, and has the SI units of watts per square meter, W/m^2.

The transfer of energy can occur as a single event called a pulse, or as a series of consecutive displacements called a train of pulses. If a train of pulses has a regularly repeating pattern, it can be described by a sinusoidal wave.

Sinusoidal Wave

A **sinusoidal wave** is a repeating pattern that gives the relative displacement of a body from its equilibrium position. It is initiated by **simple harmonic motion** and can be described completely by a single wavelength and a single frequency. A repeating pattern can be described by a mathematical equation called a **periodic function.**

Note: **Sine waves** and **cosine waves** are common sinusoidal waves.

The basic repeating pattern of any periodic function is called a cycle. One complete cycle of a sinusoidal wave has a value of 2π, because it is equivalent to a body traveling once around a circle. A sinusoidal wave is completely described by the set of characteristics listed below:

The **amplitude,** A, is the maximum displacement from the equilibrium position. The equilibrium position has an energy value of zero. The transfer of energy by the wave is measured by the displacement away from equilibrium. The maximum displacement in the positive (maximum value of the function) direction defines a part of the curve called the crest of the wave. The maximum displacement in the negative direction (minimum value of the function) identifies the trough of the wave.

Note: By convention, in graphing sinusoidal waves the equilibrium position is parallel (or coincident) with the Cartesian x-axis and generally assigned the arbitrary value of zero. It also arbitrarily coincides with the direction in which the wave is traveling. Points above this line are considered positive, and those below the line are considered negative.

The points of zero displacement are called **nodes.** These mark the points where the wave crosses the equilibrium position. In sine waves, the nodes occur at half wavelength intervals, λ/2.

The points of maximum displacement (positive or negative) are called **antinodes.** These correspond to the crests (maxima) and troughs (minima) of the wave. For sine waves, there are two antinodes in each cycle (one positive and the other negative); antinodes occur halfway between nodes.

The **phase,** Φ, of a sinusoidal wave is the relative position of its nodes (and antinodes) along the line of propagation with respect to some starting point or time.

Note: A single cycle of a sine wave starts and ends with a node and has a third node in the center of the cycle between the crest and trough. In contrast, a cosine wave starts and ends with antinodes and has an antinode in the center of the cycle. A node occurs between each pair of antinodes. A sine wave and a cosine wave are 90° out of phase with each other.

The **wavelength,** λ, is the distance between corresponding points on two successive cycles. It is generally measured from the crest of one wave to the crest of the adjacent wave, but any two corresponding points must give you the same value. The unit of wavelength is distance, which in the SI system is given in meters, m.

Frequency, v, is the number of complete cycles that passes a given point in one second. Since frequency is cycles per second, the unit of frequency is the reciprocal second, s^{-1}, also called the hertz, Hz.

The **period,** T, is the length of time required for the body to complete one cycle. The period is equal to the reciprocal of the frequency, v:

$$T = 1/v$$

The unit of the period is the second, s; that of frequency is the reciprocal second or hertz, s^{-1} = Hz.

The **velocity** (or speed), v, **of a sinusoidal wave** is equal to the product of the wavelength and the frequency:

$$v = \lambda v$$

The SI unit of speed and velocity is meters per second. The speed depends primarily on the medium the wave is traveling through. For the special case of **electromagnetic waves** traveling through a vacuum, the speed is a constant, c:

$$v = c = 3.00 \times 10^8 \text{ m/s}$$

Types of Waves

There are two broad categories of waves, mechanical waves and electromagnetic waves. They are distinguished by the source generating the wave and the medium the wave propagates through.

Mechanical Waves

Mechanical waves require a physical medium (gas, liquid, or solid) for propagation; they cannot travel through a vacuum. The velocity of a mechanical wave depends on the strength of the source and the elastic properties of the medium.

The medium must be elastic so that the disturbance can displace particles of the medium from their original or equilibrium positions. Generally, the more elastic the medium, the more easily it is disturbed and restored to its equilibrium state.

Graph of a Typical Sine Wave

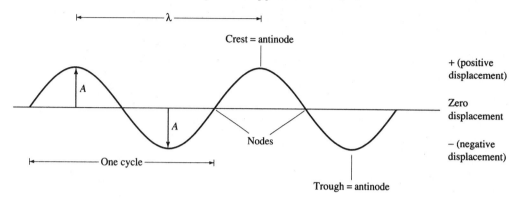

A = amplitude

The horizontal axis represents the value of the equilibrium position of the body; it corresponds to zero displacement. The vertical axis gives the arbitrarily defined displacement of the body from equilibrium. By convention, displacement above the horizontal axis is positive and that below the horizontal is negative.

Mechanical waves are most familiar and easiest to describe because they follow Newton's laws of motion.

The **velocity of a mechanical wave** is:

$v \propto$ (elasticity/inertia)$^{1/2}$

This velocity is:

1. **Directly proportional to the square root of the elasticity of the medium.**

   Elasticity is the "stiffness" of the bonds or interactions between the component particles of the medium. The greater the stiffness, the more easily (faster) the displacement will be propagated. The elastic property of the medium is given by the elastic moduli, Young's (Y), bulk (B), shear (S), or, if the medium is a string, by the Tension (T).

2. **Inversely proportional to the square root of the inertia of the medium.**

   The more massive the component particles of the medium, the slower the rate of propagation of a wave through the medium. Inertia can be measured by either the density (ρ), which is the mass per unit volume, or by the mass per unit length (μ).

Type of Wave	Speed of Wave
Sound wave in a fluid	$(B/\rho)^{1/2}$
Compressional or longitudinal waves in solids (P-waves)	$((B + 4/3\ S)/\rho)^{1/2}$
Shear or transverse waves in solids (S-waves)	$(S/\rho)^{1/2}$
Compressional waves in a thin rod	$(Y/\rho)^{1/2}$
Transverse waves on a string	$(T/\mu)^{1/2}$

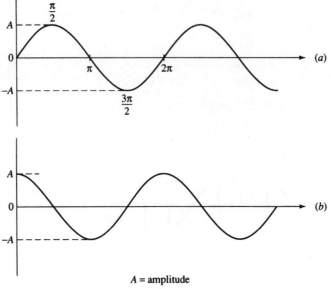

A = amplitude

Comparison of a single cycle of (a) a sine wave to that of (b) a cosine wave. Both are sinusoidal waves because of their shapes. They differ by a phase angle of 90° or one quarter of a cycle.

Electromagnetic Waves

Electromagnetic waves, also called electromagnetic radiation, EMR, or light, do not require a physical medium for propagation; they can travel through a vacuum. EMR waves consist of two vector quantities, an electric field, and a magnetic field that are mutually perpendicular. The strength of each of these fields varies sinusoidally and produces the disturbance (displacement) that changes with time and travels through space. (See Section 2.11.)

1. In a vacuum, all EMR waves travel with the same velocity, $c = 3 \times 10^8$ m/s.

2. In physical media, the speed decreases. The decrease depends not only on the medium but also on the frequency of the light; the higher the frequency of the EMR, the greater its speed is affected by any physical medium. This leads to a phenomenon called dispersion and is the explanation for rainbows.

3. Electromagnetic waves generally arise from the interaction of mutually induced electric and magnetic fields that vary sinusoidally with time.

Wave Motion

Wave motion describes

1. the relation between the displacement and the direction of propagation and

2. the relative motion of the nodes (and antinodes) with time.

Note: In mechanical waves, particles of the medium oscillate; in electromagnetic waves, the electric and magnetic fields oscillate.

Transverse Waves

In **transverse waves,** the displacement (of particle position or field strength) is perpendicular to the direction of wave propagation. Electromagnetic radiation is always propagated as a transverse wave.

Transverse Wave

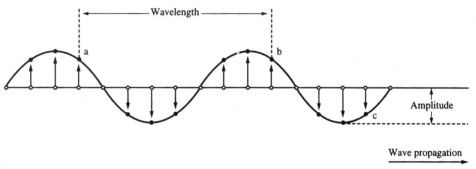

The arrows are displacement vectors for the motion of particles of the medium in mechanical waves or the field strength in electromagnetic waves.

Longitudinal Waves

In **longitudinal waves** the displacement is parallel to the direction of propagation. Most sound waves and the compressional waves in a spring are longitudinal waves.

Note: Some wave motions are a combination of both longitudinal and transverse wave motions. The motion of water waves is such a combination because the water molecules move in circular or ovoid paths; the north-south (up-down) motion is the transverse component; the east-west (right-left) motion is the longitudinal component.

Longitudinal Wave

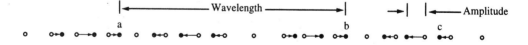

Arrows show displacement of particles of the medium.

In **traveling waves,** the nodes move. This can be described in either of two equivalent remarks:

1. The position of a particular crest (or trough) will change with time.

2. The amplitude at a fixed point will change with time.

Water waves are an example of traveling waves.

Standing Waves

In **standing waves,** the positions of the nodes and antinodes are fixed and do not change with time. Collinear waves moving in opposite directions in the medium can add vectorally to produce a wave that appears to be stationary. A vibrating violin string is an example of a standing wave.

Law of Superposition

The **law of superposition** states that if two or more waves intersect at any point, the net displacement is the sum of the individual wave amplitudes (displacements) at that point. After the point of intersection, the waves continue along their original paths unaltered by the interaction. Collinear waves interact at all points along the line of propagation.

The result of superposition is called interference, and the effect observed depends on the phases and amplitudes of the waves at the points of intersection. See Figure 1 on the following page.

1. **Constructive interference** occurs where the amplitudes have the same sign (both positive or both negative) at a given point.

    Perfect constructive interference occurs if the waves have the same phase and frequency so their antinodes coincide exactly (crests super-posed on crests, and troughs superposed on troughs).

2. **Destructive interference** occurs where amplitudes have opposite signs at a given point.

    Perfect destructive interference occurs when the waves have the same frequency but are 180° out of phase with each other so that crests are superimposed on troughs. The amplitude of the resulting wave is always less than the amplitudes of any of the individual waves being super-posed.

Note: For the special case where both waves have the same amplitude, perfect destructive interference produces complete destruction of the wave (zero amplitude at all points along the line of propagation).

Fourier's theorem states that any wave (sinusoidal or not) can be reproduced by superposing various sine waves. Most real waves are not sinusoidal (i.e., having only one wavelength and one frequency) but are the result of the superposition of several waves.

Figure 1
Interference Patterns

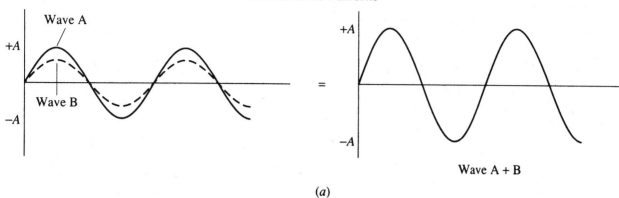

(a)

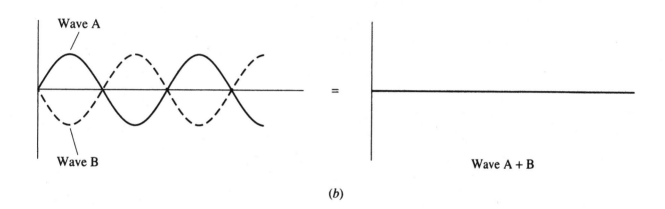

(b)

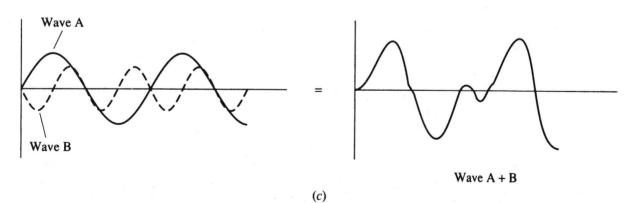

(c)

Interference patterns: (a) Perfect constructive interference. (b) Perfect destructive interference. (c) Example of a real nonsinusoidal wave resulting from superposition of two sinusoidal waves.

B. PERIODIC MOTION

In periodic motion, a body repeats a certain motion, such as oscillating about its original equilibrium position. The body keeps traveling over the same definite path in equal intervals of time. Such a repeated path is called a closed path and each complete transit of the path is called a cycle.

In order to repeat the path, the body must regularly change its velocity, always altering the direction of the motion and often the speed as well. Therefore, the body must regularly experience a net force that provides the acceleration necessary to change the velocity.

Note: All periodic functions (patterns) can be replaced by a sine wave.

Generating a Sine Wave from a Periodic Function

Circular Motion

The simplest way of generating a sine wave is by plotting the uniform (constant speed) circular motion of a body using a reference circle.

The graph of the motion is outlined below.

Uniform Circular Motion of a Body Using a Reference Circle

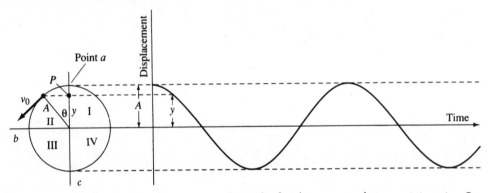

A body moves with constant speed in a circular path of radius A around some origin point, O. The horizontal axis of the sine wave graph is parallel to one of the diameters of the circle. The position of the circulating body relative to this diameter is plotted as the body moves around the circle from point *a* to point *b* to point *c*, etc., until it returns to point *a* where it repeats the cycle. The radius to the current position of the body forms the phase angle θ with the radius to the original position of the body. The amplitude of the wave is the projection of the radius onto the *y*-axis (north-south pole line) of the circular motion.

For uniform circular motion, the length of time required for the body to complete one cycle of the circle is called the period and depends on the radius of the circle, *R*, and the speed of the body, *v*:

Period = Circumference of reference circle/speed
$T = 2\pi R/v$

A circle can be divided into four quarters or quadrants that are 90° apart. These are labeled Quads I, II, III, and IV and are moving counterclockwise from point *a*.

Pendulum Motion

An ideal pendulum consists of a dense mass called a bob suspended from a fixed point by a massless and nonstretchable string. The bob is free to swing back and forth about an axis. The axis is the equilibrium position that the pendulum has when it is at rest (zero velocity).

Pendulum Motion

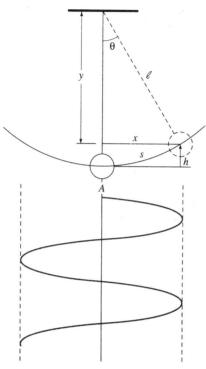

The pendulum oscillates or vibrates around its equilibrium position; the bob is displaced from the equilibrium position, $A = 0$, by an angle θ and during each quarter cycle sweeps through an arc, S. For small angles (θ), the motion of the pendulum generates a sine wave. The vertical axis is the zero displacement or equilibrium position; displacements to the right are, arbitrarily, positive and those to the left, negative.

Spring Motion

Spring motion describes the motional effect of stretching or compressing a spring. A body attached to the spring will then oscillate about the rest or equilibrium position of the spring.

Spring Motion

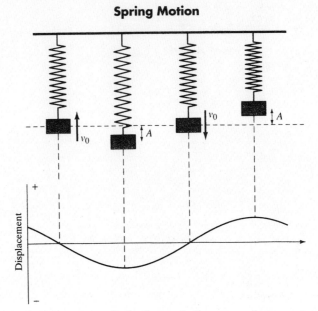

Graph of the motion of a body attached to an oscillating spring.

Simple harmonic motion, SHM, occurs when a body moves back and forth around a definite path in equal intervals of time. SHM can always be described by a sine wave. SHM is a periodic motion where the force providing the acceleration is directly proportional to the displacement of the body from its equilibrium position and always directed toward the equilibrium position. Such a force is called a restoring force and is described by Hooke's Law. The motion may be linear or angular.

Linear vibrational motion is typical of the oscillations of springs. Angular vibrational motion is typical of both circular motion and the motion of pendulums.

A body that moves with simple harmonic motion has the following characteristics:

1. The period, T, is the time required for one complete cycle of the motion. It is independent of the amplitude of the motion.

2. The frequency, ν, is the reciprocal of the period:

   $$\nu = 1/T = (k/m)^{1/2}/2\pi$$

   Note: SHM is isochronous, which means the period and frequency are independent of the amplitude of the motion. They depend only on the mass and the force constant.

3. Displacement, *d*: There are two typical cases for measuring the displacement of a simple harmonic motion:

   Case 1
   The body starts at its equilibrium position. That is, at time $t = 0$, the body has a displacement of $d = 0$ and is moving toward its maximum positive displacement (amplitude). Then, its displacement at any other time, *t*, is given by:

   $$d = A \sin 2\pi vt = A \sin \omega t$$

   A is the amplitude of the maximum displacement, and $\omega = 2\pi v$ is called the angular frequency of the motion and is used to express the frequency in radians per second instead of hertz.

   Case 2
   The body starts at its maximum displacement position. That is, at time $t = 0$, the body has a displacement of $d = A$ and is moving toward its equilibrium position (where $d = 0$). Then, its displacement at any other time, *t*, is given by:

   $$d = A \cos 2\pi vt = A \cos \omega t$$

4. The velocity, *v*, of the body at any time is given by:

   $$v = 2\pi(A^2 - d^2)^{1/2}$$

   where the value of *t* determines the value of *d*. There are two roots to the square root equation: $+v$ indicates the body is moving toward its maximum positive displacement (crest of the wave); $-v$ indicates the body is moving toward its maximum negative displacement (trough of the wave).

5. The acceleration, *a*, at any time, *t*, is given by:

   $$a = -4\pi^2 v^2 d = -(k/m)d$$

   The acceleration has its maximum value at the points of maximum displacement (positive or negative); the acceleration is zero at the equilibrium position ($d = 0$).

   Note: At the turning points where the acceleration has its maximum values, the velocity is zero because all of the energy is potential. At the equilibrium point where the acceleration is zero, the velocity has its maximum value because all of the energy is kinetic.

Motion of a Pendulum

Characteristics of the wave function:

1. **Period**
   The equation for the period of a SHM is modified for the specific case of an ideal pendulum. The displacement of the pendulum is directly proportional to its length, ℓ, and the acceleration is due only to gravity, *g*; therefore:

   $$T = 2\pi(\ell/g)^{1/2}$$

2. **Frequency**

Frequency, v, is the reciprocal of the period; therefore:

$$1/T = v = (1/2\pi)(g/\ell)^{1/2}$$

Note: The period and the frequency are independent of the mass of the pendulum.

Kinetic and Potential Energy of the Motion

At all points in the path the energy is the sum of the potential and kinetic energy terms.

1. At the points of maximum displacement, the bob of the pendulum has only potential energy, E_p = maximum, and no kinetic energy, $E_k = 0$. The velocity at these points is zero.

2. At the equilibrium position, the bob has only kinetic energy, E_k = maximum, and no potential energy, $E_p = 0$. The velocity of the bob is maximal at this point.

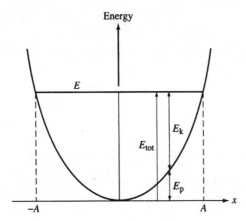

Distribution of E_p and E_k during the swing of a pendulum.

Motion of a Spring

Motion of a spring is vibrational SHM motion described by Hooke's Law.

Hooke's Law was empirically derived from observing the motion of spring systems. It states that when an elastic body such as a spring is deformed, its displacement x is proportional to the applied force. The proportionality constant is called the force constant, or **spring constant**, k, and depends on the "stiffness" of the spring. The larger the value of k, the more difficult it is to stretch or compress the spring. The Sl unit for k is the newton per meter, N/m or kg/s^2.

When the spring is deformed, it exerts a restoring force, F_r, that is always oriented toward the equilibrium position, which means it is always antiparallel to the original deforming force:

$$F_r = -kx$$

Characteristics of the Motion

There are two general descriptions, the case of a horizontal spring system and the case of a vertical spring system.

Case 1

A horizontal spring system consists of a spring attached to a mass at one end and to a vertical wall at the other.

1. At equilibrium, the distance of the mass from the wall is the rest or equilibrium length of the spring. If an applied force stretches the spring, the mass is displaced from its equilibrium position by some distance A (which equals the maximum amplitude of the resulting motion). Because of the "stiffness" of the spring, a restoring force develops that opposes the applied force. The restoring force is at a maximum at this point.

2. When the applied force is removed, the restoring force accelerates the body back toward the equilibrium position. As the body approaches the rest position, the magnitude of F_r steadily decreases.

3. However, the body has momentum, mv, upon reaching the equilibrium position and tends to "overshoot" it.

4. As the body passes the rest point, the spring is compressed, producing a restoring force in the opposite direction.

5. The restoring force is maximal at the turning point, which is the point of maximum compression.

6. Step 2 occurs in the opposite direction, accelerating the body back toward the rest position.

7. The body overshoots the rest point.

8. The cycle repeats.

Case 2

A vertical spring system consists of a spring attaching a body to a horizontal beam or ceiling. The argument describing this motion is identical to that of Case 1. The only difference is that the spring has two equilibrium lengths. The unloaded spring will have a particular equilibrium length. Loading the spring with a body produces a second equilibrium length that depends on the stiffness of the spring and on the mass of the body. The spring-mass system is then displaced from and oscillates about this latter equilibrium point.

Energy

At the turning points in the motion (maximum stretch and maximum compression), the velocity decreases to zero in prelude to reversing direction. All of the energy is potential because the kinetic energy is zero. As the body passes through the equilibrium position, the potential energy drops to zero and all of the energy is now kinetic. At positions between the rest and turning points, the energy is the sum of the kinetic and potential energy contributions.

Horizontal and Vertical Spring-Mass System

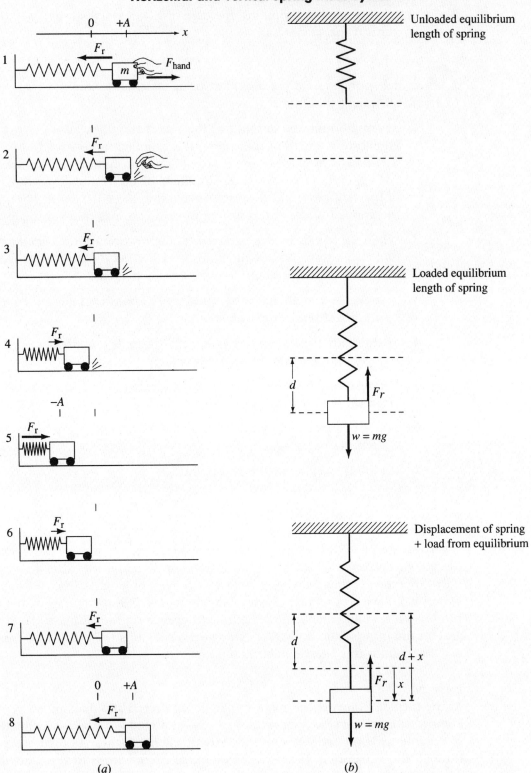

(a) The 8 steps describing the motion of a horizontal spring-mass system. (b) Motion of a vertical spring-mass system.

PRACTICE PROBLEMS

1. A simple pendulum has a period of 4.63 seconds at a place on the Earth where the acceleration of gravity is 9.82 m/s². At a different location, the period increases to 4.64 seconds. What is the value of g at this second point?

    A.   9.78 m/s²
    B.   9.82 m/s²
    C.   9.86 m/s²
    D.   Cannot be determined without knowing the length of the pendulum

2. What is the wavelength of a transverse wave with a velocity of 15 meters per second and a frequency of 5.0 hertz?

    A.   3.0 m
    B.   10 m
    C.   20 m
    D.   45 m

3. What is the optimum difference in phase for maximum destructive interference between two waves of the same frequency?

    A.   360°
    B.   270°
    C.   180°
    D.   90°

4. Standing waves can be formed if coincident waves have

    A.   the same direction of propagation.
    B.   the same frequency.
    C.   different amplitudes.
    D.   different wavelengths.

5. A pendulum with a length ℓ has a period of 2 seconds. In order for the pendulum to have a period of 4 seconds, we must

    A.   halve the length.
    B.   quarter the length.
    C.   double the length.
    D.   quadruple the length.

6. If a pendulum 12 meters long has a frequency of 0.25 hertz, what will be the period of a second pendulum at the same location if its length is 3.0 meters?

    A.   2.0 s
    B.   3.0 s
    C.   4.0 s
    D.   6.0 s

7. A pendulum clock is losing time. How should the pendulum be adjusted?

    A.   The weight of the bob should be decreased so it can move faster.
    B.   The length of the wire holding the bob should be shortened.
    C.   The amplitude of the swing should be reduced so the path covered is shorter.
    D.   None of the above.

8. A 20-kg weight is attached to a wall by a spring. A 5.0 Newton force horizontally displaces it 1.0 meter from its equilibrium position along a frictionless floor. What is the closest estimate of the period of the oscillation of the weight?

    A.   2.0 seconds
    B.   6.0 seconds
    C.   13 seconds
    D.   16 seconds

ANSWER KEY

1. A   2. A   3. C   4. B   5. D   6. A   7. B   8. C

ANSWERS AND EXPLANATIONS

1. **The correct answer is (A).** The answer can be determined easily without doing a numerical solution. Rearrange $T = 2\pi \, (\ell/g)^{1/2}$ to $Tg^{1/2} = $ constant. The period is inversely related to the square root of the acceleration due to gravity. Since T has increased, both $g^{1/2}$ and g must decrease. Choice A is the only value of g that is less than the original 9.82 m/s^2.

$$g_2 = (T_1^2 g_1 / T_2^2)$$
$$= (4.63 \text{ s})^2 (9.82 \text{ m/s}^2)/(4.64 \text{ s})^2$$
$$= 9.78 \text{ m/s}^2$$

2. **The correct answer is (A).** Wavelength is velocity divided by frequency. The formula is invariant to the type of wave involved.

$$\lambda = v/\nu = (15 \text{ m/s})/5.0 \text{ s}^{-1} = 3.0 \text{ m}$$

3. **The correct answer is (C).** Two waves are completely out of phase when their antinodes coincide so that each crest on one wave coincides with a trough on the other. This occurs when the waves differ by 180°.

4. **The correct answer is (B).** In standing waves, the nodes are stationary. This can be accomplished when two waves with the same frequency travel in opposite directions.

5. **The correct answer is (D).** In a pendulum, the period and the square root of the length are directly proportional:

$$T = 2\pi(\ell/g)^{1/2} \text{ so that } T/\ell^{1/2} = \text{constant}$$

To double the period, you must double the square root of the length. To double the square root of the length, you must quadruple the length:

$$(4\ell)^{1/2} = 4^{1/2} \, \ell^{1/2} = 2\ell^{1/2}$$

6. **The correct answer is (A).** The frequency is the reciprocal of the period: $\nu = 1/T$, so that $T = 4.0$ seconds. Period and the square root of the length are directly proportional. Therefore, the ratio of the two periods is:

$$T_1/T_2 = (\ell_1/\ell_2)^{1/2} = (12/3)^{1/2}$$
$$= 4^{1/2} = 2.0 \text{ seconds}$$

7. **The correct answer is (B).** The period of a pendulum is directly related to the square root of the length of the cord holding the bob. It is independent of the weight and amplitude.

8. **The correct answer is (C).** The force constant is: $k = |\,F\,|/|\,\Delta x\,| = 5.0 \text{ N}/1.0 \text{ m} = 5.0 \text{ N m}^{-1}$. The period is:

$$T = 2\pi(mk^{-1})^{1/2}$$
$$= 2(\pi)(20 \text{ kg}/5.0 \text{ N m}^{-1})^{1/2}$$
$$= 2\pi(2)(\text{kg m N}^{-1})^{1/2}$$
$$= 4\pi(\text{kg m N}^{-1})^{1/2} \sim 4(3)(\text{kg m N}^{-1})^{1/2}$$
$$= 12(\text{s}^2)^{1/2} = 12 \text{ s}$$

Note: N = kg m s^{-2}; therefore, kg/m N^{-1} = kg m/N = kg m s^2/kg m = s^2.

2.10 MECHANICAL WAVES: ACOUSTIC PHENOMENA

A. SOUND WAVES

Sound waves are the transmission of mechanical energy produced when a source initiates a disturbance in an elastic medium. Sound does not travel through a vacuum. Simple sound waves are sinusoidal with well-defined wavelengths, frequencies, and amplitudes.

Sonic Spectrum

The **sonic spectrum** is the range of frequencies over which "sound waves" can be propagated.

The upper limit of the spectrum is well defined. It has a maximum frequency of 10^9 Hz for gases. The value for solids and liquids is higher. The frequency of the sound depends inversely on the interparticle distance of the medium. In solids and liquids, these distances are smaller than in gases so the frequencies are higher.

The lower limit is not well defined. However, earthquakes are common low-frequency phenomena producing wavelengths in the kilometer range and corresponding frequencies in the region of 10^{-1} Hz.

Audio Range

The audio range is the region of the sonic spectrum that can be perceived by the human ear. For the average person, it covers frequencies from 20 Hz to 20,000 Hz. Frequencies above this range are called ultrasonic frequencies, and those below this range are called infrasonic frequencies.

Optional Aside

Do not confuse sound waves (which are mechanical waves) with radio or television waves (which are electromagnetic waves).

In Fluids, Sound Is Transmitted Only as Longitudinal Waves

The particles of the medium oscillate parallel to the direction of propagation of the wave. The velocity of propagation depends on the temperature, pressure, and identity of the fluid.

The relative velocity is:

$$v = (B/\rho)^{1/2}$$

where B is the bulk modulus of the fluid, and ρ is its density. B is the ratio of stress to strain in the fluid. The stress is the change in pressure, and the strain is the fractional change in volume that the stress produces:

$$B = \Delta P/(\Delta V/V)$$

The larger the magnitude of B, the more difficult it is to compress the fluid.

Optional Aside

This is a check of the units in the equation for the velocity:

$$B/\rho = (N/m^2)/(kg/m^3)$$
$$= (kg\ m/s^2)/m^2/(kg/m^3)$$
$$= (kg/s^2\ m)/(kg/m^3)$$
$$= m^2/s^2$$

$$v = (B/\rho)^{1/2}$$
$$= (m^2/s^2)^{1/2}$$
$$= m/s$$

The velocity of sound in air at 0°C and one atmosphere of pressure is 330 m/s or $\sim$ 740 miles per hour. The velocity in water under the same conditions is about four times as great, $\sim$ 1402 m/s.

Optional Aside

The density of water is $\sim$ 1000 times that of air, so we might expect sound to travel faster in air. However, $B_{water} > B_{air}$ because water is less compressible than air; therefore, $\Delta V/V$ is less for water than air for the change in pressure, ΔP. That is, the larger bulk modulus of water causes sound to have a greater velocity in the water.

The velocity of sound in fluids increases with increasing temperature at the rate of approximately 0.6 m/s per 1°C, or $\sim$ 2 ft/s °C. In air all sound waves have the same velocity at a given temperature regardless of their frequencies.

Note: Temperature affects the velocity of sound in all media. However, the effect is greatest for gases and least for solids.

In Solids, Sound Can Be Transmitted as Longitudinal Waves and as Transverse Waves

Transverse waves are possible because of the three-dimensional lattice structure of solids. This structure allows particles to move perpendicularly to the line of propagation. The restoring force for this perpendicular displacement is weak; therefore, for a given frequency the velocity of the transverse wave will be less than the velocity of the corresponding longitudinal wave.

Optional Aside

The distance from an observer to the source of an earthquake can be determined by measuring the difference in the arrival times of the transverse and the longitudinal waves generated by the source.

In solids, the velocity of a longitudinal wave is given by:

$$v = (Y/\rho)^{1/2}$$

where Y is the Young's modulus, which is analogous to the bulk modulus, B.

The larger the value of Y, the more difficult it is to compress the solid and the smaller the period of oscillation of the particles and, therefore, the greater the velocity. The velocity of sound in solids is about 15 times that of air or $\sim 5 \times 10^3$ m/s.

In solids the velocity of transverse waves is given by:

$$v = (T/\mu)^{1/2}$$

T is the tension or stiffness of the medium. μ is the mass per unit length of the medium.

B. CHARACTERISTICS OF SOUND

The characteristics of sound can be described by three physical properties: intensity, frequency, and harmonic composition. Physical properties are objective because they are quantitative and can be measured independently of the observer.

Each physical property of sound has a subjective counterpart: loudness, pitch, and timbre, respectively. Subjective properties are qualitative and cannot be measured directly; their values depend on the perceptions of the observer.

Intensity, I

Intensity, I, is the average rate per unit area (normal to the direction of propagation) at which sound energy is transferred by the sound wave. It is the ratio of power per unit area:

$$I = \text{Power}/A$$

and has the units of watts per square meter, W/m².

Intensity is more important than total energy carried by the wave because the wave spreads over larger areas as it moves away from its source so that I drops with increasing distance from the source, as shown in the figure below.

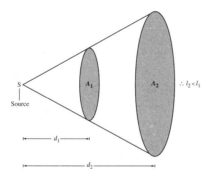

Intensity is inversely proportional to the square of the distance from its source.

For a given frequency v, the intensity I_v is directly proportional to the square of the amplitude, a, of the sound wave.

The **threshold of hearing**, I_0, is the minimum intensity of sound that is audible to the average listener. It has a value of $\sim 10^{-12}$ W/m² for sound with a frequency of $\sim 10^3$ Hz.

Sound level, β: The intensity of a sound, I, is measured with respect to the threshold of hearing. This ratio is called the sound level:

$\beta = 10 \log I/I_0$

1. The quantity, β, is called the **decibel,** dB. The range of perceptible intensities runs from a low of $I_0 \sim 10^{-12}$ W/m^2 to a high of ~ 1 W/m^2. This range covers 12 orders of magnitude; therefore, intensity is measured using the logarithm scale.

2. The threshold intensity, I_0, has a sound level value of $\beta = 0$ dB.

3. The maximum intensity, which marks the onset of pain, has a sound level of $\beta = 120$ dB.

4. The relationship between sound levels and intensities:

β (dB)	I/I_0
0	$10^0 = 1$
10	$10^1 = 10$
20	$10^2 = 100$
30	$10^3 = 1000$
•	•
•	•
120	10^{12}

5. The difference in β is constant for each change in order of magnitude of intensity. That is, β changes by 10 dB in going from an intensity of 10^0 to 10^1 and in going from 10^1 to 10^2, etc., so that for a given frequency, there is a uniform sensation to the changes in intensity.

Loudness

Loudness is an auditory sensation and depends on the perceptions of the listener. It is the listener's subjective perception of sound level.

Optional Aside

The distinction between intensity and loudness occurs because the human ear is not equally sensitive to all frequencies. Although waves with greater intensity are generally louder, higher-frequency waves do not seem as loud as lower-frequency waves of the same intensity. For example, a 20-dB sound with a frequency of 1000 Hz sounds louder than a 20-dB sound with a frequency of 100 Hz, even though both have the same intensity.

Frequency

Frequency, v, is a physical property that expresses the number of waves (cycles) per unit of time passing a given point.

Pitch
Pitch is the subjective perception of frequency and depends on the frequency the ear receives.

1. Two waves with frequencies in a ratio of 2:1 are an octave apart.

2. Major chords in music are 4 frequencies in the ratio of 4:5:6:8.

3. At frequencies greater than 3000 Hz, pitch increases with intensity of a given frequency. Increasing the intensity of a high-frequency sound makes its frequency seem even higher than it is.

4. At frequencies below 2000 Hz, pitch decreases with increasing intensity of a given frequency, so a sound seems lower as it becomes more intense.

Harmonic Components

The lowest frequency produced by a sound source is called its fundamental frequency or first harmonic. Harmonics that are whole-number multiples of the fundamental are called overtones. The second harmonic is the first overtone. It lies an octave above the fundamental and vibrates with twice the frequency of the fundamental. The third harmonic is called the second overtone. It is two octaves above the fundamental and vibrates at three times the fundamental frequency.

Timbre or Quality
Timbre, or quality, is the subjective perception of the harmonics. The number and relative intensities of harmonics present in a sound depends on the source, such as a musical instrument, producing the tones. This different combination of harmonics is what allows us to distinguish tones of the same frequency produced by different instruments.

C. PROPERTIES OF SOUND

Sound waves exhibit all the typical properties of mechanical waves.

Reflection

Waves are reflected whenever they come to a boundary or change in the medium through which they are traveling. The boundary may be obvious, such as the physical barrier of a wall; or less obvious, such as the change in the density of air produced by local changes in temperature.

For mechanical waves, the phase of the reflected wave depends on whether the boundary is "fixed" or "free."

If the boundary is fixed, the reflected wave is 180° out of phase with the initial wave. A fixed boundary is one that is fairly inelastic and does not permit the wave to be transferred through it. Most sound waves are reflected this way because they usually hit solid boundaries, such as walls.

Optional Aside

At the interface between the medium transmitting the wave and the boundary, in agreement with Newton's third law, the force of the wave on the wall is countered by an equal and opposite force produced by the wall on the medium. If the pulse of the wave first reaching the boundary exerts an upward force on the wall, the wall will exert a downward force on the medium, and the resulting reflected wave will be exactly the reverse of the incident wave.

If the boundary is free (not fixed), the reflected wave will be in phase with the initial incident wave.

Echo

An **echo** is a single reflection of a sound wave. Multiple reflections of a sound wave are called reverberations.

Optional Aside

The human ear can retain awareness of sounds for ~ 0.1 second; therefore, the ear cannot perceive all echoes or reverberations.

1. If the reflection time is greater than 0.1 second, the ear will hear the echo or reverberation.

2. If the reflection time is less than 0.1 second, the echo will not be perceived because it will be masked by the memory of the original sound.

3. For perceptible echoes to occur, the reflecting surface must be more than 16.5 meters away so that the sound will have to travel a 33-meter round trip, which takes ~ 0.1 second.

Diffraction

Sound waves can be diffracted, or bent around the corners of obstacles, so that the wave is propagated on the other side of the obstacle and not just absorbed or reflected by the obstacle. The amount of diffraction is a function of the wavelength of the sound and the width of the obstacle.

If the wavelength is $<<$ width, no diffraction will occur. The sound wave will pass through the slit unaltered.

If the wavelength is $\geq$ width, diffraction occurs. Therefore, long-wavelength sounds (low-frequency sounds), can be heard farther and more clearly than short-wavelength (high-frequency) sounds.

Doppler Effect

Doppler effect is the change in frequency or pitch produced when the source of the wave or the detector of the wave or both are in motion with respect to the medium transmitting the wave. The greater the relative speed, the greater the shift in frequency. The shift is given by:

$$\nu' = \nu[(v + v_D)/(v - v_S)]$$

where v' is the perceived frequency and v is the actual frequency. v is the velocity of the wave in the medium, v_D is the velocity of the detector, and v_S is the velocity of the source producing the sound.

- If the detector is stationary and the source is moving, the equation becomes:

$$v' = v[v/(v - v_S)]$$

- If the source is moving toward the detector, the denominator becomes $v - v_S$ so $v' > v$ and the pitch sounds higher.

- If the source is moving away from the detector, the denominator becomes $v + v_S$ so $v' < v$ and the pitch sounds lower.

- If the source is stationary and the detector is moving, the equation becomes:

$$v' = v(v + v_D)/v$$

- If the detector is moving toward the source, the numerator becomes $v + v_D$ so $v' > vv$ and the pitch sounds higher.

- If the detector is moving away from the source, the numerator becomes $v - v_D$ so $v' < v$ and the pitch sounds lower.

- If both the source and the detector are moving fairly slowly, the equation can be approximated by:

$$v' \sim v[1 \pm (v_R/v)]$$

where v_R is the relative speed between the source and the detector and is given by:

$$v_R = | v_S \pm v_D |$$

Note: Although the Doppler effect was described for sound waves, the description and equations given apply to any wave, mechanical or electromagnetic.

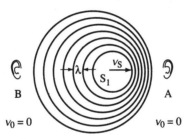

The source moves toward observer A
and away from observer B at speed v_S.

Beats

Beats are the interference pattern produced by superposing two waves of slightly different frequencies being propagated in the same direction. The amplitude of the resulting wave varies with time.

For two waves, A and B, with frequencies v_A, v_B, and periods T_A, T_B, if $v_A > v_B$ then $T_A < T_B$, and the beat frequency is:

$$v_{beat} = v_A - v_B = 1/T_A - 1/T_B$$

because $v = 1/T$.

The human ear can detect beats with a frequency of up to 6-7 Hz.

Frequencies that differ by less than 2 or 3 Hz are not perceived as beats. They are perceived as being out of tune.

At higher frequencies, it is more difficult to distinguish beats and the two frequencies merge to give the listener an average frequency:

$$\nu_{average} = 1/2(\nu_A + \nu_B)$$

Note: Although beats were described for sound waves, the description and equations given apply to any wave, mechanical or electromagnetic.

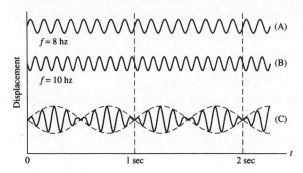

D. MUSIC

Initial and reflected waves superpose to produce standing waves in a medium with stationary nodes. The deliberate production of combinations and sequences of these standing waves that are pleasant to the ear is called music and is very subjective. Most musical instruments can be divided into two broad categories, strings and pipes.

Strings are instruments like guitars, violins, and pianos, where the source of the sound is a vibrating string that produces a compression-rarification wave in the air that is detected by the ear as sound.

The frequency of a wave produced by a string varies with the string's length, diameter, tension, and density. The relationship of frequency to these variables is summarized in the four **laws of strings:**

1. The law of lengths states that if the tension, density, and diameter of a string are held constant, the frequency is inversely proportional to the length and the change in frequency of a wave produced by the string with a change in the length of that string is given by:

   $$\nu_1/\nu_2 = \ell_2/\ell_1$$

2. The law of diameters states that if the tension, density, and length of a string are held constant, the frequency is inversely proportional to the diameter and the ratio of the frequencies of two strings with different diameters is given by:

   $$\nu_1/\nu_2 = d_2/d_1$$

3. The law of tensions states that if the length, density, and diameter of a string are held constant, the frequency is directly proportional to the square root of the tension on the string, and the change in frequency with the change in tension on the string is given by:

   $$\nu_1/\nu_2 = (F_1)^{1/2}/(F_2)^{1/2}$$

4. The law of densities states that if the length, tension, and diameter of a string are held constant, the frequency is inversely proportional to the square root of its density, and the ratio of the frequencies of two strings with different densities is given by:

$$v_1/v_2 = (\rho_2)^{1/2}/(\rho_1)^{1/2}$$

String Harmonics

Any string can be set in vibrational motion. However, to produce a standing wave, the tension in the string must be adjusted so that:

$$v = (F/\mu)^{1/2}$$

where v is the velocity of the wave in the string, F is the tension, and μ is the mass per unit of length of the string. The wavelength and frequency of the fundamental standing wave are related by $\lambda v = v$, so that:

$$v = (1/\lambda)(F/\mu)^{1/2} = \frac{v}{\lambda}$$

In most musical string instruments, the ends are fixed and the tension on the string is fixed. Waves reflected back from the fixed ends set up standing waves in the string. Since the amplitude of the wave is zero at the two fixed ends, they act as nodes. The distance between the nodes is the length of the string, ℓ, and the wavelength of the fundamental standing wave is 2ℓ:

$$\lambda = 2\ell$$

Overtones will be multiples of the fundamental:

$$v_n = nv_1$$

where n is an integer that identifies the harmonic.

$$v_n = (1/n\lambda)(F/\mu)^{1/2}$$

$$\lambda_n = \frac{2I}{n}$$

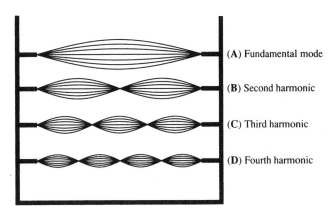

(A) Fundamental mode

(B) Second harmonic

(C) Third harmonic

(D) Fourth harmonic

Vibrational motion of the first four harmonics of a single string.

Pipes

Musical instruments that use pipes include organs and horns. In string instruments, the string vibrates first; the energy of the wave produced is then transferred to the molecules of the air and the compression-rarification air waves strike the ear. In pipes, the column of air inside the pipe is analogous to the string. It vibrates first and then transfers its energy to the air molecules outside of the pipe. A closed end of a pipe acts like a node. The wave is reflected from its fixed boundary. In contrast, an open end of a pipe acts as an antinode, a point of maximum amplitude for the wave. Because of this difference, the fundamental frequency of a closed-end pipe will be different from that of an otherwise identical open-end pipe.

Open pipes are pipes that are open to the air at both ends. This produces an air column with free boundaries at the open ends because the air is free to expand out of the pipe. The longitudinal standing waves produced are analogous to those in strings except that the positions of all the nodes and antinodes are exactly reversed. The fundamental harmonic has antinodes at each open end and a single node in the center of the pipe; the wavelength is still twice the length of the pipe:

$$\lambda = 2\ell$$

All harmonics of the fundamental tone are possible in an open-end pipe.

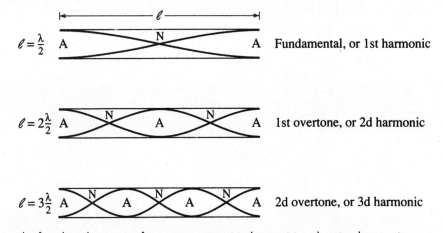

The first three harmonics for an open pipe. Nodes are N and antinodes are A.

Closed pipes are pipes with one closed end and one open end. The closed end provides a fixed boundary and the open end acts as a free boundary. A standing wave will always have a node at the closed end and an antinode at the open end. By definition, the distance between nodes is $\lambda/2$; the distance between a node and an adjacent antinode must be half this distance or $\lambda/4$. The fundamental wavelength must be four times the length of the closed-end pipe:

$$\lambda = 4\ell$$

This is twice the λ of the fundamental in an open-end pipe. Since the wavelength and the frequency of a wave are inversely proportional, the frequency of the fundamental tone in a closed-end pipe must be half that in an open-end pipe of the same dimensions.

Not all of the possible harmonics are allowed in the closed-end pipe. Standing waves occur only for odd (noneven) values of λ/4; therefore, only odd harmonics of the fundamental tone are produced in closed-end pipes.

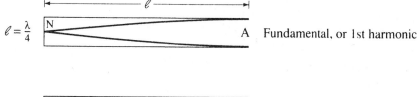

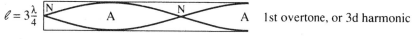

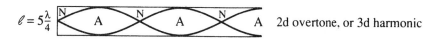

The first three allowed harmonics for a closed pipe. Nodes are N and antinodes are A.

PRACTICE PROBLEMS

1. The foghorn of a ship echoes off an iceberg in the distance. If the echo is heard 5.00 seconds after the horn is sounded, and the air temperature is −50.0°C, how far away is the iceberg?

   A. 200 m
   B. 750 m
   C. 825 m
   D. 900 m

2. What is the intensity, in W/m², of sound with a sound level of 20 dB?

   A. 10^{-12} W/m²
   B. 10^{-10} W/m²
   C. 1 W/m²
   D. 10 W/m²

3. What is the sound level of a wave with an intensity of 10^{-3} W/m²

   A. 30 dB
   B. 60 dB
   C. 90 dB
   D. 120 dB

4. A man drops a metal probe down a deep well-drilling shaft that is 3920 meters deep. If the temperature is 25°C, which is the closest estimate of how long it takes to hear the echo after the probe is dropped?

   A. 5.0 s
   B. 10 s
   C. 20 s
   D. 40 s

5. At 0°C, approximately how long does it take sound to travel 5.00 km?

   A. 15 s
   B. 30 s
   C. 45 s
   D. 60 s

6. If the speed of a transverse wave of a violin string is 12 meters per second and the frequency played is 4.0 Hz, what is the wavelength of the sound?

   A. 48 m
   B. 12 m
   C. 3.0 m
   D. 0.33 m

7. Two pulses, exactly out of phase, travel toward each other along a string as indicated below:

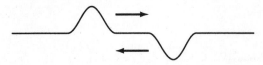

The phenomenon that occurs when the pulses meet is called

A. refraction.
B. reflection.
C. diffraction.
D. interference.

8. In which medium will the speed of sound of frequency 10^3 Hz be greatest?

A. air at 25°C
B. water at 25°C
C. gelatin at 25°C
D. iron metal at 25°C

9. If two identical sound waves interact in phase, the resulting wave will have a

A. shorter period.
B. larger amplitude.
C. higher frequency.
D. greater velocity.

10. A stereo receiver has a power output of 50 W at a frequency of 1000 Hz. If the frequency is decreased to 100 Hz, the output decreases by 10 dB. What is the power output at 10 Hz?

A. 5.0 W
B. 10 W
C. 50 W
D. 100 W

11. What is the speed of a longitudinal sound wave in a steel rod if Young's modulus for steel is 20×10^{10} N/m^2 and the density of steel is 8×10^3 kg/m^3?

A. 4.0×10^{-8} m/s
B. 5.0×10^3 m/s
C. 25×10^6 m/s
D. 2.5×10^9 m/s

12. If two frequencies emitted from two sources are 48 and 54 vibrations per second, how many beats per second are heard?

A. 3
B. 6
C. 9
D. 12

13. The frequency heard by a detector is higher than the frequency emitted by the source. Which of the statements below must be true?

A. The source must be moving away from the detector.
B. The source must be moving toward the detector.
C. The source and the detector may be moving toward each other.
D. The source may be moving away from the source.

ANSWER KEY

1. B	3. C	5. A	7. D	8. D	9. B	10. A	11. B	12. B	13. C
2. B	4. D	6. C						

ANSWERS AND EXPLANATIONS

1. **The correct answer is (B).** The normal speed of sound at 0°C in air is about 330 meters/second. The speed changes by 0.6 m/s for each change of 1°C; therefore, the speed in air at −50°C is:

   330 m/s − 50°C(0.6 m/s°C) = 300 m/s

   In 5 seconds the sound wave traveled a round trip distance of (300 m/s)(5 s) = 1500 m; therefore, the iceberg is 1500/2 = 750 meters away.

2. **The correct answer is (B).** $\beta = 10 \log I/I_0$. The threshold of hearing is 0 dB = 10^{-12} W/m². Since each 10 dB represents an order of magnitude of intensity, 20 dB is two orders of magnitude (100×) greater than the threshold intensity. This gives it an intensity of 10^{-10} W/m².

3. **The correct answer is (C).** $\beta = 10 \log I/I_0 = 10 \log (10^{-3}/10^{-12}) = 10 \log 10^9 = 10 \times 9 = 90$ dB

4. **The correct answer is (D).** There are two parts to the problem. First, you must find the length of time it takes the probe to fall to the bottom of the shaft, and then you need the amount of time it takes sound to travel back that same distance:

   $$y = \frac{1}{2}gt^2 \text{ therefore } t = (2y/g)^{\frac{1}{2}}$$
   $$t = \left(\frac{2.3920m}{9.8m/s^2}\right)^{\frac{1}{2}} = (800s^2)^{\frac{1}{2}} = 28.35$$

   The probe free falls for 28 seconds before hitting the bottom of the well.

   Next, adjust the speed of sound in air for the 25°C. The velocity of sound in air increases by about 0.6 m/s°C. At 25°C, the speed of sound is 15 degrees faster, or 345 m/s. At that speed it takes about 11 seconds for the sound to return up the shaft. The total round-trip time is 28.3 + 11 = 39.3 seconds. This makes D the closest choice. Actually, once the free-fall time of 28 seconds is determined, choices A, B, and C can be eliminated because they are less than the free-fall time alone.

5. **The correct answer is (A).** At 0°C the speed of sound in air is 330 m/s; therefore, it takes:

   $(5.00 \times 10^3 \text{ m})/(330 \text{ m/s}) \sim 15$ s

6. **The correct answer is (C).** The speed is equal to the product of the velocity and wavelength, therefore:

   $\lambda = v/v = (12 \text{ m/s})/4 \text{ s}^{-1} = 3$ meters

7. **The correct answer is (D).** By definition, two waves propagated through the same medium can be superposed to produce interference patterns.

8. **The correct answer is (D).** The frequency of the sound wave is not relevant to the question. Sound waves are fastest in solids. The stiffer the solid, the faster the propagation.

9. **The correct answer is (B).** Two waves are in phase if their crests and troughs coincide. The amplitude of the resulting wave is the algebraic sum of the amplitudes of the two waves being superposed at that point. Therefore, the amplitude is doubled.

10. **The correct answer is (A).** Choices C and D can be eliminated immediately. You must have less power than at 1000 Hz in order to get the decrease in sound level. The intensity is directly proportional to the power. A 10-dB drop is a drop of one order of magnitude. Decreasing 50 W by an order of magnitude gives 5 W.

11. **The correct answer is (B).** The relationship between speed and Young's modulus is:

$$v = (Y/\rho)^{1/2}$$
$$= (20 \times 10^{10} \text{ kg m/s}^2)/(8 \times 10^3 \text{ kg/m}^3)^{1/2}$$
$$= (25 \times 10^6 \text{ m}^2/\text{s}^2)^{1/2}$$
$$= 5 \times 10^3 \text{ m/s}$$

12. **The correct answer is (B).** $v_{\text{beat}} = v_1 - v_2 = 54 - 48 = 6$ beats

13. **The correct answer is (C).** This is the Doppler effect. Since the frequency is shifted to a higher value, the source and the detector must be getting closer together. This eliminated choices B and D. A is eliminated because it is not mandatory that the source be the device moving. The same effect is accomplished by holding the source steady and moving the detector toward it.

2.11 WAVES: LIGHT AND OPTICS

A. ELECTROMAGNETIC RADIATION

Electromagnetic radiation, EMR, has the following properties:

1. EMR can be transmitted through a vacuum with a constant speed. Unlike mechanical waves that require the presence of a physical medium, the radiant energy of heat, light, and electricity can be propagated through free space (a vacuum) in the form of electromagnetic waves.

2. The energy of an electromagnetic wave is equally divided between an electric field and a mutually perpendicular magnetic field. Both fields are perpendicular to the direction of propagation; therefore, all electromagnetic waves are transverse waves.

3. All EMR waves travel through a vacuum with the same speed, $c = 3.00 \times 10^8$ m/s, called the speed of light.

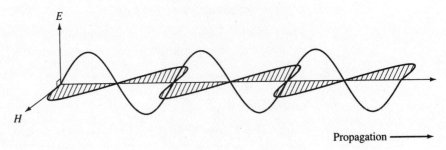

Direction of propagation of a wave along with its mutually perpendicular electric, *E*, and magnetic, *H*, fields.

Planck's Equation

The energy in the electromagnetic spectrum can be transmitted as waves or as equivalent particles called photons. A photon is a massless particle that represents a discrete quantity of energy, called a quantum of energy.

The amount of energy carried by the photon is related to the frequency or the wavelength of the electromagnetic radiation by Planck's equation:

$$E = h\nu = hc/\lambda$$

where $h = 6.63 \times 10^{-34}$ J s (called Planck's constant) and $c = 3.00 \times 10^8$ m/s is the speed of light in a vacuum.

Polarization

All electromagnetic radiation is propagated as transverse waves that travel radially outward in all directions from their source. Because the waves are transverse, they can oscillate along any of an infinite number of planes perpendicular to the line of propagation.

An unpolarized wave is one whose direction of oscillation changes randomly with time. Unpolarized waves can be polarized.

A polarized wave oscillates in only one plane. By convention, the direction of polarization is the direction of the electric field vector. Light that oscillates only in one plane is called plane polarized light.

A polarizer is a device or substance that selects only one of the possible planes and blocks all others. Polarization can only apply to transverse waves because longitudinal waves have no oscillations perpendicular to the line of propagation.

Spectral Regions

Electromagnetic radiation cannot be observed directly. In order to be detected and measured, EMR must interact with matter and change some observable property of the matter. That is, in the interaction the EMR energy is transformed into some other energy form such as kinetic, potential, thermal, chemical, electrical, etc., that can be observed and measured.

The range of energies of the electromagnetic waves make up the **electromagnetic spectrum,** which is subdivided into various regions whose energies are associated with specific types of interactions with matter.

1. **Power Wave Region**
   These waves are produced by electric generators and transferred along transmission lines. These are low-energy, long-wavelength, low-frequency waves.

2. **Radio Wave Region**
   This covers a large region of the spectrum with wavelengths of a few millimeters to approximately 10 kilometers. These include the waves that carry television and radio signals. It also includes a region called the microwave region.

   Microwave Region
   This region is at the high-energy end of the radio wave region. Both radio

and microwaves can penetrate the human body and produce local heating. At the molecular level, microwaves cause molecules to change their rates of rotation.

3. **Infrared Region**

This region starts just above the region typically used for communications (radio and microwave regions) and extends up to the low-energy end of the visible region (red light). Humans perceive IR radiation as heat. At the molecular level, IR radiation produces molecular vibrations.

4. **Optical Region**

This region has three major subdivisions: the near infrared, the visible, and the near ultraviolet. Energies in this region cause electrons to change orbitals.

5. **Ultraviolet Region**

These rays and rays of higher energy cause the ionization of atoms. This is also the region responsible for suntans and skin cancer.

6. **X-rays**

These are produced when a metal target is hit by electrons accelerated through a high voltage drop. As the electron beam approaches the atoms in the metal lattice, it is repelled by the atom's electron cloud and decelerates. Most of the kinetic energy lost by the electrons in the beam goes into increasing the thermal energy of the lattice atoms. However, approximately 1% is emitted in the form of x-rays.

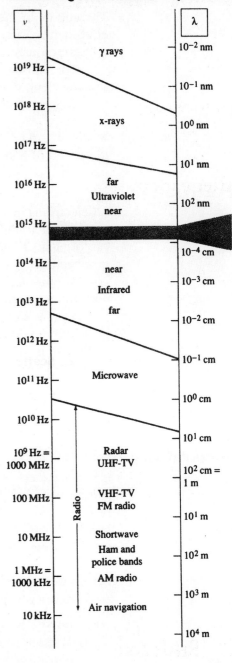

Electromagnetic Radiation Spectrum

X-rays are used to expose photographic materials. Soft tissues are more transparent to x-rays than bone; therefore, bones tend to absorb the radiation and cast their shadow on the film.

7. **Gamma Rays**

These are high-energy waves produced by radioactive nuclei.

Note: The boundaries between regions of the electromagnetic spectrum are not sharp.

B. THE VISUAL SPECTRUM

The **visual spectrum** is the region of the optical spectrum that can be perceived by the human eye. Each component wavelength is called a color. When all the colors are present in a sample, the individual components cannot be distinguished and "white light" is produced.

Light Rays

For convenience, a light wave is represented by a straight line coincident with the direction of propagation of the wave.

Attenuation of Wave Energy

When light passes from a vacuum into any material medium, or when it comes to a boundary between two media, its energy is attenuated (becomes progressively weaker) because of two effects:

1. **Absorption**
   Part of the light energy is absorbed by molecules of the physical medium it travels through and by the molecules of a boundary that it impinges upon. Generally the thermal energy of the molecules is raised by this process.

2. **Scattering**
   Part of the light energy is scattered in all directions at the boundary. A beam originally traveling in one direction is scattered along many directions. Since the total energy is constant, it is now split among a number of beams so that no scattered beam is as intense as the original beam.

The intensity of reflected light at a boundary between two media depends on the indices of refraction, n_1 and n_2, of the two media. In going from medium 1 to medium 2, the ratio of the intensity of the reflected light, I_r, to the intensity of the incident light, I_i, is given by:

$$I_r/I_i = [(n_2 - n_1)/(n_2 + n_1)]^2$$

This equation is valid for light rays that are normal to the surface (angle of incidence = 0°). Light loses about 4% of its intensity each time it is reflected from a mirror.

C. REFLECTION

Reflection occurs when light rays reach a boundary between two media and are bounced back into the original medium. The rays approaching the boundary are called the incident rays. Those bouncing off the surface are called reflected rays.

Regular reflection occurs when each incident ray produces a single reflected ray. Scattering is negligible.

Specular surfaces are highly polished boundaries that cause regular reflection of incident light. The image of a luminous object produced by a specular surface is sharp. A mirror is an example of a specular surface.

The **laws of reflection** state that:

1. The angle of incidence is equal to the angle of reflection. These angles are typically measured with respect to the normal, which is a line perpendicular to the surface at the point where the light ray strikes the surface.

2. The incident ray, the reflected ray, and the normal to the reflecting surface all lie in the same plane.

The Laws of Reflection

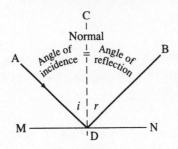

Plane surface

Normal reflection occurs when the specular surface is a smooth plane. Normals at different points on the surface are parallel with each other. Therefore, parallel incident rays will produce parallel reflection rays.

Diffusion occurs if the surface is not a smooth plane. That is, normals to various points will not all be parallel with each other. Therefore, parallel incident rays will produce nonparallel reflection rays.

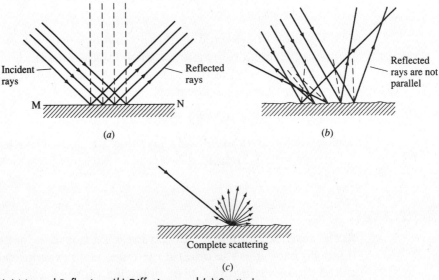

(a) Normal Reflection, (b) Diffusion, and (c) Scattering

Images Formed by Reflection

When rays from an object are reflected, they form an image of the object. The brain interprets the position of the image by following the lines of the reflected rays back to some point where they converge or appear to converge.

A **real image** is formed by rays that actually pass through the image point. The image point is the location of the image.

1. A real image can be projected onto a screen placed at the image point.

2. Real images are inverted with respect to the object.

3. Real images can either be magnified or reduced with respect to the size of the object.

A **virtual image** occurs when rays appear to diverge from the image point. The eye follows the diverging rays backward and extrapolates them to the point where they appear to meet (converge). The rays do not actually pass through the image point.

1. Virtual images cannot be projected on a screen.

2. Virtual images are erect with respect to the object.

3. Virtual images can be enlarged or reduced in size with respect to the size of the object.

Plane mirrors are flat reflecting surfaces. The image of an object in front of a plane mirror appears to be behind the mirror. Plane mirrors form virtual images because the image point is "behind" the mirror. The reflected rays never actually pass through the image point. They are reflected at the mirror surface.

Images formed by plane mirrors:

1. are virtual

2. are erect

3. are the same size as the object

4. appear as far behind the mirror as the object is in front of the mirror

5. are reversed left to right

Spherical mirrors have a curved reflecting surface.

The **center of curvature, C,** is the center of the sphere of which the mirror forms part of the surface. The radius of the sphere is called the radius of curvature, R.

The **aperture** is the portion of the sphere making up the mirror.

The **vertex, V,** is the geometric center of the mirror. This point lies within the body of the mirror, not on its surface.

The **principal axis** is the diameter of the sphere that passes from the center of curvature through the vertex.

A **normal, N,** to the surface is any radius drawn from the center of curvature to the point of incidence on the surface of the lens. The normal is perpendicular to a tangent to the surface at that point. For concave mirrors, normals are radii. For convex mirrors, normals are extensions of the radii beyond the outer surface of the sphere.

The **principal focal point, F,** is the point on the principal axis to which parallel incident rays converge, or appear to converge, after being reflected.

The **focal length, f,** is the shortest distance from the focal point to the mirror surface. The focal length of the principal focus is half the radius of curvature of the sphere.

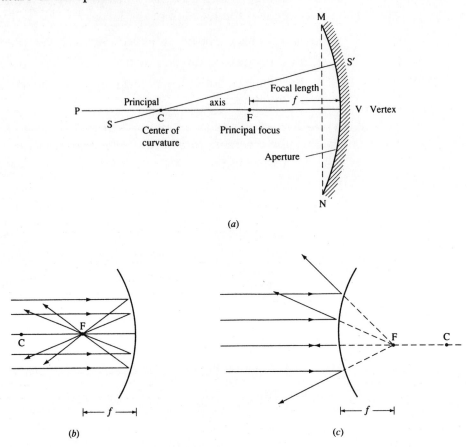

(a)

(b)   *(c)*

(*a*) Terms of spherical mirrors. Spherical surfaces and focal points for (*b*) a concave mirror and (*c*) a convex mirror.

A **concave mirror** has its reflecting surface on the inner surface of the sphere.

Concave mirrors are converging mirrors. The principal focal point lies in front of the mirror, so it has a positive focal length:

$$f = R/2$$

The image formed depends on the distance of the object from the mirror surface. There are six general cases, as illustrated in Figure 2. Light rays originally parallel to the principal axis, P, are reflected back through the focal point, F. Light rays that originally pass through the focal point are reflected back parallel to the principal axis. The point where the reflected rays intersect give the position of the resulting image.

Case 1
The object is an infinite distance away from the mirror and produces parallel incident rays. If these rays are parallel to the principal axis, they will converge at the focal point. The image will be a point at the principal focal point.

Figure 2

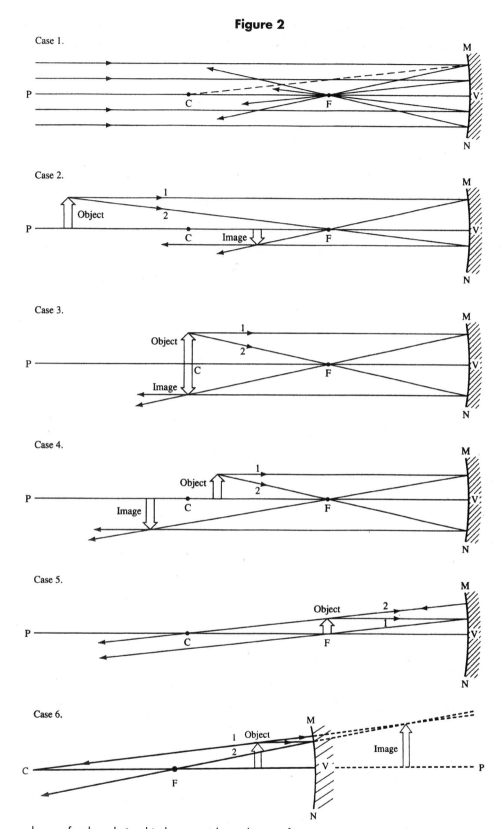

Case 1.

Case 2.

Case 3.

Case 4.

Case 5.

Case 6.

The six general cases for the relationship between object distance from concave mirror surface and the image formed.

Case 2

The object is at a finite distance beyond the center of curvature, C. The image is real, inverted, smaller than the object, and located between the principal focal point, F, and C.

Case 3

The object is at C. The image is real, inverted, the same size as the object, and located at C.

Case 4

The object is between C and F. The image is real, inverted, enlarged, and located beyond C.

Case 5

The object is at F. No image is formed. If the object were a point, all the reflected rays would be parallel.

Case 6

The object is between F and the mirror. The image is virtual, erect, enlarged, and located behind the mirror.

A **convex mirror** has its reflecting surface on the outer surface of the sphere. Incident rays that are parallel to the principal axis diverge on being reflected from the mirror surface.

Convex mirrors are diverging mirrors. The principal focus lies behind the mirror, so its focal length is negative:

$$f = -R/2$$

The image produced by convex mirrors is always virtual, erect, smaller than the object, and located "behind" the mirror between the vertex and the principal focal point. Image size increases as the object moves closer to the mirror but never becomes as large as the original object.

The mirror equation gives the position of the image formed. The equation works for both concave and convex mirrors:

$$1/f = 1/p + 1/q$$

where f is the focal length, p is the distance of the object from the mirror, and q is the distance of the image from the mirror. Remember that f is positive for concave and negative for convex mirrors.

The **magnification,** M, for any optical system, mirror or lens, is the ratio of the size of the image, S_i, to the size of the object, S_o:

$$M = S_i/S_o = -q/p$$

where q and p are the distances respectively of the image and object from the mirror.

If M is positive, the image is erect.

If M is negative, the image is inverted.

Spherical aberration is a common problem with spherical mirrors and lenses with large apertures. Parallel rays incident on the outer edges of the mirror are not reflected through the principal focal point and instead converge at points between F and the mirror surface. This decreases the clarity of the image. This aberration can be reduced or eliminated by:

1. reducing the aperture size of the mirror. Spherical aberrations are negligible for mirrors with apertures of 10° or less.

2. replacing the spherical surface with a parabolic surface.

D. REFRACTION

Refraction is the bending of light as it crosses obliquely from one medium into another. It arises from the difference in speed of light in different media. The slower the speed in a particular medium, the more the light will be bent upon entering that medium. The attenuation of speed in a given medium depends on the frequency of the light. The higher the frequency, the more the wave will be slowed.

Optional Aside

The speed of light in a transmitting medium is not the same as its speed in a vacuum. The attenuation of speed depends on a physical property of the medium called its optical density. The greater the optical density, the slower the speed of light in the medium. At the interface between two media of different optical densities, the speed of light changes and the light ray "bends" (changes direction on passing from one medium into the next). The optical density is measured by the refractive index of the medium.

Refraction Index

The **refractive index,** n, of a transparent substance is the ratio of the speed of light in a vacuum, c, to its speed in the substance, v:

$$n = c/v$$

The speed of light in air is essentially the same as it is in a vacuum, so the refractive index is sometimes defined as the ratio of the speed of light in air to that in the substance. Since v can never exceed c, n is always greater than (or equal to) one.

Snell's Law

The refractive index equation above requires that you know the speed of light in the substance in order to calculate its refractive index. This information, however, is not always easily obtainable. The physicist Snell defined the refractive index in terms of the incident and refractive angles a beam made with respect to the normal to the surface:

$$n = \sin i/\sin r = v_1/v_2$$

This is written in a more general form that allows you to compare two media:

$$\sin \theta_1 / \sin \theta_2 = v_1/v_2 = (c/n_1)/(c/n_2) = n_2/n_1$$

or

$$n_1 \sin \theta_1 = n_2 \sin \theta_2$$

Laws of Refraction

Refraction can be summarized in three laws:

1. The incident light ray, the refracted light ray, and the normal to the boundary between the two media all lie in the same plane.

2. The index of refraction for any given medium is a constant and independent of the angle of incidence.

3. A light ray passing obliquely between two media with different indices of refraction (optical densities) will be bent.

   - If the ray enters the medium with the larger index of refraction, the ray will be bent toward the normal because the light has been slowed to a greater extent.

   - If the ray enters the medium with the smaller index of refraction, the ray will be bent away from the normal because the light has been sped up.

   - For a transparent medium with parallel walls, such as a cube of glass, the path of a ray exiting from the glass back will be parallel to its path before entering the glass.

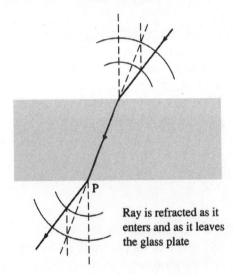

Ray is refracted as it enters and as it leaves the glass plate

Internal Reflection

When light reaches a boundary between two media with different optical densities, some of the light is reflected. The greater the angle of incidence, the greater the amount of light reflected at the boundary. For light in the medium with the greater refractive index, there will be a critical angle, θ_c, that produces an angle of refraction of 90°. Under these conditions, the light ray skims along the interface between the two media. If the angle of incidence exceeds the critical angle, the ray will be completely reflected at the boundary. This is called internal reflection. Snell's law relates the critical angle to the refractive index:

$$\sin i_c = 1/n$$

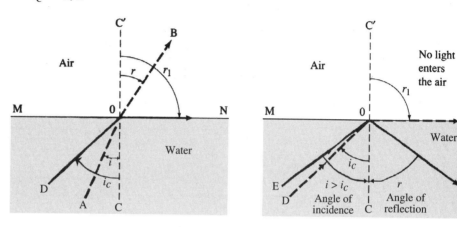

The critical angle and internal reflection.

Dispersion

Dispersion is the separation of ordinary white light into its component colors. It is a direct consequence of refraction. In a vacuum or in air, all the components travel with the same speed. When the light passes into a physical medium, light with different wavelengths will travel with different speeds and therefore get bent to different extents in a given medium. The lower the energy of the wave, that is, the longer its wavelength or lower its frequency, the less it is bent by a medium.

Prisms are solid triangles of transparent material used to disperse light. The material of the prism has a higher index of refraction than air, so light waves will be bent toward the normal on entering the prism and away from the normal on exiting the prism. Because of the angle between the two faces of the prism, the entering and exiting light rays are not parallel.

High-energy violet light is refracted to a greater extent than the lower-energy red light. The light dispersed by a standard prism will form a rainbow with red light on top and violet light on the bottom.

(*a*)

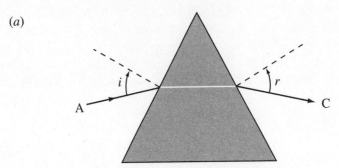

The path of a light ray through a prism

(*b*)

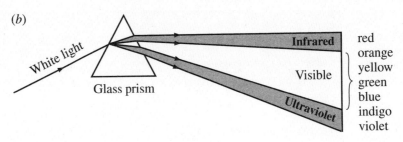

(*a*) Prism showing the relation between the entering and exiting rays. (*b*) The rainbow spectrum produced when white light is dispersed.

E. OPTICAL LENS

An optical lens is any transparent material that can be used to focus a transmitted beam of light to form an image of an object.

- Rays parallel to the principal axis will be refracted so that they converge or appear to converge at the principal focal point.

- The position of the principal focus on the axis depends on the index of refraction of the lens material. This is in contrast to spherical mirrors where the principal focus is midway between the mirror surface and the center of curvature.

- A lens can focus light because of the refractive properties of its material. Light rays go through two boundaries; one when entering the lens and the second when leaving the lens. Therefore, both surfaces of the lens must be described.

- Spherical lenses consist either of two curved, nonparallel sides, or one curved and one planar side. Each curved side will have a center of curvature.

The principal axis passes through each center of curvature for the lens. For a symmetrical lens, the radius of curvature is identical for both sides and the optical center coincides with the geometric center of the lens.

- Images formed on the same side of the lens as the object are virtual images. Images formed on the side of the lens opposite to the object are real images.

- There are two types of lenses, converging and diverging.

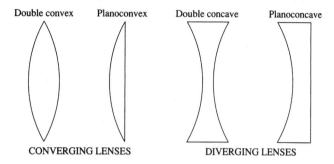

Converging Lenses

Converging lenses are thicker in the middle than at the edges. Double convex and planoconvex are examples of converging lenses. Parallel rays converge at the principal focal point. Because rays actually go through the focus, that focus is called a real focus. Real images form at a real focus. The real focus is on the opposite side of the lens from the object.

A Double Convex Converging Lens

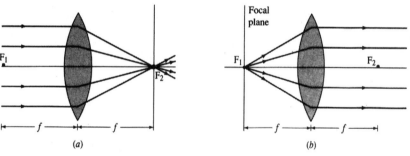

For converging lenses, the image produced depends on the location of the object. There are six cases, as illustrated in the figure on the following page. Light rays originally parallel to the principal axis of the lens are reflected through the focal point, F_2, on the opposite side of the lens. Light rays that originally pass through the focal point, F_1, emerge parallel to the principal axis on the opposite side of the lens. Light rays that pass through the intersection of the principal axis and the center of the lens pass through in a straight line. The point where the rays intersect give the position of the resulting image.

Case 1
The object is at infinity; the image formed is a point coincident with the real focal point.

Case 2
The object is more than two focal lengths away; the image is real, inverted, reduced in size, and located between F and 2F on the opposite side of the lens.

The Six Cases for Image Formation with a Converging Lens.

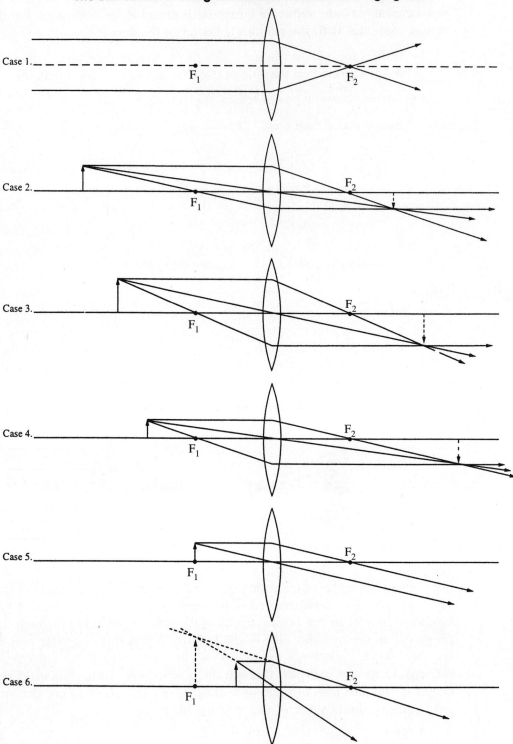

252

Case 3

The object is exactly two focal lengths away at 2F; the image is real, inverted, the same size as the object, and located at 2F on the opposite side of the lens.

Case 4

The object is between the principal and second focal point (between F and 2F); the image is real, inverted, enlarged, and located beyond 2F on the opposite side of the lens.

Case 5

The object is at the principal focus, F; no image is formed because the refracted waves are parallel to each other.

Case 6

The object is between F and the lens surface; the image is virtual, erect, enlarged, and located on the same side of the lens as the object.

Diverging Lenses

Diverging lenses are thicker at the edges than in the middle. Double concave and planoconcave are examples. Rays parallel to the principal axis are refracted and diverge on the other side of the lens. The eye follows the diverging rays and extrapolates to the point where they appear to converge. This is the principal focal point. Since no rays actually pass through this point, it is called a virtual focus. Virtual images are formed on the same side as the virtual focus.

Images formed by diverging lenses are always virtual, erect, and reduced in size.

Images Formed by Diverging Lenses

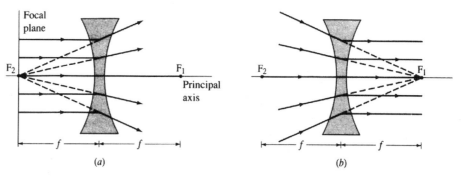

The **thin lens equation** is equivalent to the mirror equation and gives the position of the image formed with respect to the focal length and the distance of the object from the lens. The equation works for both concave and convex lenses:

$$1/f = 1/p + 1/q$$

where f is the focal length, p is the distance of the object from the lens, and q is the distance of the image from the lens.

- Remember that f is positive for converging lenses and negative for diverging lenses.

- If the sign of q is positive, the image formed is real. If the sign is negative, the image is virtual.

The magnification, M, for any optical system, mirror or lens, is the ratio of the size of the image, S_i, to the size of the object, S_o:

$$M = S_i/S_o = -q/p$$

where q and p are the distances, respectively, of the image and object from the mirror.

If M is positive, the image is erect.

If M is negative, the image is inverted.

Compound Optical Systems

Few optical instruments contain only a single lens. Most are made of a series of lenses. However, each lens in the system behaves independently, acting as if it were the only lens present. The effect of a given lens on light determines the character of the light rays (parallel, converging, diverging, etc.) that enter the next lens in the series.

PRACTICE PROBLEMS

1. Glass has an index of refraction of 1.50. What is the frequency of light that has a wavelength of 500 nm in glass?

   A. 1.00 Hz
   B. 2.25 Hz
   C. 4.00×10^{14} Hz
   D. 9.00×10^{16} Hz

2. Water has an index of refraction of 1.33. If a plane mirror is submerged in water, what is the angle of reflection if light strikes the mirror at an angle of 30°?

   A. less than 30° because the index of refraction for water is 1.33
   B. exactly 30°
   C. more than 30° because the index of refraction for water is 1.33
   D. no light is reflected because 30° is the critical angle for water

3. The index of refraction for water is 1.33 and that for glass is 1.50. A light ray strikes the water/glass boundary with an incident angle of 30.0° on the water side. Which statement is most likely true for its refracted angle in the glass?

   A. The angle of refraction is 26.3°.
   B. The angle of refraction is 34.7°.
   C. The angle of refraction is 30.0°.
   D. The angle of refraction is 60.0°.

4. Light is incident on a prism at an angle of 90° relative to its surface. The index of refraction of the prism material is 1.50. Which of the following statements is most accurate?

   A. The angle of refraction will be greater than 0° but less than 45°.
   B. The angle of refraction will be greater than 45° but less than 90°.
   C. The angle of refraction will be 0°.
   D. The angle of refraction cannot be determined from the information given.

5. White light incident on an air/glass interface is split into a spectrum within the glass. Which statement is most accurate?

   A. Red light has the greatest angle of refraction.
   B. Violet light has the greatest angle of refraction.
   C. Yellow light has the greatest angle of refraction.
   D. The color with the greatest angle of refraction cannot be determined from the information given.

6. A real object is placed 10 cm from a converging lens that has a focal length of 6 cm. Which statement is most accurate?

   A. The image is real, erect, and enlarged.
   B. The image is real, inverted, and enlarged.
   C. The image is real, erect, and reduced.
   D. The image is real, inverted, and reduced.

7. What is the focal length of a lens that forms a virtual image 30 cm from the lens when a real object is placed 15 cm from the lens?

   A. 10 cm
   B. 15 cm
   C. 30 cm
   D. 45 cm

8. What is the magnification of a lens that forms an image 20 cm to its right when a real object is placed 10 cm to its left?

   A. 0.50
   B. 1.0
   C. 1.5
   D. -2.0

9. The human eye can respond to light with a total energy of as little as 10^{-18} J. If red light has a wavelength of 600 nm, what is the minimum number of red light photons that the eye can perceive?

   A. 1
   B. 2
   C. 3
   D. 5

10. Which phenomenon occurs for transverse waves but not for longitudinal waves?

   A. reflection
   B. refraction
   C. diffraction
   D. polarization

ANSWER KEY

| 1. C | 2. B | 3. A | 4. C | 5. B | 6. B | 7. C | 8. D | 9. C | 10. D |

ANSWERS AND EXPLANATIONS

1. **The correct answer is (C).** The velocity of light in glass can be found from the definition of refractive index, $n = c/v$; wavelength and frequency are related to velocity by the general wave relation, $v = \lambda \nu$, therefore:

    $\nu = v/\lambda = c/n\lambda$
    $\quad = (3.00 \times 10^8 \text{ m/s})/(1.50)(500 \times 10^{-9} \text{ m})$
    $\quad = 4.00 \times 10^{14} \text{ Hz}$

2. **The correct answer is (B).** The law of reflection is independent of the medium involved. The angle of reflection is equal to the angle of incidence for normal reflection.

3. **The correct answer is (A).** Snell's law is:

    $\quad n_1 \sin \theta_1 = n_2 \sin \theta_2$
    $1.33 \sin 30° = 1.50 \sin \theta_2$

    Since $n_1 < n_2$, then $\sin \theta_1 > \sin \theta_2$. For $\sin 30° > \sin \theta_2$, 30° must be greater than θ_2, for which A is the only reasonable choice.

4. **The correct answer is (C).** Snell's law is $n_1 \sin \theta_1 = n_2 \sin \theta_2$. Since the incident rays are normal to the prism surface, $\theta_1 = 0°$, and $\sin 0° = 0$. Since

    $0 = n_2 \sin \theta_2$
    $\theta_2 = 0$

5. **The correct answer is (B).** The higher frequency of a light sample, the greater its energy and the faster its speed through any medium. From Snell's Law the velocity and $\sin \theta$ with respect to the normal are inversely proportional. Of the choices, violet light has the highest frequency and therefore, the highest velocity, and therefore, the greatest angle of refraction.

6. **The correct answer is (B).** The object is between one and two focal lengths from the converging lens; therefore, the image produced must be real, inverted, and enlarged.

7. **The correct answer is (C).** The distance is given by the thin lens equation, $1/f = 1/p + 1/q$. Since the image formed is virtual, the sign of q is negative. Therefore:

    $1/f = 1/p - 1/q = 1/15 - 1/30 = 1/30$

    $f = 30 \text{ cm}$

8. **The correct answer is (D).** Magnification is given by $M = -q/p = -20 \text{ cm}/10 \text{ cm} = -2.0$. The sign of q is positive because the image is real. The negative value of M means the image is inverted.

9. **The correct answer is (C).** $E = hc/\lambda = (6.63 \times 10^{-34} \text{ J s})(3.00 \times 10^8 \text{ m/s})/(600 \times 10^{-9} \text{ m}) = 3.31 \times 10^{-19} \text{ J}$. This is the energy of each red photon. The number of such photons needed to produce a total of 10^{-18} J of energy is:

    $(10^{-18} \text{ J})/(3.31 \times 10^{-19} \text{ J/photon}) \sim 3 \text{ photons}$

10. **The correct answer is (D).** Polarization can only occur with transverse waves because the motion must be perpendicular to the direction of propagation.

2.12 ELECTROSTATICS

A. ELECTRIC CHARGE

The fundamental unit of **electric charge,** e, is a scalar quantity with magnitude:

$$e = 1.6 \times 10^{-19} \, C = 1 \, esu$$

where esu is the abbreviation for electrostatic unit. In the SI system, the unit of electrical charge is the coulomb, C, defined as the total charge on a specific number of electrons:

$$1 \, C = 6.25 \times 10^{18} \, e^-$$

The whole charge on a body is given by the symbol q. It is an integer multiple, n, of the unit of electric charge:

$$q = ne$$

Electric charge is either positive or negative:

- The **proton,** p, carries the fundamental unit of positive charge, $+e$.

- The **electron,** e^-, carries the fundamental unit of negative charge, $-e$.

Do not confuse the symbol for electric charge, e, with the very similar symbol for the subatomic particle, the electron, e^- or $-_1^0 e$.

- **Ions** are atoms or molecules with a **net charge q.** The net charge on a body is the difference between the total positive charge (total number of protons) and the total negative charge (total number of electrons).

- **Electrification** is any process that produces a net electric charge on a body. It is usually produced by friction between surfaces that causes the transfer of electrons from one surface to the other.

- **Point charge:** If the net charge on a body behaves as if it were concentrated at a single point on the body, it is said to act like a point charge.

Static electricity occurs when the electric charge is stationary, confined to a body, and not moving.

Electricity is electric charge that is in motion and is not stationary.

Optional Aside

The number of protons in a nucleus is fixed and cannot be changed. The only way to change the net charge on an atom (or on any body) is to change the number of electrons present.

If electrons are removed, there are more protons in the nucleus than surrounding electrons. The ion produced has a net positive charge and is called a cation.

If electrons are added, there are more surrounding electrons than there are protons in the nucleus. The ion produced has a net negative charge and is called an anion.

Conductors are substances through which electric charge is readily transferred:

- Most **metals** are good conductors because they have loosely held valence electrons that are easily removed and free to move through the lattice of the solid's nuclei.

- **Electrolytes** are ionic compounds such as salts that dissociate into their ionic compounds in solution. It is the ions formed that conduct charge.

Insulators are substances through which electric charge is not readily transferred:

- Most **nonmetals** are insulators because they hold their valence electrons too tightly to form free electron clouds.

- **Molecular compounds** are insulators because they do not have ionic components and remain neutral when they dissolve. They are **nonelectrolytes.**

- Salts that do not dissolve cannot dissociate into their ionic components.

- The net charge, q, on a body is the difference between the total positive charge (total number of protons) and the total negative charge (total number of electrons).

B. THE LAW OF CONSERVATION OF CHARGE

This law states that net charge cannot be created or destroyed. For every unit of positive charge produced (or consumed) in an interaction, a unit of negative charge must also be produced (or consumed) so that the algebraic sum of the electric charges in any closed system remains constant.

- For reactions that convert matter to energy (or energy into matter), equal amounts of positive and negative charge are produced (or consumed).

- For reactions that redistribute or separate charge, the algebraic sum of the electric charges must remain constant. The sum of the charges on the product side of the reaction must be the same as the sum of the charges on the reactant side.

C. ELECTROSTATICS

Electrostatics is the study of stationary electric charges. The principles of electrostatics are empirical (based on experiment rather than theory). They can be summarized by eight basic observations:

1. There are only two kinds of charges, positive and negative.
2. Opposite charges exert an attractive force on each other.
3. Like charges exert a repulsive force on each other.
4. A charged body can attract (or repel) an uncharged body.
5. Electric forces act over distance and do not require physical contact between the interacting bodies. The strength of the interacting force decreases with increasing distance between the bodies. This observation leads to **Coulomb's law.**

6. When charges are separated by contact, such as rubbing two bodies together (rubber and fur), equal amounts of positive and negative charge are produced. This observation is the **Law of Conservation of Charge.**

7. The charge on a uniform solid or hollow conducting sphere is uniformly distributed over the entire surface of the body.

   - There is no net charge in the interior of the body. All charge is confined to the surface of the body.

   - The sphere exerts no force on a charged particle placed at any point inside the sphere.

   - Although the charge is actually on the surface, the sphere behaves as if all the charge is concentrated at its geometric center.

8. If the body is not a uniform sphere, the charge is still confined to its surface but the distribution varies with the curvature of the surface. Charge tends to concentrate at sharp points on the body. For example, if the body is shaped like an egg, the charge will be more concentrated at the smaller, narrower end than at the large end. (The electric field intensity is larger at sharp points.) If the concentration of charge becomes great enough, it can spontaneously discharge, producing a discharge spark as it ionizes the gas of the air around the conductor.

Coulomb's Law

Coulomb's law of electrostatics states that the force of interaction, F, between two point charges, q_1 and q_2, that are at rest is directly proportional to the product of their charges and inversely proportional to the square of the distance, r^2, between them.

$$F = kq_1q_2/r^2$$

In the SI system, the proportionality constant k has the value:

$$k = 9 \times 10^9 \text{ N m}^2 \text{ /C}^2$$

- If the force of interaction is attractive, F_{att}, the charges are opposite in sign and the sign of F_{att} is negative.

- If the force of interaction is repulsive, F_{rep}, the charges are of the same sign and the sign of F_{rep} is positive.

Optional Aside

The numerical value of k in a vacuum is 8.987×10^9 N m^2/C^2 and in air it is 8.93×10^9 N m^2/C^2. Both are approximated as 9×10^9 N m^2/C^2.

Electric Field

An **electric field** is produced by a point charge and is the region of space around that charge which can exert an electric force on any other point charge that enters the region (or field).

The **electric field intensity,** E, at any point in the field is the vector quantity that measures the force exerted on a positive test charge placed at that point:

$E = F/q$

The SI units of E are the newton per coulomb, N/C.

Since F is a vector, E is also a vector.

- For a positive test charge, the force and electric field vectors are parallel.

- For a negative test charge, the force and electric field vectors are antiparallel.

Electric lines of force are used to represent the electric field surrounding a point charge or interacting between two or more point charges. The lines have the same direction as the field. By convention, the lines originate at and point away from a positive charge; they terminate at and point toward a negative charge. Force lines are drawn so that a tangent to the line gives the direction of the electric field at that point. The intensity of the electric field is proportional to the density of the lines; that is, the number of force lines per unit area normal to the field.

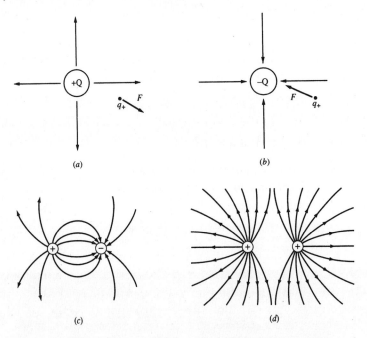

Direction of force, F, and field lines associated with (a) a positive and (b) a negative point charge. (c) Field lines between two oppositely charged bodies. (d) Field lines between two like charged bodies.

The **potential difference,** V, between two points in an electric field is the work required per unit charge to move a charge between the two points in the field:

$V = W/q$

The SI unit of potential difference is the volt, V, which is the ratio of one joule per coulomb:

$1\ V = 1\ J/C = N\ m/C$

1 volt is the potential difference between two points in an electric field if 1 joule of work is done in moving a charge of 1 coulomb between the two points.

- If work is done in moving a charge between two points, the two points are at different electric field potentials. The magnitude of the work done in moving the charge is the difference in the potential between the two points.

- If no work is done in moving a charge between two points, they must be at the same potential difference. They are equipotential. Since work is $W = Fd$, the potential can be expressed as:

$V = W/q = Fd/q$

- The electric field, E, can also be expressed in terms of the potential difference:

$E = F/q = (qV/d)/q = V/d$

The electric field intensity between two points is the ratio of potential difference between the points to their distance.

The term "potential gradient" refers to the change on potential difference per unit of distance.

Grounding

Potential difference at a point is a relative term and has meaning only with respect to the assigned value of some reference point. The Earth is considered to be a conductor with an electric potential arbitrarily assigned the value of zero. Since the Earth is so large, it acts as a limitless source of electrons; electrons can be added to or removed from the Earth without changing the planet's potential. If a conductor is connected to the Earth, electrons will move between the conductor and the Earth until the potential between them is equal. In other words, any conductor electrically connected to the Earth must also be zero potential. Such a conductor is said to be grounded.

An **equipotential line** is one where all points on the line are at the same potential energy.

An **equipotential surface** is one where all points on the surface are at the same potential energy. The potential difference between any two points on the surface is zero; therefore, no work is done in moving a test charge between two points on the surface. Equipotential surfaces are perpendicular to the lines of force.

PRACTICE PROBLEMS

1. What is the potential difference between point A and point B if 10 J of work is required to move a charge of 4.0 C from one point to the other?

   A. 0.4 V
   B. 2.5 V
   C. 14 V
   D. 40 V

2. How much work is required to move an electron between two terminals whose potential difference is 2.0×10^6 volts?

   A. 3.2×10^{-13} J
   B. 8.0×10^{-26} J
   C. 1.25×10^{25} J
   D. 8.0×10^{-13} J

3. Two electrically neutral materials are rubbed together. One acquires a net positive charge. The other must have

   A. lost electrons.
   B. gained electrons.
   C. lost protons.
   D. gained protons.

4. Which diagram best represents the electric field lines around two oppositely charged particles?

   A.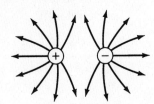

   B.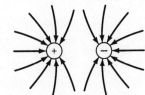

   C.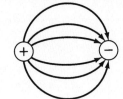

   D.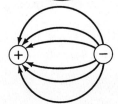

5. What is the charge on a body that has an excess of 20 electrons?

   A. 3.2×10^{-18} C
   B. 1.6×10^{-18} C
   C. 3.2×10^{-19} C
   D. 2.4×10^{-19} C

6. Two point charges, A and B, with values of 2.0×10^{-4} C and -4.0×10^{-4} C, respectively, are separated by a distance of 6.0 meters. What is the magnitude of the electrostatic force exerted on point A?

   A. 2.2×10^{-9} N
   B. 1.3 N
   C. 20 N
   D. 36 N

7. Two point charges, A and B, are separated by 10 meters. If the distance between them is reduced to 5.0 meters, the force exerted on each

   A. decreases to half its original value.
   B. increases to twice its original value.
   C. decreases to one quarter of its original value.
   D. increases to four times its original value.

8. Sphere A with a net charge of $+3.0 \times 10^{-3}$ C is touched to a second sphere B, which has a net charge of -9.0×10^{-3} C. The two spheres are then separated. The net charge on sphere A is now:

   A. $+3.0 \times 10^{-3}$ C
   B. -3.0×10^{-3} C
   C. -6.0×10^{-3} C
   D. -9.0×10^{-3} C

9. Which electric charge is possible?

   A. 6.02×10^{23} C
   B. 3.2×10^{-19} C
   C. 2.4×10^{-19} C
   D. 8.0×10^{-20} C

10. If the charge on a particle in an electric field is reduced to half its original value, the force exerted on the particle by the field is

    A. doubled.
    B. halved.
    C. quadrupled.
    D. unchanged.

11. In the figure below, points A, B, and C are at various distances from a given point charge.

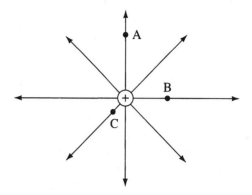

Which statement is most accurate? The electric field strength is

    A. greatest at point A.
    B. greatest at point B.
    C. greatest at point C.
    D. the same at all three points.

12. If the magnitude of the charge on two identical charged bodies is doubled, the electrostatic force between the bodies will be

    A. doubled.
    B. halved.
    C. quadrupled.
    D. unchanged.

13. The electrostatic force between two point charges is F. If the charge of one point charge is doubled and that of the other charge is quadrupled, the force becomes which of the following?

    A. $1/2F$
    B. $2F$
    C. $4F$
    D. $8F$

14. The graph that best represents the relation between the electrostatic force *F* associated with two point charges and the distance *d* separating the point charges is

A.

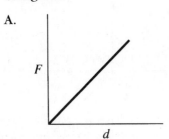

B.

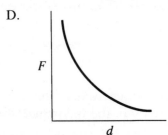

C.

D.

15. What is the amount of work done on an electron by a potential difference of 100 volts?

A. 6.25×10^{20} eV
B. 100 eV
C. 1.60×10^{-17} eV
D. 1.60×10^{-19} eV

16. Which of the following is a vector quantity?

A. Electric charge
B. Electric energy
C. Electric power
D. Electric field intensity

ANSWER KEY

1. B	3. B	5. A	7. D	9. B	11. C	13. D	15. B
2. A	4. C	6. C	8. B	10. B	12. C	14. D	16. D

ANSWERS AND EXPLANATIONS

1. **The correct answer is (B).** Potential difference between two points in an electric field is the work per unit charge required to move a charge between the two points:

   $V = W/q$ = joules/coulomb = volts

   $\quad = 10\,\text{J}/4.0\,\text{C} = 2.5\,\text{V}$

2. **The correct answer is (A).** Work is the product of the magnitude of the charge and the potential difference it is moved through:

   $W = qV = (2.0 \times 10^6\,\text{V})(1.6 \times 10^{-19}\,\text{C})$

   $\quad = 3.2 \times 10^{-13}\,\text{J}$

3. **The correct answer is (B).** Protons are fixed in the nucleus and cannot be transferred by friction. Electrons can be transferred by friction. Therefore, net charges are due to the transfer of electrons between two bodies. Conservation of charge means that if there is a net positive charge, one body must have lost electrons and the other body must have gained the electrons.

4. **The correct answer is (C).** Lines of electric force, by convention, originate on a positive charge center and terminate on a negative charge center.

5. **The correct answer is (A).** The elementary charge e is 1.6×10^{-19} C. Therefore, 20 electrons have a total magnitude of:

   $20(1.610^{-19}\,\text{C}) = 3.2 \times 10^{-18}\,\text{C}$

6. **The correct answer is (C).** Coulomb's law:

   $F = k(q_A q_B)/r^2$

   $F = (9.00 \times 10^9\,\text{N m}^2/\text{C}^2)(2.0 \times 10^{-4}\,\text{C})\,(-4.0 \times 10^{-4}\,\text{C})/(6.0\,\text{m})^2$

   $F = 720\,\text{N m}^2/36\,\text{m}^2 = 20\,\text{N}$

7. **The correct answer is (D).** From Coulomb's law, $F = k(q_A q_B)/r^2$, force is inversely proportional to the square of the distance separating the points. Decreasing the distance to half its original value means the force quadruples.

8. **The correct answer is (B).** This is an application of the law of conservation of charge. The initial net charge is:

   $(+3.0 \times 10^{-3}\,\text{C}) + (-9.0 \times 10^{-3}\,\text{C}) = -6.0 \times 10^{-3}\,\text{C}$

   The same net charge must exist after contact. The -6.0×10^{-3} C is evenly distributed between the two spheres.

9. **The correct answer is (B).** The fundamental charge is 1.6×10^{-19} C. All net charges must be integer multiples of this value.

10. **The correct answer is (B).** The electric field strength is the ratio of the force exerted on a unit charge in the field:

    $E = F/q$

    Therefore, F and q are directly proportional and linearly related.

11. **The correct answer is (C).** From Coulomb's law, force varies inversely with the square of the distance from the charge. The strength of the electric field at a point is the ratio of this force to the charge:

$$E = F/q = (k(q_1q_2)/r^2)/q$$

Therefore, E and r^2 are inversely proportional. The smaller the value of r, the smaller the value of r^2 and the greater the value of E.

12. **The correct answer is (C).** From Coulomb's law, $F = k(q_q q_2)/r^2$, force is directly proportional to the product of the two charges q_1 and q_2. If both charges are doubled, their product is quadrupled and so is the electrostatic force.

13. **The correct answer is (D).** From Coulomb's law, $F = k(q_1q_2)/r^2$, force is directly proportional to the product of the charges:

$$q_1q_2 = (2q_1)(4q_2) = 8q_1q_2$$

The product increases eightfold and so does the force.

14. **The correct answer is (D).** Force varies inversely with the square of the distance; therefore, expect a nonlinear (quadratic) decrease in F with increase in distance, d.

15. **The correct answer is (B).** The potential difference between two points is the ratio of the work done in moving the unit charge between the two points. Therefore, $W = qV$.

16. **The correct answer is (D).** A vector has magnitude and direction. The choices A, B, and C have magnitude only. The direction of the electric field vector is the same as the direction of the force.

2.13 ELECTRIC CIRCUITS

A. CURRENT

Current, I, is the rate of flow of charge through a cross-sectional area of a conductor per unit area. This flow can consist of either positive or negative charges. By convention, the direction of current flow is the direction in which the positive charges would move. This is opposite to the direction in which electrons flow.

Current = Charge/Time $I = Q/t$

The SI unit of current is the ampere, A. One ampere equals a flow rate of one coulomb, C, per second, s.

1 A = 1 C/s

Three conditions are required to produce an electric current:

1. A potential difference across part of the conductor. The potential difference or voltage or emf can be produced by a generator or by a battery. It provides the acceleration to the charges.

2. A closed path or circuit through which the charges can move. If the path is open, the flow of charge is stopped and a static charge will develop instead.

3. Carriers of charge that are free to move throughout the circuit.

Solid Conductors
The charge carriers are free electrons. Most metals are solid conductors.

Electrolytes in Solution
The carriers are the cations (positive ions) and anions (negative ions) produced by the dissociation of the electrolyte in the solvent.

Ionized Gases
Gases usually are poor conductors unless they are ionized. The carriers are ions and free electrons.

Direct Current

Direct current, dc, is produced if the direction in which the current flows is constant. Direct current is described by a line where all points are of the same sign.

Representation of Direct Current

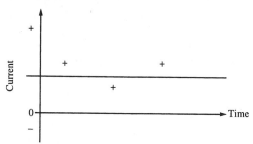

Alternating Current

Alternating current, ac, is produced if the direction in which the current flows reverses direction periodically. Alternating current is described by a sine wave that changes sign every half cycle.

Sine Wave Representation of Alternating Current

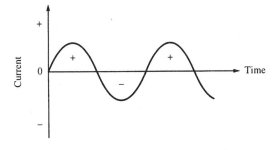

B. RESISTANCE

Resistance, R, is the opposition to the flow of charge provided by the material the current is flowing through.

The SI unit of resistance is the ohm, Ω, where $1\ \Omega = 1$ volt/ampere.

Optional Aside

Free electrons in a vacuum are accelerated by an electric field. In a conductor, however, the motion of the electrons is interrupted by frequent collisions with the fixed nuclei of the solid conductor. During the collisions, kinetic energy is transferred from the electrons to the nuclei, increasing their vibrational motion and, therefore, their temperature. Because the kinetic energy is transformed irreversibly into thermal energy, collisions are a dissipative process involving a nonconservative force.

Laws of Resistance

1. Resistance increases with increasing temperature for pure metals and most metallic alloys. Resistance decreases with increasing temperature for carbon, semiconductor materials, and most electrolytic solutions.

2. The resistance of a uniform conductor is directly proportional to the length, ℓ, of the conductor:

    R/ℓ = constant

3. The resistance of a uniform conductor is inversely proportional to its cross-sectional area, A:

    RA = constant

4. The resistance of a given conductor depends on the material of which it is composed.

Resistivity, ρ, summarizes the laws of resistance. The resistance of a uniform conductor is directly proportional to its length and inversely proportional to its area. The proportionality constant is the resistivity and depends only on the material and temperature of the conductor:

$R = \rho(\ell/A)$

The SI unit of resistivity is Ω m.

C. VOLTAGE

Voltage, V, is the potential difference across a conductor. It supplies the force that accelerates the charges so they flow.

The transformation of available energy into electrical energy is accomplished by either:

- a dynamic converter, which is a rotating machine such as a generator

- a direct converter, which has no mechanical moving parts, such as a cell or battery

Electrochemical Cells

Certain spontaneous chemical reactions, called redox reactions, involve the transfer of electrons from one reactant to another. If the two reactants are physically separated, the electrons can be transferred between them via an external circuit. The path of the current is from the reactant being oxidized, through the circuit, to the reactant being reduced. Current will flow until one of the reactants is used up. The cell must be replaced or be recharged by having the reaction reversed.

Electrodes

Generally, reactants are electrolytes, and their connections to the external circuits are called electrodes. There are two types of electrodes:

1. A cathode is the electron-rich electrode; it has a net negative charge and acts as a source of electrons, supplying them to the circuit.

2. An anode is the electron-deficient electrode; it carries a net positive charge and attracts electrons, receiving them from the circuit.

The flow of charge in a cell is unidirectional, so cells are a source of direct current. Electrons flow from the cathode, through the circuit, and into the anode. The circuit symbol for a single cell is:

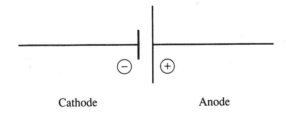

Cathode   Anode

Optional Aside

The cathode attracts the cations of the electrolyte. The anode attracts the anions.

Electromotive Force, emf ε

Electromotive force, emf, ε, of a source is the maximum energy per unit charge supplied by the source. If the circuit between cathode and anode is incomplete (open), the flow of current between them stops and the maximum potential difference, called the emf, develops across the cell. Therefore, V_{OC}, the potential difference or voltage across the cell when it is in an open circuit, is the emf of the cell:

$$V_{OC} = \varepsilon$$

The SI unit of emf is the volt, V.

The potential difference, V, across the source of emf in a closed circuit is less than the emf because of the internal resistance of the source:

$$\varepsilon = V_{OC} > V$$

Joule heating, Ir, is the heat produced by the collisions of the electrons with the nuclei and is equal to the product of the current, I, and the internal resistance, r. It occurs in all conductors, including the source of the current, the wires carrying the current, and any devices in the circuit that use the current. The thermal energy increases the rate of vibration of the nuclei around their equilibrium positions in the solid.

Internal resistance, r, is the direct result of Joule heating. As the nuclear vibrations increase in frequency and length, the chances of colliding with the electrons increases. The more an electron collides with the nuclei, the slower its progress through the conductor. That is, the resistance to the flow of charge increases as the conductor heats up.

Terminal Voltage

The irreversible or Joule heat produced by a current through a conductor produces the internal resistance. The potential difference across the electrodes or terminals of the cell is different from the emf of the cell:

$$V = \varepsilon \pm Ir$$

The terminal voltage, V, equals the emf, ε, plus or minus the Joule heat, Ir. The sign of Ir depends on the direction of current flow through the cell or battery.

1. If the cell is supplying the voltage, current flows through the circuit from its cathode to its anode. Then $V = \varepsilon - Ir$, and the terminal voltage is less than the emf. This is generally the case for all cells and batteries.

2. If the cell is being "recharged," current is being forced to flow from the anode, which is the reactant that gets reduced (gains electrons), to the cathode, whose reactant is normally oxidized (loses electrons), then $V = \varepsilon + Ir$, and the terminal voltage is greater than the emf.

3. If no current is flowing through the cell, no Joule heating can occur and $V = \varepsilon$.

A **battery** is a direct converter made up of two or more electrochemical cells connected to each other in series or in parallel or in a series-parallel combination. Batteries are therefore sources of direct current. The circuit diagram for a battery indicates the number of cells it contains. For example, the symbol for a three-cell battery is:

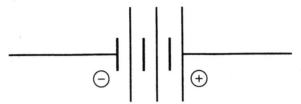

For a battery made of cells connected in a series:

- The emf of the battery equals the sum of the emfs of the individual cells.

- The current in each cell of the battery and in the external circuit are equal in magnitude to the current in the battery as a whole.

- The internal resistance of the battery equals the sum of the internal resistances of the individual cells.

For a battery of identical cells connected in parallel:

- The emf of the battery and of each cell is constant and equal to the potential difference across the external circuit.

- The current in the circuit is equal to the current in the battery, which is the sum of the currents supplied by each cell.

- The reciprocal of the internal resistance of the battery is equal to the sum of the reciprocals of the internal resistance of each cell.

D. Ohm's Law

Ohm's law of resistance states that in a closed circuit, the current, I, is inversely proportional to the resistance, R, and directly proportional to the voltage, V, of the circuit:

$I = V/R$

Note that the voltage used in Ohm's law is the terminal voltage for the source in a closed circuit. This is less than the maximum emf that occurs in the open circuit. The SI dimensions of the derived unit of resistance, the ohm, Ω, are:

$$R = V/I = (J/C)/(C/s) = (J\ s)/C^2 = (N\ m\ s)/C^2 = (kg\ m^2\ s)/(s^2\ C^2)$$
$$= (kg\ m^2/C^2\ s) = \Omega$$

1. For individual components of a circuit, R_i, V_i, and I_i are the variables.

2. Any set of components in a circuit can be replaced by a single equivalent component, and the symbols for the variables are R_{eq}, V_{eq}, and I_{eq}.

3. For the complete circuit, the total equivalent values are given as R_{tot}, V_{tot}, and I_{tot}.

E. Circuit Diagram

A circuit diagram shows the closed path available for the current to flow through.

Electric current is a mechanism for transmitting energy. A closed conducting path or loop is required if the energy is to be used outside of the source. Devices or circuit components that can use the energy to perform work are called loads or resistances.

The current at any point in a circuit is measured with an ammeter; the ammeter is always connected in series with the device it is monitoring. The circuit diagram symbol is:

 or Ⓘ

The voltage at any point in a circuit is measured with a voltmeter; the voltmeter is always connected in parallel with the device it is monitoring. The circuit diagram symbol is:

Ⓥ

Series Circuit

A **series circuit** has only one conducting path available to the current.

Typical Series Circuit

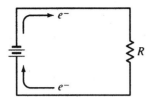

1. *Current*

   Since all current must go over the same path, its value is constant at all points in the circuit:

   $$I_{tot} = I_i$$

   The current flowing through any individual component, I_i, must be the same as the total current in the path.

2. *Voltage*

   The total voltage in the circuit is equal to the applied emf (voltage source). This is equal to the algebraic sum of the individual voltage drops across each device in the circuit:

   $$V_{tot} = emf = \Sigma\ V_i$$

3. *Resistance*

   The total resistance in the circuit is the algebraic sum of the individual components:

   $$R_{tot} = \Sigma\ R_i$$

Note: Devices in a series circuit should be rated to operate at the same current.

Parallel Circuit

A **parallel circuit** provides more than one conducting path. The circuit has two or more components connected across two common points in the circuit, and this provides the separate paths for the current.

Typical Parallel Circuit

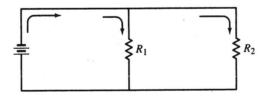

1. *Current*

   The total current is the sum of the currents in the individual branches and equal to the current supplied by the source:

   $$I_{tot} = \Sigma I_i$$

2. *Voltage*

   The potential difference is constant across all branches of the circuit:

   $$V_{tot} = V_i$$

3. *Resistance*

   The reciprocal of the total resistance is the algebraic sum of the reciprocals of the individual resistances:

   $$1/R_{tot} = \Sigma \, 1/R_i$$

   If only two resistances are connected in parallel, the equation can be rewritten as:

   $$R_{tot} = (R_1 R_2)/(R_1 + R_2)$$

   The total resistance is the ratio of the product of the two resistances over their sum.

Note: Devices in a parallel circuit should be rated to operate at the same voltage.

Compound Circuit

A **compound circuit** contains both series and parallel circuit sections. Each section can be resolved into its equivalent single R, V, and I value.

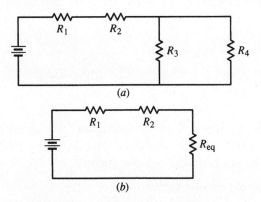

(*a*)

(*b*)

(*a*) Typical compound circuit. R_3 and R_4 are connected in parallel and can be replaced by the single equivalent resistance $R_{eq} = R_3 R_4/(R_3 + R_4)$. This resolves into circuit (*b*) where all resistances are connected in series so that $R_{tot} = R_1 + R_2 + R_{eq}$.

Kirchhoff's Laws

1. Kirchhoff's first law or branch theorem states that the algebraic sum of all currents entering and leaving any junction point in a circuit must be zero. It is based on the Law of Conservation of Charge.

2. Kirchhoff's second law or loop theorem states that the algebraic sum of all changes in potential around a closed circuit is zero. It is based on the Law of Conservation of Energy.

F. CAPACITOR

A **capacitor,** C, consists of two conductors (usually, but not necessarily, in the form of parallel plates) brought near to but not touching each other, separated by air, a vacuum, or an insulating material called a dielectric, and used to store electric charge.

The space between the two plates means the circuit is open at that point. If the capacitor is connected to a potential difference, then opposite static charges will develop on the two plates. Since the charges are at rest, each plate is an equipotential surface and a uniform electric field exists in the space between them.

Capacitance

Capacitance measures the ability of a capacitor to store electric charge. It is the ratio of the charge on either plate of a capacitor to the potential difference between them:

$$C = Q/V$$

The SI unit of capacitance is the farad, F, which equals one coulomb per volt:

$$1 \text{ F} = 1 \text{ C/V}$$

Capacitance is directly proportional to the area of each plate and inversely proportional to the distance separating them. For a parallel-plate capacitor, the proportionality constant is $[K/4\pi k]$, where K is the dimensionless **dielectric constant** of the insulator and k is the constant in Coulomb's law:

$$C = \frac{K}{4\pi k}\left(\frac{A}{d}\right)$$

A large capacitance is produced by:

1. a large plate area.

2. an insulator with a high dielectric constant.

3. a small distance between the plates.

Dielectric

A **dielectric** is the insulating material between the two plates of the conductor. The nature of the dielectric medium changes the capacitance.

The **dielectric constant,** K, is the ratio of the capacitance when the plates are separated by the insulator to the capacitance when they are separated by a vacuum:

$$K = C_{\text{diet}}/C_{\text{vac}}$$

K is a dimensionless number that ranges from 1 to 10 for most common dielectric materials.

The net effect of a dielectric between the plates is to lower the potential gradient of the electric field between the plates.

Capacitors in Circuits

In Series
The charge is constant and the voltage drop across each capacitor is:

$$V_i = Q/C_i$$

Therefore,

$$V_{tot} = \Sigma \, V_i = Q \, \Sigma \, 1/C_i$$

And the reciprocal of the total capacitance is the sum of the reciprocals of the individual capacitances:

$$1/C_{tot} = \Sigma \, 1/C_i$$

In Parallel
The voltage is constant and the individual charge on each capacitor is:

$$Q_i = C_i V$$

Therefore,

$$Q_{tot} = V\Sigma C_i$$

And the total capacitance is the sum of the individual capacitances:

$$C_{tot} = \Sigma C_i$$

G. ELECTRIC WORK, POWER, AND ENERGY

Work is required to move a charge Q through a potential difference V. The amount of charge moved is given by the product of the current and the time:

$$W_{el} = QV = ItV$$

Joules = coulomb volts = ampere second volt

The work is equal to the amount of energy given up by the charge in moving through the circuit. From **Joule's law,** the heat produced in a conductor is directly proportional to the resistance, the square of the current, and the time the current is maintained:

$$W_{el} = I^2Rt$$

Power is work per unit time:

$$P_{el} = W_{el}/t = IV$$

The equation gives the power dissipated or developed as a charge moves through a circuit.

Using Ohm's law, power can be expressed as:

$$P = IV = I^2R = V^2/R$$

The unit of power is the watt, W.

Electric Energy

Electric energy is the product of the power consumed by the device and the time during which the device operates:

$$E_{el} = Pt = W_{el}$$

The unit of electrical energy is usually given as kilowatt hours, kWh.

H. ALTERNATING CURRENT

In the United States, house current is 120 volts ac. The instantaneous or maximum voltage varies from $+170$ V to -170 V during each cycle.

The effective value equals the square root of the mean of the maximum value and is therefore called the root mean square or rms value. It is the maximum value divided by $2^{1/2}$.

For an ac source, the effective value is the number of amperes, which for a given resistance produces heat at the same average rate as the same number of amperes of steady, direct current.

Root mean square current, I_{rms}, is the effective ac current:

$$I_{rms} = I_{max}/2^{1/2} = 0.707 I_{max}$$

Root mean square voltage, V_{rms}, is the effective ac current:

$$V_{rms} = V_{max}/2^{1/2} = 0.707 V_{max}$$

PRACTICE PROBLEMS

1. In a solid metal conductor, electric current is the movement of

   A. electrons only.
   B. protons only.
   C. nuclei.
   D. electrons and protons.

2. What is the current in the circuit shown below?

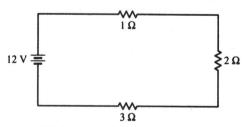

   A. 0.5 A
   B. 2.0 A
   C. 6.0 A
   D. 12 A

3. The ratio of the potential difference across a conductor and the current moving through the conductor is called the

   A. resistance.
   B. conductance.
   C. capacitance.
   D. electric potential.

4. For a circuit with constant resistance, which graph represents the relation between current and potential?

A.

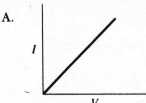

B.

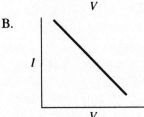

C.

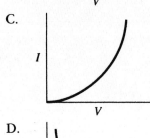

D.

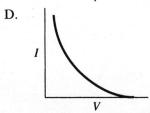

5. If the length of a conducting wire is doubled, the resistance of the wire will be

A. quartered.
B. halved.
C. doubled.
D. quadrupled.

Questions 6 and 7 are based on the following circuit diagram:

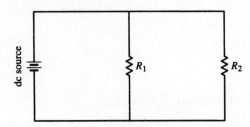

6. If R_1 = 2.0 Ω and R_2 = 6.0 Ω, what is the total resistance of the circuit?

A. 1.5 Ω
B. 4.0 Ω
C. 8.0 Ω
D. 12 Ω

7. If the potential of a dc source is 5.0 volts, and R_2 = 10 Ω, what must be the potential difference across R_2?

A. 0.50 V
B. 2.0 V
C. 5.0 V
D. 50 V

8. Current in an ionized gas sample depends on

A. cations only.
B. anions only.
C. free electrons only.
D. cations, anions, and free electrons.

9. The rate at which electrons pass a given point in a conductor is called the

A. resistance.
B. electric current.
C. charge.
D. potential difference.

10. If all the components of an electric circuit are connected in series, the physical quantity that is constant at all points in the circuit must be the

A. voltage.
B. current.
C. resistance.
D. power.

11. The current through a conductor is 3.0 A when it is attached across a potential of 6.0 V. How much power is used?

   A. 0.50 W
   B. 2.0 W
   C. 9.0 W
   D. 18 W

12. A 12 Ω load is connected across a 6.0 V dc source. How much energy does the load use in half an hour?

   A. 1.5×10^{-3} kWh
   B. 2.0×10^{-3} kWh
   C. 3.0×10^{-3} kWh
   D. 12×10^{-3} kWh

13. A current of 20.0 A flows through a battery with an emf of 6.20 V. If the internal resistance of the battery is 0.01 Ω, what is the terminal voltage?

   A. 1.24 V
   B. 6.00 V
   C. 6.40 V
   D. 31.0 V

14. Devices A and B are connected in parallel to a voltage source. If the resistance of A is four times as great as the resistance of B, then the current through A must be

   A. twice as great as that in B.
   B. half as great as that in B.
   C. four times as great as that in B.
   D. one fourth as great as that in B.

15. What happens to the resistance of a wire if its cross-sectional area is doubled?

   A. *R* is doubled.
   B. *R* is halved.
   C. *R* is quadrupled.
   D. *R* is quartered.

16. If the power produced by a circuit is tripled, the energy used by the circuit in 1 second will be

   A. multiplied by 3.
   B. divided by 3.
   C. multiplied by 9.
   D. divided by 9.

17. What must be the reading in the ammeter A for the circuit section shown?

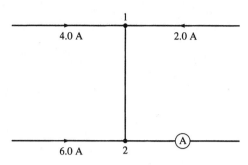

   A. 0 A
   B. 6.0 A
   C. 8.0 A
   D. 12 A

18. The two plates of a conductor are oppositely charged. What is the relationship among the intensities at the locations A, B, and C?

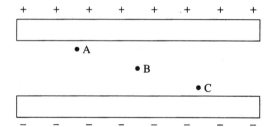

   A. Greater at A than at B
   B. Greater at B than at C
   C. Equal at A and C but less at B
   D. Equal at all three locations

19. What is the current in a wire if the flow of charge is 5.0 coulombs per 0.50 seconds?

   A. 1.0 A
   B. 2.5 A
   C. 5.0 A
   D. 10 A

20. For components connected in series, which quantity must be constant?

   A. Current
   B. Voltage
   C. Resistance
   D. Power

ANSWER KEY

1. A	3. A	5. C	7. C	9. B	11. D	13. B	15. B	17. D	19. D
2. B	4. A	6. A	8. D	10. B	12. A	14. D	16. A	18. D	20. A

ANSWERS AND EXPLANATIONS

1. **The correct answer is (A).** In a solid metal conductor, the positions of the atoms are fixed in the lattice and the electrons are free to move.

2. **The correct answer is (B).** The three resistors are connected in series so $R_{tot} = \Sigma R$ = 6 Ω. From Ohm's law, $V_{tot}/R_{tot} = I_{tot}$ = 12 V/6 Ω = 2 A.

3. **The correct answer is (A).** Ohm's law.

4. **The correct answer is (A).** Ohm's law. V and I are directly proportional and linearly related. R is the slope of the curve.

5. **The correct answer is (C).** Resistance is directly proportional to length and inversely proportional to the cross-sectional area of the conductor. If the area remains constant, then doubling the length will double the resistance.

6. **The correct answer is (A).** The resistors are in parallel so:

$$R_{eq} = R_1 R_2/(R_1 + R_2) = 12 \ \Omega^2/8 \ \Omega = 1.5 \ \Omega$$

7. **The correct answer is (C).** For a parallel circuit, the potential difference is the same across all branches of the circuit.

8. **The correct answer is (D).** Conductivity in solids is due to free electrons; in electrolytic solutions, it is due to ions; in ionized gases, it is due to both ions and free electrons.

9. **The correct answer is (B).** Definition of current.

10. **The correct answer is (B).** A series circuit has only one path for current so it must be the same at all points in the circuit.

11. **The correct answer is (D).** Power = VI = 18 W

12. **The correct answer is (A).** The energy used by a load is the product of the power it uses per unit time and the length of time it is operated:

$$E = W = Pt = V^2 t/R$$
$$= (6.0 \ V)^2 (0.50 \ h)/12 \ \Omega$$
$$= 1.5 \times 10^{-3} \ kWh$$

13. **The correct answer is (B).** The Ir drop across the battery is the Joule heat produced:

$$Ir = (20 \ A)(0.01 \ \Omega) = 0.20 \ V$$

Since the battery is producing current and not being recharged, the terminal voltage will be less than the emf by the Joule heat produced. This eliminates choices C and D immediately:

$$V = E - Ir = 6.20 \ V - 0.20 \ V = 6.00 \ V$$

14. **The correct answer is (D).** Ohm's law. For constant V, I and R are inversely proportional and linear. If R increases by four times, then I must be divided by four.

15. **The correct answer is (B).** Resistance is inversely proportional to the area; double the area and you reduce the resistance by half.

16. **The correct answer is (A).** Power is the rate of using energy, $W = Pt$. Work and power are directly proportional and linear.

17. **The correct answer is (D).** Kirchhoff's law says the current entering a junction must equal the current leaving the junction. The current entering junction 1 is 6.0 A, so the current entering junction 2 is 12 A and the current leaving 2 and going through the ammeter is 12 A.

18. **The correct answer is (D).** The intensity of the electric field between the plates of a capacitor is uniform.

19. **The correct answer is (D).** Current is the rate of flow of charge past a given point in 1 second.

20. **The correct answer is (A).** Ohm's law.

2.14 MAGNETISM

A. MAGNETIC FIELD AND MAGNETIC FORCE

Magnetic field, B, also called the **magnetic induction**, is a force field generated by a free-moving charged particle or the movement of electrons in a bar magnet.

Magnetic force, F_B, is the force exerted on a charged particle, q, moving with velocity, v, through a uniform magnetic field, **B**. It is defined by the vector cross product:

$$F_B = qv \times B$$

This means that the vectors F_B, v, and **B** are mutually perpendicular to each other.

The relationship can be determined using the **right-hand rule**.

- Point the thumb in the direction of v and the fingers in the direction of **B**.

- The palm of the hand will face the direction of F_B if the particle has a positive charge and it will face away from F_B if the particle has a negative charge.

The magnitude of F_B is given by:

$$F_B = qvB \sin\theta$$

where θ is the angle between the direction of the magnetic field and the direction in which the particle is traveling.

- If v and **B** are parallel to each other, $\sin\theta = \sin 0 = 0$ and no force is exerted on the particle by the magnetic field.

- If v and **B** are perpendicular to each other, $\sin\theta = \sin 90 = 1$ and the maximum force is exerted on the particle by the magnetic field.

The SI unit for magnetic field strength is the tesla, T, or newton/ampere-meter, N/Am. Smaller magnetic fields are measured in cgs units of gauss, G, where:

$$1 \text{ T} = 10^4 \text{ G}$$

The magnetic field strength at the Earth's surface is approximately 10^{-4} T or 1 G. That of an average electromagnet is about 1.5 T.

B. COMPARISON OF MAGNETIC AND ELECTRIC FIELDS AND FORCES

The association of F_B with the magnetic field, **B**, is similar to the association of the electric force, F_E, with the electric field, E. However, there are several important differences:

- The magnetic force is perpendicular to the magnetic field, while the electric force is always parallel to the electric field.

- The magnetic force can only act on a moving charged particle. The electric force can act on either moving or stationary charged particles.

- Because the magnetic force acts perpendicularly to the direction the particle is traveling, it does no work on the particle. The electric force is parallel to the motion of the particle and, therefore, does work in moving the charged particle.

- Electric charges are either positive or negative. Magnetic monopoles do not exist. A magnet always has both a North and a South pole. Lines of force go from the North pole to the South pole.

C. CIRCULAR MOTION OF A CHARGED PARTICLE IN A UNIFORM MAGNETIC FIELD

Because the magnetic force, F_B, is perpendicular to the velocity vector of the charged particle, F_B can act as a centripetal force, F_c, on the charged particle causing it to move in a circular path. Equating:

$$F_c = ma_c = mv^2/r$$

and

$$F_B = qv\mathbf{B}$$

gives the radius of the circular path followed by the charged particle:

$$r = mv/q\mathbf{B}$$

D. MAGNET FIELD ASSOCIATED WITH CURRENT IN A STRAIGHT WIRE

The current in a conducting wire produces a magnetic field. The field forms a series force line in concentric circles around the wire:

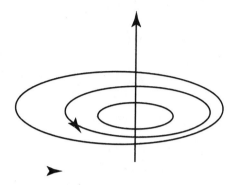

To find the direction of the field, apply the right hand rule:

- Point your thumb in the direction of the current in the wire.

- Curl your fingers around the wire. This is the direction of the magnetic field.

For two parallel wires:

- If they are carrying current in the same direction, the direction of the magnetic fields between them will be going in opposite directions and will attract each other. The wires will move toward each other.

- If they are carrying current in opposite directions, the direction of the magnetic fields between them will be going in the same direction and will repel each other. The wires will move apart.

PRACTICE PROBLEMS

1. Two wires, A and B separated by a distance d, carry currents i_A and i_B in opposite directions.

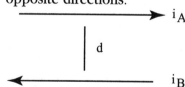

Which statement is true? The magnetic field, B, produced by the current in wire A in turn produces

A. a net force on both wire A and wire B.
B. no net force on either wire A or wire B.
C. a net force on wire A only.
D. a net force on wire B only.

2. Which derived unit below is equivalent to the SI unit for magnetic field strength, the tesla, T?

A. Nm/A
B. NA/m
C. N/Am
D. Am/N

3. What is the magnitude of the force acting on a particle of charge 1C traveling with a velocity of 1 m/s in a direction parallel to a magnetic field of 1 T?

A. 0 N
B. 0.5 N
C. 1 N
D. 2 N

4. A charged particle q moves horizontally through a magnetic field as shown:

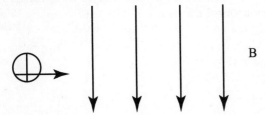

The force experienced by the particle will be:

A. $\perp$ to v and $\parallel$ to B
B. $\parallel$ to v and to B
C. $\perp$ to v and $\perp$ to B
D. $\parallel$ to v and $\parallel$ to B

5. Two ions, X^- and Y^{2-}, are analyzed in a mass spectrometer. They travel at the same velocity. Ion X^- has twice the mass of ion Y^{2-}. Which statement is true?

A. The radius of the path of X^- will be half that of Y^{2-}.
B. The radius of the path of X^- will be twice that of Y^{2-}.
C. The radius of the path of X^- will be four times that of Y^{2-}.
D. The radius of the path of X^- will be the same as that of Y^{2-}.

6. What is the expression for the momentum, p, of a charged particle going through a mass spectrometer?

A. $p = qr\mathbf{B}$
B. $p = qm\mathbf{B}$
C. $p = qv^2$
D. $p = qv\mathbf{B}$

7. Two parallel conducting wires carry current in opposite directions. When the wires are viewed looking down from the top, which statement is true?

A. The two wires will attract each other because both magnetic fields are counterclockwise.
B. The two wires will repel each other because both magnetic fields are counterclockwise.
C. The two wires will attract each other because one magnetic field is clockwise while the other is counterclockwise.
D. The two wires will repel each other because one magnetic field is clockwise while the other is counterclockwise.

ANSWER KEY

1. D	2. C	3. A	4. C	5. C	6. A	7. D

ANSWERS AND EXPLANATIONS

1. **The correct answer is (D).** The magnetic field produced by a current in a wire has no effect on the current that produced it. It effects the current in nearby wires.

2. **The correct answer is (C).** Solve $F = qv\mathbf{B}$ for **B** and substitute the units:

   $\mathbf{B} = F/qv = $ N/Cm/s $ = $ N/(C/s)m $ = $ N/Am

3. **The correct answer is (A).** $F = qv \sin\theta$. $\sin\theta = \sin 0 = 0$. The particle would feel the maximum magnetic force if it traveled perpendicularly to the field.

4. **The correct answer is (C).** From the cross product relationship $\mathbf{F} = qv \times \mathbf{B}$, **F**, v, and B are mutually perpendicular.

5. **The correct answer is (C).** $r = mv/q\mathbf{B}$ becomes $r_x = m_x/q_x = 2m_y/q_x = 2m_y/1 = 2m_y$ and $r_y = m_y/q_y = m_y/2 = (1/2)m_y$. Therefore, r_x is four times that of r_y.

6. **The correct answer is (A).** From $F_c = F_B$ we get $mv^2/r = qvB$. Momentum is $p = mv = qrB$.

7. **The correct answer is (D).** Use the right hand rule on each wire. Looking down each wire from top to bottom, the concentric circles of each magnetic field are going in opposite directions. Therefore the direction of the fields in the space between the wires points in the same direction.

2.15 ATOMIC AND NUCLEAR STRUCTURE

A. STRUCTURE OF THE NUCLEUS

Nucleons are the subatomic particles found in the nucleus: the protons and the neutrons. The number and ratio of the nucleons can only be changed by nuclear processes, not by general chemical reactions.

Note: Electrons are extranuclear particles because they are outside of the nucleus. The number of electrons associated with an atom can be changed readily by chemical processes.

The **atomic number,** Z, is the number of protons in the nucleus; it determines the identity and, therefore the properties, of the atom. All atoms of the same element have the same atomic number.

The **mass number,** A, is the sum of the number of protons and neutrons in the nucleus of an atom. The neutrons affect the mass of the nucleus but not any nonmass-related properties.

Isotopes

Isotopes are atoms of the same element that have different numbers of neutrons in the nucleus. Except for mass, the properties of isotopes of the same element are identical.

The **atomic weight,** AW, of an element is the average atomic mass of the atoms of the element and reflects the relative abundance of the isotopes of the element.

Nuclides are nuclear species. Isotopes are nuclides that have the same number of protons (and therefore the same atomic number) but different numbers of neutrons (and therefore different mass numbers).

The element symbol $^A_Z X$ represents a given isotope of a given element, X. The superscript gives the mass number and the subscript, the atomic number.

For example, the two isotopes of copper are $^{63}_{29}Cu$ and $^{65}_{29}Cu$. Each has 29 protons in the nucleus. ^{63}Cu also has 34 neutrons per nucleus, giving it a total of $29 + 34 = 63$ nucleons. Isotope ^{65}Cu has two more neutrons than ^{63}Cu.

Optional Aside

The nucleus contains almost all of the mass of the atom. The resting mass of an electron is $m_e = 9.11 \times 10^{-31}$ kg. It takes about 1876 electrons to equal the mass of one proton or neutron. Therefore, the contribution of electrons to the atomic weight is negligible. The heaviest known element is atomic number 109. Its 109 electrons are equivalent to less than 5 percent of the mass of a single nucleon.

Mass Defect

The AW of a given individual atom should equal the mass of all the protons and neutrons in the nucleus. The resting mass of a proton is $m_p = 1.6726 \times 10^{-27}$ kg and that of a neutron is $m_n = 1.6750 \times 10^{-27}$ kg.

$$AW = m_p(\text{number of protons}) + m_n(\text{number of neutrons})$$

The actual weight is generally less than this value. The difference is called the **mass defect.** The defect arises because energy must be expended by the nucleus to overcome the repulsion of the protons for each other. This energy is provided by converting some of the mass of the nucleus into energy. The transformation is given by Einstein's equation:

$$E = mc^2$$

Intranuclear Forces

Each nuclide is held together by three forces that act to overcome the repulsions due to the like nuclear charges:

1. The nuclear interaction is a very strong but short-ranged force that binds the nucleons together.

2. Electronic interaction is smaller in magnitude and increases in importance with increasing numbers of protons.

3. Weak interaction is the weakest of the three forces and is responsible for β-decay nuclear processes.

Note: There is a fourth force, the gravitational interaction, which is the weakest force and not significant in nuclear physics.

B. NUCLEAR PROPERTIES

About 1500 nuclides are known. Of these, approximately 300 are stable. The remaining 1200 are unstable (all nuclei above $Z = 83$ are unstable). They are called radionuclides.

Radionuclides are **radioactive.** They spontaneously undergo nuclear decay processes to form more stable nuclei. The decay processes can include emission or capture of particles or the emission of electromagnetic radiation.

Half-life, $\tau_{1/2}$, is the time required for half of a sample of a given radionuclide to undergo radioactive decay.

Decay is a random process; therefore it is not possible to predict if or when a given nuclide will decay. However, the half-life gives the probability that any particle will decay. The original nuclide is called the *parent*, and the new nuclide formed after the decay process is called the *daughter*.

If T is the period of the half-life, then at some initial time $t_0 = 0$, there will be N_0 nuclei. At time $t = T$ there will be only half as many of the original nuclei left, $N_0/2$. At $t = 2T$, there will be half of $N_0/2$ left, or $N_0/4$, etc.

The change in the number of parent nuclei present, ΔN, in a given time interval Δt depends on the number of nuclei initially present, N_0, and the **decay constant,** λ:

$$\Delta N = -\lambda N_0 \Delta t$$

The negative sign appears because the number of nuclei is decreasing, so ΔN is always negative.

The equation can also be expressed as

$$\ln N - \ln N_0 = -\lambda t \quad \text{or} \quad N/N_0 = e^{-\lambda t}$$

where $e = 2.718$, the base of natural logarithms. The last equation has the advantage that it clearly shows radioactive decay as an exponential process.

The decay constant is related to the half-life by:

$$\lambda = \ln 2/\tau_{1/2} = 0.693/\tau_{1/2}$$

A short half-life means a large decay constant. λ has the units of reciprocal seconds, s^{-1}.

The **activity** of a sample is the rate of decay, usually measured as disintegrations per second. It is the product of the decay constant and the number of nuclei present:

$$\text{activity} = \lambda N$$

The activity must decrease with time because N decreases with time.

Conservation of Energy and Mass
The total number of particles (atomic number and mass number) must remain the same.

$$^{238}_{92}U \rightarrow \,^{234}_{90}Th + \,^{4}_{2}\alpha$$

The Uranium-238 isotope undergoes decay, giving off the helium nucleus. The resulting element must contain the remaining protons and neutrons not emitted:

Mass # = 238 − 4 = 234
Atomic # = 92 − 2 = 90

α-Decay

α-particles are bare helium nuclei, $^4_2He^{+2}$, or $^4_2\alpha$, with a net charge of positive 2.

In α-decay, the parent nuclide reduces its nuclear size by two protons and two neutrons. The daughter is a new nuclide of a different element, having an atomic number two less than that of the parent. The element underwent a transmutation into a different element.

α-decay occurs in nuclides that are unstable because their nuclei are too large:

$$^{228}_{90}Th \rightarrow {}^4_2\alpha + {}^{224}_{88}Ra$$

Thorium is transmuted into radium. Conservation requires that the total number of protons and the total number of neutrons be identical on both sides.

Once formed, the α-particles readily react with any available electrons to produce neutral helium atoms.

α-particles have only short-range penetration and are easily stopped by a sheet of paper or by a few centimeters of air.

They are always emitted with the same kinetic energy.

Optional Aside

The strong interaction that holds nucleons together is short ranged, while the coulombic repulsion of protons toward each other has unlimited range (although it does drop off with the square of the distance between the interacting particles). As the size of the nucleus increases, the number of protons increases and the magnitude of the repulsive force becomes comparable and eventually exceeds the strong interaction. At this point, the nucleus is too large to be stable.

β-Decay

β-particles are high-speed electrons, $^0_{-1}e-$ or $^0_{-1}\beta$. They have greater penetration than a-particles and can penetrate thin metal sheets. They are stopped by a millimeter of lead or several centimeters of flesh.

β-particles are emitted with variable kinetic energies. In β-decay, a neutron disintegrates into a proton that remains in the nucleus and an electron that is emitted as the β-particle. The resulting daughter has a Z that is increased by one and an A that remains the same (because a neutron is replaced by a proton so the total number of nucleons is unchanged).

$$^{14}_6C \rightarrow {}^{14}_7N + {}^0_{-1}\beta$$

β-decay occurs in nuclei that have too many neutrons relative to the number of protons present.

Positron Emission

This is an analog of β-decay that involves emission of the electron antiparticle, the positron $_{+1}^{0}e$.

Emission of a positron is accomplished by the conversion of a proton into a neutron. Z decreases by one and A remains unchanged.

$$_{7}^{13} \rightarrow {}_{6}^{13}C + {}_{+1}^{0}e$$

This occurs in a nucleus that has too many protons relative to the number of neutrons present.

Neutrino, ν

The kinetic energy of beta and positron particles occurs because both processes can also form a massless, uncharged particle called the neutrino. It functions to carry away energy without a change in mass.

Since the actual decay process can form two particles, the decay energy can be divided between the pair in any combination. Therefore, beta and positron particles have variable kinetic energies when emitted.

β-decay can occur for either a free neutron or for one in the nucleus:

$$_{1}^{0}n \rightarrow {}_{1}^{1}p + {}_{+1}^{0}e + \nu$$

Positron emission can occur only for protons in the nucleus but not for free protons:

$$_{1}^{1}p \rightarrow {}_{0}^{1}n + {}_{+1}^{0}e + \nu_{\text{anti}}$$

(The energy particle released is actually an antineutrino.)

Electron capture is the equivalent of positron emission. Z decreases by one and A remains the same. A proton captures an electron and forms a neutron and a neutrino:

$$_{1}^{1}p + {}_{-1}^{0}e \rightarrow {}_{0}^{1}n + \nu$$

γ-Decay

γ-rays are high energy electromagnetic quanta or photons.

γ-rays are neutral and massless, which make them similar to X-rays. However, their wavelengths are typically less than 1/100 those of X-rays.

The emission of γ-rays reduces the energy of the nucleus without changing the number of protons and neutrons. This is the only decay process discussed that does not result in a transmutation of the nuclide.

γ-rays are much higher in energy than either α- or β-particles and, therefore, have greater penetration.

Fission and Fusion Reactions

The binding energy per nucleon that holds the nucleons together in the nucleus is greatest in intermediate-sized nuclei. Very light and very heavy nuclei have lower binding energies per nucleon ratios and are unstable.

In nuclear **fission**, a heavy nucleus splits into two lighter nuclei after absorbing a neutron. In the process, several other neutrons are emitted so that a chain reaction is established:

$$^{235}_{92}U + ^{1}_{0}n \rightarrow ^{140}_{541}Xe + ^{94}_{38}Sr + 2\ ^{1}_{0}n + \text{energy}$$

In nuclear **fusion**, two light nuclei fuse to form a single, heavier nucleus. The binding energy per nucleon of the daughter is less than that of the parents. The difference in binding energies is released in the reaction:

$$^{2}_{1}H + ^{3}_{1}H \rightarrow ^{4}_{2}He + ^{1}_{0}n + \text{energy}$$

PRACTICE PROBLEMS

1. The main force responsible for holding the nucleons together in a nuclide is

   A. coulombic force.
   B. nuclear force.
   C. electronic force.
   D. gravitational force.

2. In the nuclear equation below, X represents

   $$^{22}_{11}Na \rightarrow ^{22}_{10}Ne + ^{0}_{1}X$$

   A. an α-particle.
   B. a β-particle.
   C. a positron.
   D. a γ-photon.

3. What is the value of the mass number of the daughter nuclide in the equation below?

   $$^{34}_{15} \rightarrow ^{A}_{Z}S + ^{0}_{-1}e$$

   A. 14
   B. 15
   C. 33
   D. 34

4. What is the atomic number of the daughter nuclide in the following reaction?

   $$^{30}_{15}P \rightarrow ^{A}_{Z}Si + ^{0}_{+1}e$$

   A. 14
   B. 16
   C. 30
   D. 31

5. If $^{13}_{7}N$ has a half-life of about 10.0 minutes, how long will it take for 20 grams of the isotope to decay to 2.5 grams?

   A. 5 min
   B. 10 min
   C. 20 min
   D. 30 min

6. A certain radionuclide decays by emitting an α-particle. What is the difference between the atomic numbers of the parent and the daughter nuclides?

   A. 1
   B. 2
   C. 4
   D. 6

7. What is the difference in mass number between the parent and daughter nuclides after a β-decay process?

A. −1
B. 0
C. 1
D. 2

8. Which species has no net charge?

A. α-particle
B. electron
C. proton
D. neutrino

9. A nitrogen atom has 7 protons and 6 neutrons. What is its atomic mass number?

A. 1
B. 6
C. 7
D. 13

10. Which is an isotope of $^{182}_{63}X$?

A. $^{182}_{62}X$

B. $^{182}_{64}X$

C. $^{180}_{63}X$

D. $^{180}_{62}X$

11. Which reaction is a fission reaction?

A. $^3_1H + ^1_1H \rightarrow ^4_2He + energy$

B. $^{35}_{17}Cl + ^1_1H \rightarrow ^{32}_{16}S + ^4_2He$

C. $^{235}_{92}U + ^1_0n \rightarrow ^{140}_{54}Xe + ^{94}_{38}Sr + 2^1_0n + energy$

D. $^9_4Be + ^4_2He \rightarrow ^1_0n + ^{12}_6C$

12. In the following equation, what is X?

$^{14}_7N + ^4_2He \rightarrow ^{17}_8O + X$

A. a proton
B. a positron
C. a β-particle
D. an α-particle

13. What is the number of neutrons in $^{140}_{54}Xe$?

A. 54
B. 86
C. 140
D. 194

14. Radon gas, Rn, has a half-life of 4 days. If a sample of Rn gas in a container is initially doubled, the half-life will be

A. halved.
B. doubled.
C. quartered.
D. unchanged.

15. A radionuclide decays completely. In the reaction flask, only helium gas is found. The decay process was probably

A. β-decay.
B. α-decay.
C. γ-decay.
D. positron emission.

16. What is the half-life of a radionuclide if 1/16 of its initial mass is present after 2 hours?

A. 15 min
B. 30 min
C. 45 min
D. 60 min

17. The half-life of $^{22}_{11}Na$ is 2.6 years. If X grams of this sodium isotope are initially present, how much is left after 13 years?

A. $\dfrac{X}{32}$

B. $\dfrac{X}{13}$

C. $\dfrac{X}{8}$

D. $\dfrac{X}{5}$

ANSWER KEY

1. B	3. D	5. D	7. B	9. D	11. C	13. B	15. B	16. B	17. A
2. C	4. A	6. B	8. D	10. C	12. A	14. D		

ANSWERS AND EXPLANATIONS

1. **The correct answer is (B).** Definition.

2. **The correct answer is (C).** The superscript indicates $_1^0X$ is a massless particle. The subscript indicates it carries a $+1$ charge. This fits the description of the positron (the antiparticle of the electron).

3. **The correct answer is (D).** The mass number is A. Conservation of matter means:

    $34 = A + 0$. Therefore, $A = 34$.

4. **The correct answer is (A).** The atomic number is Z. Conservation of charge means:

    $15 = Z + 1$. Therefore, $Z = 14$.

5. **The correct answer is (D).** It will require several half-lives to get the amount involved. Choice A is eliminated because it is less than one half-life. Similarly, choice B is eliminated because it is exactly one half-life.

    In every 10-minute period, half of the nuclei will decay and, therefore, the mass will decrease to half its previous value. After the first 10 minutes, only 10 grams will remain. After the second 10-minute interval, only 5 grams will remain. After the third, only 2.5 grams. It takes three 10-minute half-lives to reach 2.5 grams so the time required is 30 minutes.

6. **The correct answer is (B).** An α-particle is a $_2^4$He helium nucleus. In α-decay, two protons are effectively removed.

7. **The correct answer is (B).** β-decay emits a high energy electron, $_{-1}^0e$. In the process, a neutron decays into a proton plus the emitted electron. The number of nucleons remains unchanged, with the proton replacing the neutron in the sum of nucleons.

8. **The correct answer is (D).** By definition.

9. **The correct answer is (D).** The mass number is the sum of neutrons and protons $= 6 + 7 = 13$ nucleons.

10. **The correct answer is (C).** Isotopes of an element have the same atomic number but different numbers of neutrons and, thus, different mass numbers. The atomic number of X is 63.

11. **The correct answer is (C).** In a fission reaction, a heavy nucleus absorbs a neutron and splits into two lighter-weight nuclei. The process releases other neutrons and energy and can support a chain reaction.

12. **The correct answer is (A).** The conservation of matter means the mass number of X must be 1:

$14 + 4 = 17 + Z$; therefore, $Z = 1$

and the atomic number is 1:

$7 + 2 = 8 + A$. Therefore, $A = 1$.

This is the description of a proton, $^{1}_{1}p$.

13. **The correct answer is (B).** The number of neutrons is the mass number minus the atomic number: $\Sigma(n + p) - \Sigma p = 140 - 54 = 86$.

14. **The correct answer is (D).** The half-life is a constant that depends on the identity of the nuclide, not on the amount of nuclide present.

15. **The correct answer is (B).** The α-particle is the helium nucleus. Each α-particle then acquires two electrons to form a neutral helium atom.

16. **The correct answer is (B).** In every half-life, the mass decreases to half its previous value:

$1/16 = 1/2^4$

It takes four half-lives to decay down to 1/16 the original mass. Each must be 30 minutes long since the entire process takes two hours.

17. **The correct answer is (A).** In 13 years, there will be 5 half-lives of 2.6 years each ($5 \times 2.6 = 13$). The mass decreases to $1/2^5 = 1/32$ its original value.

CHAPTER 3

Physical Sciences Sample Exam

TIME: **85** MINUTES   **77** QUESTIONS

Directions: This test includes 10 sets of questions related to specific passages (62 questions) and 15 shorter, independent questions. The passages represent all four format styles that you may see on the MCAT (Information Presentation, Problem Solving, Research Study, and Persuasive Argument). Explanatory answers immediately follow the test.

Passage I (Questions 1–5)

Theory 1. Early in the twentieth century, many chemists believed that the stability of the methane molecule, CH_4, could be explained by the "octet" rule, which states that stability occurs when the central atom, in this case carbon, is surrounded by 8 "valence," or outer, electrons. Four of these originally came from the outer electrons of the carbon atom itself, and four came from the four surrounding hydrogen atoms (hydrogen was considered to be an exception to the rule, since it was known to favor a closed shell of two electrons, as helium has).

According to the octet rule, neither CH_3 nor CH_5 should exist as stable compounds, and this prediction has been borne out by experiment.

Theory 2. While the octet rule predicted many compounds accurately, it also had shortcomings. The compound PCl_5, for example, is surrounded by 10 electrons. The greatest shock to the octet rule concerned the "noble gases" such as krypton and xenon, which have eight electrons in their atomic state and therefore should not form compounds, since no more electrons are needed to make an octet. The discovery in 1960 that xenon could form compounds such as XeF_4 forced consideration of a new theory, which

held that (a) compounds can form when electrons are completely paired, either in bonds or in nonbonded pairs; (b) the total number of shared electrons around a central atom can vary and can be as high as 12; and (c) the shapes of compounds are such as to keep pairs of electrons as far from each other as possible.

For example, since sulfur is surrounded by 6 electrons in the atomic state, in the compound SF_6 it acquires 6 additional shared electrons from the surrounding fluorines for a total of 12 electrons. The shape of the compound is "octahedral," as shown below, since this configuration minimizes the overlap of bonding pairs of electrons.

1. According to Theory 1, the compound CH_2Cl_2

   A. should have 8 electrons surrounding the carbon atom.
   B. cannot exist since the original carbon atom does not have 8 electrons.
   C. should have 8 electrons surrounding each hydrogen atom.
   D. requires more electrons for stability.

2. According to Theory 1, the compound XeF_4

   A. exists with an octet structure around the xenon.
   B. should not exist since the xenon is surrounded by more than eight electrons.
   C. will have similar chemical properties to CH_4.
   D. exists with the xenon surrounded by 12 electrons.

3. The atom boron has three outer electrons. In bonding to boron, a fluorine atom donates one electron. The BF_3 molecule is known to exist. Which of the following is true?

   A. BF_3 is consistent with Theory 1.
   B. The existence of BF_3 contradicts Theory 2.
   C. According to Theory 2, the structure of BF_3 is a pyramid:

   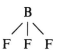

   D. According to Theory 2, the structure of BF_3 is triangular and planar:

   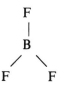

4. A scientist seeking to explain why Theory 2 has more predictive power than Theory 1 might argue that

   A. 8 electrons represent a "closed shell."
   B. while 8 electrons represent a "closed shell" for some atoms, for others the closed shell may be 6, 10, or 12.
   C. it is incorrect to assume that a given atom always has the same number of electrons around it.
   D. CH_4 is not as important a compound as XeF_4.

5. Theory 2 could be undermined by evidence

   A. of the existence of SF_4.
   B. of the existence of XeF_5.
   C. showing that CH_4 was more stable that XeF_4.
   D. of molecules with stable octets.

Passage II (Questions 6–13)

Among the simplest molecules are those formed from two identical atoms in the first rows of the periodic table. Bond strengths and bond lengths in these molecules vary considerably but can be predicted from molecular orbital theory.

Table 1 gives properties of several homonuclear diatomic molecules and molecular ions. A dash (—) indicates that a species does not exist as a stable entity.

Table 1

Molecule	Bond Length (Å)	Bond Energy (kJ/mole)
H_2^+	1.06	256
H_2	0.741	432
He_2^+	1.08	322
He_2	—	—
Li_2	2.67	110
B_2	1.59	274
C_2	1.24	603
N_2	1.10	942
O_2	1.21	494
Cl_2	1.99	239
Cl_2^+	1.89	415
Ne_2	—	—

Figure A shows the energy levels in these molecules.

Figure A

(a) Li_2 through N_2 (b) O_2 and F_2

6. According to Table 1, for how many stable, neutral molecules is the bond length under 1.50Å, and the bond energy greater than 450 kJ/mol?

   A. 0
   B. 1
   C. 2
   D. 3

7. Which of the following trends does Table 1 illustrate?

   A. Bond length increases with molecular weight.
   B. Within a period, bond energy increases along the period.
   C. Within a period, bond length varies inversely with bond energy.
   D. Atoms that fail to form diatomic molecules have an odd number of valence electrons.

8. Consider the stable neutral molecule/positive ion pairs shown in Table 1. Which statement is generally true?

   A. Removing an electron from a molecule X_2 to form X_2^+ lowers both the bond energy and the bond length
   B. Removing an electron from a molecule X_2 to form X_2^+ lowers the bond energy and increases the bond length
   C. Removing an electron from a molecule X_2 to form X_2^+ raises the bond energy and decreases the bond length
   D. None of the above.

9. Suppose that the bonding in N_2 is represented by the Lewis structure

   :N:::N:

   and in O_2 by the structure

   :Ö::Ö:

   Suppose also that triple bonds as shown in Lewis structures can be taken to be shorter than double bonds. Then the Lewis structures are

   A. consistent with the data shown in the table.
   B. consistent with the bond energy data, but inconsistent with the bond length data.
   C. consistent with the bond length data, but inconsistent with the bond energy data.
   D. inconsistent with both the bond length data and the bond energy data.

10. According to Figure A, the molecular orbital diagram, what is the bond order of Li_2?

    A. 0
    B. $\frac{1}{2}$
    C. 1
    D. 2

11. According to Figure A, why does He_2 not exist as a stable molecule?

    A. Its bond order is only $\frac{1}{2}$.
    B. It would have a bond order of 0.
    C. It has no bonding electrons in orbitals deriving from atomic $2s$ orbitals.
    D. A stable molecule may not use σ^* orbitals for bonding.

12. Table 1 shows instances where the addition of electrons to a molecule resulted in decreased stability. Figure A shows that for the example of N_2 to O_2, the effect is explained as follows:

    A. The extra electrons are placed in bonding orbitals.
    B. The extra electrons are placed in antibonding orbitals.
    C. The extra electrons go into a combination of bonding and anti-bonding orbitals.
    D. Since electrons repel one another, adding them to a molecule invariably is destabilizing.

13. The trend by which bond length appears to correlate inversely with bond energy might be explained by noting which of the following?

    A. Higher-energy electrons prefer to be close together.
    B. Higher bond energy corresponds to more electrons, and each electron requires a given amount of space.
    C. Since higher bond energy corresponds to a greater number of electrons in the space between the nuclei, these electrons will tend to pull the nuclei toward each other.
    D. Since higher bond energy corresponds to a greater number of electrons in the space between the nuclei, these electrons will tend to pull the nuclei away from each other.

Passage III (Questions 14–19)

By formally defining "half reactions," we can predict the spontaneity of actual reactions, which can be thought of as proceeding through a pair of half reactions. The table below gives the standard reduction potential of selected half reactions. Half reactions are arranged with the most spontaneous first.

Reaction	$E°$ (volts)
$F_2 + 2e^- \ 2F^-$	2.87
$Cr_2O_7^{2-} + 14H^+ + 6e^-$ $\rightarrow 2Cr^{3+} + 7H_2O$	1.33
$Br_2 + 2e^- \rightarrow 2Br^-$	1.09
$Ag_+ + e^- \rightarrow Ag$	0.80
$Fe^{3+} + e^- \rightarrow Fe^{2+}$	0.77
$Cu^{2+} + 2e^- \rightarrow Cu$	0.34
$Cu^{2+} + e^- \rightarrow Cu^+$	0.15
$H^+ + e^- \rightarrow [1/2] \ H_2$	0.00
$Pb^{2+} + 2e^- \rightarrow Pb$	−0.13
$Ni^{2+} + 2e^- \rightarrow Ni$	−0.25
$Zn^{2+} + 2e^- \rightarrow Zn$	−0.76

14. How many spontaneous oxidation reactions are shown on the table?

    A. 0
    B. 3
    C. 4
    D. 7

15. How many cells with a measured voltage greater than 1.50 v can be made using standard half cells with the half reactions listed?

    A. 6
    B. 13
    C. 15
    D. 17

16. Suppose that under a new system of reporting half-potentials, the value of 0.00 is to be assigned to the reduction of Cu^{2+} ion to copper metal. Under this system, $E°$ for the reduction of F_2 would have what value?

    A. 2.53 v
    B. 2.72 v
    C. 3.02 v
    D. 3.21 v

17. Using values in the table, calculate $E°$ for the reaction $Pb^{2+} + Cu \rightarrow Pb + Cu^{2+}$.

    A. 0.21 v
    B. −0.21 v
    C. 0.47 v
    D. −0.47 v

18. A student finds an old chemistry textbook that expresses half-potentials as *oxidation* potentials; e.g., potentials for a reaction such as $Fe \rightarrow Fe^{2+} + 2e^-$. If the reduction potential table were converted to an oxidation potential table, with the highest potentials on top, which of the following would be true?

    A. The F_2/F^- reaction would be listed first.
    B. The Cu^{2+}/Cu reaction would be above the Cu^2/Cu^+ reaction.
    C. The Zn^{2+}/Zn reaction would be above the H^+/H_2 reaction.
    D. The Ni^{2+}/Ni reaction would be below the H^+/H_2 reaction.

19. Based on the information in the reduction potential table, a spontaneous reaction will occur when

    I. copper metal is dropped into HNO_3.
    II. metallic lead is dropped into HNO_3.
    III. bromine gas is bubbled through a solution of $Pb(NO_3)_2$.

    A. I only
    B. II only
    C. III only
    D. I and II only

Passage IV (Questions 20–27)

While researching the solubility of various lead salts, an investigator decides to try a new way to graph the results. Although a chart of anion concentration against cation concentration usually shows a hyperbola or a similar curve, her choice of axes produces the straight lines shown below:

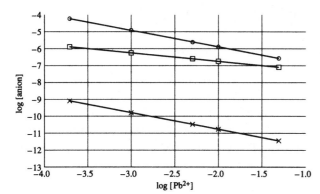

Key to anions:
—•— [SO_4^{2-}]   —▣— [OH^-]   —✖— [CO_3^{2-}]

Solubilities of lead salts.

20. For a given concentration of lead ion, which anion has the lowest concentration?

A. SO_4^{2-}
B. OH^-
C. CO_3^{2-}
D. Cannot be determined

21. What is the approximate value of [CO_3^{2-}] when log [Pb^{2+}] = 1.75?

A. -7
B. -11
C. 10^{-7}
D. 10^{-11}

22. The absolute value of Δlog (anion)/Δlog [Pb^{2+}] is

I. the same for SO_4^{2-} and OH^-.
II. about twice as great for OH^- as for SO_4^{2-}.
III. about the same for SO_4^{2-} and CO_3^{2-}.

A. I only
B. II only
C. III only
D. I and II only

23. Since the lowest curve is a straight line, we may say that:

A. [CO_3^{2-}] decreases linearly as [Pb^{2+}] decreases.
B. [CO_3^{2-}] increases linearly as [Pb^{2+}] increases.
C. log [CO_3^{2-}] decreases linearly as log [Pb^{2+}] decreases.
D. log [CO_3^{2-}] increases linearly as log [Pb^{2+}] decreases.

24. The slope of the lowest curve is closest to which of the following?

A. $-\dfrac{1}{2}$
B. $\dfrac{1}{2}$
C. -1
D. 1

25. Which of the following might explain the difference in the slopes of the top two curves?

A. K_{sp} is higher for $PbSO_4$ than for $Pb(OH)_2$.
B. The fact that there are 2 OH^-'s to every Pb^{2+} leads to a different graph for $Pb(OH)_2$ than for $PbSO_4$.
C. $PbSO_4$ is more soluble than $Pb(OH)_2$.
D. None of the above.

26. Consider the application of LeChatelier's Principle to the dissociation of $PbSO_4$:

$$PbSO_4(s) = Pb^{2+} + SO_4^{2-}$$

Which of the following is consistent with the data shown on the graph?

A. The graph agrees with LeChatelier's Principle since as $[PbSO_4]$ increases, $[Pb^{2+}]$ increases.

B. The graph agrees with LeChatelier's Principle since as $[Pb^{2+}]$ increases, $[SO_4^{2-}]$ increases.

C. The graph agrees with LeChatelier's Principle since as $[Pb^{2+}]$ increases, $[SO_4^{2-}]$ decreases.

D. The graph is inconsistent with LeChatelier's Principle since as $[Pb^{2+}]$ increases, $[SO_4^{2-}]$ decreases.

27. Since for $Pb(OH)_2$, $K_{sp} = [Pb^{2+}][OH^-]^2$,

A. $\log K_{sp} = (\log [Pb^{2+}])(\log [OH^-])^2$
B. $\log K_{sp} = (\log [Pb^{2+}])/(\log [OH^-])^2$
C. $\log K_{sp} = \log [Pb^{2+}] + 2\log [OH^-]$
D. $\log K_{sp} = (\log [Pb^{2+}])^3$

Passage V (Questions 28–34)

The study of equilibrium allows us to determine whether a reaction will proceed. The calculation uses the equilibrium constant, which can be derived from the standard free energy change. The study of reaction rates is essential if we are to determine the speed with which a reaction proceeds.

A chemist *predicts* that a reaction in which reactant A is converted to products B and C will proceed according to Figure 1.

Figure 1

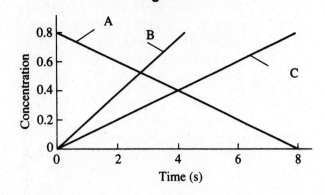

The chemist then *measures* the concentrations of the three species against time, and obtains the results shown in Figure 2.

Figure 2

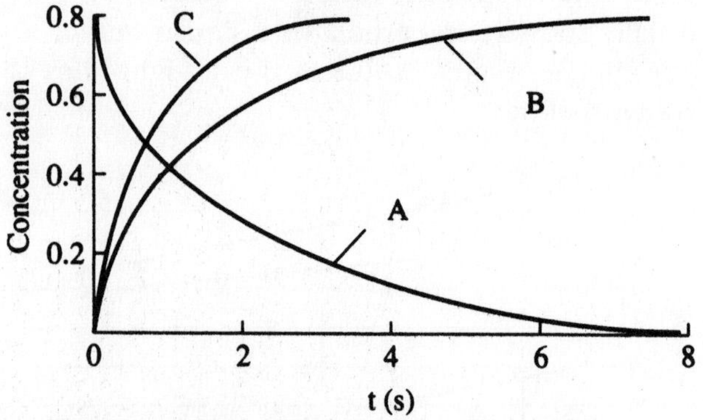

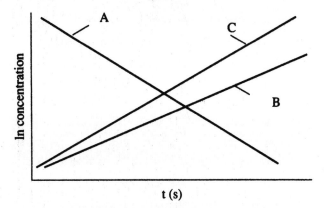

In order to determine the rate law for the reaction, the chemist replots the data as shown in Figure 3.

Figure 3

28. Using Figure 1, when $C_A = C_B$, what does C_C approximately equal?

A. $0.5C_A$
B. C_A
C. $C_A - C_B$
D. $C_A + C_B$

29. As the reaction in Figure 1 proceeds, the total pressure of all species

A. decreases.
B. stays the same.
C. increases.
D. increases, then decreases.

30. Which of the following summarizes the reaction graphed in Figure 1?

A. $A + B \rightarrow C$
B. $A \rightarrow B + C$
C. $A \rightarrow 2B + C$
D. $A \rightarrow B + 2C$

31. Which of the following expresses the rate of the reaction graphed in Figure 1?

A. $-dC_A/dt = k$
B. $-dC_A/dt = k[A]$
C. $-dC_A/dt = k[B]$
D. $-dC_A/dt = k[B][C]$

32. Compared to Figure 1, which predicted the concentrations over time, the initial rate of appearance of B in Figure 2 is

A. lower.
B. the same.
C. higher.
D. sometimes lower, sometimes higher.

33. Based on Figure 2, the total pressure at 1 s is closest to

A. 0.3
B. 0.5
C. 1.3
D. 1.8

34. Which of the following best describes the fit of the data in Figure 3 to the chemist's initial prediction?

A. The predicted kinetics were 0th-order; the experimental kinetics were in agreement.
B. The predicted kinetics were first-order; the experimental kinetics were in agreement.
C. The predicted kinetics were 0th-order; the experimental kinetics were first-order.
D. The predicted kinetics were first-order; the experimental kinetics were second-order.

Passage VI (Questions 35–39)

Reaction 1

A chemist obtains the kinetic data shown for the following reaction, where S is a "substrate," N a "nucleophile," and X a "leaving group."

$$SX + N \rightarrow SN + X$$

[SX]	[N]	Relative Rate
0.05	0.05	1.20
0.05	0.10	2.40
0.10	0.05	2.40
0.10	0.10	4.80
0.15	0.15	10.80

Reaction 2

Next, the chemist obtains data for a second reaction, where the substrate, nucleophile, and leaving group are all different:

$$S'X' + N' \rightarrow S'N' + X'$$

[S'X']	[N']	Relative Rate
0.005	0.10	16
0.005	0.15	16
0.0075	0.5	24
0.015	0.30	48

Finally, the chemist investigates the effect of the nucleophile for each of the two reactions. Her results follow:

Nucleophile	Rate of Reaction 1	Rate of Reaction 2
CH_3OH	very slow	Changing nucleophiles had no effect on rate
H_2O		
$Cl-$	↓	
NH_3		
$Br-$	moderate	
$OH-$		
$I-$	↓	
$SH-$		
	very fast	

35. In Reaction 1, the relative rate varies

    I. linearly with the concentration of SX.
   II. linearly with the concentration of the nucleophile.
  III. inversely with SX.

    A. I only
    B. II only
    C. III only
    D. I and II only

36. In Reaction 2, increasing the concentration of N' while holding $S'\,X'$ constant

    A. can either increase or decrease the relative rate.
    B. increases the relative rate.
    C. decreases the relative rate.
    D. has no effect on the relative rate.

37. The rate of Reaction 1 is best expressed by which of the following?

    A. rel. rate = 0.05[SX] + 0.05[N]
    B. rel. rate = 0.05[SX]
    C. rel. rate = 480[SX]
    D. rel. rate = 480[N][SX]

38. The rate of Reaction 2 is best expressed by which of the following?

    A. rel. rate = 0.005[S′X′] + 0.10[N′]
    B. rel. rate = 0.005[S′X′]
    C. rel. rate = 1600[S′X′]
    D. rel. rate = 3200[S′X′]

39. The chemist decides that "better" nucleophiles (i.e., those that enhance the rate)

    I. tend to be found in the conjugate acid form of a species rather than the conjugate base.
   II. have a central atom that is located toward the lower end of a group (column) in the Periodic Table.
  III. have a central atom located to the right side of the Periodic Table.

    A. I only
    B. II only
    C. III only
    D. II and III only

Passage VII (Questions 40–43)

A student draws the following graphs based on different sets of data. The graphs drawn are:

A.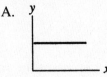

B.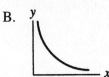

C.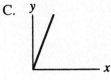

D.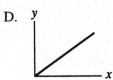

40. The graph that shows a body in equilibrium, with the ordinate representing velocity and the abscissa representing time, is

    A. Graph A.
    B. Graph B.
    C. Graph C.
    D. Graph D.

41. The graph that has axes representing velocity and time and that represents the motion with the largest acceleration is

    A. Graph A.
    B. Graph B.
    C. Graph C.
    D. Graph D.

42. Which graph best represents a motionless body?

    A. Graph A with axes of distance vs. time
    B. Graph A with axes of velocity vs. time
    C. Graph B with axes of acceleration vs. time
    D. Graph B with axes of velocity vs. time

43. If all the graphs have axes of distance vs. time, which one represents motion with the smallest constant nonzero velocity?

   A. Graph A
   B. Graph B
   C. Graph C
   D. Graph D

Passage VIII (Questions 44–47)

A 700-N person pushes a 900-N box 5.00 meters up a 15.0-meter-long ramp in 3.00 seconds. At that point on the ramp, the box is 3.00 meters above the ground. The frictional force for the box on the ramp is 100 N.

44. How much power was required to move the box?

   A. 1167 W
   B. 1500 W
   C. 500 W
   D. 584 W

45. What is the potential energy gained by the box?

   A. 2.70×10^3 J
   B. 1.50×10^4 J
   C. 2.65×10^4 J
   D. 3.54×10^4 J

46. What is the minimum force the person must apply to the box to get it moving?

   A. 100 N
   B. 900 N
   C. 540 N
   D. 640 N

47. What is the minimum force required to keep the box where it is without sliding down the ramp?

   A. 100 N
   B. 640 N
   C. 540 N
   D. 440 N

Passage IX (Questions 48–51)

A student wants to make a musical instrument using a hollow tube and a glass of water. She tests her idea on a single unit. The tube is suspended in the water in the glass. A portion of the tube, length X, is above the water line. The remaining portion, length Y, is below the water line.

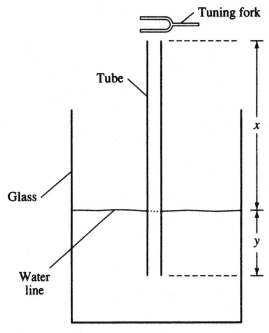

She strikes a tuning fork, holds it over the mouth of the tube, and adjusts the tube's height until the sound is loudest.

48. What is the wavelength of the fundamental frequency of the sound produced by the tube?

   A. 2X
   B. 4X
   C. 2Y
   D. 4Y

49. When the tube is adjusted to make the sound louder, the wave property illustrated is

   A. polarization.
   B. beats.
   C. resonance.
   D. refraction.

50. The wavelength of the sound that is refracted into the water at the air-water boundary is

A. less than 2*Y*.
B. greater than 4*X*.
C. between 2*X* and 4*X*.
D. exactly 4*Y*.

51. The sound wave created by the tuning fork has a wavelength equal to which of the following?

A. one complete period of vibration for the tuning fork
B. one half the period of vibration for the tuning fork
C. one quarter the period of vibration for the tuning fork
D. twice the period of vibration for the tuning fork

Questions 52–77 are independent of any passage and independent of each other.

52. A student draws four small-diameter tubes labeled A through D placed in a reservoir of water.

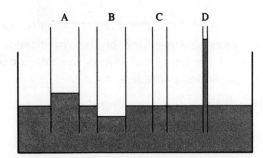

Which two tubes in the drawing correctly illustrate the expected behavior of water?

A. A and D
B. B and C
C. A and C
D. C and D

53. A musician produces a certain note on a flute. If the musician blows harder, what happens to the sound wave associated with the note?

A. Its speed increases.
B. Its frequency increases.
C. Its frequency decreases.
D. Its amplitude increases.

54. How long will it take sound to reach an observer who is 2200 feet away from the source if the speed of sound in air is approximately 1100 feet per second?

A. $\frac{1}{2}$ second
B. 1 second
C. 2 seconds
D. 4 seconds

55. A ball is thrown vertically upward with a velocity of 40.0 m/s. What will be the height of the ball after 5.00 seconds?

A. 8.00 m
B. 77.5 m
C. 200 m
D. 322 m

56. Three children weighing 40 lb, 60 lb, and 80 lb, respectively, want to balance a 14-foot-long seesaw, pivoted at its center. The 80-lb child sits 2 ft from the left end of the seesaw. The 60-lb child sits 2 ft from the right end of the seesaw. Where must the 40-lb child sit?

A. 1.0 ft to left of pivot
B. 2.5 ft to right of pivot
C. 2.5 ft to left of pivot
D. 5.0 ft to right of pivot

57. A 50-N box is set in motion. The coefficient of static friction is 0.50 and the coefficient of kinetic friction is 0.20. What is the difference between the force needed to initiate motion and the force needed to maintain motion?

A. 10 N
B. 15 N
C. 25 N
D. 125 N

58. If air pressure is 14.7 lb/in^2, what is the total force exerted on one side of an 8½ × 11-inch sheet of paper?

A. 63.6 lb
B. 137 lb
C. 6.36×10^3 lb
D. 1.37×10^3 lb

59. What is the electric current produced when a charge of 120 coulombs flows through a wire with a diameter of 2 cm in one minute?

A. 1 ampere
B. 2 amperes
C. 3 amperes
D. 4 amperes

60. The iodine isotope $^{131}_{53}I$ decays to form the Xenon isotope $^{131}_{54}Xe$. What else results from this reaction?

A. An α-particle is emitted.
B. A positron is absorbed.
C. A positron is emitted.
D. A β-particle is emitted.

61. A pendulum of length L has a period of 0.5 second. To increase the period to 1.0 second, the length of the pendulum must be

A. doubled.
B. quadrupled.
C. halved.
D. quartered.

62. The effect of β-particle emission is to produce a daughter nuclide that has

A. increased its atomic number by one.
B. decreased its atomic number by one.
C. increased its mass number by one.
D. decreased its mass number by one.

63. Which of the following is not a correct empirical formula?

A. $Ca_3(SO_4)_2$
B. C_6H_{12}
C. Na_2S
D. N_2O_5

64. For those atoms in the first column of the Periodic Table that form stable positive ions, the ion usually has a considerably smaller radius than the neutral atom. What explains this effect?

A. The outer electron(s) effectively screen the nuclear charge.
B. The ion has a smaller nuclear charge.
C. The neutral atom has a greater nuclear charge.
D. The neutral atom has an outer electron in an orbital of higher "n" than the ion.

65. A gaseous air pollutant is found to have a mole fraction of 3×10^{-6} in the atmosphere. What is its partial pressure in atm if the barometric pressure is 1.00 atm?

A. 10^{-6}
B. 3×10^{-6}
C. 6×10^{-6}
D. $760 \times (3 \times 10^{-6})$

66. Which of the following results in a spontaneous reaction in water?

I. addition of a weak base to a strong base
II. addition of a weak acid to a strong base
III. addition of a weak base to a strong acid

A. I only
B. II only
C. III only
D. II and III only

67. A reaction is found to have an equilibrium constant of 0.06 at a temperature of 298K and a pressure of 1.0 atm. It can be concluded that at these conditions

I. $\Delta H° > 0$
II. $\Delta S° > 0$
III. $\Delta G° > 0$

A. I only
B. II only
C. III only
D. I and II only

68. In the following reaction, which is (are) true?

$$H_2S + 2NO_3^- + 2H^+ \rightarrow S + 2NO_2 + 2H_2O$$

I. H_2S is oxidized.
II. H_2S is the oxidizing agent.
III. NO_3^- is reduced.

A. I only
B. II only
C. III only
D. I and III only

69. A compound contains 5.9% hydrogen and 94.1% oxygen. What is its empirical formula?

A. HO
B. H_2O
C. H_2O_2
D. H_6O_{94}

70. The reaction

$$Ag^+ + Fe^{2+} \rightarrow Ag + Fe^{3+}$$

proceeds spontaneously. If a galvanic cell is constructed with Ag^+/Ag as one half cell and Fe^{3+}/Fe^{2+} as the other, the silver electrode will be

A. the cathode, positive.
B. the cathode, negative.
C. the anode, positive.
D. the anode, negative.

71. The nuclear reaction

$$_1^2H + _1^3H \rightarrow _2^4H + _0^1 + energy$$

is an example of what type of reaction?

A. α-decay
B. fission
C. fusion
D. β-decay

72. Monochromatic light passes through two parallel slits in a screen and falls on a piece of film. The pattern produced is an example of

A. interference and reflection.
B. interference and diffraction.
C. refraction and diffraction.
D. diffraction and polarization.

73. Which of the following distances is shortest?

A. 0.456×10^4 cm
B. 4.56×10^4 m
C. 0.456 km
D. 4.56×10^6 mm

74. A 70-kg man exerts a force of 20 N parallel to the surface of an incline while pushing a 50-N crate 10 meters up the incline. The incline is not frictionless. Which statement best describes the change in potential energy of the crate?

A. The E_p of the crate increases by less than 200 J.
B. The E_p of the crate increases by more than 200 J.
C. The E_p of the crate increases by less than 500 J.
D. The E_p of the crate decreases by less than 500 J.

75. Which of the following statements is most accurate for the system of object and concave mirror illustrated below?

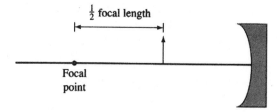

A. The image is larger than the object, inverted, and real.
B. The image is larger than the object, upright, and virtual.
C. The image is smaller than the object, upright, and real.
D. The image is smaller than the object, inverted, and virtual.

76. A 50-kg probe lands on a planet that has a mass that is twice as great as that of Earth and a radius that is twice as large as that of Earth. What is the gravitational force experienced by the probe?

A. The same as on the Earth.
B. Half that on Earth.
C. Twice that on Earth.
D. Four times that on Earth.

77. What happens to the kinetic energy of a body if its speed is tripled?

A. The kinetic energy decreases to 1/9 its original value.
B. The kinetic energy decreases to 1/3 its original value.
C. The kinetic energy increases to 9 times its original value.
D. The kinetic energy increases to 3 times its original value.

ANSWER KEY

Physical Sciences Sample Exam

1. A	11. B	21. D	31. A	41. C	51. A	61. B	71. C
2. B	12. B	22. C	32. C	42. A	52. A	62. A	72. B
3. D	13. C	23. D	33. C	43. D	53. D	63. B	73. A
4. B	14. B	24. C	34. C	44. A	54. C	64. D	74. A
5. B	15. C	25. B	35. D	45. C	55. B	65. B	75. B
6. D	16. A	26. C	36. D	46. D	56. B	66. D	76. B
7. C	17. D	27. C	37. D	47. D	57. B	67. C	77. C
8. D	18. C	28. A	38. D	48. B	58. D	68. C	
9. A	19. B	29. C	39. D	49. C	59. B	69. A	
10. C	20. C	30. C	40. A	50. B	60. D	70. A	

ANSWERS AND EXPLANATIONS

1. **The correct answer is (A).** The core idea of the octet rule is that the central atom, in this case carbon, has 8 shared electrons. This question requires critical reading of the question.

   The original atom itself usually has fewer than 8 electrons (so B is incorrect), and the passage explains that hydrogens themselves cannot have octets (so C is wrong).

2. **The correct answer is (B).** Either by familiarity with Xe and F, or by reference to the table in the text, a reader can see that 12 electrons are shared in this compound, limiting the choices to B or D. But Theory 1 only allows 8 electrons, so D is ruled out, leaving B as the correct response. This question requires the reader to examine the relationship of the passage to the conclusion given.

3. **The correct answer is (D).** The compound has 6 electrons, so it violates Theory 1 and fits Theory 2; thus A and B are ruled out. The reader is left with a choice between two structures. Since the text says that Theory 2 dictates the structure that keeps electrons farthest apart, the choice should be D. This question requires the reader to examine the relationship of the passage to the conclusion, and is particularly difficult because it asks the reader to think about a concept—alternate structures—only mentioned briefly in the passage.

4. **The correct answer is (B).** This answer is in fact a short restatement of Theory 2. C looks similar, but is incorrect, since it implies variability within the same atom rather than among different ones. A denies the importance of Theory 2, contradicting the sense of the question, and D contradicts the idea of greater predictive power, suggesting as it does that some experimental data are unimportant, without giving a reason. This question requires that a reader generalize from the given information.

5. **The correct answer is (B).** Theory 2 could be proven wrong by a compound having more than 12 electrons surrounding a central atom; this compound has 13. A and D are facts that fit within Theory 2, and C relates compounds fitting Theories 1 and 2 but not threatening the second theory. This question requires that a reader generalize from the information given.

6. **The correct answer is (D).** First find the molecules that have energies greater than 450 kJ/mol; then rule out those that are too long; then rule out ions. Those remaining are C_2, N_2, and O_2.

7. **The correct answer is (C).** Look at a series where the bond energy increases; e.g., Li_2 through O_2. The bond length steadily decreases.

8. **The correct answer is (D).** For example, B is true for the hydrogen ion/neutral pair, while C is true for the chlorine pair.

9. **The correct answer is (A).** According to the dot structure, N_2 has a triple bond and O_2 has a double bond; the bond energy for N_2 in the chart is also greater than for O_2. The chart shows N_2 to have a shorter bond length than O_2.

10. **The correct answer is (C).** Two electrons in a bonding orbital (one from each of the separate Li $2s$ atomic orbitals) give a single bond.

11. **The correct answer is (B).** The two $1s$ electrons on each helium atom fill both the σ $1s$ and the σ^* $1s$ orbitals, resulting in a net bond order of zero.

12. **The correct answer is (B).** N_2 has its highest electrons in bonding π orbitals. The two additional electrons necessary to form O_2 go into π^*x and π^*y orbitals, which are antibonding.

13. **The correct answer is (C).** Choice A predicts the correct effect, but lacks a sound reason. Choice C combines the fact that electrons in bonding orbitals tend to be between the nuclei with the observation that coulombic attraction will pull both nuclei toward the electrons in the bond, shortening the internuclear distance.

14. **The correct answer is (B).** Spontaneous oxidation half-reactions are those whose reduction E°'s are less than zero.

15. **The correct answer is (C).** Combine the first reaction with each of the others (10 cells). Then combine the bottom reaction with the second, third, fourth, and fifth (4 cells). Finally, combine the second reaction with the next-to-last reaction (1 cell).

16. **The correct answer is (A).** Here we are lowering the value of $E°$ for the Cu^{2+}/Cu cell (not the Cu^{2+}/Cu^+ reaction) by 0.337 v. We must lower all the other $E°$ values by the same amount.

17. **The correct answer is (D).** $E° = -0.13 - (0.34) = -0.47$ v

18. **The correct answer is (C).** A table of oxidation potentials would have an order that is the reverse of a table of reduction potentials. Only C reflects such a reverse order.

19. **The correct answer is (B).** Calculated potentials are:

   I. $0 - 0.34 = -0.34$ v

   II. $0 - (-0.13) = 0.13$ v

   III. no reaction; no reducing agent (e.g., Pb metal) is present

20. **The correct answer is (C).** For any value of lead ion (on the x-axis), the value of log $[CO_3^{2-}]$ is the lowest of the three anions. (Note that the y-axis shows "log [anion]"—not "[MS]log [anion]," as in a pH chart—so that descending on the y-axis means going toward lower values of the anion concentration.

21. **The correct answer is (D).** Choose the line nearest the bottom; read up from "-1.75" and read to the left to "-11." Since the y-axis is "log [anion]," this value implies that $[CO_3^{2-}] = 10^{-11}$.

22. **The correct answer is (C).** The question asks for slopes. The slopes of the top and bottom lines are about equal. II would be correct if it said "about $\frac{1}{2}$ as great . . ."

23. **The correct answer is (D).** Rule out choices A, B, and C because they do not describe inverse relationships between the two ions. Answer D correctly describes a negatively sloping line.

24. **The correct answer is (C).** For instance, take the horizontal change from -2.75 to -1.8, for which the vertical change is from -10 to -11. Then $(\Delta y)/(\Delta x) = (-1)/(.95) = -1.05$.

25. **The correct answer is (B).** The slopes for the sulfate and carbonate salts are similar, while the slope for the hydroxide is lower. One common feature of the sulfate and carbonate salts of lead is that each has one cation to one anion, where in the hydroxide there are two anions to one cation.

26. **The correct answer is (C).** LeChatelier's Principle states that a stress on one side of the equation pushes the equilibrium in the direction that best relieves the stress. Response "C" is consistent with LeChatelier's Principle and with the data on the graph. Response "A" is ruled out since the graph does not mention solid $PbSO_4$ (the amount of which would not, at any rate, affect the equilibrium).

27. **The correct answer is (C).** This expression uses the correct rules for logarithms of products and exponents.

28. **The correct answer is (A).** Find the point where the curves for A and B cross and drop down to the line for C.

29. **The correct answer is (C).** Pressure increases. If the product were only C, the total pressure would remain unchanged (e.g., at 8 s, A is gone but C has A's initial value). But B is produced as well.

30. The correct answer is (C). The slopes of A and C are equal in magnitude, though not in their signs, but the slope of B is twice that of C.

31. The correct answer is (A). The rate of disappearance of A is a constant since the graph for A is a straight line.

32. The correct answer is (C). The slope of B is very high, close to 0 s.

33. The correct answer is (C). $P = 0.3 + 0.5 + 0.5 = 1.3$

34. The correct answer is (C). Note that if a concentration of a given species rises or falls linearly over time, then the reaction must be 0th-order with respect to that species; i.e., its rate of change is unaffected by the amount of the species present. But if the *log* of the concentration of the species is linear over time, then the reaction is 1st-order with respect to that concentration.

35. The correct answer is (D). Doubling either concentration while holding the other constant results in a doubling of the relative rate.

36. The correct answer is (D). Note rows 1 and 2. The change in rate from row 3 to row 4 is due only to substrate; see rows 2 and 3.

37. The correct answer is (D). For example, use the derived rate law with values from row 1 to get k.

38. The correct answer is (D). For example, use the derived rate law, where there is no dependence on the concentration of the nucleophile with row 1 to get k.

39. The correct answer is (D). Note that SH^- promotes the reaction better than does OH^-, and I^- better than Cl^-.

40. The correct answer is (A). A body in equilibrium has constant velocity if it is in motion (and zero velocity if it is stationary). In graph A, the value of the velocity is constant, that is, the slope of the curve is zero.

41. The correct answer is (C). For acceleration in the same direction as the motion, the velocity increases at a uniform rate. The constant slope of the velocity versus time graph gives the acceleration. The greater the acceleration, the greater the slope.

42. The correct answer is (A). Choices C and D can be eliminated immediately because they have a slope. The slope on graph A is zero. Choice B is eliminated because it shows the velocity as constant but not necessarily zero. If the axes are distance and time, then graph A represents no change in position (no motion).

43. The correct answer is (D). If the velocity is low, the slope of the distance versus time curve is low because the distance covered in any unit of time is small.

44. The correct answer is (A). Power is the rate of doing work: $P = W/t$ where the work is force times distance:

$$P = \frac{Fd}{t}\frac{(700\ \text{N})(5.00\ \text{m})}{3.00\text{s}} = 1167\ \text{W}$$

A quick estimate is given by

$$P = \frac{(7 \times 10^2\ \text{N})(5\ \text{m})}{3\text{s}} = \frac{35 \times 10^2\ \text{W}}{3} \approx 12 \times 10^2\ \text{W}$$

The choice closest to this value is A.

45. **The correct answer is (C).** E_p = mgh ~ (900 N) (10 m/s²)(3 m) = 2.7 × 10⁴ J

The closest choice is C, 2.65 × 10⁴ J.

46. **The correct answer is (D).** The person is counteracting two forces, the force of friction and the component of the weight of the box parallel to the surface of the ramp.

$$\frac{\text{parallel component}}{\text{wgt}} = \frac{\text{hgt. of plane}}{\text{length of plane}}$$

$$\text{parallel component} = \frac{3.00 \text{ m}}{5.00 \text{ m}} \times 900 \text{ N} = 540 \text{ N}$$

The total force to be overcome is 540 N + 100 N = 640 N.

47. **The correct answer is (D).** The force of friction helps prevent the box from sliding down the ramp. The force required to keep the box where it is is equal in magnitude but opposite in direction to the component of the mass of the box that is parallel to the surface of the ramp, minus the frictional force.

F = 540 N − 100 N = 440 N

48. **The correct answer is (B).** The tube behaves like a closed-end pipe, so there is a node at the water end and an antinode at the opposite or air end of the tube. The length of the air column is one-fourth the wavelength of the fundamental tone: $\frac{\lambda}{4} = X$.

49. **The correct answer is (C).** Resonance occurs when the vibration of one system (tuning fork) sets up sympathetic vibrations on a nearby system (air column in tube). The second system must have a natural frequency close to that of the first vibrating system. Adjusting the tube height adjusts the wavelength, and thus the frequency of the air column, until it meets the condition for resonance.

50. **The correct answer is (B).** The wavelength of the sound depends on length of the air column producing the sound and is independent of any other medium into which it is transmitted. At the boundary between the air and the water, the speed of sound changes, but its frequency does not. Since $V = \lambda v$, wavelength and speed are directly proportional. The speed of sound in a liquid is typically faster than it is in a gas. In order for the frequency to remain constant at the higher speed, we expect a shift to longer wavelengths.

51. **The correct answer is (A).** By definition, a complete vibration or period covers one wavelength.

52. **The correct answer is (A).** Water rises by capillary action because it "wets" the glass. The water in the tubes should therefore be higher than the level in the reservoir. This eliminates tubes B and C and therefore choices B, C, and D. Choice A is correct because the smaller the diameter of the tube, the higher the water will rise.

53. **The correct answer is (D).** Choice A is eliminated because the speed of all sound waves in air is constant, and independent of frequency and amplitude. Choices B and C are eliminated because the speed is constant, the wavelength dependent on the length of the air column in the flute is also constant; therefore the frequency cannot change. The increase in energy increases the amplitude of the wave.

54. **The correct answer is (C).** Since distance covered equals the product of the speed and the time, then:

$$t = \frac{d}{v} = \frac{2200 \text{ ft}}{1100 \text{ ft/s}} = 2 \text{ s}$$

55. **The correct answer is (B).** $d = v_0 t + \frac{1}{2} at^2$ where the initial velocity $v_0 = 40$ m/s and the acceleration is due to gravity so that $a = -g = -9.8$ m/s^2. The negative sign occurs because the acceleration is opposite to the initial direction of motion.

$$d = \left(40 \frac{\text{m}}{\text{s}}\right)(5 \text{ s}) + \left(-4.9 \frac{\text{m}}{\text{s}^2}\right)(5\text{s})^2$$
$$= 200 \text{ m} - 122.5 \text{ m} = 77.5 \text{ M}$$

This answer is easily estimated by rounding the acceleration to 10 m/s^2 so that $1/2 \, at^2$ becomes $(1/2)(10 \text{ m/s}^2)(5 \text{ s})^2 = 125$ m and d is approximately 200 m $- 125$ m $= 75$ m which is closest to choice B.

56. **The correct answer is (B).** At equilibrium, the sum of the clockwise torques must equal the sum of the counter-clockwise torques. The two heavier children each sit 5 ft from the pivot point as indicated below and produce torques rotating in opposite directions.

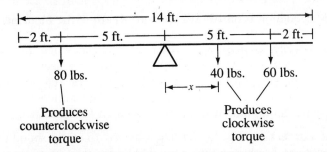

The 40-lb child must sit on the same side of the seesaw as the 60-lb child, at a distance of x ft to the right of the pivot. This eliminates choices A and C immediately. Choice D is eliminated because this would form a coupled moment and equilibrium would require that there be 80 total pounds 5 ft to the right of the pivot, but the two children together have a weight of 100 lbs. This leaves B as the only reasonable answer. Confirm this by doing the calculation:

$$(80 \text{ lb})(5 \text{ ft}) = (40 \text{ lb})(x\text{ft}) + (60 \text{ lb})(5 \text{ ft})$$
$$400 \text{ ft-lb} = 40(x \text{ ft-lb}) + 300 \text{ ft-lb}$$
$$x \text{ ft} = \frac{(400 - 300) \text{ ft-lb}}{40 \text{ lb}} = 2.5 \text{ ft}$$

57. **The correct answer is (B).** $F_{\text{initiating}} = (\mu_s)\text{Wgt.}$ and $F_{\text{maintaining}} = (\mu_k)\text{Wgt}$

$$F_i - F_m = (\mu_s - \mu_k)\text{Wgt} = (0.50 - 0.20)(50 \text{ N}) = 15 \text{ N}$$

58. **The correct answer is (D).** You can save time by estimating the expected answer.

Force = Pressure × Area where Pressure = P = 14.7 lb/in^2 ~ 15 lb/in^2 (the area is estimated as 9 in. × 11 in. = 99 in.^{2} ~ 100 in.^{2}).

$$F \sim \left(15\frac{lb}{in.^2}\right)(100 \text{ in.}^2) = 1.5 \times 10^3 \text{ lb}$$

The best choice is D. Confirm the calculation as:

$$F = \left(14.7\frac{lb}{in.^2}\right)(93.5 \text{ in.}^2) = 1.37 \times 10^3 \text{ lb}$$

59. **The correct answer is (B).** Electric current, I, is the total charge per unit of time:

$I = Q/t$ = 120 C/60 s = 2 amperes

The diameter of the wire is not necessary to this calculation.

60. **The correct answer is (D).** The reaction is

$$^{131}_{53}I \rightarrow {}^{131}_{54}Xe$$

The other particle is emitted, not absorbed. This eliminates choice B. By conservation of matter and charge, X must be ^0_1X which corresponds to a beta emission.

61. **The correct answer is (B).** For a simple pendulum, the period is T and is directly proportional to the square root of the length:

$$T = 2\pi\sqrt{L/g} \text{ so that } \frac{T}{\sqrt{L}} = \frac{2\pi}{\sqrt{g}}$$

To double the period, the length must be quadrupled so that its square root is doubled:

$$\sqrt{4L} = 2\sqrt{L}$$

62. **The correct answer is (A).** Emission of an electron from a nucleus occurs when a neutron disintegrates into a proton and the emitted electron. Since the mass of the neutron and the proton are approximately the same, the mass number remains unchanged. The neutron is replaced by a proton, so the atomic number increases by one.

63. **The correct answer is (B).** The formula is not in the simplest numeric ratio. It should read "CH_2."

64. **The correct answer is (D).** The electron in the neutral atom occupies an s orbital of higher n than the valence electrons of the positive ion. The valence electron of the neutral atom will stay, on average, farther from the nucleus than the inner electrons.

65. **The correct answer is (B).** Use $P_i = X_iP_T = (2 \times 10^{-6}) \times (1.00)$.

66. **The correct answer is (D).** Mixing two bases will not result in a reaction that proceeds to a great extent since neither readily furnishes H^+. But if an acid is mixed with a base, *as long as at least one is strong,* the reaction will go essentially to completion.

67. **The correct answer is (C).** Since $K < 1$, the reaction is not spontaneous. Because $\Delta G° = -RT\ln K$, we conclude that $\Delta G° > 0$. Although $\Delta H°$ and $\Delta S°$ combine to determine $\Delta G°$, we lack information to determine the sign of either of them.

68. **The correct answer is (C).** The oxidation state of sulfur increases from -2 to 0. Note that since H_2S is oxidized, it must be the *reducing* agent. Since the oxidation state of N in NO_3^- drops from 7 to 4, NO_3^- is reduced.

69. **The correct answer is (A).** Assume a 100-g sample for convenience. It will contain 5.9 g H, or 5.9 mol. It will also contain 94.1 g oxygen, or $94.1/16 = 5.9$ mol. Thus the ratio of H to O is 1:1. (The *molecular* formula—but not the empirical one—is likely to be H_2O_2.)

70. **The correct answer is (A).** Since Ag^+ is reduced at the silver electrode, that electrode is the cathode. Since electrons flow spontaneously toward that electrode, it must be positively charged.

71. **The correct answer is (C).** In fusion reactions, two light mass nuclei combine to produce a heavier nucleus. Choice B is eliminated because no nucleus was split into less massive nuclei. Choice D is eliminated because a β-particle is essentially an electron and no particles occur in the reaction shown. Choice A is eliminated because β-particle decay generally is not accompanied by the emission of a neutron.

72. **The correct answer is (B).** The light passing through each slit is diffracted (bent), and the two resulting beams overlap on the film to form interference patterns.

73. **The correct answer is (A).** To compare the figures, replace the prefixes by their exponential equivalents and rewrite each number in scientific notation. Therefore, each becomes:

   A. $0.456 \times 10^4 \times 10^{-2}$ m $= 4.56 \times 10^1$ m
   B. 4.56×10^4 m is already in scientific notation
   C. 0.456×10^3 m $= 4.56 \times 10^2$ m
   D. $4.56 \times 10^6 \times 10^{-3}$ m $= 4.56 \times 10^3$ m

74. **The correct answer is (A).** Since the crate is moving up the incline, the potential energy is increased. This eliminates choice D immediately. The potential energy cannot be determined explicitly since the vertical rise of the incline is unknown. However, the amount of work performed can be calculated.

   $W = Fd = (20$ N$)(10$ m$) = 200$ J

   The work was used to overcome friction and to raise the object. If the incline were frictionless, all of the work would have gone into producing potential energy. This sets an upper limit of 200 J on the increase in E_p.

75. **The correct answer is (B).** The image appears to be "inside" the mirror, so the image is always virtual. This eliminates choices A and C immediately. Choice D can be eliminated because mirror images are always upright. Choice B is confirmed by tracing the rays.

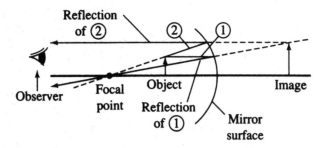

Rays parallel to the horizontal axis are reflected back through the focal point (Ray 1). Rays whose backward extrapolation would pass through the focal point are reflected parallel to the horizontal (Ray 2). The eye follows the lines of these rays back into the mirror, where they appear to converge. The result is an enlarged, upright, virtual image.

76. **The correct answer is (B).** The force of gravitational attraction is given by:

$$F_{grav} = \frac{Gm_1m_2}{r^2}$$

where G is the universal gravitational constant. The mass of the planet is $2m_1$. The radius of the planet is $2r$, so

$$F_{planet} = \frac{G2m_1m_2}{(2r)^2} = \frac{G2m_1m_2}{4r^2} = \frac{Gm_1m_2}{2r^2}$$

The gravitational force on the planet will be half that experienced on the Earth.

77. **The correct answer is (C).** Kinetic energy is: $E_k = 1/2 \ mv^2$. The kinetic energy is directly proportional to the square of the velocity (or speed). If the speed is multiplied by 3, the E_k must be multiplied by $3^2 = 9$.

Unit Two

VERBAL REASONING

CHAPTER 4

How to Answer
Verbal Reasoning Questions

The Verbal Reasoning section of the MCAT includes selections from the sciences, social sciences, and humanities. Each exam has nine reading passages: three in science, three in social science, and three in humanities. Reading passages range from 250 to 850 words, with most passages averaging 500 to 600 words. Each passage is followed by six to ten multiple-choice questions.

The questions are based on information gained from reading the passage. Questions fall into the following four categories:

1. **Comprehension**
   This type of question tests your ability to understand information given in the reading selection.

2. **Evaluation**
   This type of question asks you to look at the material presented in the reading passage and evaluate the reliability of the information as it relates to the argument being presented.

3. **Application**
   This type of question requires you to take the information in the article and apply it to a different situation.

4. **Incorporation of New Information**
   This type of question asks you to reevaluate the argument presented in the reading passage in light of new information.

The Verbal Reasoning section is not intended to assess prior knowledge in the subject areas from which the readings are gathered, but rather to measure your ability to understand, evaluate, and apply information presented in the form of reading passages. The readings chosen are intentionally picked because they are obscure and you are not likely to have read them before. No prior knowledge in either the sciences, social sciences, or humanities is required to be successful on this section of the exam.

You are expected to read nine passages and answer 60 questions in 85 minutes. This works out to about 1 minute and 25 seconds to answer each question if the reading takes no time at all. If you figure an average time of only $2\frac{1}{2}$ minutes per passage, the total reading time comes to 22.5 minutes. If this is subtracted from the 85 minutes allowed for this section, you actually have only 62.5 minutes to answer the 60 questions, or about 55 seconds per question. Just to attain the reading speed needed to complete the articles in $2\frac{1}{2}$ minutes each will take much practice.

4.1 TIPS FOR IMPROVING YOUR SPEED IN ANSWERING THE QUESTIONS

1. Many students find reading the questions before reading the passage to be very helpful.

    *   By reading the questions first, you'll have a better idea of what to look for when you read the passage.

    *   Read the first sentence of a paragraph and then decide whether to go ahead and read the paragraph. Usually, if the first sentence of a paragraph does not concern any of the topics discussed in the questions, then that paragraph will probably not contain any answers to the questions.

    *   In this situation, it may be a good idea to skim the paragraph rather than read it. If, while skimming the paragraph, you notice information that does apply to one or more of the questions, you can stop skimming the paragraph and read it.

    *   This method can be effective in reducing the time spent on each passage. At first, this method may seem awkward. But by practicing as you prepare for the MCAT exam, you can learn to use it effectively.

        NOTE: This method does not work for everybody. If, after you have practiced using this method, it does not seem to be effective, don't use it on the actual exam.

2. Learn to read articles for information without allowing yourself to become involved in the article.

    *   The more involved you become in the article, the slower you will read the article. Many of the articles chosen for the MCAT exam are interesting. However, you must avoid the temptation to think about the article except to answer the questions being asked.

    *   Keep in mind that you are not reading for enjoyment but for information. The more you practice reading for information, the more successful you will be on the exam.

    *   You must discipline your mind to look only for answers to the questions. When you are doing practice readings, stop reading and start all over again if you notice that your mind is beginning to wander or that you are beginning to think about the implications of the article beyond the immediate questions that you must answer.

4.2 WHAT MAKES A GOOD READER

To be successful on the MCAT Verbal Reasoning section, you must

1. **Understand the Main Idea of the Article**
    There is almost always at least one question for each reading that requires you to demonstrate your understanding of the main idea of the article. Therefore, as you finish each practice reading passage, ask yourself, "What is the main idea?"

2. **Pay Attention to Detail**
   Questions on the Verbal Reasoning section often focus on what may seem to be small details.

3. **Understand the Difference Between What Is Inferred, Implied, and Stated**
   Many questions on the Verbal Reasoning section of the MCAT ask you to differentiate between appropriate inference and inappropriate inference. You may be asked to differentiate between what can reasonably be implied from an article and what cannot. You may also be asked whether something was stated in an article or implied.

4. **Understand the Logic that the Author of the Article Is Using to Make His or Her Argument**
   Follow the logic even if you do not think that the author's argument holds up.

5. **Understand the Author's Point of View**
   Make sure that you don't misinterpret the author's argument. It is easy to confuse your points of view with the author's.

6. **Understand the Main Idea of Each Paragraph and How that Paragraph Relates to Both the Preceding Paragraph and the Following Paragraph**
   Many questions will ask you to demonstrate your understanding of the relationship between the main ideas of different paragraphs.

4.3 TYPES OF MCAT VERBAL REASONING QUESTIONS

The following is a list of typical questions you can expect to find on the Verbal Reasoning section of the MCAT:

1. **Main Idea Questions**
   These questions test your comprehension of the theme of the article.

2. **Purpose Questions**
   These questions probe your understanding of the author's reason for writing the article.

3. **Inference Questions**
   These questions require that you understand the logic of the author's argument and to then decide what can be reasonably inferred from the article and what cannot be reasonably inferred from the article.

4. **Supporting Evidence Questions**
   These questions ask you to identify the evidence the author uses to support his or her argument. Most of the articles used on the MCAT are argumentative and, as the reader, you must train yourself to identify the evidence.

5. **Analysis of Information Questions**
   These questions may require you to analyze relationships between given and implied information. You will be asked not only to understand the way the author uses different pieces of information but also to evaluate whether the author has built sound arguments.

6. **Effect of New Information Questions**

    You will be given new information in the context of questions and then asked how this new information affects the author's original argument.

7. **Synthesis of Concepts and Ideas Questions**

    You will be asked to determine which statement best expresses the author's arguments or conclusions.

8. **Implication Questions**

    You will be asked questions that require you to make judgments about what would follow if the author is correct in his or her argument or what a particular discovery might lead to.

The following section presents a sample of each kind of article that appears on the MCAT, together with examples of the kinds of questions you will be asked. At the end of the section you will find the correct answers for the questions and explanations of why each answer is correct.

Example I

The Rhinegold's malignity seems to have leaped from Valhalla's legendary realm to the sphere of humans. Wieland Wagner was to have produced *Der Ring des Nibelungen* in Geneva, with the gifted young Christian Vochting conducting; both died within a year of each other, Vochting this past November. Undaunted, the Grand Theatre's director, Herbert Graf, met the first challenge by producing *Das Rheingold* himself, conceiving both stage effects and costumes. The second problem was solved through the courtesy of Rudolf Bing, who lent Metropolitan conductor Ignace Strasfogel for the emergency. Then there was the formidable hurdle of molding in three weeks a green cast (only John Modenos as Alberich having been in *Das Rheingold* before) and a green orchestra, the opera not having been played in Geneva for 40 years.

The result was an admirable production of six performances in January and February. Through adroit lighting, Graf emphasized the characters without resorting to the starkness of the modern Bayreuth stage. A film projection on a fine-net screen seemed to submerge the audience in the Rhine's rippling current; also through film, Valhalla was projected in the background as a massive but nebulous bastion of stone blocks. For clangorous Nibelheim's obscurity, a large shaft of rock sufficed. In long

robes, with cuirass-like decor, the gods lent visual warmth in rich blue, Nile green, and saffron; Loge's flame-red cape glistened with flecks of gold; and the giants wore garb of vertical gray slabs, suggesting their Valhalla.

An exceptionally homogeneous cast included the mature mezzo of Sandra Warfield as Frica, the ringing soprano of Jeanne Cook as Freia, and the somewhat light baritone of Ramon Vinay as an imperious Wotan. Glade Peterson's flickering, mercurial Loge was a delight. Portraying the giants were lumbering Franz Petri and Manfred Schenk, with Modenos and Fritz Peter as Alberich and Mimme, and Michel Bouvier and Thomas Page as Donner and Froh. Strasfogel made *Das Rheingold* stirringly eloquent, and at the end he, Graf, and the cast were rewarded with shouts of enthusiasm.

1. The reviewer explains that one of the difficulties in putting together the performance was that it had not been done in Geneva in

    A. 10 years.
    B. 100 years.
    C. the winter.
    D. 40 years.

2. The reviewer's opinion of the performance was that

   A. it was ruined by the deaths of the two key people.
   B. in spite of the deaths of the two key people, the performance went well.
   C. the performance was neither good nor bad.
   D. using film in the background was an inappropriate idea.

3. The reviewer comments that

   A. the cast was new and untrained when it was assembled.
   B. the actors did not get along well, which weakened the performance.
   C. the conducting and the singing did not go well together.
   D. the acting was good, but the singing was poor.

4. The reviewer implies that the singer who added the least to the production was

   A. Glade Peterson.
   B. Ramon Vinay.
   C. Sandra Warfield.
   D. John Modenos.

5. Who took over after the death of the two key people involved in the opera's production?

   A. Ramon Vinay
   B. Herbert Graf
   C. Sandra Warfield
   D. Rudolf Bing

6. On the basis of the article, it would be reasonable to assume that its author

   A. had never seen the opera before.
   B. was extremely familiar with the opera and had positive feelings about it.
   C. was very familiar with the opera but did not like it.
   D. had some knowledge of the opera prior to seeing it performed, but learned most of what he knew from seeing this performance.

Example II

There is evidence that the usual variety of high blood pressure is, in part, a familial disease. Since families have similar genes as well as similar environments, familial diseases could be attributable to shared genetic influences, shared environmental factors, or both. For some years, the role of one environmental factor commonly shared by families, namely dietary salt (i.e., sodium chloride), has been studied at Brookhaven National Laboratory. These studies suggest that chronic excess salt ingestion can lead to high blood pressure in man and animals. Some individuals, however, and some rats consume large amounts of salt without developing high blood pressure. No matter how strictly all environmental factors were controlled in these experiments, some salt-fed animals never developed hypertension, whereas a few rapidly developed very severe hypertension followed by early death. These marked variations were interpreted to result from differences in genetic constitution.

By mating in successive generations only those animals that failed to develop hypertension from salt ingestion, a resistant strain (the "R" strain) has been evolved in which consumption of large quantities of salt fails to influence the blood pressure significantly. In contrast, by mating only animals that quickly develop hypertension from salt, a sensitive strain (the "S" strain) has also been developed.

The availability of these two strains permits investigations not heretofore possible. They provide a plausible laboratory model on which to investigate some clinical aspects of the human prototypes of hypertension. More important, there might be the possibility of developing methods by which genetic susceptibility of human beings to high blood pressure can be defined without waiting for its appearance. Radioactive Sodium 22 was an important tool in working out the characteristics of the sodium chloride metabolism.

1. On the basis of this article, one could infer that the main difference between S rats and R rats is

   A. how much salt each strain consumes.
   B. the difference in rates of the development of hypertension between strains.
   C. each strain of rats' ability to deal with stress.
   D. the ability of each strain to digest salt.

2. The main point of the article is that

   A. only environmental factors are important when studying high blood pressure.
   B. environmental factors alone do not fully explain incidences of high blood pressure within different families.
   C. salt is bad for some people, but not for others.
   D. salt has been correlated to high rates of hypertension.

3. The purpose of breeding two distinct strains of rats was to

   A. better understand environmental stress factors in high blood pressure.
   B. better understand how social structure contributes to high blood pressure.
   C. improve the clinical study of genetic differences in salt ingestion.
   D. use the rats as a model to develop strains of high- and low-salt ingestion in humans.

4. According to this article, the common variety of high blood pressure can be caused by

   A. too much stress at work.
   B. mostly environmental factors.
   C. genetic factors.
   D. basically consuming too much salt.

5. According to the article, which of the following is one indication that there is an important genetic component to high blood pressure?

   A. High blood pressure tends to run in families.
   B. Studies on rats show that when rats who develop high blood pressure are bred with other rats who have high blood pressure, their offspring tend to develop high blood pressure.
   C. Humans without family histories of high blood pressure rarely develop high blood pressure.
   D. High blood pressure is unknown among rats that have not been developed to produce high blood pressure.

6. One of the most important potential results of the research being done on these two strains of rats is

   A. a better understanding of how salt is ingested into a rat's body.
   B. the ability to identify which humans are most likely to develop hypertension.
   C. a better understanding of how family life affects high blood pressure.
   D. the ability to determine how the stress of captivity affects the rates of hypertension among rats.

7. If high blood pressure has a genetic component, it would be reasonable to infer which of the following?

   A. Humans should no longer worry about their diet as it pertains to high blood pressure.
   B. It would be a waste of time for people with high blood pressure to try to reduce their stress level to reduce their blood pressure.
   C. Weight would not be an important factor in the development of high blood pressure.
   D. We might be able to develop a prenatal test that would detect a tendency toward high blood pressure.

8. If this research were to continue in the future, we might recommend that children who had a genetic tendency to develop high blood pressure

   A. be given a special low-salt diet from birth.
   B. plan on living a shorter life, based on their families' tendencies to develop high blood pressure.
   C. not be allowed to marry each other.
   D. be excluded from the program established to breed a strain of humans who exhibit a low tendency to develop high blood pressure.

Example III

Two hundred years after enactment of the Virginia Statute for Religious Freedom, questions continue to be raised about the separation of church and state in this country. Such questions have most recently addressed issues relating to prayer in the schools, tax exemptions for parochial institutions, clerical advocacy of specific political policies, and secular humanism.

Because of the current intensity of interest in the relationship between church and state and in the continuation of the unbroken tradition of scholarship on the statute, the Virginia Foundation for the Humanities and Public Policy sponsored a symposium in September 1985 that brought together noted scholars in religion, political science, philosophy, and history—among them J. G. A. Pocock, Martin Marty, Walter Berns, and Richard Roty—and members of the public in a discussion of the relationship between the American political tradition and the principles articulated in the Virginia statute. Symposium participants examined the origins of the statute, its historical influence and interpretation, and its relevance and implications for society today.

Thomas Jefferson's Bill for Establishing Religious Freedom, which passed through the Virginia legislature through the legislative skill of James Madison, became the basis for the constitutional guarantees of religious freedom in the First Amendment. Jefferson's words expressed the principle of freedom of thought that was to rest at the foundation of the American republic. The enactment of the Virginia statute marked the first time in thirteen centuries of Western history that a law ended religious persecution, exclusion, and compulsion. It also established the radical separation of church and state. Because the statute contributed to the spread of popular religions and helped to open the door of the new nation to the diverse religious groups of Europe, the Virginia Statute for Religious Freedom is one of the essential documents defining not only the law but also the culture of this country.

In Pocock's view, the Virginia statute successfully legislated both the freedom of the religious sect from the established religion and the freedom of the liberal state from either. It should seem then that the statute goes a little way . . . toward establishing a kind of unitarian universalism—the religion of free inquiry—not as the official religion of American society, but as that most easily recognized by that society's magistracy and values; and at the same time words regarding the Pentecostal sects as a kind of loyal opposition.

As a background and tone-setting document, the statute is typical of founding texts that lie behind present-day debates over "who owns America," said Martin Marty of the University of Chicago in discussing the statute's importance. If one part of society sees separation of church and state as necessary to securing liberty of conscience, another part sees it (especially the Supreme Court's "acceptance of belief-as-religion") as contributing to the elimination of theism from the public educational system and to the entrenchment of secular humanism in its place.

"Toleration of religious differences, for most Americans, has not meant indifference to religion," said Walter Berns of the American Enterprise Institute. "By separating church and state, Americans consigned religion to the private sphere or, more precisely, to the care of private institutions, but they have traditionally seen reason to provide public support—on a nondiscriminatory basis—for those institutions." And, he predicted, because they retain the support of the people, such laws will continue to be passed by state legislatures, "the Supreme Court to the contrary notwithstanding."

Jefferson himself described the country he was trying to create as "an experiment." Rorty believes that if that experiment fails, our descendants will not necessarily learn either a philosophical or a religious truth from that failure. They will simply know what to look for while constructing the next experiment. "Even if nothing else survives from the age of the democratic revolutions," he said, "perhaps our descendants will still remember that social institutions can be viewed as experiments in cooperation rather than as attempts to embody a universal and a historical order. It is hard to believe that this memory would not be worth having."

1. According to the article, the Virginia law that guaranteed freedom of religion was used as a model for which constitutional amendment?

   A. First
   B. Second
   C. Third
   D. Fourth

2. One could infer from the article that the author supports

   A. some aspects of the law that established freedom of religion but opposes other parts of the law.
   B. the concept of freedom of religion, but believes the Supreme Court has gone too far in its interpretation of what freedom of religion constitutes.
   C. both the concept of freedom of religion and its interpretation.
   D. the concept of the Virginia law, but believes the law needs to be updated for the modern world.

3. According to Pocock's view, the Virginia law on freedom of religion established which two important principles?

   A. Freedom for organized religion and freedom for religious competition
   B. Freedom for people to practice whatever religion they choose and freedom from establishment of a government religion
   C. Freedom of religious sects to establish themselves separately from religion and freedom of the liberal state from both established religion and religious sects
   D. Freedom for people to choose not to participate in any religion and the right of religious groups not to be taxed by the government

4. According to the author, some current issues that involve separation of church and state are

A. federal laws outlawing segregation in private schools, church rules forbidding birth control, and clerics running for political office.

B. the right of certain religious groups not to allow their members to join the armed services, the state's right to confiscate religious property, and the teaching of sex education in the public schools.

C. whether a sect has the same protection under the Constitution as a religion, whether religious groups should be involved in censoring art, and whether religious groups have the right to support political candidates.

D. whether we should have school prayer, whether parochial schools should be tax-exempt, and whether it is appropriate for clerics to be advocates of political issues.

5. Rorty points out that Jefferson's bill was an experiment in

A. social cooperation.

B. providing a universal and historical order.

C. preserving a democratic revolution.

D. maintaining a uniform religion in the United States.

6. The separation of church and state in America has not ensured which one of the following?

A. Toleration of religious differences

B. Lack of a tradition of public support to private institutions with religious affiliation

C. Passage of similar laws in state legislatures due to the public's support

D. Complete freedom from governmental control and interference

ANSWER KEY

Example I		Example II		Example III	
1. D	4. B	1. B	5. B	1. A	4. D
2. B	5. B	2. B	6. B	2. C	5. A
3. A	6. B	3. C	7. D	3. C	6. B
		4. C	8. A		

ANSWERS AND EXPLANATIONS

Example I

1. **The correct answer is (D).** The answer to this question is based on the following statement from paragraph 1: ". . . the opera not having been played in Geneva for 40 years."

2. **The correct answer is (B).** The answer to this question is based on the following statement from paragraph 2: "The result was an admirable production, given six performances in January and February."

3. **The correct answer is (A).** The answer to this question is based on this statement from paragraph 1: "Then, there was the formidable hurdle of molding in three weeks a green cast . . . and a green orchestra. . . ."

4. **The correct answer is (B).** This answer is inferred from the following statement in paragraph 3: "An exceptionally homogeneous cast included the mature mezzo of Sandra Warfield as Frica, the ringing soprano of Jeanne Cook as Freia, and the somewhat light baritone of Ramon Vinay as an imperious Wotan."

5. **The correct answer is (B).** The answer to this question is based on the following statement from paragraph 1: "Undaunted, the Grand Theatre's director, Herbert Graf, met the first challenge by producing *Das Rheingold* himself. . . ."

6. **The correct answer is (B).** It is clear from his description of the opera and of the actors that he both likes the opera and is quite familiar with it.

Example II

1. **The correct answer is (B).** The answer to this question can be inferred from the following statement found in paragraph 2: "By mating in successive generations only those animals that failed to develop hypertension from salt ingestion, a resistant strain (the 'R' strain) has evolved in which consumption of large quantities of salt fails to influence the blood pressure significantly. In contrast, by mating only animals that quickly develop hypertension from salt, a sensitive strain (the 'S' strain) has also been developed."

2. **The correct answer is (B).** The answer to this question is based on the following statements found in paragraph 1 and on the general discussion in the article as a whole: "Some individuals, however, and some rats consume large amounts of salt without developing high blood pressure. . . . These marked variations were interpreted to result from differences in genetic constitution."

3. **The correct answer is (C).** The answer to this question is based on the following statement from paragraph 3: "The availability of these two strains permits investigations not heretofore possible. They provide a plausible laboratory model on which to investigate some clinical aspects of the human prototypes of hypertension."

4. **The correct answer is (C).** The answer to this question is found in the following statement in paragraph 1: "Some individuals, however, and some rats consume large amounts of salt without developing high blood pressure. No matter how strictly all environmental factors were controlled in these experiments, some salt-fed animals never developed hypertension whereas a few rapidly developed very severe hypertension followed by early death. These marked variations were interpreted to result from differences in genetic constitution."

5. **The correct answer is (B).** The answer to this question can be inferred from the following statement from paragraph 2: "In contrast, by mating only animals that quickly develop hypertension from salt, a sensitive strain (the 'S' strain) has been developed."

6. **The correct answer is (B).** The answer to this question is found in the following statement from paragraph 3: "More important, there might be the possibility of developing methods by which genetic susceptibility of human beings to high blood pressure can be defined without waiting for its appearance."

7. **The correct answer is (D).** The answer to this question can be inferred from the statement used to explain the answer to Question 6.

8. **The correct answer is (A).** The answer to this question is based on the following statement found in paragraph 3: ". . . there might be the possibility of developing methods by which genetic susceptibility of human beings to high blood pressure can be defined without waiting for its appearance."

Example III

1. **The correct answer is (A).** The answer to this question is based on the following statement from paragraph 3: "Thomas Jefferson's Bill for Establishing Religious Freedom which passed through the Virginia legislature . . . became the basis for the constitutional guarantees of religious freedom in the First Amendment."

2. **The correct answer is (C).** The answer to this question can be inferred from the fact that the author does not give any criticism of the concept of separation of church and state and by the fact that he closes the article with a positive quote on the concept of church and state. The following statement from paragraph 7 is an example of the positive direction of the article to the separation of church and state: "'Even if nothing else survives from the age of democratic revolutions,' he said, 'perhaps our descendents will still remember that social institutions can be viewed as experiments in cooperation rather than as attempts to embody a universal and historical order. It is hard to believe that this memory would not be worth having.' "

3. **The correct answer is (C).** The answer to this question is based on the following statement from paragraph 4: "In Pocock's view, the Virginia statute successfully legislated both the freedom of the religious sect from the established religion and the freedom of the liberal state from either."

4. **The correct answer is (D).** The answer to this question is found in the following statement from paragraph 1: "Such questions have most recently addressed issues relating to prayer in the schools, tax exemptions for parochial institutions, clerical advocacy of specific political policies. . . ."

5. **The correct answer is (A).** The answer to this question can be inferred from the following statement in paragraph 6: ". . . perhaps our descendants will still remember that social institutions can be viewed as experiments in cooperation. . . ."

6. **The correct answer is (B).** The answer to this question is found in the following statement in paragraph 6: "By separating church and state, Americans consigned religion to the private sphere . . . but they have seen reason to provide public support—on a nondiscriminatory basis—for those institutions."

CHAPTER 5

Verbal Reasoning Sample Exam

Although the actual Verbal Reasoning section of the MCAT exam has been reduced to 60 questions, for the purposes of practice we have left our Verbal Reasoning tests at 65 questions.

TIME: 85 MINUTES   65 QUESTIONS

Directions: There are nine passages in this test. Each passage is followed by questions based on its content. After reading a passage, choose the one best answer to each question. Correct and explanatory answers follow the test.

Passage I (Questions 1–7)

The reasons people give for choosing a job in the field of aging vary a great deal. Among the most common are these:

The rewards of satisfaction. It's sometimes hard to tell whether the worker or the client gains more from the exchange. People who hold jobs in this field say that they learn a great deal from older adults about human nature and enduring values. They almost always emphasize how much they enjoy working with older people. This often reflects personal experience—a close relationship with grandparents is frequently cited as a reason young people are drawn to the field, while middle-aged persons may become interested through awareness of their own aging.

The stimulation of challenge. The field of aging is a pioneering specialty, and opportunities abound to make a difference in older people's lives. Workers in this field have an opportunity to dispel myths and stereotypes, to suggest new ways of doing things, and to promote growth and development late in life. Many people are in the field because so much needs to be done.

The availability of opportunity. Public and private funds have poured into this field for more than 20 years, supporting program expansion as well as considerable change in the way health, housing, transportation, and other services are provided to older adults. The Older Americans Act of 1965 and other legislation have spurred federal and state expenditures in planning and development, direct services, and gerontological education and training. Today, the Older Americans Act fosters a billion-dollar social services program and a structure of administrative and advocacy organizations at the federal, state, and local levels. Public support for aging programs is expected to continue, and private support seems likely to expand. The continued growth of the older population is the single most important factor in the proliferation of job opportunities in the field of aging. The number of Americans over the age of 65 has been rising rapidly for several decades and currently stands at about 30 million. By the year 2000, it will exceed 36 million. The oldest segment of our population—those over 85 years of age—is growing most rapidly of all. The impending growth in the number of Americans in their eighties and nineties is bound to produce a sharp increase in the need for health, housing, long-term care, and social services in the years ahead.

Endless possibilities. A casual encounter with someone in the field, experience as a student intern or volunteer, a job opening, the availability of financial aid for gerontology students—all are typical first steps on the road to a career in the field of aging.

1. The Older Americans Act was passed in which of the following years?

    A. 1965
    B. 1973
    C. 1980
    D. 1988

2. According to the author, which of the following is one of the most common reasons people give for working in the field of aging?

    A. The growth in the number of elderly people
    B. The reward of satisfaction
    C. Good income opportunities
    D. The ability to move from field to field

3. By the year 2000, the number of people in the United States over the age of 65 is expected to be

    A. between 20 million and 25 million.
    B. 30 million.
    C. 36 million.
    D. over 36 million people.

4. According to the article, the fastest growing segment of the elderly population is the group that is

    A. between 65 and 75.
    B. between 70 and 80.
    C. between 75 and 85.
    D. over 85.

5. According to the author, which one of the following is true?

    A. Both public and private support for the aging are likely to remain the same.
    B. Public support for programs that serve the aging is likely to continue and private support is likely to increase.
    C. Although public support for programs that serve the aging is likely to continue, private support is likely to decrease.
    D. Both public and private support for programs that serve the aging are likely to increase.

6. All of the following are cited as means of entering the field of serving the aging EXCEPT:

    A. college training in gerontology.
    B. a chance encounter with someone in the field.
    C. volunteer work.
    D. fear of growing old.

7. It would be reasonable to interpret the author's attitude toward careers in the field of aging as

    A. very positive.
    B. neutral.
    C. slightly negative.
    D. very negative.

Passage II (Questions 8–15)

Neutrinos offer an opportunity to measure events that take place inside the sun. Neutrinos are uncharged and, for all practical purposes, massless particles of matter; they very rarely react with anything. A single neutrino can pass through the entire sun with only one chance in a billion of being stopped. Their theoretical properties, however, including a fractional one-half spin quantum number, make them detectable. Even though their brief half-life would lead many to decay in transit, a measurable flux of neutrinos created in the interior of the sun and sent in the direction of Earth should arrive at Earth-based neutrino counters.

Since the number of neutrinos produced varies with the temperature of the specific thermonuclear reaction, scientists counting emitted neutrinos should be able to draw significant conclusions about the reactions taking place in the sun's core. But actually counting these elusive particles is another problem. Not even the most elaborate neutrino traps—including one buried deep below the Earth's surface in the Homestake Mine in South Dakota by Raymond Davis of Brookhaven National Laboratory and his colleagues—have found enough neutrinos to match the number predicted by classical theories of the solar interior.

Many ingenious reasons have been proposed to explain this "neutrino deficit." The measuring instruments may be inadequate. Or, perhaps, at the extreme of astronomers' imaginings, a "sink" of some sort in the sun is altering most of the neutrinos before they can escape. Even the global solar oscillations have been suggested as an explanation: If such oscillations really rock through the sun quickly, perhaps in as short a period as an hour, they could be moving energy out from the center of the sun fast enough to cool the thermonuclear furnace and reduce the production of neutrinos.

But whatever the final explanation, the apparent neutrino deficit suggests some hard, fundamental questions. "Since stellar astronomy relies fundamentally on an understanding of the sun, the solar neutrino question could shake the very foundation of astrophysics," says Beverly Lynds, assistant director of Kitt Peak National Observatory near Tucson, Arizona.

"The lack of solar neutrinos indicates that something is wrong. Is it with our theory of the sun's structure or with that of atomic reactions? If it is the model of the sun," she concludes, "then the whole theory of stellar evolution could be wrong."

8. Which one of the following statements is true?

   A. Scientists have found more neutrinos than they expected.
   B. Scientists have found as many neutrinos as they expected.
   C. Scientists have found far fewer neutrinos than were expected.
   D. Scientists, on some occasions, have found more neutrinos than expected and, on other occasions, fewer neutrinos than expected.

9. The number of neutrinos produced, according to the article, varies based on which one of the following factors?

   A. The size of the thermonuclear reaction
   B. The temperature of the thermonuclear reaction
   C. The number of electrons produced during the thermonuclear reaction
   D. The number of protons produced during a thermonuclear reaction

10. According to the article, which of the following best explains the "neutrino deficit"?

   A. Usage of measuring instruments that are highly refined and reliable
   B. A condition in the sun that affects neutrinos before they escape from the sun
   C. The reduction in neutrino production due to the moon's increased velocity at periodic times of the year
   D. The unusually slow oscillation of solar movements in the sun's center

11. The article points out that one theoretical property of neutrinos that makes them detectable is their

   A. ability to interact noticeably with other particles.
   B. massive size in groups.
   C. one-half spin quantum number.
   D. activity in the sun's core.

12. Neutrinos are defined by which of the following?

   I. Positively charged particles
   II. Negatively charged particles
   III. Chargeless particles

   A. I only
   B. I and II only
   C. III only
   D. II and III only

13. Beverly Lynds, assistant director of the Kitts Peak National Observatory, states that the solar neutrino question could shake the foundations of which one of the following disciplines?

   A. Astrophysics
   B. Stellar astronomy
   C. Astronomy
   D. Nuclear physics

14. According to Beverly Lynds, the lack of solar neutrinos could be an indication that something is wrong with which one of the following theories?

   A. The theory of stellar evolution
   B. The role of gravity in the universe
   C. Theory of atomic reactions
   D. Electromagnetic theory

15. According to the article, neutrinos would be useful for measuring which of the following?

   A. Activity going on in the Earth's core
   B. Activity going on in the sun
   C. The energy released in a nuclear fusion reaction
   D. The attraction between protons and electrons

Passage III (Questions 16–21)

The Russian laws of war state the obvious: The nation that is better prepared to wage war militarily, politically, economically, and psychologically will win. Correlation of forces, a conceptual comparison of the relative strengths of potential enemies, is an integral dynamic contained within Russian doctrinal philosophy. It is used to set national goals, and determines the appropriate form of struggle to meet those goals. Since the correlation of forces is such a key Russian doctrinal concept, the United States intelligence community must understand its influence on Russian decision-making policies.

War is not the primary objective of Russian political strategy. The goal of Russian politics is to create and maintain favorable economic and political conditions. The Russians prefer to achieve this objective peacefully—by forcing appeasement upon the enemy; they bargain from a position of strength whenever possible. Thus, the correlation of forces is used to determine when that position of strength exists, and when it is strong enough to achieve their goal without resorting to armed conflict.

This general estimate of the situation is usual in all political and military decision-making processes, but its inherent "scientific" application in policy making is distinctly Russian. Based on the gathered data, the Russians determine if the correlation of forces is favorable, unfavorable, or nearly equal. Consequently, they decide which form of struggle to use, ranging from diplomacy to general war.

The ideal Russian strategy is a favorable correlation of forces. Under these conditions, the Russians expect to attain their goals without resorting to war. They hope to influence the enemy to concede that they would have more to gain by negotiating than by fighting. The Russians will then bargain from a position of strength. This tactic is clearly evident in the post-World War II partitioning of Europe.

When methods of lesser risk are not likely to achieve their goals, the Russians will use the correlation theory to determine the risks involved in using armed forces. If the potential gain outweighs the risk, the Russians will use their armed forces as the quickest and most reliable means possible—but only when the correlation of forces indicates that major enemies will be unlikely or unable to intervene militarily. Their theory was accurate in Hungary, Czechoslovakia, and Afghanistan.

If they believe the correlations of forces are unfavorable, the Russians will either reset the goal at a more attainable level, or choose a form of struggle below that of a state of war, such as subversion, sabotage, colonial rebellion, or proxy war. To the Russians, these armed conflicts pose little political risk and are useful when diplomacy fails.

There is a risk of war when the correlation of forces is nearly equal. Under this condition, Russian decision makers have three options:

- Reset the goal to a level attainable by diplomacy, which changes the correlation of forces;

- Subjectively lower the correlation of forces to *unfavorable* and choose a supplementary form of struggle;

- Subjectively raise the correlation of forces to *favorable* and attempt to bargain from a position of strength.

The Russians believe that a scientific application of the correlation of forces will prevent the nation from being drawn into a war they will lose. They are therefore unlikely to take the risks involved in subjectively raising the correlation of forces. Case in point: the Cuban missile crisis.

The greatest risk of war occurs when the correlation of forces is inaccurately determined. When each of two adversaries believes it has a more favorable correlation of forces than the other, war is virtually inevitable. Each side will attempt to force appeasement on the enemy. Almost ironically, just as disagreement on their relative strengths will most likely lead to war, the war will end when the two sides agree on their relative strengths as the outcome of the war becomes obvious.

The Russians take pride in their ability to correctly assess their relative strength using the correlation of forces, and in their ability to

manipulate the forces used in the correlation. Their long-term goals include efforts to constantly shift the correlation in their favor. They are confident in their ability to use the laws of war to achieve their goals without becoming involved in a general war. They have far less faith in the policy makers of the west.

16. Based on the article, which one of the following would be a reasonable assumption about Russian foreign policy?

   A. The Russians believed that the West was much more rational about foreign policy than was Russia.
   B. The West used the same methods for calculating the risk of war as the Russians did.
   C. The Russians believed that the West was less rational about calculating their foreign policy than the Russians were.
   D. The Russians were more willing to risk war than the West was.

17. The author defined the correlation of forces as which one of the following?

   A. A conceptual comparison of relative strength of potential enemies
   B. The balance of power
   C. An imbalance of military power
   D. A balance of military power, but not of economic power

18. According to the author, the risk of war was greatest under which of the following conditions?

   A. The correlation of forces was equal.
   B. One side had a clear advantage over the other.
   C. Both sides were weak, but one side was weaker than the other.
   D. The correlations of forces was inaccurately determined.

19. Which one of the following is NOT an example of Russia's use of military force in circumstances where it believed that military force was the only way to obtain its goals and that other major powers would not or could not intervene?

    A. Afghanistan
    B. China
    C. Hungary
    D. Czechoslovakia

20. The article points out that Russian political strategy was to

    A. use armed conflict whenever possible.
    B. create and maintain favorable economic and political conditions by forcing appeasement upon the enemy.
    C. avoid armed conflict in all situations.
    D. make allies with small neighboring countries and to intimidate larger, more powerful countries.

21. Based on the information in the article, which of the following conditions would have been most likely to inspire Russia to wage war?

    A. A strong Russia and a weak adversary
    B. A weak Russia and a strong adversary
    C. An adversary that is equal in power to Russia
    D. A threat to a Russian ally

Passage IV (Questions 22–28)

At last it is out—the *Encyclopedia of Southern Culture*, a ten-year project involving more than 800 scholars and writers. By the time the encyclopedia rolled off the binders at the University of North Carolina Press, it had taken more than twice the time spent fighting the Civil War.

Although the focus is on the eleven states of the Confederacy, this volume goes wherever Southern culture is found, from outposts in the middle Atlantic states to pockets of Chicago and Bakersfield.

. . . The book attempts to keep fresh the memories of a distinctive way of life—a little like sitting a spell and visiting with a culture that links Huey Long and Mahalia Jackson, Scarlett O'Hara and Hank Aaron, the Bible Belt and [Walt] Disney World. Indeed, the 1,200 entries range from Aaron to Zydeco; they cover *Gone With the Wind*, Tennessee Williams, Rednecks, Belles and Ladies, Catfish, Charleston, Bluegrass, Rosa Parks, and Martin Luther King, Jr.

In the foreword, *Roots* author Alex Haley—himself an entry—writes: "Out of the historic cotton tillage sprang the involuntary field hollers, the shouts, and the moanin' low that has since produced such a cornucopia of music, played daily, on every continent . . .

"Equally worldwide is Southern literature. Writers took the oral traditions of the South—the political rhetoric, preaching, conversational wordplay, and lazy-day storytelling—and converted them into art." For Haley, what makes the encyclopedia special is the personal experiences that researchers—including historians, literary critics, anthropologists, theologians, politicians, psychologists, lawyers and doctors, folklorists, university presidents, newspaper reporters, magazine writers, and novelists—have brought to it. "They walked and talked with the sharecropper farmers, the cooks, the quiltmakers, the convicts, the merchants, the fishermen, and all the others who make these pages a volume of living memories."

Co-editors Charles Reagan Wilson and William Ferris work out of the Barnard Observatory on the campus of the University of Mississippi, which houses the Center for the Study of Southern Culture. Although the observatory has three towers from which astronomers could gaze at the heavens, it has no telescopes. It has, however, become the human lens through which scholars have sought the essence of the South. The editors deliberated about various definitions of culture and eventually adapted that of anthropologist Clifford Geertz: "An historically transmitted pattern of meaning embodied in symbols, a system of inherited conceptions expressed in symbolic forms."

"The South historically has been our most isolated, our most intense regional experience," says Ferris, who has been director of the Center since 1979 and is living proof that you can go home again. Ferris was born on a farm on Route 1 in Vicksburg, where they grow soybeans and cattle. Although he left to teach American folklore and Afro-American culture at Yale, and to make records and documentary films, he is now firmly home.

Ferris believes folklore is the key to understanding Mississippi's great artists. "It is the key to William Faulkner, Eudora Welty, Richard Wright, B. B. King. Unless we accept that, we are alienated from who we are," he says. Mississippi is especially inspired for its talkers, he says; nobody can make a point without telling a story. "In Faulkner, the characters are always talking and Faulknerian style reflects the voices he grew up with."

The volume is organized around 24 thematic sections, covering such topics as Black Life, Mythic South, History and Manners, Religion, Violence, and Women's Life. "What we end up with are many Souths," says Wilson. "There is the geographical South. There is the South outside the South, which includes not only expatriate writers but southern black communities in northern cities. And then there is also the South of *Roots* and Faulkner and the blues. You cannot deal with one and not the other."

. . . The editors argued that Southerners have a stronger sense of regionalism than people anywhere else in America—akin to the Basques in Spain, the Kurds in the Middle East, the French in Canada. In choosing some 250 persons for the biographical sketches, Wilson says they selected those whose works transcended a particular field or those not found in research works, such as quilter Harriet Powers and painter Clementine Hunter.

The two editors wrote dozens of articles themselves. From Wilson come pieces about the southern funeral and Reconstruction. From Ferris come entries on Leadbelly, voodoo, and one of his specialties, mules. . . . The entries on food would make a volume by themselves. Tom Rankin of the Southern Arts Federation contributed the lore about Moon Pies. Created 70 years ago by the Chattanooga Bakery, they consist of two big cookies held together by a marshmallow, originally coated with chocolate. Moon Pies became a cultural phenomenon during the Great Depression along with RC Cola®, when each cost a nickel and together comprised what Rankin terms the "10-cent lunch. . . ."

. . . In advance of its publication, the Press received letters like the one from . . . a gentleman in California, "Moved from the South to California. There is no culture here, so rush us a copy."

22. According to the article, *The Encyclopedia of Southern Culture* covers all of the following topics dealing with southern life EXCEPT:

    A. oral traditions, storytelling, and anecdotes.
    B. philosophy, science, and environmentalism.
    C. origins of food fads such as the Moon Pie.
    D. biographical sketches on selected individuals.

23. The author is suggesting that the common bond shared by Faulkner, Welty, and Wright in their writings stems from the influence of

    A. folklore and the oral tradition of storytelling.
    B. folklore's emphasizing the supernatural.
    C. important musical geniuses such as B. B. King.
    D. having been born in Mississippi.

24. The focus of the encyclopedia is on

   A. the Confederate states only.
   B. the South and any area in the United States where Southern culture can be found.
   C. the rural areas of the South only.
   D. the cultural centers of the South.

25. The article compares the American Southerners' intense sense of regionalism to that of the

   A. Basques in Spain.
   B. Maoris in the South Pacific.
   C. Kikuyu in Kenya.
   D. Igorots of the Philippines.

26. According to the article, the foundation of Southern literature includes

   I. Storytelling, legends, and folk tales.
   II. Religious preaching.
   III. Local gossip and rumor.

   A. I only
   B. I and II only
   C. I and III only
   D. III only

27. The production of the *Encyclopedia of Southern Culture* involved

   A. 20 years of research.
   B. as many years as the Civil War.
   C. more than 1,200 writers and editors.
   D. more than 800 scholars and writers.

28. The article implies that the editors of *The Encyclopedia of Southern Culture* regard the South as a

   A. monolithic cultural region.
   B. multiplicity of cultural, social, and political blendings in a specific region.
   C. homogeneous culture.
   D. bastion of significant literary contributions.

Passage V (Questions 29–34)

Of the many explanations put forth over the years to explain neural-behavioral adaptability, virtually every one has been felled by subsequent experimental evidence. If some proved more durable than others, it was often because they appeared able to resolve the apparent paradox of change in a fixed system.

One of these was the "reverberating loop" or "dynamic change" hypothesis derived from anatomical studies by Rafael Lorente de No of the Rockefeller University, back in the 1930s. He discovered that neurons in the brain were often interconnected in the form of closed chains. This observation suggested to Lorente de No, Norbert Wiener, and others that neural activity—memory and learning, for instance—could be sustained by the circulation or reverberation of electrical signals within closed loops of neurons. The theory was attractive because it explained a durable modification of brain function without requiring change of any kind in cell-to-cell connection. The theory suggested that these looping signals were the files, the data bank, of memory.

Recent work in neurophysiology, however, has called the reverberating hypothesis into serious question. For one, it has been shown that, loop or no loop, neurons do more than excite other neurons. They can also inhibit; through the control they exercise on the passage of chemical neurotransmitters—the conveyors of signals from cell to cell—the synapses, where nerve cell meets nerve (or muscle) cell, can squelch as well as fire a nerve impulse. What initially appeared to be a self-excitary closed circuit might just as easily contain one or more inhibitory connections that could block the further transmission of a signal.

Such realizations as these cast a dark shadow over the loop hypothesis. What obliterated it was the realization that memory persists even in the face of such extreme trauma to the brain as cooling or epileptic seizures. Certainly such shocks would be expected to interrupt the reverberation within a closed-loop memory file. A more durable function for Lorente de No's well-documented neural loops has not been advanced. Nevertheless, information storage is no longer accepted as its function.

29. The anatomical studies of brain neurons in the 1930s suggested that neurons were

    A. capable of transmitting electrical signals.
    B. capable of storing information.
    C. interconnected in closed loops.
    D. endowed with a multiplicity of stimuli.

30. The writer implies that

    A. while recent research in the field of neuro adaptivity has discredited past theories, we still have much to learn to have a complete understanding.
    B. though past theories on neuro transmission were incorrect, we now have a complete understanding of how neurons work.
    C. though research has discredited many past theories on neural behavior adaptivity, new research has given us a complete understanding of the process.
    D. while some recent experiments seem to have cast doubt on the closed loop theory of neuro adaptivity that was developed in the 1930s, he believes that new research will reaffirm the closed-loop theory.

31. Recent research has shown that neurons are capable of

    A. performing only the task of storing memory as evidenced by de No's research.
    B. exciting and inhibiting nerve impulses.
    C. transmitting signals to the brain.
    D. adapting to different stimuli.

32. The "reverberating loop" hypothesis

    A. was disproved by the work of Rafael Lorente de No and Norbert Wiener.
    B. derived from anatomical studies by Rafael Lorente de No.
    C. is still the best explanation of information storage.
    D. has never been questioned.

33. According to the author, the early theory of neural loops in the brain suggested to scientists that neurons did which of the following?

    A. Transmitted nerve impulses to the body
    B. Served to store information
    C. Protected neurons in the brain
    D. Provided communication to either side of the brain

34. The article suggests that over the years, explanations for neural-behavioral adaptability have

    A. fluctuated within the field of science.
    B. persisted in spite of later experimental evidence.
    C. been discredited by subsequent studies.
    D. created divided opinions on the reliability of such research.

Passage VI (Questions 35–41)

"Turn on the television around Easter and at least one station will be airing Cecil B. DeMille's *The Ten Commandments*," says SUNY–Brockport film historian Sumiko Higashi. "Despite his later reputation for commercial schlock, DeMille's early silent films, produced in the teens, were artistic expressions of some of America's most urgent social concerns. Immigration to this country peaked during those years and DeMille's stories of ethnic, class, and sexual conflict appealed to the public during an era of progressive reform. Critics also reacted favorably to his early films and described them as dramatic, imaginative, and technically superior."

Higashi examined personal papers, correspondence, film scripts, trade journals, scrapbooks, and newspaper and magazine clippings to document a period in DeMille's career—after the legitimate stage and before the formula spectacles—when the man whose posing set the tone for acting and dressing like a director was noted for serious and artistic films.

"DeMille was one of the most popular and commercially successful filmmakers ever," says Higashi, "yet all but his biblical spectacles have faded from memory. With respect to visual style, the historical epics have a dated look. His films are not featured in revival houses or, with the exception of *The Cheat*, included in the canon of works studied in film courses.

"After the early twenties, DeMille's work became formulaic. The films usually made money and even set records at the box office, but they ceased to be interesting except to film buffs with a contemporary camp sensibility."

In 1913, DeMille was 32, unsuccessful, and nearly broke. Jesse L. Lasky, a vaudeville producer, and his brother-in-law Samuel Goldfish (later Goldwyn) had lost most of their money in a failed replica of the Folies Bergeres. Undaunted, the three decided to pool what little capital they had left in an even riskier venture— film. Lasky, Goldfish, DeMille, and Arthur Friend, a fourth partner, formed the Jesse L. Lasky Feature Play Company (named after Lasky, who was best known) to produce feature-length films.

Once in Hollywood, DeMille set up a studio in a barn that is today preserved in Los Angeles as a site of early filmmaking. DeMille brought to the industry an ability to recognize a good story, attention to detail, and the courage to think big. The Lasky Company's first production, a western called *The Squaw Man*, became an instant hit and was hailed by the critics as an example of superior filmmaking.

Almost from the beginning, critics raved about "Lasky lighting" and the "Lasky look," a reference to the use of modeled and high-contrast lighting to achieve dramatic effects. Director DeMille had assembled a first-rate crew, including Alvin Wyckoff and David Belasco's art director, Wilfred Buckland. At first DeMille edited his own film, but in the teens he established a long and fruitful relationship with cutter Anne Bachens. Also notable among his staff was scenarist Jeanie Macpherson.

In 1915, he achieved international acclaim on the release of *The Cheat*, a film in which a socialite who has lost club funds in a stock market gamble accepts $10,000 from a Japanese merchant to avoid ruinous disclosure. She agrees to "pay the price," but in a scene that electrified the public and critics alike, the merchant seizes

the socialite and brands her with his trademark when she reneges. A psychological bombshell, *The Cheat* won acclaim among French critics and solidified the reputation of the Lasky Company as a producer of first-rate feature films. And, for his remarkably subtle portrayal of the merchant in contrast with the exaggerated posturing traditional to melodrama, the Japanese actor Sessue Hayakawa became a star.

Although *The Cheat* is still widely recognized, "noteworthy silents such as *Kindling*, which realistically portrayed class division, tenement life, and lack of opportunity for the poor, are ignored by today's film scholars," Higashi says. "DeMille's early films deal with social issues about class and ethnic distinctions with sensitivity as well as ambivalence." *Chimmie Fadden Out West* and *The Heart of Nora Flynn* depict lower-class Irish in a favorable light compared with the established rich. *Rose of the Rancho* and *Girl of the Golden West* . . . are positive portrayals of Spanish-speaking Americans.

"Although he was a pioneer in a revolutionary new medium," notes Higashi, "DeMille remained influenced by the theatrical tradition of nineteenth-century melodrama, specifically its emphasis on spectacle for the purposes of didacticism. Straddling the Victorian Age and the modernism of the twentieth century, he disseminated the values of a consumer culture within the moralizing framework familiar to audiences he came to know during innumerable tours of the country as an actor."

By the late teens, DeMille moved from films dealing with social issues to pictures that portrayed the stylish and ostentatious consumption of high society. . . . During the twenties . . . entertainments designed for an increasingly consumer-oriented society, DeMille's Jazz Age films legitimized conspicuous consumption. He had discovered the formula that would produce one box-office smash after another in the form of society spectacles and biblical epics.

35. Which one of the following was Lasky's first production of a western movie?

    A. *Chimmie Fadden Out West*
    B. *Rose of the Rancho*
    C. *The Squaw Man*
    D. *Girl of the Golden West*

36. The first film for which Cecil B. DeMille won international acclaim was

    A. *Rose of the Rancho.*
    B. *Chimmie Fadden Out West.*
    C. *Girl of the Golden West.*
    D. *The Cheat.*

37. Cecil B. DeMille's first studio was located in a

    A. barn in Hollywood.
    B. small study in Astoria Queens.
    C. barn in Stony Brook.
    D. warehouse in downtown Los Angeles.

38. While Cecil B. DeMille is often remembered as a producer of schlock movies, the author of this article has made a reasonable argument for which of the following?

    A. Cecil B. DeMille was one of the great filmmakers of all time.
    B. Most of Cecil B. DeMille's movies were of poor quality but his biblical classics will be remembered as great movies.
    C. Many of Cecil B. DeMille's later works were movies not worth remembering, but several of his early films addressed important social issues and were valuable to the development of movies.
    D. Most of Cecil B. DeMille's early films were of poor quality, but many of his later works will be remembered for a long time.

39. The author states that Cecil B. DeMille was strongly influenced by which of the following nineteenth-century traditions?

    A. Slapstick
    B. Melodrama
    C. Musicals
    D. Minstrel shows

40. The article implies that one of Cecil B. DeMille's most remembered films is

    A. *The Ten Commandments.*
    B. *The Cheat.*
    C. *Kindling.*
    D. *Girl of the Golden West.*

41. Which of the following characterize DeMille's contribution as a filmmaker prior to the twenties?

    I. Innovative, highly creative films with dramatic techniques and close attention to the plot
    II. A positive sensitivity toward social and political issues often emphasizing a sympathetic attitude toward ethnic groups
    III. Spectacular films that appealed to mass audiences interested in opulence and luxury

    A. I and II only
    B. I and III only
    C. II only
    D. III only

Passage VII (Questions 42–48)

It has been said that when California sneezes, the rest of the United States catches cold. Certainly, since the California State Board of Education's adoption of a bold new kindergarten through twelfth-grade history and social science framework, there has been interest from throughout the country.

Key questions have been raised. Will the framework become the turning point for social studies reform, perhaps even a new national model? Or, as some skeptics postulate, will California falter and find itself unable to put the change into classrooms by the September 1990 deadline?

Everything "is right on schedule," according to Bill Honig, California's superintendent of public instruction. New textbooks are being created to meet an April 1990 textbook submission deadline. Although publishers are close-mouthed because of the highly competitive nature of textbook publishing, McGraw-Hill's western regional manager, Bill Jarret, says his company is developing texts at the K−6 or K−8 level and will be ready.

Textbook analyst Harriet Tyson is more dubious about the situation and points out that publishers generally want to sell their books to several states. "Aside from Arizona [which adopted a similar framework in 1988], I don't know of any states willing to tear up their syllabi and teach to the California model."

McGraw-Hill looks at it differently. Says Jarrett: "We are not publishing a California edition or for the California framework. We publish for a national market. We hope to find these texts meet the needs of social studies curriculums in other cities and states, too."

No one disputes that California has clout with the textbook industry. One of the "text-book adoption states," it comes up with a list of recommended texts from which many of the state's school systems exclusively buy. With 1,025 school systems serving 4.5 million children, California purchases 11 percent of the textbooks sold in the United States. The state historically runs neck-and-neck with Texas as the largest (or second largest) purchaser of textbooks in the nation, spending in excess of $200 million annually.

What California is requesting from textbook publishers at this point is a change in the way history and social science texts are written.

Among the distinguishing characteristics of the new California framework are its focus on the chronological study of history as a story well told; its urging of a sequential curriculum in which major historical events and periods are studied in depth; its encouragement to teachers to present controversial issues honestly within their historical context; and its acknowledgment of the importance of religion in human history.

The state is calling for texts that will mesh with the resequenced curriculum. Diane Ravitch, one of the framework's drafters and a professor of history at Teacher's College, Columbia University, says the new instructional materials should be characterized by "vivid narrative accounts of American history and world history," "well-written biographies," and "content-rich materials including enriching literature and primary source materials."

To accomplish this, most publishers will have to research and write completely new texts. At the same time, California's requested changes are in line with what textbook reformers have been calling for for years.

42. The writer implies that

    A. California will lead the nation in a new approach to history and social science.

    B. California has isolated itself educationally from the rest of the country by introducing a new curriculum in history and social science.

    C. California has asked publishers to design the impossible.

    D. California has ignored the interest of other states in going ahead with the new curriculum.

43. According to the article, California purchases

   A. 1,025 textbooks per year.
   B. 4.5 million textbooks each year.
   C. only McGraw-Hill textbooks.
   D. 11 percent of all textbooks sold in the United States.

44. According to the article, California has adopted a bold new curriculum emphasizing which of the following subjects?

   I. Social Science
   II. English
   III. History

   A. I only
   B. I and II only
   C. II and III only
   D. I and III only

45. According to the author, it would be reasonable to infer that educational reformers would

   A. be supportive of California's new curriculum.
   B. have no opinion of the new curriculum until it has been implemented.
   C. be opposed to the new California curriculum.
   D. support some aspects of the new curriculum while opposing other aspects.

46. Based on the article, it would be reasonable to assume that publishers would be more willing to design textbooks for the new California curriculum if which one of the following were true?

   A. California were clearer about what it wants in the new textbooks
   B. Publishers had more freedom to decide what should go into the new textbooks
   C. Other states adopted frameworks similar to California's
   D. There were more competition in the textbook industry

47. Based on information from the article, the two top states for buying textbooks are California and

   A. Utah.
   B. Florida.
   C. Arizona.
   D. Texas.

48. Which one of the following is a characteristic of the new California framework?

   A. An emphasis on only historical figures to show the importance of history
   B. A focus on the chronological study of history as a well-told story
   C. A study of major historical events and periods based on the teacher's knowledge and expertise
   D. A presentation of controversial issues within their historical framework at the teacher's discretion

Passage VIII (Questions 49–55)

When speaking of dictionaries, most people think immediately of Samuel Johnson or Daniel Webster. But the making of dictionaries was a popular intellectual pursuit long before then. Actually, the earliest dictionaries are almost as old as writing itself. When the Sumerians first put reed stylus to clay in Mesopotamia (modern-day Iraq), they found an immediate need for dictionaries.

During much of Sumerian history, the land of Sumer was bilingual. Akkadian (with its more familiar dialects of Babylonian and Assyrian) was spoken alongside Sumerian. As a consequence, it was not long before Akkadian translations were added to the Sumerian word lists, and this resulted in the first bilingual dictionaries. Later, when Sumerian was dying as a spoken language, the Babylonian scribes added pronunciation guides to the Sumerian in some of these bilingual lexical lists. These ancient dictionaries are of great value today because Akkadian and Sumerian are both long dead. Although we might have a chance at learning Akkadian because it is a Semitic language with close relatives in Arabic and Hebrew, without these ancient dictionaries, we would probably never completely understand Sumerian, which has no known linguistic affinities.

The lexicographical traditions established in ancient Mesopotamia were eventually passed on to Western Europe via the classical world. Indeed, the plethora of modern dictionaries can be attributed to the fruitfulness of these ancient roots. Dictionaries are useful. They teach spelling, pronunciation, the meaning of words, the subtleties of words, the history of language, and many other things. We are introduced to dictionaries at a very early age and spend the rest of our natural lives consulting them. Although we tend to think of dictionaries only as language aids—tools to help us understand our own or someone else's language—that is only the tip of the iceberg. . . . Our major means of communication with one another is through language, and language is what dictionaries are about. It is very difficult to think of any tool that is consulted more frequently than the dictionary, and not just by lexicographers.

Dictionaries are of special importance to those who study ancient civilizations. Our only contact with these long dead peoples are through their archaeological artifacts and their written legacy. Because there are no native informants to help with the languages, the meanings and nuances of words must be learned through the context in which they were used. Similar or parallel passages in the literature are invaluable for getting at the meaning of a word or phrase. Synonyms and antonyms help to illuminate the nuances of words and to refine definitions.

The current thinking in lexicography, at least in ancient Near Eastern studies, is to attempt to expand the time gap between new editions of dictionaries of dead languages by producing comprehensive dictionaries of those languages. These comprehensive dictionaries do more than provide lists of words and their definitions. These dictionaries give examples of words in their original, contextual usage. For each word, all or at least all significant occurrences of the word are cited in the dictionary in the original sentence or phrase where they

occurred, together with a translation and bibliographical citation. . . .

Comprehensive dictionaries have many virtues, not the least of which is longevity. When the user of such a dictionary finds or edits a new document, the dictionary can be consulted; and the words, sentences, or phrases in the new document can be compared with what is already known. . . . Because a comprehensive dictionary contains virtually all of the evidence available at the time of its publication, it is easily kept up to date and remains a useful tool for a very long time . . . and can often retain its usefulness for centuries. . . . It is beyond question that dictionaries are one of the most important tools at the disposal of the humanist . . .

49. According to the article, which of the following are some virtues of comprehensive dictionaries for scholars in the humanities?

I.   A reputable resource of words, phrases, and sentences to consult when finding or editing a new document

II. An invaluable tool containing useful evidence that is kept up to date

III. An important means to verify histories of an ancient civilization

A.   I and II only
B.   II and III only
C.   II only
D.   III only

50. As stated by the author, the land of Sumer was bilingual through most of its history. The two languages spoken in Sumer were

A.   Sumerian and Akkadian.
B.   Babylonian and Assyrian.
C.   Akkadian and Babylonian.
D.   Sumerian and Assyrian.

51. The article refers to several ancient civilizations, including the

    A. Babylonians and the Sumerians.
    B. Sumerians and the Hittites.
    C. Babylonians and the Phoenicians.
    D. Egyptians and the Phoenicians.

52. The article states that dictionaries teach all of the following EXCEPT:

    A. spelling.
    B. the meaning of words.
    C. the history of language.
    D. the development of prefixes and suffixes.

53. According to the article, lexicographical traditions were first established in

    A. Mesopotamia.
    B. Babylon.
    C. Europe.
    D. Iran.

54. According to the article, which of the following helps to illuminate nuances of words and refine definitions?

    A. Homonyms
    B. Prefixes and suffixes
    C. Synonyms and antonyms
    D. Root words and root meanings

55. The author states that when most people think of dictionaries, they immediately think of

    A. the Sumerians.
    B. the ancient Greeks.
    C. Aristotle and Plato.
    D. Samuel Johnson and Daniel Webster.

Passage IX (Questions 56–65)

Nothing ever being quite as simple as it might seem, there are still many unresolved questions surrounding the evolution of life. One such question concerns the Earth's atmosphere and its gaseous composition.

"Due in large part to volcanic outgassing," says Henrich Holland, a Harvard professor of geochemistry, "the early atmosphere was heavily [made up of] carbon dioxide, with perhaps no more than one percent free oxygen. That was between two and three billion years ago." But analysis of rocks and minerals indicated that this changed around two billion years ago, as photosynthetic organisms devoured the carbon dioxide and released oxygen.

Some scientists have proposed that metazoans could not have developed until there were sufficient levels of oxygen in the atmosphere, both for these advanced organisms to breathe and to shield them from the lethal ultraviolet rays of the sun. This critical level was, according to one view, reached at about the time the Cambrian era began—some 600 million years or so ago—and, in fact, was the event that brought about the Cambrian explosion of life forms.

J. William Schopf, a professor of paleobiology and geophysics at the University of California at Los Angeles (UCLA), agrees that an oxygenic atmosphere is necessary for metazoans to exist, but he contends that it was also necessary for their eukaryotic predecessors. He argues that considerable amounts of free atmospheric oxygen had already built up around two billion years ago, citing a variety of geologic data to support his claim. As in other areas relevant to paleobiology, the last word on this issue is yet to be heard.

Paleobiology is a field in ferment; it is not at all unusual for there to be wide divergence of opinions and interpretations among the people active at such a stage in any discipline. Each of these researchers has particular investigations which he intends to carry out and which will yield, each hopes, data that will resolve hanging questions.

Schopf plans to use the proceeds of a National Science Foundation's Alan T. Waterman award to enable him to assemble an interdisciplinary team, including geologists, chemists, biologists, paleobiologists, and others, from universities around the world. Only such a team, he holds, can successfully attack the array of unanswered paleobiological questions directly. The prize money, he says, will be used for travel and salary expenses of the team members.

"There are still a lot of gaps in the [paleobiological] record," Schopf says. "With the right people, I think we'll be able to fill them in. But in the end, it comes down to the material that you have to work with. The rocks," he says, "are the court of last resort."

56. According to the author, the Earth's atmosphere three billion years ago was probably made up mostly of which of the following gases?

    I. Carbon dioxide
    II. Hydrogen
    III. Oxygen

    A. I only
    B. I and II only
    C. I and III only
    D. II and III only

57. The author states that the first life forms to develop on the Earth were

    A. metazoans.
    B. protozoans.
    C. plants.
    D. viruses.

58. Professor J. William Schopf will use his grant to

    A. pursue advanced geochemistry study under Henrich Holland at Harvard.
    B. assemble the best paleobiologists in the United States to study the origin of life.
    C. pay travel and salary expenses for an interdisciplinary team of scientists to study the evolution of life.
    D. encourage greater cooperation between paleobiologists and geophysicists.

59. According to Henrich Holland, the atmosphere of three billion years ago came into existence largely because of which one of the following?

    A. The gravitational pull of the Earth attracting gases to form an atmosphere
    B. Climatic cooling
    C. Development of plant life
    D. Volcanic outgassing

60. The article states that the Cambrian era began

    A. three billion years ago.
    B. one billion years ago.
    C. 600 million years ago.
    D. 60 million years ago.

61. The author states that the atmosphere probably changed around two billion years ago because

    A. volcanic action subsided on the Earth's surface.
    B. plants had developed and were changing the atmosphere by performing photosynthesis.
    C. simple oxygen (O_2) was being transformed into ozone (O_3).
    D. solar radiation was affecting the atmosphere.

62. One theory discussed in the article says that the metazoans' need for oxygen makes it most likely that they came into existence

    A. three billion years ago.
    B. two billion years ago.
    C. one billion years ago.
    D. 600 million years ago.

63. J. William Schopf argues which one of the following?

    A.   There was very little atmospheric oxygen two billion years ago.

    B.   There was considerable free flowing atmospheric oxygen in the Earth's atmosphere two billion years ago.

    C.   While there was minimal oxygen in the Earth's atmosphere, there was enough to support many life forms.

    D.   Life did not exist on Earth two billion years ago.

64. Based on the article, it would be reasonable to assume the author believes which of the following?

    A.   Most of what is known about the origins of life is already well understood.

    B.   Metazoans did not develop until 500 million years ago.

    C.   We have much to learn about the origins of life.

    D.   Research in the field of paleobiology has not been done with scientific accuracy.

65. According to the article, the argument that metazoans came into existence more than 600 million years ago is based on which of the following statements?

    A.   While metazoans did need a high level of oxygen in the atmosphere, so did their eukaryotic predecessors.

    B.   Metazoans did not need as much oxygen as scientists had previously thought.

    C.   The atmosphere of the Earth is much older than previously assumed and the level of oxygen in the atmosphere therefore would have increased to sufficient levels to support metazoans much earlier than 600 million years ago.

    D.   Metazoans developed 600 million years before eukaryotics.

ANSWER KEY

Verbal Reasoning Sample Exam

1. A	11. C	21. C	31. B	41. A	51. A	61. B
2. B	12. C	22. B	32. B	42. A	52. D	62. D
3. D	13. A	23. A	33. B	43. D	53. A	63. B
4. D	14. A	24. B	34. A	44. D	54. C	64. C
5. B	15. B	25. A	35. C	45. A	55. D	65. A
6. D	16. C	26. B	36. D	46. C	56. A	
7. A	17. A	27. D	37. A	47. D	57. A	
8. C	18. A	28. B	38. C	48. B	58. C	
9. B	19. B	29. C	39. B	49. A	59. D	
10. B	20. B	30. A	40. A	50. A	60. C	

ANSWERS AND EXPLANATIONS

1. **The correct answer is (A).** The answer to this question is based on a statement in paragraph 4: "The Older Americans Act of 1965 and other legislation have spurred federal and state expenditures in planning and development, direct services, and gerontological education and training."

2. **The correct answer is (B).** The answer to this question is supported by statements in paragraph 1 and paragraph 2: "The reasons people give for choosing a job in the field of aging vary a great deal. Among the most common are these:" (paragraph 1) and "The rewards of satisfaction . . ." (paragraph 2).

3. **The correct answer is (D).** The answer to this question is found in paragraph 4: "By the year 2000, it [the number of Americans over 65] will exceed 36 million."

4. **The correct answer is (D).** The answer to this question is found in paragraph 4: "The oldest segment of our population—those over 85 years of age—is growing most rapidly of all."

5. **The correct answer is (B).** The answer to this question is based on this statement in paragraph 4: "Public support for aging programs is expected to continue, and private support seems likely to expand."

6. **The correct answer is (D).** The answer to this question can be inferred by finding support for A, B, and C in the following statements in paragraph 5: "Endless possibilities. A casual encounter with someone in the field (B), experience as a student intern or volunteer (C), . . . the availability of financial aid for gerontology students (A)—all are typical first steps on the road to a career in the field of aging." There is no mention of D.

7. **The correct answer is (A).** This answer is inferred from several statements throughout the article including the following. In paragraph 2 there is the reference to "the rewards of satisfaction." Also in paragraph 2 are these statements: "People who hold jobs in this field say that they learn a great deal from older adults about human nature and enduring values. They almost always emphasize how much they enjoy working with older people." In paragraph 3, it is mentioned that "opportunities abound to make a difference in older people's lives" and "an opportunity to dispel myths and stereotypes, to suggest new ways of doing things, and to promote growth and development late in life." Paragraph 4 points out: "There is the availability of opportunity (since) the impending growth in the number of Americans in their eighties and nineties is bound to produce a sharp increase in the need for health, housing, long-term care, and social services in the years ahead."

8. **The correct answer is (C).** The answer to this question is found in the following statement from paragraph 2: "Not even the most elaborate neutrino traps . . . have found enough neutrinos to match the number predicted by classical theories of the solar interior."

9. **The correct answer is (B).** The answer to this question is found in the following statement in paragraph 2: "Since the number of neutrinos produced varies with the temperature of the specific thermonuclear reaction. . . ."

10. **The correct answer is (B).** The answer to this question is implied by the following statement found in paragraph 3: ". . . a 'sink' of some sort in the sun is altering most of the neutrinos before they can escape."

11. **The correct answer is (C).** The answer to this question can be found in the following statement in paragraph 1: "Their theoretical properties, however, including a fractional one-half spin quantum number, do make them detectable."

12. **The correct answer is (C).** The answer to this question is found in the following statement in paragraph 1: "Neutrinos are uncharged. . . ."

13. **The correct answer is (A).** The answer to this question is found in the following statement in paragraph 4: "Since stellar astronomy relies fundamentally on the understanding of the sun, the solar neutrino question could shake the very foundations of astrophysics."

14. **The correct answer is (A).** The answer to this question is found in the following statement in paragraph 5: "If it is the model of the sun," she concludes, "then the whole theory of stellar evolution could be wrong."

15. **The correct answer is (B).** The answer to this question is found in the following statement in paragraph 1: "Neutrinos offer another opportunity to measure events taking place inside the sun."

16. **The correct answer is (C).** The answer is inferred from a number of statements in the article. In paragraph 2 are these statements: "War is not the primary objective of Russian political strategy. The goal of Russian politics is to create and maintain favorable economic and political conditions. The Russians prefer to achieve this objective peacefully—by forcing appeasement upon the enemy. . . ." From paragraph 10 are the following statements: "The Russians take pride in their ability to correctly assess their relative strength using the correlation of forces, and in their ability to manipulate the forces used in the correlation . . . They are confident in their ability to use the laws of war to achieve their goals without becoming involved in a general war. They have far less faith in the policy makers of the west."

17. **The correct answer is (A).** The answer to this question is supported by the following statement in paragraph 1: "Correlation of forces, a conceptual comparison of the relative strengths of potential enemies, is an integral dynamic contained within Russian doctrinal philosophy."

18. **The correct answer is (A).** The answer to this question is found in paragraph 7: "There is a risk of war when the correlation of forces is nearly equal."

19. **The correct answer is (B).** The answer to this question is based on ruling out choices A, C, and D as these choices are supported by statements in paragraph 5 leaving choice C as the only answer. The statements that support A, C, and D are the following: "If the potential gain outweighs the risk, the Russians will use their armed forces as the quickest and most reliable means possible—but only when the correlation of forces indicate that major enemies will be unlikely or unable to intervene militarily. Their theory was accurate in Hungary, Czechoslovakia, and Afghanistan."

20. **The correct answer is (B).** The answer to this question is supported by statements in paragraph 2: "The goal of Russian politics is to create and maintain favorable economic and political conditions. The Russians prefer to achieve this objective peacefully—by forcing appeasement upon the enemy. . . ."

21. **The correct answer is (C).** The answer to this question can be inferred from several statements in paragraph 9: "The greatest risk of war occurs when the correlation of forces is inaccurately determined. When two adversaries believe they each have a more favorable correlation of forces, war is virtually inevitable."

22. **The correct answer is (B).** The answer to this question is based on ruling out choices A, C, and D. They are supported by statements found in the article leaving choice B as the remaining answer since there are no statements to support it. From paragraph 5 comes the statement: "Equally worldwide is Southern literature. Writers took the oral traditions of the South—the political rhetoric, preaching, conversational wordplay, and lazy-day storytelling—and converted them into art," which supports choice A. The statement that supports choice C is in paragraph 11: "Tom Rankin of the Southern Arts Federation contributed the lore about Moon Pies . . . (which) became a cultural phenomenon during the Great Depression. . . ." Choice D is supported by a statement in paragraph 10: "In choosing some 250 persons for the biographical sketches, Wilson says they selected those whose works transcended a particular field or those not found in research works. . . ."

23. **The correct answer is (A).** The influence of folklore was stressed in the writings of these authors.

24. **The correct answer is (B).** The answer to this question is found in paragraph 2: "Although the focus is on the eleven states of the Confederacy, this volume goes wherever Southern culture is found, from outposts in the middle Atlantic states to pockets of Chicago and Bakersfield."

25. **The correct answer is (A).** The answer to this question is found in paragraph 10: ". . . The editors argued that Southerners have a stronger sense of regionalism than people anywhere else in America—akin to the Basques in Spain, the Kurds in the Middle East, the French in Canada."

26. **The correct answer is (B).** The answer to this question is supported by the following statement found in paragraph 5: "Writers took the oral traditions of the South—the political rhetoric, preaching, conversation wordplay, and lazy-day storytelling—and converted them into art."

27. **The correct answer is (D).** The answer to this question is found in the following statement from paragraph 1: "At last it is out—the *Encyclopedia of Southern Culture*, a ten-year project involving more than 800 scholars and writers."

28. **The correct answer is (B).** The answer to this question is implied by the following statements found throughout the article: ". . . The book . . . links Huey Long and Mahalia Jackson, Scarlett O'Hara and Hank Aaron, the Bible Belt and [Walt] Disney World" (paragraph 3); ". . . this volume goes wherever Southern culture is found, from outposts in the middle Atlantic states to pockets of Chicago and Bakersfield" (paragraph 2). These statements are from paragraph 9. "'What we end up with are many Souths,' says Wilson. 'There is the geographical South. There is the South outside the South, which includes not only expatriate writers but Southern black communities in northern cities. And then there is also the South of *Roots* and Faulkner and the blues. You cannot deal with one and not the other.'"

29. **The correct answer is (C).** The answer to this question is supported by the following statements in paragraph 2: "One of these was the 'reverberating loop' or 'dynamic change' hypothesis derived from anatomical studies by Rafael Lorente de No of the Rockefeller University, back in the 1930s. He discovered that neurons in the brain were often interconnected in the form of closed chains . . . and . . . that neural activity . . . could be sustained by the circulation or reverberation of electrical signals within closed loops of neurons."

30. **The correct answer is (A).** The answer is based on the first paragraph in which the author states: "Of the many explanations put forth over the years to explain neural-behavioral adaptivity, virtually every one has been felled by subsequent experimental evidence."

31. **The correct answer is (B).** The answer to this question is supported by the following statements in paragraph 3: "For one, it has been shown that loop or no loop, neurons do more than excite other neurons. They can also inhibit. . . ."

32. **The correct answer is (B).** The answer to this question is found in paragraph 2: "One of these was the 'reverberating loop' or 'dynamic change' hypothesis derived from anatomical studies by Rafael Lorente de No. . . ."

33. **The correct answer is (B).** The answer to this question is based on a statement in paragraph 2: "The theory suggested that these looping signals were the files, the data bank, of memory."

34. **The correct answer is (A).** The answer to this question is inferred from the following statements in paragraph 1: "Of the many explanations put forth over the years to explain neural-behavioral adaptability, virtually every one has been felled by subsequent evidence. If some proved more durable than others, it was often because they appeared able to resolve the apparent paradox of change in a fixed system."

35. **The correct answer is (C).** The answer to this question is found in paragraph 6: "The Lasky Company's first production, a western called *The Squaw Man*, became an instant hit and was hailed by the critics as an example of superior filmmaking."

36. **The correct answer is (D).** The answer to this question is found in paragraph 8: "In 1915 [DeMille] achieved international acclaim on the release of *The Cheat*, a film in which a socialite who has lost club funds in a stock market gamble accepts $10,000 from a Japanese merchant to avoid ruinous disclosure."

37. **The correct answer is (A).** The answer to this question is based on a statement in paragraph 6: "Once in Hollywood, DeMille set up a studio in a barn that is today preserved in Los Angeles as a site of early filmmaking."

38. **The correct answer is (C).** The answer to this question is supported by statements in paragraph 1: "Despite his later reputation for commercial schlock, DeMille's early silent films, produced in the teens, were artistic expressions of some of America's most urgent social concerns. . . . DeMille's stories of ethnic, class, and sexual conflict appealed to the public during an era of progressive reform. Critics also reacted favorably to his early films and described them as dramatic, imaginative, and technically superior."

39. **The correct answer is (B).** The answer to this question is found in the following statement from paragraph 10: "'Although he was a pioneer in a revolutionary new medium,' notes Higashi, 'DeMille remained influenced by the theatrical tradition of nineteenth-century melodrama, specifically its emphasis on spectacle for the purposes of didacticism.'"

40. **The correct answer is (A).** The answer to this question is based on the two following statements. The first statement is found in paragraph 1 and the second statement is in paragraph 3. "Turn on the television around Easter and at least one station will be airing Cecil B. DeMille's *Ten Commandments*." "'DeMille was one of the most popular and commercially successful filmmakers ever,' says Higashi, 'yet all but his biblical spectacles have faded from memory.'"

41. **The correct answer is (A).** The answer to this question is inferred from statements found in paragraphs 1 and 9. From paragraph 1 come the following statements: ". . . DeMille's early silent films, produced in the teens, were artistic expressions of some of America's most urgent social concerns. Immigration to this country peaked during those years and DeMille's stories of ethnic, class, and sexual conflict appealed to the public during an era of progressive reform. Critics also reacted favorably to his early films and described them as dramatic, imaginative, and technically superior." From paragraph 9 comes this statement: " . . . noteworthy silents such as *Kindling*, which realistically portrayed class division, tenement life, and lack of opportunity for the poor, are ignored by today's film scholars. . . . DeMille's early films deal with social issues about class and ethnic distinctions with sensitivity as well as ambivalence."

42. **The correct answer is (A).** This answer is correct based on a statement in the first paragraph quoted here. "It has been said that when California sneezes the rest of the United States catches cold." This statement clearly implies a strong leadership role for California.

43. **The correct answer is (D).** The answer to this question is based on the following statement found in paragraph 6: ". . . California purchases 11 percent of the textbooks sold in the United States."

44. **The correct answer is (D).** The answer to this question is based on the following statement found in paragraph 1: ". . . California State Board of Education's adoption of a bold new kindergarten through twelfth-grade history and social science framework. . . ."

45. **The correct answer is (A).** The answer to this question is based on the following statement found in paragraph 10: "At the same time, California's requested changes are in line with what textbook reformers have been calling for for years."

46. **The correct answer is (C).** The answer to this question is based on the following statement found in paragraph 4: "Textbook analyst Harriet Tyson is more dubious about the situation and points out that publishers generally want to sell their books to several states."

47. **The correct answer is (D).** The answer to this question is based on the following statement found in paragraph 6: "The state historically runs neck-and-neck with Texas as the largest (or second largest) purchaser of textbooks in the nation. . . ."

48. **The correct answer is (B).** The answer to this question is based on the following statement found in paragraph 8: "Among the distinguishing characteristics of the new California framework are its focus on the chronological study of history as a story well told. . . ."

49. **The correct answer is (A).** The answer to this question is supported by the following statements found in paragraph 6: "When the user of such a dictionary finds or edits a new document, the dictionary can be consulted; and the words, sentences, or phrases in the new document can be compared with what is already known. . . . Because a comprehensive dictionary contains virtually all of the evidence available at the time of its publication, it is easily kept up to date and remains a useful tool for a very long time. . . ."

50. **The correct answer is (A).** The answer to this question can be found in paragraph 2: "During much of Sumerian history, the land of Sumer was bilingual. Akkadian (with its more familiar dialects of Babylonian and Assyrian) was spoken alongside Sumerian."

51. **The correct answer is (A).** The answer to this question is implied by statements in paragraph 2: "Akkadian (with its more familiar dialects of Babylonian and Assyrian) was spoken alongside Sumerian. . . . Later, when Sumerian was dying as a spoken language, the Babylonian scribes added pronunciation guides to the Sumerian. . . ."

52. **The correct answer is (D).** The answer to this question is based on ruling out choices A, B, and C, leaving choice D as the remaining answer. Choices A, B, and C are supported by the following statements in paragraph 3: "Dictionaries are useful. They teach spelling, pronunciation, the meaning of words, the subtleties of words, the history of language, and many other things. . . ."

53. **The correct answer is (A).** The answer to this question is found in paragraph 3. "The lexicographical traditions established in ancient Mesopotamia were eventually passed on to Western Europe via the classical world."

54. **The correct answer is (C).** The answer to this question is supported by the following statement in paragraph 4: "Synonyms and antonyms help to illuminate the nuances of words and to refine definitions."

55. **The correct answer is (D).** The answer to this question is based on the following statement in paragraph 1: "When speaking of dictionaries, most people think immediately of Samuel Johnson or Daniel Webster."

56. **The correct answer is (A).** The answer to this question is supported by the following statement in paragraph 2: "Due in large part to volcanic outgassing . . . the early atmosphere was heavily [made up of] carbon dioxide, with perhaps no more than one percent free oxygen."

57. **The correct answer is (A).** The answer to this question can be inferred from the following statement in paragraph 4: "J. William Schopf, a professor of paleobiology and geophysics at the University of California at Los Angeles (UCLA), agrees that an oxygenic atmosphere is necessary for metazoans to exist. . . ."

58. **The correct answer is (C).** The answer is based on the following statements in paragraph 6: "Schopf plans to use the . . . award to . . . assemble an interdisciplinary team, including geologists, chemists, biologists, paleobiologists, and others, from universities around the world. . . . The prize money . . . will be used for travel and salary expenses of the team members."

59. **The correct answer is (D).** The answer to this question is supported by the following statement in paragraph 2: "Due in large part to volcanic outgassing," says Henrich Holland, a Harvard professor of geochemistry, "the early atmosphere was heavily [made up of] carbon dioxide . . . between two and three billion years ago."

60. **The correct answer is (C).** The answer to this question is found in paragraph 3. ". . . the Cambrian era began—some 600 million years or so ago—and, in fact, was the event that brought about the Cambrian explosion of life forms."

61. **The correct answer is (B).** The answer to this question is based on the statement found in paragraph 2. "But analysis of rocks and minerals indicated that this changed around two billion years ago, as photosynthetic organisms devoured the carbon dioxide and released oxygen."

62. **The correct answer is (D).** The answer to this question is based on several of the following statements in paragraph 3: "Some scientists have proposed that metazoans could not have developed, until there were sufficient levels of oxygen in the atmosphere. . . . This critical level was, according to one view, reached at about the time the Cambrian era began—some 600 million years or so ago. . . ."

63. **The correct answer is (B).** The answer to this question is supported by a statement in paragraph 4. "He argues that considerable amounts of free atmospheric oxygen had already built up around two billion years ago. . . ."

64. **The correct answer is (C).** The answer to this question can be inferred from the following statement from paragraph 1: "Nothing ever being quite as simple as it might seem, there are still many unresolved questions surrounding the evolution of life."

65. **The correct answer is (A).** The answer to this question is based on the following statement found in paragraph 4: "J. William Schopf . . . agrees that an oxygenic atmosphere is necessary for metazoans to exist, but he contends that it was also necessary for their eukaryotic predecessors."

Unit Three

WRITING SAMPLE

The MCAT includes a 60-minute writing sample, which requires you to respond to two essay topics. The writing sample section of the MCAT is designed to assess your writing skills in the following areas:

- Development of a central idea

- Synthesis of concepts and ideas

- Cohesive and logical presentation of ideas

- Clear writing, following accepted practices of grammar, syntax, and punctuation, consistent with timed, first-draft composition

Each exam will provide a specific statement that will require an expository response. Essay statements will not pertain to the technical content of biology, chemistry, physics, or mathematics; the medical school application process or reasons for the choice of medicine as a career; social or cultural issues not in the general experience of MCAT examinees; or religious or other emotionally charged issues.

In the writing sample section of the MCAT, you will be asked to respond to a statement that provides an opinion; states a philosophy; or discusses a principle that relates to a general area of interest in business, politics, history, art, or ethics. You will be expected to incorporate in your essay three writing tasks. All three tasks must be addressed in an essay that is clear and organized. The following are the three tasks:

1. Explain or interpret the statement as thoroughly as possible.

2. Explore the meaning of the statement by providing a circumstance, example, or situation that contradicts the sentiment of the given situation. Thus, a viewpoint opposite to the one presented in the statement must be described, using a concrete example that can be either real or hypothetical.

3. Discuss how the conflict between the given statement and its opposition (as presented in the second writing task) might be resolved. In this task, you must apply your understanding of the statement to a more general problem of policy, choice, or evaluation raised by the conflict between the given statement and the opposing viewpoint.[1]

---

[1] Reprinted by permission from the MCAT Student Manual Information on the 1991 MCAT, preliminary version published by the Association of American Medical Colleges.

Keep in mind that your score is based on the thoroughness of your response in addressing all three tasks and the clarity of your ideas. Your essay should be coherent and unified, reflecting your skill at writing a fully developed, logical essay that makes use of related, concrete examples.

It is important that your writing on both topics reflect your ability to offer reasonable explanations within the required framework of also responding to the three tasks. It is a good idea to review each task carefully to ensure that you understand what each task requires in your essay. The following chapters offer suggestions in practicing your essay writing and a quick review of grammar.

CHAPTER 6

Writing Skills Review

6.1 BASIC SKILLS

Writing under pressure provokes anxiety, particularly if you are a science major who devoted little time to developing your writing style. Writing clear, concise, well-organized essays for the MCAT is important. The information provided in this chapter should be useful in helping you to review your knowledge of essay writing and improve your own writing skills.

WRITING FOR QUANTITY

The essay section of the MCAT involves producing a writing sample within a given time period. If you have not recently taken courses that require a minimum of writing, you may need to work on writing for quantity as well as for quality. Your goal here should be the ability to produce a two-page essay in fifteen minutes. Try this sample exercise.

Sample Writing Exercise

Write for exactly fifteen minutes on a topic or issue of your choice. Think through your topic for a few minutes. Then write as though you are writing a letter to a friend who is interested in what you think without worrying about the mechanics of writing. The following are some sample topics from which you can choose:

1. Discuss an important problem that adult men and women face in today's society.

2. Present some methods useful for coping with stress.

3. Discuss how good eating habits and exercise are instrumental in keeping one's body fit.

At the end of fifteen minutes, examine what you have produced. You should have written approximately two pages. If you wrote less than that, you need to write more for quantity before you work on quality. It is important to remember that writing is a skill that responds to practice. The more often you write, the easier it becomes.

If you were unable to write two pages in fifteen minutes, work on improving your writing fluency by doing "The Fifteen-Minute Exercise" described below. If you easily covered two pages in fifteen minutes, then proceed to section 6.2, "Practice Writing for the MCAT."

The Fifteen-Minute Exercise

Use a clock to time yourself for the fifteen-minute exercise. Write on one topic for no more than fifteen minutes each day. Concentrate on a topic or issue and not on a list of what you did on a given day. Stop at the fifteen-minute limit even if you become involved in what you are writing. The next time, you can always pick up where you left off if the topic seems compelling.

This exercise should be done each day until you can easily fill two pages in fifteen minutes. Concentrate on writing in complete sentences but do not worry about your sentence structure in terms of syntax, grammar, spelling, or organization. Just keep your ideas flowing and your hand moving steadily across the page. If it helps to imagine yourself writing to your friend, try that tactic.

Remember to be consistent in writing for fifteen minutes every day until you reach your goal of two pages. For each successive fifteen-minute period, try to increase the amount of writing you produce. After a week or so you should begin to see an improvement in your writing fluency and an increase in the amount you can write in the given time. Naturally, writing on a topic or issue about which you have strong convictions is much easier than writing on a topic you care little about. Nevertheless, even if you do not like writing on a particular topic, pretending that you do may be helpful in accomplishing your goal.

When you can cover two pages easily in a fifteen-minute period, you are ready to go on to the next section of this chapter.

WRITING FOR QUALITY

Writing is a complex process that does not come easily to even the most skilled writer. The common assumption about writing on essay exams is the mistaken belief that a good essay must be free of all grammatical errors. This is not true. The most important measure of an essay's success is the quality of its content. A good essay contains clear ideas and examples to support the author's point of view.

Brainstorming for a few minutes on a specific topic or issue helps you think about various ideas on which to focus your writing. This step involves writing down everything that comes to mind about the subject. Your purpose here is to decide on a direction for your essay and to organize your thoughts into a logical outline.

The second step involves writing a first draft following the outline generated in the brainstorming stage. Next, read over your first draft to see if you have made your thinking clear to another person. Often what seems very clear to you is incomprehensible to someone else. At this point, it helps to have someone read your essay.

You want this reader to be interested first in your thinking. If your writing presents good ideas and communicates them persuasively, readers may overlook your mechanical errors. However, if your writing fails to persuade the reader to accept your point of view, the reader may assume that his or her lack of interest is due to your failure to correct mechanical errors.

WRITING EFFECTIVELY

Once you are writing fluently, you should begin to analyze your writing for its effectiveness.

Look carefully at how you organize your essay. Be sure to write on the topic and to focus on it consistently throughout your essay. Provide your central idea, the thesis. Put your major ideas in an effective order. Make sure your reasoning is logical and that your ideas are presented clearly. Remember to be consistent in developing your ideas through explanation and detail with sufficient examples that reinforce your point of view.

Check your paragraph development. Every paragraph should be unified, coherent, and well developed. Each sentence should relate to the paragraph's central idea. Look to see if the sentences presented are in an effective order with adequate transitions between sentences and paragraphs.

Look at your sentence structure. Include a mixture of long, short, and middle-length sentences, varying sentences from simple to complex so your essay has a smooth, connected effect. Provide sentences that are clear in meaning. Avoid beginning your sentences with the same kind of grammatical structure.

Examine your diction. Use concise word choices to be more effective. Watch for clauses and sentences in the passive voice. The active voice usually makes your writing more direct and forceful. Avoid being wordy and repetitive—a sure sign that you have run out of ideas.

In writing your essay, keep the following points in mind:

1. Determine what the topic is asking.

2. Answer all parts of the question.

3. Provide a well-formulated thesis.

4. Make sure your point of view is serious and logical with ideas supported by sufficient reasoning and examples.

6.2 PRACTICE WRITING FOR THE MCAT

DEVELOPING THE TOPIC

1. **Plan Your Time and Answer**
   Try to provide yourself with sufficient time to understand your topic. Take a few minutes to plan your time and answer even if you are under severe time pressure. Jot down the main points you intend to make as you think through your response or make quick scratch outlines. Having this list of main points as a working plan can help you focus on what you are writing and produce a better-organized essay.

2. **Identify the Topic**
   Read the topic carefully. Discuss the topic without digressing to related areas unless they are called for. Remember, you are expected to provide clear, concise, and accurate statements without wandering from the topic. Don't redefine the topic to suit yourself. Write on the topic as it is given.

3. **State Your Thesis**
   State your thesis in the first paragraph. Make sure the paragraphs that follow support your thesis. If you have a paragraph that does not seem to relate to your thesis, then that paragraph does not belong in your essay.

4. **Write the Introduction**
   Your introductory paragraph should alert the reader to the topic you are writing on. The first paragraph should be a guide to the rest of the essay.

5. **Support Your Reasoning with Adequate Explanation and Examples**
   Make sure your discussion of ideas is both logical and sensible. Include examples that can best illustrate your point of view.

6. **Keep Your Audience in Mind**
   Your tone should be as serious and reasonable as the audience you are addressing. The reader does not know you in the way an instructor might. Therefore, the use of humor is likely to be misunderstood and out of place. Since you are writing a formal essay, use formal English. Refrain from using slang, as it is inappropriate in such writing.

HOW TO DIVIDE THE 30 MINUTES

The following is a model to use when allocating the thirty minutes you have to write each MCAT essay:

1. Spend the first 5 to 7 minutes thinking about the topic and organizing your essay.

2. Spend the next 16 to 20 minutes writing your essay.

3. Spend the final 5 to 7 minutes going over your essay. Use this time to check for both structural and grammatical errors.

REVIEW OF ESSAY FORM

The usual essay form is a five-paragraph essay.

The introductory paragraph contains the thesis statement that tells the reader what the essay is about. The thesis statement can be at the beginning, in the middle, or at the end of the first paragraph. The introductory paragraph also presents several main ideas the author will discuss in the body of the essay.

The body of the essay follows the introductory paragraph. It consists of three consecutive paragraphs that support the thesis statement previously presented. Each paragraph has a topic sentence that introduces the main idea of the paragraph. This sentence is usually the first or second sentence in the paragraph. Each paragraph provides the reader with specific, clear details and appropriate examples to substantiate the writer's point of view.

A concluding paragraph summarizes the essay by restating the thesis statement and by drawing together the arguments made in the essay. New ideas should not be introduced in the concluding paragraph.

ESSAY STRUCTURE

Here is a diagram of the structure of a five-paragraph essay. Keep in mind that your essay does not necessarily have to adhere strictly to this structure. The diagram does, however, provide you with an example of an appropriate essay form.

> 1st paragraph
> contains thesis sentence
>
> 2nd–4th paragraphs
> contain specific ideas writer develops to support thesis sentence
>
> 5th paragraph
> concluding paragraph

PROOFREADING YOUR ESSAY

Proofreading what you have written is an important and necessary part of good essay writing. At this point, you become the editor of your essay. You should try to give yourself five minutes at the end of the timed period to proofread your essay. Once you have proofread for content, you should proofread for any mechanical errors such as punctuation, grammar, and spelling. Clarify any illegible scribbles you made. Illegible handwriting is not only taxing for the reader but can also result in your essay receiving a lower score. You will not have time to recopy your essay nor will you be expected to do so; but you are expected to correct your writing.

Most students are familiar with the kinds of grammatical errors they tend to make. You may already know you have trouble with pronouns or that you often write fragments instead of complete sentences. If you have problems with misspelling, it pays to either have learned how to spell the word or to use an equivalent substitute when your memory fails you. It can be difficult to spot mechanical errors in your own prose. Proofreading for mechanical errors has to be performed as a separate task for a writer.

6.3 A QUICK REVIEW OF GRAMMAR

The following section has been provided to help you review certain rules of grammar, as well as common grammatical errors students tend to make when writing under timed conditions.

PUNCTUATION RULES

1. **Apostrophe (')**

    The apostrophe is used

    a.   To indicate possession.

    Bob's hat, Burns' poems, Jones's houses,

    Note: Use apostrophe only (without the s) for certain words that end in s:

    1. When s or z sound comes before the final s

        Moses' journey, Cassius' plan

    2. After a plural noun

        girls' shoes, horses' reins

The following examples show where to place the apostrophe:

Example: These (ladie's, ladies') blouses are on sale. The apostrophe means "belonging to everything left of the apostrophe."

ladie's means "belonging to ladie" (no such word)

ladies' means "belonging to ladies" (correct)

Example: These (childrens', children's) coats are size 8. One cannot say "belonging to childrens" (childrens'); therefore, children's (belonging to children) is correct.

Also Note:

1. When two or more names comprise one firm, possession is indicated in the last name.

   Lansdale, Jackson, and Roosevelt's law firm
   Sacks and Company's sale

   Note: ours, yours, his, hers, its, theirs, and whose—all are possessive but have no apostrophe.

2. In a compound noun, separated by hyphens, the apostrophe belongs in the last syllable—*father-in-law's.*

   Note: The apostrophe is omitted occasionally in titles:

   Teachers College, Actors Equity Association

   Note: The plurals of compound nouns are formed by adding the s (no apostrophe, of course) to the first syllable: I have three *brothers-in-law.*

   The apostrophe has the following two other uses besides indicating possession:

   1. For plurals of letters and figures

      three d's, five 6's

   2. To show that a letter has been left out

      let's (for let us)

2. **Colon [:]**

   The colon is used in the following instances:

   a. After such expressions as "the following," "as follows," and their equivalents

      Example: The sciences studied in high schools are as follows: biology, chemistry, and physics.

   b. After the salutation in a business letter

      Example: Gentlemen:

      Dear Mr. Gregory:

   Note: A comma is used after the salutation in a friendly letter.

   Dear John,

3. **Comma [,]**

Use the comma in writing just as you use a pause in speaking. Students often become uncertain about the rules for using commas. Try not to overuse the comma in your sentences. Here are some specific situations in which a comma is used:

a. Direct address

Example: Mrs. Smith, has the parcel arrived?

b. Apposition

Example: Dr. Jones, our family doctor, prescribed the medicine.

c. Parenthetical expressions

Example: She was unable, however, to get him to sign the form.

d. Closing a letter

Example: Sincerely,

Yours truly,

e. Dates, addresses

Example: September 5, 1989

New York, New York

f. Series

Example: We had an appetizer, salad, steak, and coffee for dinner.

g. Phrase or clause at beginning of sentence, when the phrase is long.

Example: When the bus rolled to a stop a few feet away, we all ran to board it.

h. Separating clauses of long sentences

Example: We realized we would have to wait in the line, but getting into the exhibit was worth the wait.

i. Clearness

Example: After praying, the clergyman finished the service.

j. Direct quotation

Example: Mrs. Smith happily announced, "What a wonderful idea."

k. Modifier expressions that do not restrict the meaning of the thought which is modified

Example: Air travel, of which many people are still afraid, is an essential part of our way of life.

4. **Dash [—]**

The dash is about twice as long as the hyphen. It is used as follows:

a. To break up a thought

Example: There are five—remember I said five—good reasons to refuse their demands.

b. Instead of parentheses

Example: A beautiful horse—Black Beauty is its name—is the hero of the book.

5. **Exclamation Mark [!]**

   The exclamation mark is used after expressions of strong feeling.

   Example: Ouch! I hurt my thumb.

6. **Hyphen [-]**

   The hyphen divides a word.

   Example: mother-in-law

   Note: When written out, numbers from twenty-one through ninety-nine are hyphenated.

7. **Parentheses [( )]**

   a. Parentheses set apart parts of a sentence that are not absolutely necessary to its completeness.

      Example: I was about to remark (this may be repetition) that we must arrive there early.

   b. Parentheses are also used to enclose figures, letters, and dates in a sentence:

      Example: Shakespeare (1564–1616) was a great dramatist.

      The four forms of discourse are a) narration, b) description, c) exposition, d) argument.

8. **Period [.]**

   The period is used:

   a. After a complete thought unit

      Example: The section manager will return shortly.

   b. After an abbreviation

      Example: English Dept.

9. **Question Mark [?]**

   The question mark is used after a request for information:

   Example: When do you leave for lunch?

10. **Quotation Marks [" "]**

    Quotation marks are used as follows:

    a. To enclose what a person says directly

       Example: "No one could tell," she said, "that it would occur."

    b. To set off a title of a short story

       Example: Have you read "The Necklace"?

11. **Semicolon [;]**

The semicolon is used infrequently. It should be avoided where a comma or a period will suffice. Following, however, are the most common uses of the semicolon:

a. To avoid confusion with numbers

Example: Add the following: $1.25; $7.50; and $12.89.

b. Before explanatory words or abbreviations—that is, namely, e.g., etc.

Example: You should include a lot of fruit in your new diet; e.g., apples, pears, melons, and bananas.

Note: The semicolon goes before the expression "e.g." A comma follows the expression.

c. To separate short statements of contrast

Example: War is destructive; peace is constructive.

SENTENCE FRAGMENTS

Write *whole sentences.* Remember, a group of words must make a complete thought. If it does not, the words are a *sentence fragment.*

Read each sentence you write separately. Each sentence should have a subject and a verb to be complete.

Most fragments can be corrected in one of two ways:

1. Add the fragment to a sentence close by.

Example: We usually eat dinner late in the evening. Because we have a long ride home from work.

Correction: We usually eat dinner late in the evening because we have a long ride home from work.

Example: When they entered the restaurant, the waiter informed them. That there would be at least a thirty-minute wait. And that tonight the place was especially crowded.

Correction: When they entered the restaurant, the waiter informed them that there would be at least a thirty-minute wait and that tonight the place was especially crowded.

2. Turn the fragment into a sentence by adding a subject, a verb, or both.

Example: Jessica enjoys shopping for clothes. For example, trying on outfits and buying those looking well on her.

Correction: Jessica enjoys shopping for clothes. For example, she tries on outfits and buys those that look well on her.

RUN-ON SENTENCES

Such sentences are usually two sentences run together with no punctuation or with only a comma. Check your sentences. If you have run together two or more sentences, they should be punctuated to show they are clearly separate ideas.

A run-on sentence with no punctuation is called a *fused* sentence.

Example: David spent all last night studying for his biology final exam he felt tired and sleepy the next day.

Correction: David spent all last night studying for his biology final exam. He felt tired and sleepy the next day.

A run-on sentence with a comma is called a *comma splice.*

Example: John insisted that the cashier had given him the wrong change, he decided to bring it to her attention.

Correction: John insisted that the cashier had given him the wrong change. He decided to bring it to her attention.

ERRORS IN SUBJECT–VERB AGREEMENT

In standard English, the verb and the subject of a sentence must agree with each other. If the subject is one person, place, or thing, then the verb must also be singular

Example 1: John laughs every time he hears that story.

Example 2: The beach looks so inviting for sunbathing.

Example 3: The bus unloads passengers at the terminal.

Each subject is one: one person (John), one place (the beach), and one thing (the bus). The -s added to the verbs indicates that each verb is also singular. Since the subjects and the verbs are both singular, they are said to agree with each other.

Here are examples of plural (more than one) subjects and verbs:

Example 1: John and Susan laugh every time they hear that story.

Example 2: Vermont and Massachusetts are New England states.

Example 3: The buses always head toward the terminal.

Each of these subjects is more than one: two people named John and Susan, more than one place, and more than one bus. Usually, verbs that end in -s are singular and verbs that do not end in s are plural.

ERRORS IN VERB TENSES

A verb in a sentence expresses time and existence. Tense is expressed through changes in verb forms and endings (such as runs, running, ran; laughs, laughing, laughed) and the use of auxiliaries (had gone, will have gone; had used, had been using).

You should be able to effectively manage your use of verb tenses by knowing what tenses to use and what they do. Look over the following examples of the basic verb forms (including the progressive forms) in the present, past, and future for the active voice:

Simple Tenses	Example	Purpose
Present	I work	To tell what is happening or can happen now
Past	I worked	To tell what has happened in the past at a specific time
Future	I will work	To tell what may happen in the future
Present Progressive	I am working	To tell what is happening now
Past Progressive	I was working	To tell something happening in the past
Future Progressive	I will be working	To tell that a future action will continue for some time

Perfect Tenses	Example	Purpose
Present Perfect	I have worked	To tell something that has happened more than once in the past
Past Perfect	I had worked	To tell what had already happened before another event
Future perfect	I will have been working	To tell what will have happened by some particular time in the future

Remember to keep your tenses consistent. To avoid confusing or distracting your readers, try not to switch them.

PRONOUN USAGE

A pronoun is a word such as *I, you, he, she, it,* or *they* that is used in place of a noun: John was happy that *he* (that is, *John*) had finished the job.

Pronouns can cause special problems of reference. One such problem occurs when a pronoun refers to an indefinite antecedent.

Example: The contracts were not initialed by the writers, so we are sending *them* back. (What is being sent back? The writers or the contracts?)

Correction: We are sending back the contracts because *they* were not initialed by the writers.

Another problem of pronoun reference occurs when the pronoun used could refer to more than one antecedent.

Example: After David spoke to Harry on the telephone, *he* forgot that *he* was leaving town later than planned. (Who forgot and who was leaving?)

Correction: After David and Harry spoke on the telephone, David forgot that Harry was leaving town later than planned.

As a general rule, the antecedent of a pronoun must appear—not merely be implied—in the sentence. Moreover, the antecedent should be a specific word, not an idea expressed in a phrase or clause. *It*, *which*, *this*, and *that* are the pronouns that can lead meaning astray. Too often, these pronouns refer to an idea that is clear to the writer only, leaving readers thoroughly confused.

Example: Although the doctor operated at once, *it* was not a success and the patient died.

Correction: Although the doctor performed the *operation* at once, *it* was not a success and the patient died.

Or Although the doctor operated at once, the *operation* was not a success and the patient died.

Example: Mr. Roberts has recently been promoted. *This* brings him greater responsibility and will probably mean longer hours for him.

Correction: Mr. Roberts has recently received *a promotion*. His new position brings greater responsibility and probably longer hours.

CHAPTER 7

Sample Student Essays

This section offers several samples of student essays written during timed practice sessions. None have been corrected. Most students are interested in seeing essays considered acceptable or not acceptable in passing the written section of the MCAT exam. Often, reading someone else's essay on a timed topic will enable you to be more critical of your own work.

The essays in this section are responses to topics that are similar to those offered On the MCAT exam, and each essay was written in thirty minutes, as on the exam.

Each student essay presented is evaluated according to the criteria used to score MCAT writing samples as provided by the 1991 preliminary version referred to at the early part of this book. Keep in mind that the essays are judged on whether all three writing tasks have been addressed and on the overall effectiveness of the essay. A few mistakes are expected with an essay written under timed conditions, but the overall quality of an entire essay provides the basis for the score.

SCORING THE MCAT ESSAY

Each of your essays will be read and scored by two different readers according to an alphabetical score that will range from J to T. Your essay will be considered as a unit without separable aspects. A single alphabetical score is assigned to an essay based on the quality of the writing as a whole.

Keep in mind that you are not asked to agree or disagree with the statement. You can do so if you wish within the framework of your essay. However, essays are not scored on whether your position is valid. Your essay will be scored on its response to the three tasks explained in Chapter 6. The depth and thoroughness with which you explain the meaning of the initial statement, the first task, and the degree to which you explore its meaning in responding to the second and third tasks will be assessed and a numerical score assigned to the essay.

Each essay is judged on its overall effectiveness after the readers determine whether all three writing tasks have been addressed. Mistakes are expected on essays because candidates are writing under timed conditions. Minor grammatical errors will not overly affect the paper's evaluation. The thoroughness, depth, and clarity of ideas presented in the essay will determine your score.

Listed on the next page are the explanations for the alphabetical scoring assigned to essays. Terms such as "passing" and "failing" do not apply, as essays are graded in comparison to other essays. In the alphabetical scoring, each letter represents 8 to 10 percentile points.

J   These essays reflect obvious problems with organization of ideas and mechanics, making the language very difficult to follow. Alternatively, the essays may entirely fail to address any of the tasks.

K   These essays demonstrate marked problems with organization and mechanics that result in language that is occasionally difficult to follow. The essays seriously neglect or distort two of the writing tasks while attempting to address one writing task.

L   These essays demonstrate marked problems with organization and mechanics that result in language that is occasionally difficult to follow. The essays seriously neglect or distort one of the writing tasks while attempting to address two writing tasks.

M   These essays present only a minimal treatment of the topic despite a response to each of the three tasks. They may show some clarity of thought but may be simplistic. Problems in organization may be evident. The essays demonstrate a basic control of vocabulary and sentence structure, but the language may not effectively communicate the writer's ideas.

N   These essays address all three writing tasks but present only a moderate treatment of the topic. They show clarity of thought but may lack complexity. The essays demonstrate coherent organization, although some digressions may be evident. The writing shows an overall control of vocabulary and sentence structure.

O   These essays address all three writing tasks and present a substantial treatment of the topic although they are not as thorough or as effectively organized as the R and S papers. They show some depth of thought, coherent organization, and control of vocabulary and sentence structure.

P   These essays show slightly more development of ideas and the use of more complex vocabulary than the O essays.

Q   These essays address all three writing tasks and present a thorough treatment. They demonstrate depth and complexity of thought, focused and coherent organization, and control of vocabulary and sentence structure.

R   These essays are very similar to Q essays, although tighter control of organization and vocabulary are more evident.

S   These essays fully address all three tasks by presenting a thorough exploration of the topic. They demonstrate depth and complexity of thought, focused and coherent organization, and a superior control of vocabulary and sentence structure.

T   These essays fully address all three tasks by presenting a thorough exploration of the topic. They demonstrate depth and complexity of thought, focused and coherent organization, and a superior control of vocabulary and sentence structure. A T essay is considered a perfect essay, and T grades are almost never given.

7.1 STUDENT RESPONSES TO STATEMENT 1

STATEMENT 1

Consider this statement:

> A life spent making mistakes is not only more honorable but more useful than a life spent doing nothing.

Write a unified essay in which you perform the following tasks. Explain what you think the above statement means. Describe a specific situation in which a life of making mistakes is not more useful than á life doing nothing. Discuss what you think determines whether a life making mistakes is more useful than a life doing nothing.

Essay 1

The statement "A life spent making mistakes is not only more honorable but more useful than a life spent doing nothing" illustrates one aspect of living. During life, either a person can take the easy route and do nothing or a person can take a more challenging road. The latter makes mistakes but at the same time moves forward while the former is stuck in one situation.

Mistakes constitute a normal existance. To some extent, every person makes mistakes. By challenging the mind, it forces a person to explore unknown situations. This leads to the possibility of either achieving the goal perfectly or possibly making a mistake. When the latter occurs, the person learns and could apply this knowledge to progress one's life for the better. Consequently, a life that has mistakes is more useful.

A life spent doing nothing is not necessarily a literal translation but instead a comparison. "Doing nothing" can also be taken to mean a person always performing the same task as for instance, a factory worker. In this job, the labor involved is repetitious and does not take thinking into account. Thus, the possibility for mistakes is decreased dramatically. This type of situation is not challenging and it resembles a life that is considered not as useful.

The meaning of this statement indicates that although people make mistakes, such mistakes can be overlooked. Learning also takes place while making mistakes so the next situation that resembles the first will be performed or handled in a similar manner. If someone does not do anything meaningful with life, which includes making mistakes, then the life could be considered not as useful.

Life involves a process of learning. This naturally accounts for mistakes but only if the person takes challenges. If no challenges are proposed, then the person not only does not make mistakes but remains stagnant spending a life doing nothing. A life spent making mistakes helps the person learn and prosper and helps make the life more honorable, thus making the life more useful.

Explanation of Essay 1—Q-Level Essay

The essay focuses clearly on the topic defined in the statement and fully addresses each of the three writing tasks in the statement. Paragraphs 1 and 2 respond to the first task (Explain what you think the statement means), Paragraph 3 addresses the second task (Describe a specific situation in which a life doing nothing is less honorable and useful), and Paragraphs 4 and 5 respond to the third task (Discuss what you think determines whether a life spent making mistakes is more honorable and useful than a life doing nothing).

The essay presents a thoughtful analysis of both the statement and the implications of the statement. The explanation of the statement is provided in the first two paragraphs with a thorough discussion of the meaning. Following this discussion, Paragraph 3 describes a situation that would seem to be the opposite of the statement. Paragraphs 4 and 5 resolve, or synthesize, these opposing ideas through a focused discussion on the third task linking it with the first task.

The paper is unified, coherent, and organized. Ideas are clearly conveyed, and the paragraphs are developed and interrelated. Transitions between paragraphs are appropriate (paragraphs 2 and 3). Generalizations are explained with varying levels of specificity as needed (sentences in paragraph 2).

The writing is clear and controlled. There is variety in sentence structure (compare the shorter, direct sentences in paragraph 1 with the more complex sentences in paragraph 3) and in word choice (the sentences in paragraph 2). Although the paper contains some minor errors (such as a vague pronoun in the sentence "This leads to the possibility of either achieving the goal perfectly or possibly making a mistake."—paragraph 2), they do not mar the overall effectiveness of the paper.

Essay 2

The quotation "A life spent making mistakes is not only more honorable but more useful than a life spent doing nothing" means mistakes in life is something to learn from, because for every mistake one makes, something new is learn. The word "honorable" in the quote means proud. Because, eventhough, one tried to achieve something and made a mistake along the way is better than not trying at all. Besides, making mistakes and learning from them will allow a person to gain confidence in approaching other problems or avoiding new mistakes.

For example, applying to Medical School is a very difficult process, and to become a doctor is even more difficult. Because of this, some people do not even bother in trying to become a doctor. Those individuals, who at least try, learned more about the process of applying to Medical School, themselves, and what it takes to become a doctor. Where as someone, who never tried, will be something that did affect them at all. The person who never tried will have a different concept about the difficult work of a doctor and might regret in the future not to have at least tried.

Making mistakes is human, but doing something about ones mistakes is more important. A life without mistakes is senseless and monotonous which might lead to nothing at all. Making mistakes is more useful because life then becomes a challenge. Once this challenge is overcome, then we can help others who are facing a similar situation. Consequently, the main factor that determines that life is useful making mistakes is oneself. Because, sometimes people continue making the same mistakes and never learning anything out of it.

In conclusion, mistakes sometimes will distinguish a person's life because he will have learned from his mistakes. A person who has done nothing will learn nothing.

Explanation of Essay 2—N-Level Essay

The paper addresses each of the three writing tasks. Paragraph 1 responds to the first task, Paragraph 2 responds to the second task, and Paragraph 3 responds to the third task. However, the paper as a whole approaches the topic with a general explanation.

Although the paper responds to the tasks, it lacks sufficient depth in its explanation to provide a thorough, organized, and complex response. The ideas discussed in each paragraph are generalized and are not adequately linked to one another (for example, the abrupt transition between Paragraph 2 and 3). The example provided in Paragraph 2 is not an appropriate illustration for the second task.

Usage and style are somewhat competent but demonstrate some problems. In the first paragraph, for example, there are several errors such as the misspelling in the phrase ". . . something new is learn" and the failure to separate the words "even though." There is some variety in sentence structure (the sentence, "A life without mistakes is senseless and monotonous which might lead to nothing at all" in paragraph 4). However, there are a number of awkwardly worded sentences, such as, "Where as someone, who never tried, will be something that did affect them at all" in paragraph 2.

The most obvious improvements needed in this paper are in the areas of development and control of basic mechanics. A more controlled analysis of the statement and its implications would benefit the essay and strengthen the discussion in the paper. Perhaps a brief review of grammar usage and an accurate, careful proofreading of the essay may help the writer in the future to present a more polished response.

7.2 STUDENT RESPONSES TO STATEMENT 2

STATEMENT 2

Consider this statement:

The truth is found when men are free to pursue it.

Write a unified essay in which you perform the following tasks. Explain what you think the above statement means. Describe a specific situation in which the truth is not found when men are free to pursue it. Discuss what you think determines whether men can discover the truth when allowed to do so.

Essay 1

"The truth is found when men are free to pursue it" is a quotation that exemplifies two issues: one of truth and the other of freedom. Truth can be defined as what a society considers to be "right." To improve or maintain a healthy society is a foundation on which "truth" can be established. Freedom then can be defined as not being restricted to attain the "truth" in this case. Having the liberty to search and pursue one's goals to better society is a premise on which "freedom" is based.

What "truth" is has to be established. An example could consist of analyzing evidence from an investigation. One must ask questions to find out the purpose or meaning of this evidence. In order to do this, one must question witnesses. Some might think that this action infringes on one's personal rights but in actuality the answers would lead to determining the truth.

Contrarily, criminals are in jail because what they thought was the "truth" was actually against the popular society's opinion. If they had the opportunity to search for truth through freedom, then the efforts are generally by some unlawful means. The society does not benefit. What the criminal's results are cannot be considered "truth."

Having the freedom to pursue the truth is relative. If society benefits, then the truth is worthy. So the freedom to pursue it is allowed. When an investigator asks questions to find out the truth, few consider it as an invasion of privacy; rather, society approves of these actions. Too much freedom is harmful. A criminal exemplifies this action. He or she has crossed the boundary of determining truth. Society does not benefit so the criminal's freedom must be prohibited.

The guidelines for determining truth from non-truth rest on society's interpretation. If the result is positive, then it is truthful. When the opposite results, then it is taken as non-truth. Freedom, then, is a measurement by which society will permit an individual to pursue the truth. So, when truth can be found, men should be free to pursue it because society, in general, will benefit.

Explanation of Essay 1—R-level Essay

This essay, similar to the first essay for Statement 1, focuses on the statement and addresses each of the three writing tasks. The writer defines two terms in the initial statement ("truth" and "freedom" in Paragraph 1), which also reflects the thoroughness of the response throughout the paper. The depth of thought in the essay can be seen through the two effective examples provided that help explore the statement and its opposition—the example of questioning witnesses in an investigation that leads to the truth (Paragraph 2) and the curtailment of freedom for criminals who seek truth through unlawful means (Paragraph 3). The paper effectively synthesizes its ideas in the final paragraphs (4 and 5) by making the example given in the second writing task (i.e., a situation where truth is not found when men are free to pursue it) the focus of the discussion of the third task.

The paragraphs in the essay are well organized, thorough, and related to one another. The emphasis placed on definition in the first paragraph is carried throughout the response by the writer's attention to further detail by an explanation of ideas expressed as well as the effectiveness of sentence structure (compare Paragraphs 4 and 5). The level of writing is controlled and effective, demonstrating the writer's ability to use language appropriately and skillfully.

Essay 2

According to the statement, if given the freedom to do so, man can find the "truth." This is to say that if we are given free reign to pursue whatever avenue of interest we have, we will discover facts that were previously unknown to us. The discoverers of many of today's conveniences were not barred from their pursuit of inventing the automobile, the lightbulb, and others.

However, the success of fact-finding ventures does not necessarily hinge upon the freedom to do so. People throughout history, who have been hindered by the dictates of their government, have continued their search in spite of the shroud of secrecy they must employ. Da Vinci explored the secrets of the human body despite the taboos of the time on the cutting up human bodies for exploration.

Freedom to pursue one's interest is indeed advantageous and does help catalyze the discovery of such "truths." Many of the innovations of today in the sciences, such as more hardy strains of plant life and animals used for food, helps improve our standards of living. However, freedom is not essential to success.

What is essential to the success of your pursuit is relentlessness. A dedication to finding the truth is what arms the inventor/the scientist in his quest. Dedication to hurdle obstacles before him and find the elusive truth is what fuels his society forward. Freedom is a conveneience to the truly dedicated.

Explanation of Essay 2—M-Level Essay

This paper addresses each writing task clearly, has paragraphs that are well organized, and provides effective transitions between paragraphs (for example, 1 and 2). Word choice and sentence structure seem competent. The writing overall reflects a strong fluency despite a general focus on explaining the statement and its implications.

However, the ideas contained in the paper are not as complex and their implications not as thoroughly explored as in the preceding R-level paper. Examples provided (in Paragraphs 2 and 3) are not described in sufficient detail and are somewhat simplistic. Paragraph 4, which addresses the third writing task, does not sufficiently resolve, or synthesize, the opposing views developed in Paragraphs 2 and 3. Therefore, the last paragraph fails to bring the paper to a successful conclusion, since the ideas are not sufficiently detailed or fully expressed.

The most useful improvement needed in this paper is a further development of the ideas presented. Each paragraph briefly focuses on the ideas presented. For instance, the writer offers a general explanation of the statement and of the examples in Paragraphs 1 and 2 without fully developing the ideas. Although the essay provides a clear, coherent tone and a unified order, further attention to detail and thorough explanation of ideas would have boosted the paper's overall effectiveness.

7.3 STUDENT RESPONSES TO STATEMENT 3

STATEMENT 3

Consider this statement:

Nothing succeeds like the appearance of success.

Write a unified essay in which you perform the following tasks. Explain what you think the above statement means. Describe a specific situation in which something does not succeed despite an appearance of success. Discuss what you think determines whether something does succeed like the appearance of success.

Essay 1

"Nothing succeeds like the appearance of success" is an illustration of a statement by which people follow in order to encourage themselves. If the outcome of "success" is known to be true, then attempting a new project becomes much easier. "Success" can be defined as the level one needs to achieve in order to be satisfied. When the result is not the desired one, then it can be inferred as being "unsuccessful," which thus makes the statement not true.

The amount of time and dedication devoted for studying for an exam can generally be used as an indication as to how much one will perform. There usually is a positive correlation between the two. For example, the more time spent studying, the better the grade will be, thus serving as an indication of success. In some instances, this is not true. Even though some people may study many hours, they cannot perform at the level that another may perceive as being sufficient to attain success in the form of a good grade. Thus, this situation would contradict the statement because the means of achieving success by studying a lot despite still failing would discourage someone from pursuing this mode of action.

The most obvious criteria that could be used in determining this situation as true or not is the personal fulfillment of the task involved. If the gratification from performing is perceived as successful, then it will be considered as "success." Likewise, when the work involved far outweighs the benefits, then the situation will be interpreted as not successful. Thus, other means will be searched out to achieve success. Sometimes external factors could influence success. Some circumstances could dictate whether or not, despite all other signs of success, this success will appear. So, determining whether success is true or not depends on more than one factor.

The appearance of success results from various factors. Sometimes they are controlled so success can be predicted. Yet other times, even when all signs indicate success, it does not result. Overall, the statement "nothing succeeds like the appearance of success," holds true for most cases.

Explanation of Essay 1—R-Level Essay

The paper focuses clearly on the statement and fully addresses each of the three writing tasks in the item. Paragraph 1 responds to the first task thoroughly by the writer's decision to define the term "success," Paragraph 2 provides a detailed description of a specific situation, and Paragraphs 3 and 4 respond to the third task.

The paper presents a thoughtful analysis of the statement and the implications of the statement. The explanation of the statement is examined in Paragraph 1. Paragraph 2 focuses on a detailed explanation of an opposite situation. Paragraph 3 brings the statement into conflict with an example that would seem to contradict it and creates a foundation for Paragraph 4 to resolve, or synthesize, the opposing ideas in its conclusion.

The paper conveys its ideas in a unified, logically connected manner. The paragraphs are clearly and appropriately organized and are related to one another. There are appropriate transitions between paragraphs (e.g., Paragraphs 2 and 3).

Overall, the writing is clear and controlled. There is variety in word choice and sentence structure (compare complex and simple sentences found in Paragraphs 1 and 2). The depth of thought and complexity of ideas produce an effectively written paper.

Essay 2

According to the statement, acting or dressing as if you were a successful individual can fool those around you. If you are dressed in expensive clothing or act as if you are affluent, people generally assume that you are who you project. In other words, the observers also buy into the illusion you have created around yourself and treat you according to what they perceive you to be. However, the illusion of success is a hard task to sustain. Appearances can be deceiving, but they can also be seen through by the observant. Simply looking the part does not automatically endow you with abilities you do not have normally.

In the case of a novice skier, the possession of all the most up-to-date equipment and the latest fashion accessories will not compensate for his lack of talent and skill. He may look good on the ski lift, but in likelihood, he will do his version of a human snowball on his way down the slopes. Simply appearing like you belong on the ski patrol does not necessarily equate success. Though false appearances may work in the ski lodge, they will not work when you actually have to perform.

The illusion of success hinges on brevity. If your meeting is brief and superficial, false appearances will carry through successfully. However, when there is a requirement to perform or interact more deeply, appearance quickly becomes meaningless.

Looking good for that interview may initially impress your interviewer. But illusions are quickly shattered and first opinions change once you open your mouth and what is said belies the appearance. Clothes may make the man, but his inner substance when revealed can dispel the initial illusion.

Explanation of Essay 2—Q-Level Essay

While this paper addresses each writing task, it demonstrates the required skills less effectively than the preceding R-level response but more clearly than the N-level essay that accompanies Statement 1. Each task is clearly addressed and, especially in responding to the first writing task, uses more detail than that contained in the N-level paper. The paragraphs are well organized and the transitions between paragraphs are not abrupt. Word choice and sentence structure seem competent and at a higher level than in the N-level paper. Overall, the paper provides a general focus on explaining the statement and its implications.

On the other hand, the level of complexity of ideas is not as thoroughly explored as in the preceding R-level paper. For instance, the example of the novice skier is simplistic as a response to the second writing task (Paragraph 2). The writer addresses the third writing task, but fails to provide a sufficient resolution, or synthesis, of the opposing views given in Paragraphs 1 and 2. What appears to be a generalization of ideas in Paragraphs 3 and 4 does not allow for a successful conclusion to the paper. Thus, the ideas in the last two paragraphs are not sufficiently related to what has come before.

This paper could benefit from a further depth of thought in its complexity and more emphasis on detail, particularly in Paragraphs 3 and 4. The brevity of these paragraphs prevents the writer from fully developing the third task beyond the most general level. The thoroughness and detail evident in Paragraph 1, if applied to the rest of the paper, would raise the entire composition up to the level of the first paragraph and qualify the paper for a higher score.

7.4 STUDENT RESPONSES TO STATEMENT 4

STATEMENT 4

Consider this statement:

There must be more to life than having everything.

Write a unified essay in which you perform the following tasks. Explain what you think the above statement means. Describe a specific situation in which life seems lessened by not having everything. Discuss what you consider to be a balance between the two situations.

Essay 1

There must be more to life than having everything. The statement means that having "everything" does not lead to a meaningful life.

One of the great misconceptions of todays society is that they equate physical possessions with happiness.

There are many people who have millions of dollars and yet are unhappy. These people might be lacking health, or might be very lonely; therefore it can be said that there are aspects to a meaningful life which transcend physical possessions.

Even if one does have "everything"—health, money, love—I feel the true test is to use these recourses wisely in a form beneficial to ones fellow man.

Explanation of Essay 1—L-Level Essay

Although this essay is an attempt to respond to the three tasks, the overall brevity of the explanation reflects a lack of complexity, depth, and seriousness in tone. This essay neglects to deal with all three tasks sufficiently and effectively. The generalized explanation of the statement in addressing all three areas underscores the major weakness of the essay.

In addition to the essay's failure to respond to the tasks adequately, there are some errors in grammatical usage and in spelling. For example, an apostrophe is missing in the word "todays" in the second paragraph and again in the word "ones" in the essay's last paragraph. In the last paragraph, "recourses" probably represents a spelling error rather than an error of usage, but either way it highlights a failure of proofreading. Such errors, however, are minor in contrast to the overall weakness of the essay's treatment of the writing tasks. Improving the essay by a more thorough development of its response to each task and thereby improving the current essay's explanation would be an important strategy. What is presented is a very limited view of the student's writing skills. The essay would benefit considerably from expanded explanations, specific supporting details, and concrete examples.

Essay 2

In our capitalistic society, quality of life is defined in relatively narrow terms. We tend to equate material health with a successful life. The statement, there must be more to life than having everything suggests that we have the ability to experience success through mechanisms that transcend those commonly associated with success. Having everything given to you can at first seem quite appealing. However, after careful consideration one can come to the conclusion that this may a lability rather than an asset. Consider the "poor little rich kid"—this image illustrates the disadvantage of being afforded certain amenities, privileges, etc. without experience the effort to attain them. A child born into this predicament might certainly enjoy luxurious surrounding, pampered care and a superlative education. However it might be interesting to consider what they do not gain from such an experience. For example, a child who is so pampered and protected might never be allowed the opportunity to fail and gain the insight and strength necessary to transcend the failure and make it into an ultimate success. They may not be allowed to acquire a sense of themselves—who they are in relation to the world. They may not have a developed sense of their attributes, perspectives, strengths and liabilities—because they are only told how wonderful they are in terms of their familial relations. This, I assert is a superficial and false mechanism in helping to shape, mold and enhance a child's development.

If given every opportunity without the experience of having to develop discipline, persistence and determination—these essential qualities for success may never become rooted in their personality. There is no impetus to develop these characteristics because they do not seem to serve any necessary function. No matter what an individual endeavors to accomplish, the possibility of failure exists. In order to achieve ultimate success, we must learn to handle failure—by not becoming paralyzed by it or becoming despondent to the point of giving up. The strength that is needed comes from a knowledge and belief in your ability and the persistence to continue in the face of adversity. While persistence is essential, the ability to identify and isolate shortcomings and develop strategies that effectively address them is also important. In my opinion, these and other related skills are acquired through real life experiences—replete with mixtures of success, disappointment and disillusionment. Artificial success can be achieved within a pampered context, where everything is made less competitive, more sensitive and less consistent with life in the real world. But what happens to the individual who is nurtured in such an environment when he is forced to confront real life issues in a societal context? Without adequate preparation, the "poor little rich kid" will be overwhelmed and rendered ineffective to cope with the experiences and problems he will confront. He will lack the necessary tool to analyze and deal with situations outside his narrow perspective.

Life is meaningless if you have everything if you are so concentrated in yourself and your immediate surroundings that you cannot imagine sharing you resources in the world in order to make a positive impact. What good is everything if you are too intimidated or selfish to apply the knowledge and resources that you have? How can you appreciate the benefits of your knowledge?

Having and sharing your resources however substantial means infinitely more than keeping those resources locked in a mental suitcase in an ivory tower. Being successful goes beyond the individual, it is an individuals contribution to society that measures true success.

Explanation of Essay 2—S-Level Essay

Very few of the sample student essays evaluated for this edition achieved this score. This particular essay is exceptional by virtue of the student's thorough explanation of the statement, the complexity of ideas presented, and the student's writing skills. One criticism that might be made recognizes that the response to the third writing task seems abbreviated in contrast to the responses to the first two writing tasks. There are a number of mechanical errors, many of which may be overlooked in consideration of the time pressure under which the essay must be organized and written. In this essay there are errors of spelling, such as "lability" instead of "liability" in the first paragraph; agreement discrepancies, such as a "child . . . they"; and a lack of a punctuation mark, an apostrophe, in the word "individuals" in the last paragraph. There are also run-on sentences. For example, the first one in paragraph 3 is one very long run-on sentence, "Life is meaningless if you have everything if you are so concentrated in yourself and your immediate surroundings that you cannot imagine sharing you [sic] resources in the world in order to make a positive impact." The sentence can be changed to two separate sentences by eliminating the word *if*. Another sentence is a comma splice. It reads, "Being successful goes beyond the individual, it is an individuals contribution to society that measures true success." In this case, the clauses should be separated to show they are two clear ideas.

Unlike the L-level essay addressing the same statement, this essay is well organized, fluent, and complex in its treatment of ideas and demonstrates a superior control of vocabulary.

CHAPTER 8

Writing Sample Practice Exam

Using what we have discussed so far, apply your writing skills to the following sample topic from the writing sample section of the MCAT exam. Give yourself the full 30 minutes to write on each statement in order to complete this exercise. Keep in mind the tips provided about developing your topic. Give yourself adequate time to proofread sufficiently.

SAMPLE STATEMENT 1

Consider the following statement:

No person is free who is not his or her own master.

> **Directions:** In 30 minutes, write a unified essay in which you perform the following tasks:
>
> Explain what you think the above statement means. Describe a specific situation in which it is possible to *not* be free and be a master of oneself. Discuss what you think determines when a person can be free and his or her own master.

SAMPLE STATEMENT 2

Consider this statement:

Familiarity breeds contempt.

> **Directions:** In 30 minutes, write a unified essay in which you perform the following tasks:
>
> Explain what you think the above statement means. Describe a specific situation in which familiarity does not breed contempt. Discuss what you think determines whether or not familiarity breeds contempt.

REFERENCES

For a more detailed description of information, please consult the following recommended sources:

Keys for Writers. 3rd ed. Raimes, Ann. Houghton, Mifflin: Boston, 2002.

The Little, Brown Handbook. Fowler, H. Ramsay, Jane E. Aaron, and Kay Limburg. Addison Wesley Longman, Inc.: New York, 2001.

The Scott, Foresman Handbook for Writers. Hairston, Maxine, John J. Ruszkiewicz, and Christy Friend. HarperCollins: New York, 2001.

Unit Four

BIOLOGICAL SCIENCES

INTRODUCTION

Your knowledge and understanding of fundamental concepts in biology and biologically related chemistry (topics in organic chemistry) will be assessed using questions based on specific "science problems." Rather than simply "recalling" facts (as students were asked to do in previous years on a Science Knowledge Test), you will be asked to "apply" your knowledge, as well as "evaluate" and "synthesize" information presented to you in a variety of formats.

On some problems, you will be asked to interpret quantitative data presented in an assortment of tables, graphs, and other figures. Other problems may provide you with an equation or flow chart or passage from which you will be asked questions. You may also be presented with a set of experiments or case study. Problems may combine two or more biology and chemistry concepts.

You will primarily be asked to demonstrate your reasoning and problem-solving skills. These include the abilities to recognize a) logical sequences, b) cause-and-effect relationships, c) valid versus invalid conclusions, and d) extraneous or irrelevant information to the questions at hand. You should also be able to e) integrate information, f) derive new information from that which is given, g) draw conclusions from information, and h) make generalizations from one situation to another.

Passage formats will include:

- **Information Presentation**
  Information is presented in the form of a textbook or journal article. Questions test understanding and evaluation of the given information and ability to use the information in different ways.

- **Problem Solving**
  Passages describe problems in biology or organic chemistry. Questions ask you to determine the probable cause of a particular situation, event, or phenomenon, as well as ask you to select methods of solving the problem.

- **Research Study**
  Questions determine your understanding of a project after you are presented with methods, results, and rationales for the project.

- **Persuasive Argument**
  Different perspectives are presented to express a viewpoint or opposing viewpoints. Questions will determine your understanding and ability to evaluate the validity of the viewpoints.

The test will include 10 problem sets of 5 to 10 questions each (62 questions), and 15 single-question problems. This latter group will be short, i.e., perhaps one paragraph, or one graphic, ending with a question. In all cases (problem sets and individual problems), questions will be multiple choice.

The following review material is intended to provide a topic-by-topic framework that can help you determine how to arrange your preparation time. Terms in bold print are included in a list of key words at the end of each section. Please keep in mind that all Practice Problems, Sample Exams, and Practice Exams provide additional review materials. The Answers and Explanations sections will often provide "mini-lessons" that further develop topics previously discussed in the review text.

CHAPTER 9

Biology

9.1 MOLECULAR BIOLOGY

A. BIOLOGICAL MOLECULES

Many biological molecules are large **polymers** consisting of long chains of similar subunits linked together. The individual subunits or "building blocks" of such polymers are called **monomers.** Polymers are synthesized by linking monomers together in **condensation reactions,** also referred to as **dehydration syntheses** (a water molecule is removed as two monomers are bonded together). When the larger molecule is split into its component subunits, a **hydrolysis** reaction is involved (links between monomers are broken while a water molecule is added: a hydrogen to one monomer, and a hydroxyl group to the other monomer).

Dehydration Synthesis and Hydrolysis

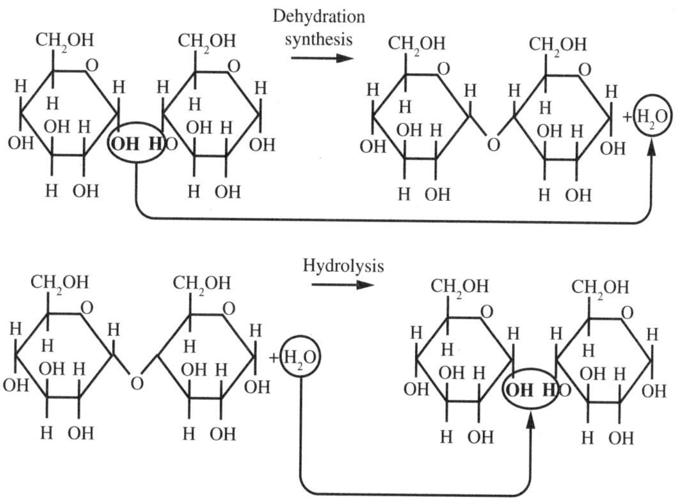

Carbohydrates

Carbohydrates are the primary energy molecules used by living things. They include sugars, as well as various storage and structural components found in living organisms. Categories of carbohydrates include:

Monosaccharides (single sugars), which are the basic monomers of all carbohydrates. These include glucose, fructose, galactose, ribose, and deoxyribose. Monosaccharides can also provide the carbon framework from which other types of organic molecules can be synthesized (fats, amino acids, etc.).

Disaccharides (double sugars) consist of two monosaccharides linked together and include sucrose, maltose, and lactose. Disaccharides can be functional as such, they may be broken down to monosaccharides for use as energy sources, or used to construct larger polysaccharide carbohydrates.

Polysaccharides contain many monosaccharides linked together and can serve as storage molecules of monomers to be used later (starch and glycogen), as well as a variety of structural materials found in cells and tissues (cellulose, chitin, and components of bone matrix).

Lipids

Lipids include a large variety of molecules that are insoluble in water. They can function as energy-storage molecules, structural and support molecules, and in a diverse range of physiologically important processes. Categories of lipids include:

Fats (triglycerides) serve as important energy-storage molecules. They consist of two basic subunits, one **glycerol** molecule linked to three **fatty acids** (by dehydration synthesis). Fats can also provide protection and insulation within the organism.

Phospholipids are similar to fats except they consist of two fatty acids bonded to a glycerol molecule rather than three. A phosphate-containing chain replaces the third fatty acid. Phospholipids are important components of cellular membranes. **Glycolipids** are also important membrane components. They have a carbohydrate portion attached to glycerol along with two fatty acids.

Steroids do not contain glycerol and fatty acids. Instead, they consist of four interconnected rings of carbon atoms with functional groups attached. Cholesterol is a steroid found in cell membranes and is needed to synthesize other important steroids, such as the hormones testosterone, estrogen, and aldosterone, as well as structural lipids like myelin.

Types of Lipids

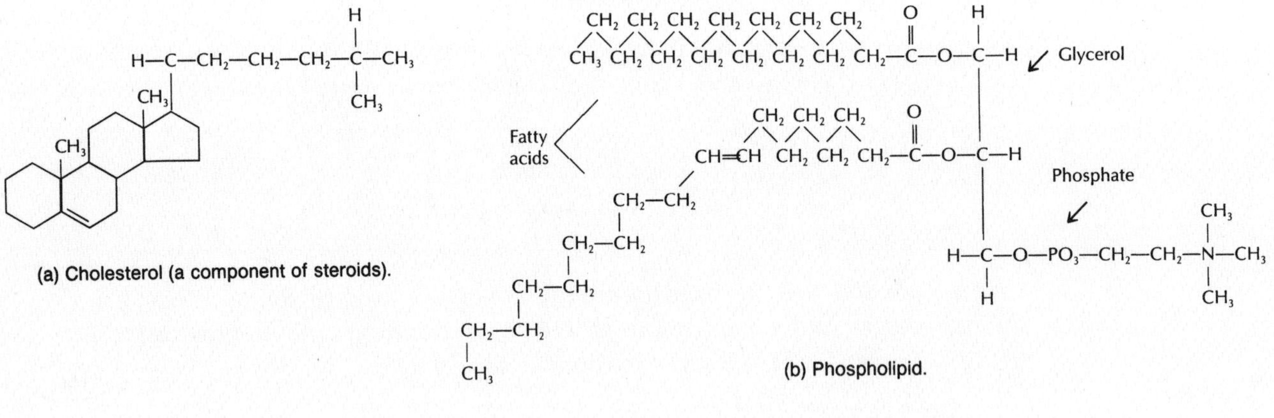

(a) Cholesterol (a component of steroids).

(b) Phospholipid.

Protein Structure

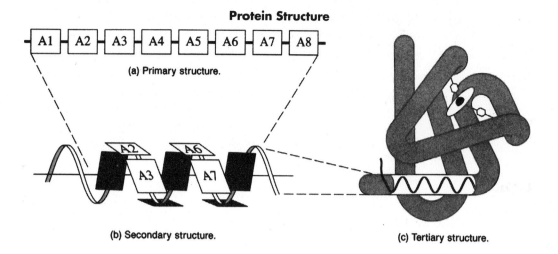

(a) Primary structure.

(b) Secondary structure.

(c) Tertiary structure.

Proteins

Proteins make up more than 50 percent of the dry weight of most living organisms. They are polymers constructed using subunits called **amino acids** (20 different amino acids can be synthesized into an almost endless variety of combinations, resulting in an enormous variety of proteins). The amino acids are linked (by dehydration synthesis) to form **peptide bonds.** Proteins may consist of one or more **polypeptide** chains. These chains can range in length from approximately 50 amino acids to a few thousand amino acids. Proteins have a **primary structure** based on their specific linear sequence of amino acids. They can also have a **secondary structure** of regular repeating patterns like coils (alpha-helix) or folds (pleated sheet) within the linear sequence; a **tertiary structure** of irregular bends and contortions along each chain; and a **quaternary structure** due to interactions among chains, when more than one polypeptide makes up the final three-dimensional structure of the molecule. The shape of a protein can be affected by environmental conditions such as temperature, pH, and salt concentrations. Proteins help perform many vital functions in living systems. For example, they can serve as molecules of movement (actin and myosin), support (collagen), transport (hemoglobin), defense (antibodies), coordination (hormones like insulin and growth hormone) and as catalysts (enzymes) to efficiently regulate the chemical reactions needed to maintain life itself.

Amino Acids Forming a Peptide Bond

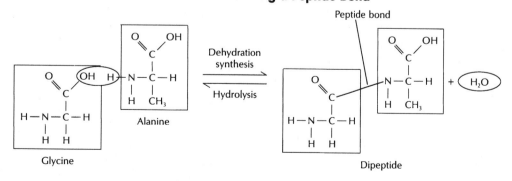

Nucleic Acids

Nucleic acids are the molecules from which the hereditary material of life is made. Both DNA (deoxyribonucleic acid) and RNA (ribonucleic acid) are polymers made of subunits called **nucleotides.** The nucleotide sequences within nucleic acids help determine the specific amino acid arrangements of all proteins made by an organism. Each nucleotide itself consists of three components: a 5-carbon sugar (either ribose or deoxyribose), a phosphate group, and a nitrogenous base. The nitrogenous bases can either be "double-ringed" **purines** (adenine and guanine) or "single-ringed" **pyrimidines** (cytosine, thymine, or uracil).

An important substance related to the nucleotides is the energy molecule **ATP** (adenosine triphosphate), which consists of the nitrogenous base adenine and the 5-carbon sugar ribose attached to three phosphate groups.

Nucleic Acid Components

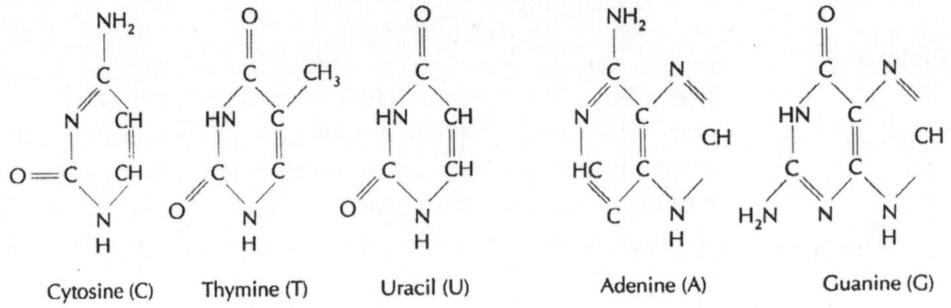

Cytosine (C)   Thymine (T)   Uracil (U)

(*a*) Pyrimidine bases.

Adenine (A)   Guanine (G)

(*b*) Purine bases.

Adenine (a purine base)

Adenosine

Phosphate group

Ribose (a 5-carbon sugar)

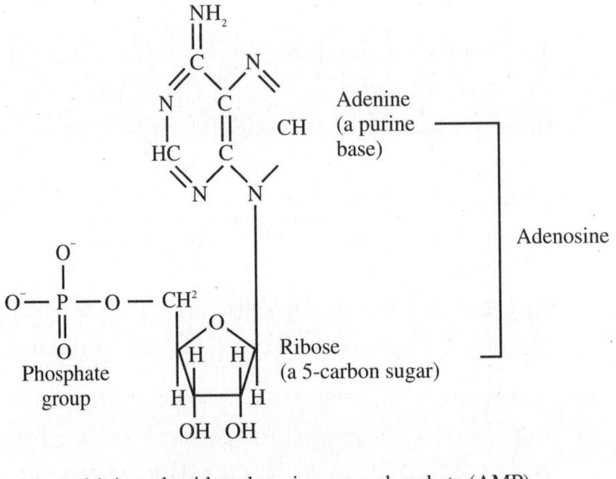

(*c*) A nucleotide, adenosine monophosphate (AMP).

Enzymes

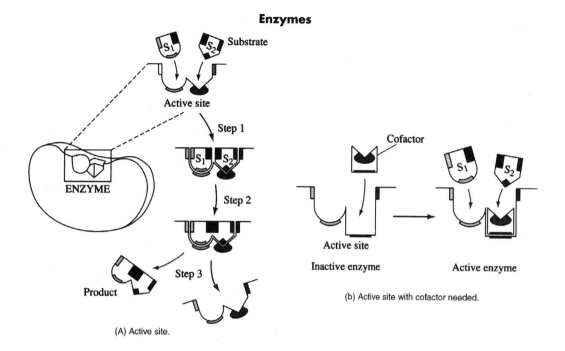

(A) Active site.

(b) Active site with cofactor needed.

B. PROTEINS AS ENZYMES

Enzymes are proteins acting as catalysts that regulate the rate of chemical reactions without being used up or consumed themselves. For reactions to proceed, reactants or **substrates** must absorb energy to break existing chemical bonds **(activation energy)**. Enzymes can reduce the amount of activation energy needed by attaching to the substrate(s) in such a way that bonds can easily be broken (as in catabolic reactions) and/or by orienting substrates to each other so that new bonds can readily form (as in anabolic reactions).

Enzymes have a distinctive **active site** at which they combine with their specific substrates to form **enzyme-substrate complexes.** These active sites are often grooves or pockets in which the substrate(s) fit. Since the enzyme's active site specifically fits only particular substrate(s), it follows that only specific reactions involving those substrates can be catalyzed by that enzyme. Because enzymes are proteins, the precise shape and position of the active site may be altered as environmental conditions affecting the entire protein molecule change. Therefore, the efficiency and activity level of an enzyme can also be affected by conditions such as temperature, pH, and salt concentration **(enzyme specificity).** In some cases, enzyme function is aided by separate substances (ions, vitamins, and other organic molecules) called **cofactors** or **coenzymes** (if the substance is organic).

When an enzyme combines with its substrate(s), the enzyme often changes its shape slightly to "embrace" the substrate(s) and improve the fit even further **(induced fit).** However, **inhibitors** may resemble the normal substrate and occupy the active site. **Noncompetitive inhibitors** may combine with the enzyme at another site, but in so doing, alter the shape of the enzyme such that the active site no longer "fits" the normal substrate. Some enzymes are **allosteric** in that they have an active conformation or shape and an inactive conformation.

When an inhibitor combines at a site on an enzyme that causes the enzyme to take its inactive conformation, this is called **allosteric inhibition.** Often an enzyme can be inhibited by the **product** of the reaction it has just catalyzed, acting as an allosteric inhibitor. This is referred to as **feedback inhibition.** It can regulate a reaction so that the production of a certain molecule can be limited to times when it is needed.

Enzyme Inhibition

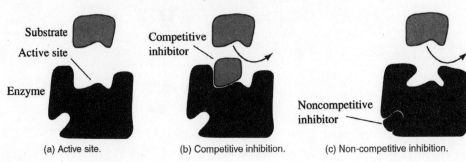

(a) Active site.   (b) Competitive inhibition.   (c) Non-competitive inhibition.

C. CELLULAR METABOLISM

ATP

Adenosine triphosphate **(ATP)** is the main energy molecule used in living cells. The breaking (hydrolysis) of the bond holding the third phosphate onto the molecule (producing ADP, **adenosine diphosphate,** and a loose phosphate) releases energy that can be used by cells to carry out their normal energy-requiring tasks such as active transport, movement, and even the anabolism of new molecules. The resynthesis of ATP from ADP and phosphate is constantly necessary, and **oxidative phosphorylation** (by chemiosmosis) during cellular respiration is the major source of ATP production in living cells. Cellular respiration includes glycolysis, the Krebs cycle, and the electron or hydrogen transport chain, and results in the production of 36 ATP molecules for the cell.

Glycolysis

Glycolysis is a 9-step sequence of reactions (in the cytosol) involving the metabolism (by oxidation) of glucose into two 3-carbon molecules of **pyruvic acid** (pyruvate). Two molecules of NAD+ are reduced in the process. Respiratory oxygen plays no role in glycolysis **(anaerobic)** and two ATP molecules are gained via **substrate-level phosphorylation** (a phosphate is transferred directly from an organic molecule to ADP).

Glycolysis

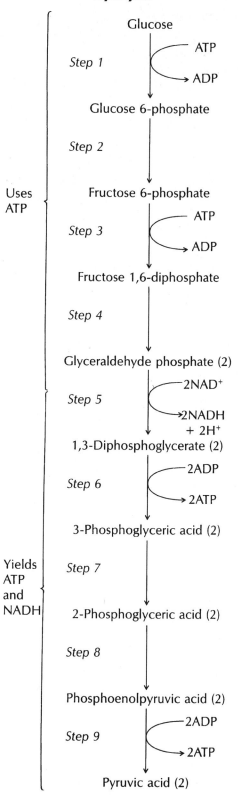

Krebs Cycle

In the mitochondrial **matrix,** each pyruvic acid is converted to one carbon dioxide molecule and the 2-carbon molecule, **acetyl-CoA,** which then enters the **Krebs cycle.** Acetyl-CoA combines with the 4-carbon molecule, oxaloacetic acid, to form the 6-carbon molecule, citric acid. The citric acid is broken down in a step-wise fashion to a 4-carbon molecule, which eventually results in the reformation of oxaloacetic acid. Carbon dioxide is released (three per pyruvate molecule) and the electron acceptors NAD and FAD are reduced to NADH and $FADH_2$, respectively. Two additional ATP molecules are gained via substrate-level phosphorylation.

The Krebs Cycle

Electron Transport Chain

Hydrogens and their electrons (from NADH and $FADH^2$ in the previous stages) are passed to the **electron transport chain** along the inner membranes of the mitochondria **(cristae).** Here, a series of electron carriers (including the **cytochrome** proteins) alternately accept and then pass the electrons (redox reactions) until respiratory oxygen serves as the final acceptor (forming water). Thirty-two ATP molecules are gained during this oxidative phosphorylation of ADP by **chemiosmosis.** Chemiosmosis in brief: During the flow of electrons, hydrogen ions accumulate in the space between the inner and outer mitochondrial membranes, forming a concentration gradient. As they flow back across channels of the inner membrane into the matrix, they activate the synthesis of ATP from ADP by **ATPase** or ATP synthase.

Electron Transport Chain

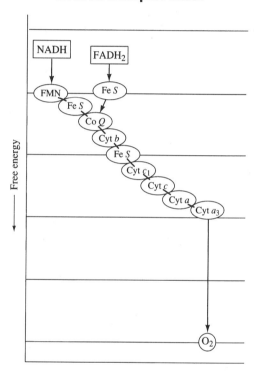

Fermentation

Fermentation (anaerobic respiration) can occur in some organisms in the absence of respiratory oxygen. Since oxygen is not available to serve as the final hydrogen and electron acceptor molecule, the Krebs cycle, and electron transport chain cannot proceed (and the majority of ATP molecules cannot be produced). Instead, after glycolysis, the pyruvic acid itself may serve as the hydrogen acceptor (forming lactic acid, as in human muscle cells), or a derivative of pyruvic acid may serve in this manner (forming ethyl alcohol or acetic acid, as in some yeast and bacterial species).

Other molecules such as lipids and proteins can also be used in cellular respiration. Molecules such as glycerol, fatty acids, and amino acids can each be converted to one or more of the intermediates along the biochemical pathways of cellular respiration **(gluconeogenesis).**

Gluconeogenesis

Glycerol can be converted to pyruvic acid, fatty acids can be converted to acetyl-CoA (via **beta-oxidation**), and amino acids can be converted to pyruvic acid, acetyl-CoA, or alpha-ketoglutaric acid (a molecule in the Krebs cycle). In order to utilize amino acids as substitutes for glucose in any of these ways, the amino group ($-NH_2$) must first be removed by the liver (**deamination**).

D. NUCLEIC ACIDS AND PROTEIN SYNTHESIS

The structure of DNA allows information to be stored and serves as a template for its own replication. Thus, information can be passed from generation to generation, making DNA the molecule of inheritance.

DNA Structure

DNA is a polymer of nucleotides. Each nucleotide contains a phosphate group, the 5-carbon sugar deoxyribose, and one of four nitrogenous bases: **adenine, guanine** (purines), **cytosine,** or **thymine** (pyrimidines). Most DNA molecules contain two such chains (double-stranded) extending in opposite directions (antiparallel) forming a double-helix. The deoxyribose-phosphate portion is on the outside of the helix and the bases face inward. Opposing base pairs are bonded together (hydrogen bonding) inside the helix. Adenine on one chain can only bond with thymine on the opposing chain. Similarly, guanine can only pair with

DNA Structure

cytosine **(complementary base-pairing).** Thus, the amounts of adenine and thymine are approximately equal in a DNA molecule, as are the amounts of cytosine and guanine **(Chargaff's Rule).** Since bases can bond together only in specific ways, the nucleotide sequence of one strand can determine the nucleotide sequence of the opposing, complementary strand. Each sequence of three DNA nucleotide bases represents the "genetic code" **(triplet code)** for one amino acid to be added during protein synthesis.

DNA Replication

Before mitosis and meiosis (during Interphase), the double-stranded DNA molecules that make up the chromosomes (along with **histone proteins**) uncoil, and each single strand serves as a template or model from which a complementary strand (half molecule) is synthesized. Thus, replication is **semiconservative.** Each new double-helix contains one "old" strand and one "new" complementary strand. Enzymes such as **helicases** (help uncoil the double-helix), **DNA polymerase** (helps put new DNA nucleotides in place), and **DNA ligase** (helps link new segments of DNA, **okazaki fragments,** to each other to make a whole new strand) are involved in DNA replication. DNA polymerase places the DNA nucleotides of each new strand into position in a 5′ to 3′ direction. Therefore, one strand **(leading strand)** is synthesized continuously, while the other strand **(lagging strand)** must be synthesized in segments (okazaki fragments).

Semiconservative Replication

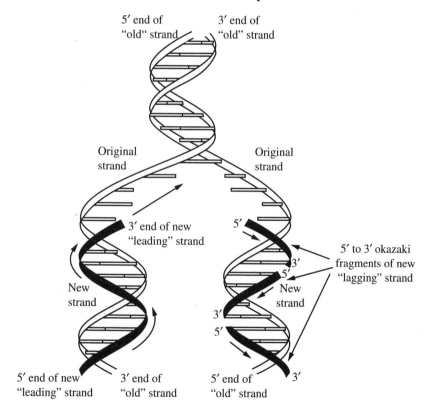

RNA Structure

RNA is also a polymer of nucleotides, but is usually single-stranded (one poly-nucleotide chain). Each nucleotide consists of a phosphate group, the 5-carbon sugar ribose, and one of four nitrogenous bases: adenine, guanine (purines), cytosine, or **uracil** (pyrimidines). Uracil is "equivalent" to thymine, in that it is complementary to adenine. There are three types of RNA, each made as a complementary copy of a nucleotide sequence on chromosomal DNA, and each serving an important role in protein synthesis. Messenger RNA **(mRNA)** carries the genetic instructions from the nucleus to the cytoplasm and serves as a template for the sequence of amino acids that is to be constructed. Transfer RNA **(tRNA)** molecules bring the appropriate amino acids into place at the assembly site, the ribosomes. Ribosomes are made, in part, of ribosomal RNA **(rRNA).**

Protein Synthesis, Transcription

During **transcription,** mRNA is made in the nucleus, using one of the DNA strands of the double-helix as a template (after the double-helix uncoils). Synthesis of the mRNA nucleotide chain is catalyzed by **RNA polymerase,** beginning at a **promoter site** on the DNA where the "gene" starts, and ending at a termination nucleotide sequence farther along the DNA. The resulting mRNA molecule will leave the nucleus and attach to a ribosome in the cytoplasm, where its sequence of nucle-otides will serve as instructions for the amino acid sequence to be synthesized. The nitrogenous bases of every three consecutive mRNA nucleotides will serve as a code **(codon)** for each amino acid to be added. There is a "start" or **initiator codon** (AUG), and three "stop" or **terminator codons** (UAA, UAG, and UGA).

Transcription

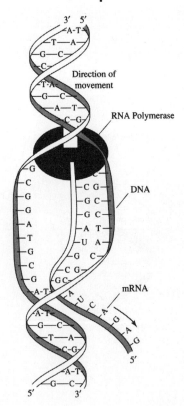

In eukaryotes, the mRNA molecule may be "processed" so that **introns** (noncoding regions) may be removed and **exons** (real coding regions) can then be spliced together before translation.

Protein Synthesis, Translation

Initiation of **translation** begins in the cytoplasm, as tRNA molecules attach to their specific amino acids (**amino acid activation** catalyzed by **aminoacyl-tRNA synthetase**). The first amino acid (methionine) is brought to the **P site** of the ribosome, its tRNA lines up with the first codon of mRNA (AUG) by means of three nucleotide bases on the bottom of the tRNA molecule (**anticodon**) that are complementary to that specific codon, and the two **ribosomal subunits (large and small)** combine. The second tRNA molecule brings its amino acid and lines up with the second mRNA codon (anticodon to codon) at the A site of the

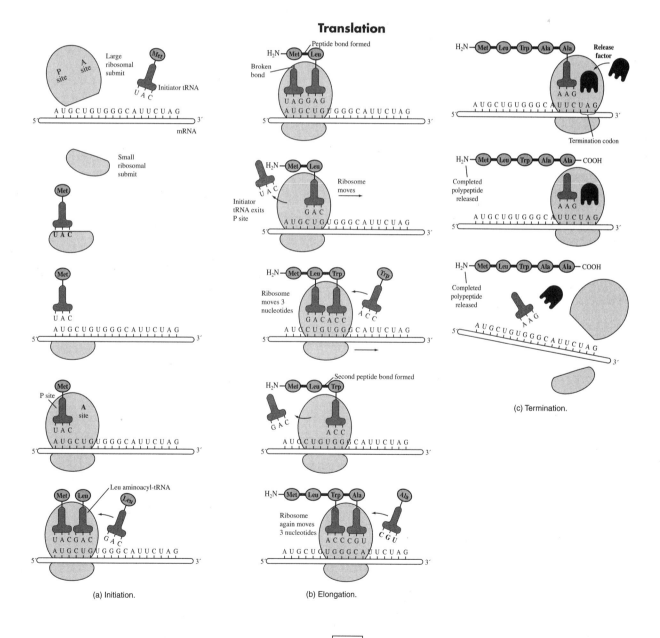

Translation

(a) Initiation.

(b) Elongation.

(c) Termination.

ribosome. During the next stage, **elongation**, the enzyme **peptidyl transferase** catalyzes the formation of a peptide bond between the first amino acid at the P site and the newly arrived amino acid at the A site. This enzyme also detaches the first tRNA from its amino acid at the P site as the tRNA at the A site carrying the growing polypeptide chain (now two amino acids in length) shifts, or translocates, from the A site to the vacated P site. The mRNA and ribosome shift so that the third mRNA codon becomes associated with the now empty A site. The third tRNA then brings its amino acid to the A site and lines up with the mRNA, anticodon to codon. Peptidyl transferase again forms a peptide bond between the newly arrived amino acid at the A site and the polypeptide chain held at the P site. The elongation cycle continues until one of the terminator codons (UAA, UAG, or UGA) is reached along the mRNA at the A site. A water molecule is then added to the existing polypeptide chain instead of an amino acid, the completed polypeptide is released from its tRNA at the P site, and the ribosomal subunits dissociate from each other. This last stage is called **termination.** The polypeptide chain may then be altered before becoming functional.

PRACTICE PROBLEMS
MOLECULAR BIOLOGY

1. The basic monomers for synthesizing carbohydrates include

   A. glucose, lactose, and glycerol.
   B. glucose, lactose, and sucrose.
   C. glucose, fructose, and glycogen.
   D. glucose, galactose, and fructose.

2. After a meal, fats (triglycerides) can be synthesized by which of the following processes?

   A. anabolizing three fatty acids and glycerol by hydrolysis
   B. catabolizing three fatty acids and glycerol by hydrolysis
   C. anabolizing three fatty acids and glycerol by dehydration
   D. catabolizing three fatty acids and glycerol by dehydration

3. How many peptide bonds will have to be formed during the translation of a protein containing 50 amino acids?

   A. 1
   B. 2
   C. 49
   D. 50
   E. 51

4. The molecule, adenosine monophosphate, can be found in

   A. DNA only.
   B. RNA only.
   C. both DNA and RNA.
   D. neither DNA nor RNA.

5. Insulin is a very small protein containing 51 amino acids in two chains linked together by disulfide bridges. What level of complexity best describes this protein?

   A. primary structure
   B. secondary structure
   C. tertiary structure
   D. quaternary structure

6. Purines are double-ringed nitrogenous bases, while pyrimidines are single-ringed bases. Which of the following must be true?

   A. In a double-stranded molecule of DNA, there will normally be an equal number of purines and pyrimidines.

   B. In a single-stranded molecule of RNA, there will normally be an equal number of purines and pyrimidines.

   C. In a double-stranded molecule of DNA, there will normally be twice as many pyrimidines as purines.

   D. In a single-stranded molecule of RNA, there will normally be twice as many pyrimidines as purines.

7. Magnesium and calcium are essential to the proper functioning of numerous enzymes in a variety of reactions. The term that best describes their role is

   A. essential amino acids.
   B. coenzymes.
   C. cofactors.
   D. catalysts.

8. Each pyruvic acid produced during glycolysis eventually leads to the production of how many molecules of carbon dioxide?

   A. 2
   B. 3
   C. 4
   D. 6

9. The products formed during the electron transport chain include

   A. ATP and water.
   B. ATP and carbon dioxide.
   C. ATP, water, and oxygen.
   D. ATP, carbon dioxide, and water.
   E. ATP, carbon dioxide, water, and oxygen.

10. What do NAD, FAD, and the cytochromes all have in common?

   A. Each is reduced.
   B. Each is oxidized.
   C. Each is reduced and oxidized.
   D. Each acts as an oxygen carrier.

11. Substance A is produced during a reaction catalyzed by Enzyme B. As the concentration of Substance A increases, it binds to Enzyme B, causing it to change its shape and become inactive. This is an example of

   I. feedback inhibition only
   II. allosteric inhibition only
   III. competitive inhibition only

   A. I and II
   B. I and III
   C. I, II, and III

12. During replication, DNA ligase would be expected to be most active at the

   A. leading strand
   B. lagging strand
   C. both strands
   D. site where the double helix uncoils

13. During which stage(s) of translation is the enzyme, peptidyl transferase, active?

   I. initiation
   II. elongation
   III. termination

   A. I and II
   B. II and III
   C. I, II, and III

14. Fill in the blanks with the correct numbers. Each mRNA codon represents _____ DNA nucleotide(s) and _____ amino acid(s).

   A. 3, 1
   B. 3, 3
   C. 1, 1
   D. 1, 3

15. If the nucleotide sequence for a particular amino acid is CTA on the DNA template strand, what is the nucleotide sequence of the anticodon on the tRNA molecule responsible for bringing that amino acid to the ribosome?

A. GAT
B. GAU
C. CUA
D. CAU

16. What would you expect to happen during translation if an exon in the middle of a gene has mutated from GTT to ATT?

A. The complete protein will be translated normally.
B. The protein will terminate prematurely.
C. The protein will never terminate.
D. The protein will never start.

ANSWER KEY

1. D	3. C	5. D	7. C	9. A	11. A	13. B	15. C
2. C	4. B	6. A	8. B	10. C	12. B	14. A	16. B

ANSWERS AND EXPLANATIONS

1. **The correct answer is (D).** Glucose, galactose, and fructose are all carbohydrate monomers (monosaccharides), whereas lactose and sucrose are disaccharides; glycerol is a building block for synthesizing triglycerides (fats); and glycogen is already a large polysaccharide carbohydrate.

2. **The correct answer is (C).** Anabolism ("building up" or synthesis) of glycerol and three fatty acids by dehydration will produce a triglyceride (fat). Catabolism ("breaking down" or decomposition) does not build anything. Hydrolysis refers to a specific catabolic process by which larger molecules are broken down to smaller units, while a water molecule is added (−H is added to one small unit, while −OH is added to the other).

3. **The correct answer is (C).** A peptide bond forms between each amino acid in a protein (polypeptide) chain. If there are 50 amino acids, the first peptide bond will be between #1 and #2, followed by 48 similar bonds as the other 48 amino acids are added.

4. **The correct answer is (B).** Adenosine monophosphate consists of adenine, ribose, and one phosphate group. Ribose is the 5-carbon sugar found only in RNA nucleotides. Deoxyribose is the pentose found in all DNA nucleotides.

5. **The correct answer is (D).** When more than one chain of amino acids is present in a protein, their interaction reflects quaternary structure. The fact that insulin is a "small" protein may mislead students into incorrectly choosing choice A (primary structure), which refers to the protein chain's sequence of amino acids.

6. **The correct answer is (A).** The purine adenine, on one strand of DNA, can only bond to the pyrimidine thymine on the complementary strand. Similarly, the purine guanine can only bond to the pyrimidine cytosine. Since there must be one purine for each pyrimidine, only choice A can be correct. Because RNA is usually single-stranded (no complementary strand), each nitrogenous base in the chain is independent of every other base, and there need not be a 1:1 ratio. The fact that purines have "double rings" and pyrimidines have "single rings" is totally irrelevant to the question!

7. **The correct answer is (C).** Molecules that are needed to assist enzymes are usually considered either cofactors or coenzymes. Since calcium and magnesium are inorganic, they are referred to as cofactors. Organic molecules such as certain vitamins would be referred to as coenzymes. Only the enzymes themselves are considered catalysts.

8. **The correct answer is (B).** Each pyruvic acid produces one carbon dioxide as it is converted to acetyl-CoA, and then two more carbon dioxides form as the acetyl-CoA is further broken down during the Krebs cycle. Although six carbon dioxide molecules result from the cellular respiration of glucose, the question refers to the number of carbon dioxides resulting from the breakdown of *each pyruvic acid.*

9. **The correct answer is (A).** Only ATP (32 molecules) and water (6 molecules) result from the electron transport chain. Carbon dioxide production is associated with the Krebs cycle (see above), and oxygen is only *consumed* during cell respiration (oxygen is produced during photosynthesis!).

10. **The correct answer is (C).** NAD, FAD, and the cytochromes are all hydrogen acceptors (electron acceptors) that first accept (reduction) and then pass along (oxidation) their hydrogens (or electrons). None of these molecules act as "oxygen carriers." Oxygen is the final hydrogen (or electron) acceptor in the electron transport chain.

11. **The correct answer is (A).** When the presence of a substance prevents an enzyme from further catalyzing the reaction that produced that substance, this is called feedback inhibition. In addition, when a substance binds to an enzyme in a place other than its active site, in a way that causes the inactivation of the enzyme, this is called allosteric inhibition. Competitive inhibition occurs when a substance binds to an enzyme's active site so that its normal substrate cannot bind there.

12. **The correct answer is (B).** DNA ligase is needed to combine the okazaki fragments formed during replication of the lagging strand of DNA. Since the leading strand is synthesized continuously, the ligase enzyme is not needed. The "uncoiling" of DNA's double-helix is accomplished by helicase enzymes.

13. **The correct answer is (B).** Peptidyl transferase is needed to a) attach a newly arrived amino acid at the ribosome's P site to the existing chain of amino acids already present at the A site, b) detach the tRNA holding the amino acid chain at the A site, once the chain has been attached to the tRNA at the P site, and c) attach the water molecule to the amino acid chain at the P site when a terminator codon is reached. The first two functions are part of elongation, while the third function is part of termination.

14. **The correct answer is (A).** One mRNA codon consists of *three* RNA nucleotides transcribed from three DNA nucleotides. Each "triplet" codon then represents one amino acid to be added to the protein during translation.

15. **The correct answer is (C).** If the template strand of DNA has the nucleotide sequence CTA, then the mRNA codon transcribed from this sequence will be GAU. The anticodon of the tRNA molecule must be complementary to the codon; thus, CUA.

16. **The correct answer is (B).** Exons are protein-coding sequences in the genetic material. The DNA nucleotide sequence, GTT, would be transcribed to produce the mRNA sequence CAA (this codon calls for the amino acid, glutamine, to be inserted into the protein being translated). If the DNA sequence mutated from GTT to ATT, the "new" mRNA codon would be UAA, which is one of the three terminator (STOP!) codons. The protein, therefore, would end prematurely.

9.2 CELLULAR BIOLOGY

A. EUKARYOTIC CELLS AND THEIR ORGANELLES

The cell is the basic unit of life. Living things are made of cells and cells arise from pre-existing cells (Cell Theory). Cells have an outer **plasma membrane** that forms a boundary around a semifluid cytoplasm **(cytosol)** which contains numerous **organelles** responsible for performing many of the cell's functions.

The nucleus—the control center of the cell—is surrounded by a double membrane or **nuclear envelope** with pores (nuclear pores). The nucleus contains chromatin material in the form of **chromosomes** made primarily of DNA, RNA, and proteins, which carry the genetic information. Sequences of nucleotides along the DNA represent the organism's "genes," which serve as templates during mRNA transcription. The **nucleolus** is a region in the nucleus at which **ribosomes** are synthesized.

In the cytoplasm, ribosomes are the sites at which the translation of the mRNA transcript is carried out; i.e., amino acids are linked together during the synthesis of the cell's proteins. Ribosomes may be found individually in the cytoplasm, in groups **(polysomes),** or associated with the membrane of another organelle, the **endoplasmic reticulum** (ER). The ER is a network of internal membranes that allows communication and transport between different regions of the cell. **Rough ER** (with ribosomes on the membrane) is associated with the synthesis and transport of plasma membrane proteins and proteins for export or secretion. **Smooth ER** (no ribosomes attached) is associated with the synthesis and transport of various lipids and carbohydrates, and the detoxification of certain harmful molecules. The **Golgi complex** is a series of membranous sacs that also

Eukaryotic Cell (Animal)

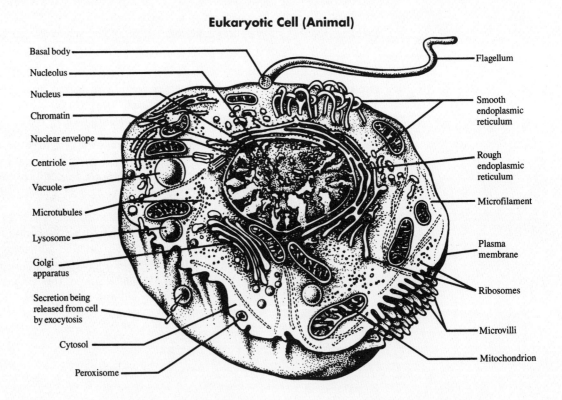

serves as a site for the synthesis of various large molecules. However, it primarily stores, sorts, modifies, combines, and packages for export many products made by the ER. **Lysosomes** contain digestive enzymes and help break down substances in the cell, as well as worn-out cellular structures. **Vacuoles** are membrane-bound storage organelles that can also take in and help break down particles and substances by **phagocytosis** (a form of **endocytosis**), or expel things by **exocytosis. Microbodies** are membrane-bound sacs containing enzymes specialized in the metabolism of particular molecules. **Peroxisomes** break down toxic substances such as hydrogen peroxide, while **glyoxysomes** (plants only) break down fats to sugars. **Centrioles** play a role in cellular reproduction (mitosis). **Mitochondria** are membranous organelles in which aerobic cellular respiration takes place (Krebs cycle and electron transport chain) and where most of the cell's ATP is synthesized. **Microtubules** and **microfilaments** serve as the cytoskeleton, in that their arrangement helps support the cell, influences the cell's shape and its ability to move. **Cilia** and/or **flagella** may be present to move cells (sperm cells have a flagellum) or move things past cells (mucous membranes may be ciliated to trap foreign particles and move them outward).

Plant cells are eukaryotic cells that have other organelles as well. **Plastids** containing pigments, or **chloroplasts,** are the sites in which photosynthesis takes place. A rigid **cell wall** made primarily of cellulose is also present. Vacuoles are much larger than in animal cells, and centrioles are absent.

B. THE CELL MEMBRANE AND TRANSPORT MECHANISMS

Cell or plasma membranes consist of phospholipids in a bilayered arrangement. Proteins can be embedded through the membrane **(integral proteins)** or occur only on the surface **(peripheral proteins).** Carbohydrates may be attached to some of the proteins and lipids on the outer surface, acting in part, as receptor sites, in cell-to-cell recognition or cell adhesion. Components can drift and change

Cell Membrane (Fluid-Mosaic Model)

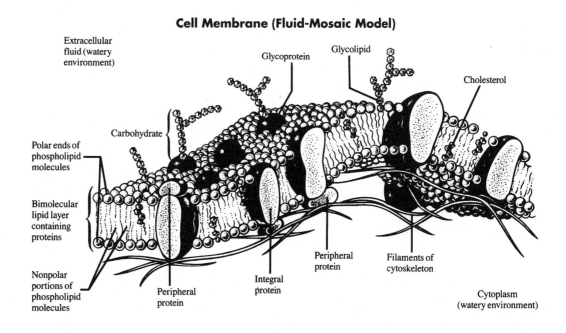

position **(Fluid-Mosaic Model).** Membrane channels also exist to help maintain a membrane potential (see Section 9.2.D).

Cell membranes are selectively permeable. Methods of transport across the membrane include the following:

- **Diffusion**

  Diffusion is the random movement of a substance, without any energy expenditure by the cell, from a region where the substance is more concentrated to where it is less concentrated.

- **Osmosis**

  Osmosis is a specialized form of diffusion where water molecules move from where they are more concentrated to where they are less concentrated (from an area containing less solute to an area containing more solute).

- **Facilitated Diffusion**

  Faciliated diffusion requires a specific carrier protein to help a substance diffuse across the membrane.

- **Active Transport**

  Active transport also involves a carrier protein. However, substances can be moved in this manner from low concentration to high. This requires energy expenditure (ATP) by the cell. Phagocytosis and exocytosis are other ways that substances can be moved into or out of cells.

Cellular Junctions

Cells in contact can have specialized sites that allow strong connections and rapid communication, and influence the passage of materials between each other. Animal cells can have **desmosomes, tight junctions,** and **gap junctions,** while plant cells have **plasmodesmata.**

Desmosomes hold cells together strongly, while still allowing substances to pass freely. **Tight junctions** seal cells together so tightly that the passage of substances is severely limited. **Gap junctions** connect and provide intercellular pores for rapid communication between adjacent cells. The **plasmodesmata** found between the cell walls of plants are channels connecting the cytoplasm of adjacent cells so that ions and molecules can pass from cell to cell.

C. CELL REPRODUCTION (MITOSIS)

The asexual reproduction of eukaryotic somatic cells involves the replication and subsequent distribution of chromosomes **(karyokinesis)** followed by the division of the cytoplasm **(cytokinesis).** Thus, two daughter cells are formed, genetically identical to each other and to the initial cell that underwent mitosis. **Diploid** organisms have two sets of chromosomes, with a specific number of chromosome types per set. Thus, diploid organisms have two of each chromosome type. These pairs, or **homologous chromosomes,** are similar in structure and carry genes affecting the same traits. At conception, one of each pair of homologous chromosomes was received from each parent in **haploid gametes** (sex cells with one set of chromosomes: sperm and ovum).

Mitosis

Interphase → Early prophase → Late prophase

Centrioles (two pairs)
Chromatin
Nucleolus
Plasma membrane
Nuclear envelope

Pair of Centrioles
Chromosome, consisting of two sister chromatids
Aster
Centromere

Spindle pole
Fragments of nuclear envelope
Kinetochore fibers

Metaphase → Anaphase → Telophase and cytokinesis

Spindle
Metaphase plate
Daughter chromosomes
Cleavage furrow

In humans there are 23 pairs of homologous chromosomes for a total of 46 chromosomes in each **somatic cell** (body cell). The 23rd pair is referred to as the **sex chromosomes,** which are either homologous (XX in females) or non-homologous (XY in males). The other 22 pairs are referred to as **autosomes.**

The actual mitotic cycle is preceded by **interphase,** a time in the cell's life cycle during which growth and normal metabolism occur, as well as preparation for replication **(G1),** chromosomes are replicated **(S),** and preparation for cell division takes place **(G2).** During this time, chromosomes are uncoiled and not visible **(chromatin).** After replication, each copied chromosome condenses and first becomes visible as two identical **chromatids** attached at the **centromeres.** This early stage of mitosis is called **prophase.** Also during prophase, the nuclear membrane breaks down, the **mitotic spindles** and **asters** form (associated with centrioles in animal cells), and then move to opposite poles of the cell. During **metaphase,** all replicated chromosomes (two chromatids) line up randomly along the center of the cell **(metaphase plate).** At **anaphase,** the centromeres divide and the mitotic spindles help pull sister chromatids apart toward opposite poles of the cell. Interactions between the chromatids and spindle occur at a region called **kinetochore.** During **telophase,** a nuclear membrane again forms at each pole around each set of chromosomes, the spindle disappears, and chromosomes uncoil. Cytokinesis then occurs starting with a **cleavage furrow** (in animal cells) or **cell plate** (plant cells). The **telomere,** at the tip of each chromosome, is associated with normal chromosome activity during mitosis, including the number of times a cell can undergo replication.

D. EUKARYOTIC TISSUES

Groups of specialized cells and their intercellular material working to perform a specific function together form a tissue. Specialized animal tissues include the following:

- **Epithelial Tissue**
  Epithelial tissue covers the outside of the body and individual organs, and lines the inside of organs and cavities. It covers, protects, and is capable of secretion and absorption. Very little intercellular material is present. Single-layered tissues are referred to as **simple epithelium,** whereas such tissues with more than one layer are called **stratified epithelium.** Square cells are **cuboidal,** rectangular cells are **columnar,** and flat, irregular cells are **squamous** epithelial cells.

- **Connective Tissue**
  Connective tissue joins other tissues together and helps support the body and its organs. It has a variety of cells dispersed throughout much intercellular material. Cells include **fibroblasts, macrophages, adipose cells, and mast cells.** Intercellular material consists of fibers and matrix, and can range from the hardness of bone to the fluid consistency of blood plasma. Fibers can be strong (collagen) and/or flexible (elastin). Connective tissues include areolar (loose), dense fibrous, bone, cartilage, blood, and lymph.

- **Muscle Tissue**
  Muscle tissue is composed of excitable cells **(muscle fibers)** surrounded by a membrane called the **sarcolemma** and specialized in their ability to contract. Such tissues include skeletal (voluntary or striated) muscle, smooth (involuntary) muscle, and cardiac muscle. A **sarcomere** is a repeating segment of muscle tissue (within **myofibrils**) that contains the protein filaments **actin** and **myosin** in a very regular arrangement. In a muscle cell at rest, myosin cross-bridges are blocked from attaching to actin by the presence of a complex of the proteins **troponin** and **tropomyosin.** When muscle cells are depolarized by motor neurons, calcium is released from sacs of **sarcoplasmic reticulum,** the troponin-tropomyosin complex releases the actin filaments to bind with calcium, and the myosin cross-bridges come in contact with actin at the **active site.** Here, ATP is broken by ATPase, energy is released, the cross-bridges swivel, and actin filaments slide toward each other. This shortens the sarcomere, resulting in contraction (see "Muscle System" in section 9.4.C).

- **Nervous Tissue**
  Nervous tissue consists of excitable cells **(neurons)** specialized in their ability to conduct and transmit impulses, and other supportive cells (glial cells or **neuroglia**). Neurons have a **soma** or cell body, one or more processes that conduct impulses toward the soma **(dendrites),** and one or more processes that conduct impulses away from the soma **(axons).** Some axons are covered by a fatty **myelin sheath** produced by glial cells called **Schwann cells.** The myelin sheath has gaps called **nodes of Ranvier.** Together the myelin and nodes of Ranvier help accelerate impulses. The site at which neurons meet is referred to as a **synapse.**

Parts of a Neuron

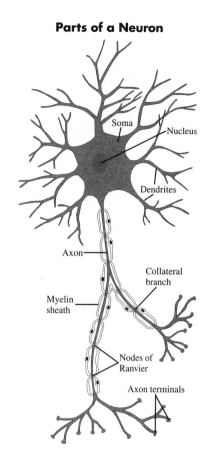

The outer membranes of neurons (like that of all cells) are surrounded by fluid. There is an unequal distribution of ions inside and outside the membrane (more Na+ outside, more K+ inside, and more negatively charged proteins inside) resulting in a **resting potential.** The inside of a neuron is more negatively charged than the outside and this difference (−70mv) is maintained, in part, by a **Na+/K+ pump** that actively transports Na+ out of the cell and K+ into the cell. An **action potential** (the origin of an impulse) is caused by a stimulus that alters the permeability of the membrane, allowing Na+ to rush inside the cell. This **depolarization,** or reversal of charge (now more positive inside and more negative outside), spreads down the axon causing a chemical **neurotransmitter** to be released from vesicles at the **axon endings** into the synapse. The neurotransmitter crosses the synapse and stimulates the next neuron (or muscle cell) in the circuit, causing it to depolarize, and so on (see neuromuscular junction in section 9.4.C). **Repolarization** involves: 1) the release of K+ from inside the neuron to the outside in order to return the positive charge to the outside of the membrane (return to resting potential), and 2) the Na+/K+ pump's activity to restore the proper ion concentrations to both the inside and outside of the membrane (Na+ pumped back out, K+ pumped back in).

Membrane Potentials

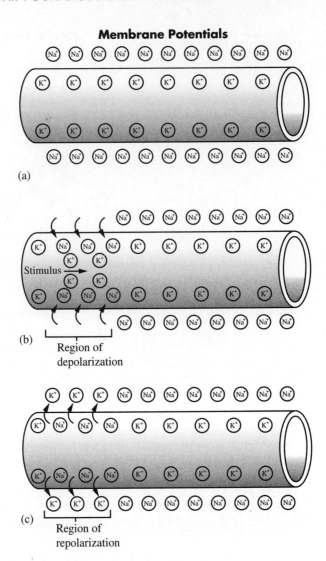

(a)

Stimulus →

(b)

Region of
depolarization

(c)

Region of
repolarization

- **Specialized Plant Tissues**

  Specialized plant tissues include three main types. **Dermal tissue,** or **epidermis,** forms an external layer of closely packed cells that helps protect, secrete, and absorb (similar to epithelial tissue in animals). **Vascular tissue** provides both support and transport. Two kinds are **xylem** tissue, which helps transport water and minerals, and **phloem** tissue, which helps transport food and other organic molecules. **Parenchyma tissue** consists of mostly unspecialized cells that can develop support, synthesis, and storage functions.

PRACTICE PROBLEMS
CELLULAR BIOLOGY

1. Which of the following organelles are not associated with the breakdown of potentially harmful substances?

   A. lysosomes
   B. peroxisomes
   C. smooth ER
   D. rough ER

2. Which of the following structures do not play a role in the movement of cells or the movement of materials past cells?

   A. centrioles
   B. flagella
   C. cilia
   D. microtubules and microfilaments

3. Cell A is hypotonic to Cell B. In which direction will there be more of a tendency for water to move between these cells?

   A. A to B
   B. B to A
   C. equal net movement in both directions
   D. no net movement in either direction

4. The nephrons of the kidney filter glucose from the blood while wastes are being removed. The nephron tubules then have the responsibility of reabsorbing the glucose molecules back into the circulation. The reabsorption of glucose by the kidney tubules would be expected to proceed by which of the following?

   A. osmosis
   B. diffusion
   C. facilitated diffusion
   D. active transport

5. Which tissue type would you expect to find in the walls of the nephron tubules?

   A. epithelium
   B. connective tissue
   C. involuntary muscle tissue
   D. neurons

6. In which organelle would proteins be modified by adding a carbohydrate component to the amino acid chains in order to form a glycoprotein?

   A. rough ER
   B. smooth ER
   C. Golgi complex
   D. mitochondria

7. Chromosomes are visible during mitosis and meiosis when they condense and are tightly coiled. Yet, they cannot be seen as distinct units at other times in the cell cycle when their chromatin material is uncoiled. What reason best explains this phenomenon?

   A. They must uncoil to reveal genetic sequences during protein synthesis.
   B. They must uncoil to reveal all DNA sequences during replication.
   C. They must be tightly coiled for them to be moved around during cell reproduction.
   D. All of the above

8. In human cells undergoing mitosis, how many chromatids are present during anaphase?

   A. 22
   B. 23
   C. 44
   D. 46
   E. 92

9. Depolarization takes place when _____ ions enter the cell from the outside, whereas repolarization begins when _____ ions leave the cell from the inside.

   A. K+, Na+
   B. K+, K+
   C. Na+, Na+
   D. Na+, K+

10. Which type of cell would not be expected to be found in connective tissue?

A. adipose cells
B. squamous cells
C. mast cells
D. fibroblasts

11. Before depolarization of a muscle cell, where will calcium ions primarily be found?

A. In extracellular fluid just outside the sarcolemma.
B. In the axon endings of a motor neuron.
C. In the intracellular fluid just inside the sarcolemma.
D. In the sarcoplasmic reticulum.

12. The proteins primarily responsible for preventing contraction in a resting muscle cell are

A. myosin and troponin.
B. myosin and tropomyosin.
C. troponin and tropomyosin.
D. myosin and actin.

13. Which type of cellular connection would you expect to find *between cells* lining the intestines?

A. desmosomes
B. tight junctions
C. gap junctions
D. plasmodesmata

ANSWER KEY

1. D	3. A	5. A	7. D	9. D	11. D	13. B
2. A	4. D	6. C	8. E	10. B	12. C	

ANSWERS AND EXPLANATIONS

1. **The correct answer is (D).** Rough ER is primarily responsible for synthesizing membrane proteins and secretory proteins. Peroxisomes break down hydrogen peroxide and other toxins, smooth ER plays a role in drug detoxification, and lysosomes break down various molecules that originate inside and outside the cell.

2. **The correct answer is (A).** Centrioles are associated with the spindle fibers that help move chromatids to opposite poles *within the cell* during the anaphase and telophase stages of mitosis and meiosis. Flagella and cilia can propel individual cells (sperm cells and paramecium, respectively), ciliated cells can move materials along (ciliated mucous membranes), and microtubules and microfilaments form the cytoskeleton of cells. The rearrangement of this cytoskeleton plays a role in the changes in shape and movement of cells like the amoeba and phagocytotic white blood cells.

3. **The correct answer is (A).** If Cell A is hypotonic to Cell B, it has less solutes than Cell B. With less solutes, Cell A must have more water than Cell B. Therefore, water will move (by osmosis) from where there is more water to where there is less water (A to B). Answer C only applies after the percentages of water have equalized in both cells. Answer D is never true because molecules are constantly in random motion based on their own kinetic energy.

4. **The correct answer is (D).** Since the amount of glucose filtered out of the blood is significantly less than the total amount of glucose remaining in the blood, the reabsorption of glucose involves moving it from where there is less (the urinary filtrate) to where there is more (circulation). This would require active transport and the expenditure of ATP.

5. **The correct answer is (A).** The walls of nephrons primarily consist of epithelial cells that carry out the various processes occurring in the kidney: filtration, reabsorption, and secretion. Connective tissue cannot carry out such processes, and nerve and muscle activities play no role in this aspect of urinary function.

6. **The correct answer is (C).** The rough ER is where proteins are made, whereas the smooth ER is where carbohydrates and/or lipids can be made. However, it is in the Golgi complex that two such components would be modified, combined, and packaged into a functional glycoprotein. The mitochondria could provide the ATP to carry out some of this work, but the work itself would take place in the Golgi complex.

7. **The correct answer is (D).** Clearly, precise DNA sequences must be revealed during transcription of genes, as well as during the complete replication of each DNA strand. In this "uncoiled" condition, the chromosomes cannot be seen as distinct units. In contrast, to move chromosomes around within the cell during prophase, metaphase, anaphase, and telophase would be virtually impossible if they remained uncoiled!

8. **The correct answer is (E).** All 46 chromosomes have been replicated during interphase, resulting in 92 chromatids. During anaphase, the 92 chromatids have been divided into two sets of 46, and are moving toward opposite poles. However, the two daughter cells have not yet been formed. Therefore, all 92 are still present in the original undivided cell.

9. **The correct answer is (D).** The passage of Na+ into the cell from outside is what causes the reversal of the resting potential from (+) outside the membrane and (−) inside the membrane to (−) outside and (+) inside (depolarized state). The release of K+ from the inside at the onset of repolarization then helps return the cell membrane to its resting potential.

10. **The correct answer is (B).** Squamous cells are flat, irregularly shaped epithelial cells. All the other choices (adipose cells, mast cells, and fibroblasts) are specialized cells found in connective tissues.

11. **The correct answer is (D).** Calcium is stored in the sarcoplasmic reticulum until depolarization. Choice B is incorrect because it is the neurotransmitter substance that leaves the axon endings of the motor neuron. This neurotransmitter disturbs the muscle cell membrane, causing Na+ to move inside from the extracellular fluid. Thus, choice A is also incorrect. Choice C is incorrect because it is K+ that moves from the intracellular fluid to the outside.

12. **The correct answer is (C).** The troponin-tropomyosin complex binds to actin when a muscle cell is at rest so that the myosin heads (cross-bridges) cannot make contact with the active site along the actin. When calcium is released from the sarcoplasmic reticulum, the troponin-tropomyosin complex will shift to bind with calcium, thus allowing contact between the myosin heads and actin that is necessary for contraction to occur.

13. **The correct answer is (B).** Only tight junctions could prevent the unwanted passage of substances from the intestinal lumen into the blood or into the abdominopelvic cavity. The movement of materials from the intestinal lumen to the blood can only take place *across* cell membranes (via osmosis, diffusion, active transport, etc.) rather than *around* or *between* cells. The other cellular connections all allow some free passage of materials around and between cells.

9.3 MICROBIOLOGY

A. PROKARYOTIC CELLS: BACTERIA*

Prokaryotic cells are present in organisms belonging to the kingdom Prokaryota (formerly Monera: the bacteria and blue-green algae).

Prokaryotic Cell Structure

Prokaryotic cells lack true nuclei and membrane-bound organelles. Ribosomes are smaller than in eukaryotes. Most prokaryotes are single-celled organisms but some

Comparison of Prokaryotic* and Eukaryotic Cells

Structure	Prokaryote	Animal Cell	Plant Cell
Plasma membrane	Yes	Yes	Yes
Cell Wall	Yes	No	Yes
Nucleus	Lacks nuclear envelope	Bounded by nuclear envelope	Bounded by nuclear envelope
Chromosomes	One continuous DNA molecule	Multiple, consisting of DNA and much protein	Multiple, consisting of DNA and much protein
Ribosomes	Yes (smaller)	Yes	Yes
Endoplasmic reticulum	No	Usually	Usually
Golgi apparatus	No	Yes	Yes
Lysosomes	No	Often	Some vacuoles function as lysosomes
Peroxisomes	No	Often	Often
Glyoxysomes	No	No	Common
Vacuoles	No	Small or none	Usually one large vacuole in mature cell
Mitochondria	No	Yes	Yes
Plastids	No	No	In many cell types (include chloroplasts in photosynthetic cells)
Cilia or flagella	Simple flagella	Complex ("9 + 2" arrangement)	Present on sperm of some plants
Centrioles	No	Yes	No

* A relatively new kingdom, Archaea, includes organisms formerly considered bacteria, whose molecular structure, biochemistry, and habitats differ from typical prokaryotes.

occur in groups or as small multicellular forms. The cells are approximately 1/10 to 1/100 of the volume of eukaryotic cells. A single, circular chromosome ("naked" DNA with few proteins) is usually located in the **nucleoid,** a central region not enclosed by a membrane. **Plasmids** (small rings of bacterial DNA) inside the cell can replicate independently and can confer additional characteristics (antibiotic resistance, metabolic specializations, etc.). The outer plasma membrane may have inner folds for metabolic functions, and is surrounded by a rigid cell wall made of **peptidoglycan,** which provides protection, and helps maintain the cell's shape and osmotic balance. Bacteria may move via flagella and axial filaments, or glide on secretions of slime.

Bacterial Classification
Bacteria can be classified by their shape (round: **coccus;** rod-shaped: **bacillus;** spiral-shaped: **spirillum**), their grouping patterns (pairs: **diplo-;** chains: **strepto-;** clusters: **staphylo-**), the staining characteristics of their cell walls (**gram+** or **gram−**), and their metabolic requirements.

Bacterial Metabolism

Metabolically, most bacteria are **heterotrophic saprobes** (get nourishment from dead organic material). However, some are photosynthetic **autotrophs,** chemosynthetic autotrophs, or **symbionts** (in relationship with other organisms). Most are aerobic, but some are **facultative anaerobes** (can carry out respiration without oxygen if necessary) or **obligate anaerobes** (can only carry out respiration anaerobically).

Bacterial Reproduction

Asexual reproduction occurs by **binary fission** (replication of the chromosome, followed by equal division of the cell into two parts). Genetic recombination can take place by **conjugation** (a cell of one mating type directly transfers genetic material to a cell of a different mating type), **transformation** (fragments of DNA released by one cell may be assimilated by another cell), or **transduction** (a virus or bacteriophage transfers a piece of DNA from a former host, along with its own DNA, into a new host).

Conjugation in Bacteria

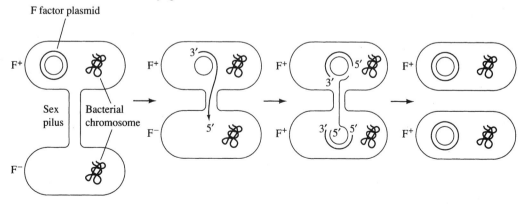

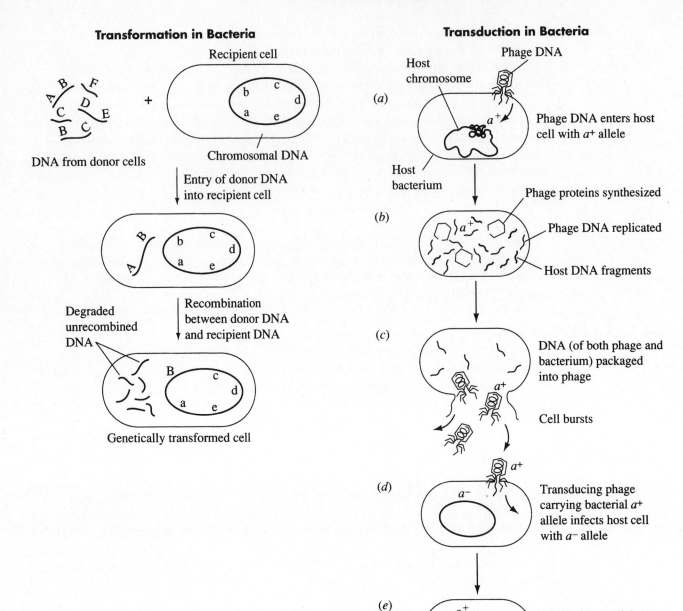

Transformation in Bacteria

Transduction in Bacteria

B. VIRUSES

Viral Structure

Viruses are noncellular particles or **virions** (much smaller than bacteria) consisting of DNA or RNA enclosed by a protein shell or **capsid.** Some are even smaller than ribosomes, and only the largest can be seen with a light microscope. Viruses are parasites that require the enzymes and much of the metabolic machinery of the host to translate their own genetic material and replicate copies of themselves. Animal viruses can be covered with an "envelope" that is partly or completely acquired from the host cell's membrane, which then eases viral entry and exit from the host.

Viruses: Lytic and Lysogenic Cycles

Phage DNA

Phage attaches
to host cell and
injects DNA.

Occasionally, the prophage
may excise from the bacterial
chromosome.

Phage
particle
(virion)

Bacterial
chromosome

Many cell
divisions

LYTIC CYCLE

LYSOGENIC CYCLE

Cell lyses, releasing
phage virions.

Phage DNA
circularizes

Lysogenic bacterium
reproduces normally.

or

Prophage

New phage DNA and
proteins are synthesized
and assembled into virions.

Phage DNA integrates within the bacterial
chromosome by recombination (crossing
over), becoming a prophage.

Bacteriophage Life Cycle

Bacteriophages are viruses that infect bacteria. They attach to the host cell, their tail sheath contracts—injecting viral DNA into the host—viral enzymes destroy or repress the host cell's DNA, and the host cell's metabolic machinery is used to make new viral DNA and protein parts that are then assembled into new virions. The phage produces **lysozyme**, an enzyme that disrupts the host's cell wall, and the new virions are released to infect other host cells. This sequence is referred to as the **lytic cycle**, and such phages that kill their host cells are **virulent**. An alternative sequence involves the incorporation of the viral DNA into the host cell's chromosome (the inserted viral genome is a **prophage**). Most of the viral genes remain inactive during this **lysogenic cycle** and such phages are called **temperate** viruses. As the bacterial host replicates normally, the viral DNA is also copied and becomes part of each new bacterial cell. The phage can revert to the lytic cycle at any time.

C. Fungi

The kingdom Fungi consists of eukaryotic organisms that are primarily multicellular and heterotrophic and have cell walls. They digest their food outside their bodies and then absorb it through their cell walls and cell membranes. Fungi can exist as saprobes, parasites, or symbionts.

Generalized Structure

Most multicellular fungi (such as molds and mushrooms) have branches or **hyphae** in a network or mass called a **mycelium.** The hyphae of some fungi may be divided into cells by **septa,** while other forms may have hyphae without septa (**coenocytic**).

Fungal Anatomy

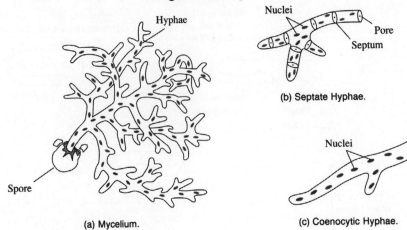

(a) Mycelium.

(b) Septate Hyphae.

(c) Coenocytic Hyphae.

Generalized Reproductive Pattern

Asexual reproduction occurs via haploid **spores** that germinate in the appropriate environment, grow into branching hyphae, and eventually form the mycelium. Most of the life cycle is thus **haploid** (one set of chromosomes). Under appropriate conditions, genetic recombination can occur when spores from hyphae of different mating strains fuse (conjugation) to form a temporary diploid stage. This is followed by meiosis, producing new haploid spores, hyphae, and mycelia. Yeasts are unicellular forms that can reproduce asexually by **budding** or fission, as well as by sexually produced spores.

PRACTICE PROBLEMS
MICROBIOLOGY

1. Bacteria can replicate human genes after specific segments of human DNA have been introduced into the bacterial cell using viruses as vectors. This type of "recombinant DNA" technology applies knowledge gained from studying which of the various forms of sexual reproduction occurring in bacteria?

   A. transformation
   B. transduction
   C. binary fission
   D. conjugation

2. Which organelles are not found in bacterial cells?

   A. endoplasmic reticulum
   B. mitochondria
   C. chloroplasts
   D. All of the above.

3. How does the genetic material in prokaryotes usually differ from that in eukaryotic cells?

   A. the number of chromosomes
   B. the shape of chromosomes
   C. the material in chromosomes
   D. all of the above

4. Which of the following microorganisms act as decomposers vital to the ecological health of our planet?

   A. prokaryotes
   B. fungi
   C. plants
   D. A and B
   E. A, B, and C

5. A rod-shaped bacterial species that is usually arranged in chains of cells would be called

    A. staphylococcus.
    B. streptococcus.
    C. diplobacillus.
    D. streptobacillus.

6. Certain bacteria in the soil and in the root nodules of plants called legumes are unique in that they can convert nitrogen gas in the air into ammonia. Without nitrogen fixation, the first step in the nitrogen cycle, other living organisms would be unable to synthesize

    A. proteins.
    B. nucleic acids.
    C. ATP.
    D. A and B.
    E. A, B, and C.

7. Shingles, a disorder localized in the host's nerve cells, results from the reactivation of the same viral species that previously caused chicken pox in that individual. This situation, involving a "latent" virus in human cells, is analogous to which of the following in bacterial cells?

    A. temperate phages
    B. lytic phages
    C. transformation using plasmids
    D. all of the above

8. Which of the following would you expect to find on the outside of a virally-infected bacterial cell?

    A. RNA
    B. lysozyme
    C. capsid
    D. DNA

ANSWER KEY

1. B   2. D   3. D   4. D   5. D   6. E   7. A   8. C

ANSWERS AND EXPLANATIONS

1. **The correct answer is (B).** Only transduction involves the viral transfer of a DNA segment from one bacterium to another. Transformation occurs when DNA fragments released from a destroyed bacterial cell into the medium are incorporated into another bacterium. Conjugation involves the direct exchange of genetic material between two bacterial cells. Binary fission is an asexual form of reproduction.

2. **The correct answer is (D).** All the choices are membrane-bound organelles. Since bacteria have prokaryotic cells, no membrane-bound organelles are present. The functions carried out by endoplasmic reticulum, mitochondria, and chloroplasts in eukaryotes take place in the cytoplasm of prokaryotes.

3. **The correct answer is (D).** Eukaryotes usually have linear-shaped chromosomes in pairs. Their chromosomal material includes DNA, RNA, and proteins. Prokaryotes usually have single, circular chromosomes made primarily of DNA.

4. **The correct answer is (D).** Both prokaryotes and fungi have many species that are saprobes or decomposers. Plants, which rely on photosynthesis for their food molecules, are "producers" (autotrophs).

5. **The correct answer is (D).** Bacilli are rod-shaped, while cocci are round. Different species have cells arranged in pairs (diplo-), chains (strepto-), and clusters (staphylo-).

6. **The correct answer is (E).** By converting nitrogen gas from the air into a form that can eventually be utilized by plants (ammonia must later be converted to nitrates by nitrifying bacteria), nitrogen-fixing bacteria provide a means for all living things to synthesize nitrogen-containing molecules. These include proteins (which contain amino acids), nucleic acids (which contain the nitrogen bases adenine, guanine, cytosine, thymine, or uracil), and ATP (which contains adenine).

7. **The correct answer is (A).** Temperate phages remain latent in the genetic material of the host cell indefinitely, until they become reactivated and cause the lysis (lytic cycle) of the host cell. Transformation using plasmids (choice C) refers to a method used in recombinant DNA technology.

8. **The correct answer is (C).** Viral infection occurs when the virus attaches to the outside of the host cell and then injects its genetic material (DNA or RNA) inside (leaving its protein coat or capsid *outside*). Lysozyme is an enzyme produced after infection that disrupts the host's cell wall from the inside and allows the release of newly assembled virions.

9.4 VERTEBRATE ORGAN SYSTEMS

A. INTEGUMENTARY SYSTEM

The skin has many functions, including protection and various aspects of homeostasis such as water and salt balance and temperature regulation. It also contains neural structures (receptors) designed to detect changes in the environment.

Epidermis

The outer layer, or **epidermis,** is composed of stratified epithelium. Beneath the stratified epithelium is a non-living **basement membrane** with a mitotically active layer of cells attached (stratum germinativum or stratum basale). These cells undergo mitosis in order to replace surface cells that have died and have been

The Skin

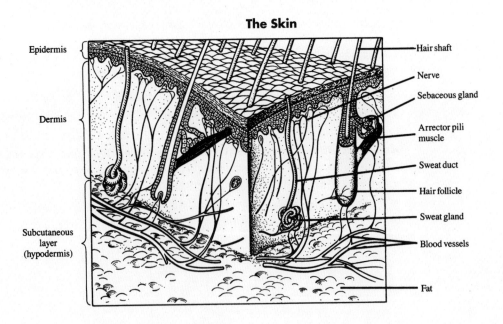

Epidermis

Dermis

Subcutaneous layer (hypodermis)

Hair shaft

Nerve

Sebaceous gland

Arrector pili muscle

Sweat duct

Hair follicle

Sweat gland

Blood vessels

Fat

worn away by contact with the external environment. Special cells of the epidermis produce **keratin,** a protein that helps prevent water loss. Other cells (**melanocytes**) produce the pigment **melanin,** which helps absorb, and thereby prevent damage, due to ultraviolet radiation from sunlight.

Dermis

The **dermis** contains various tissues and important structures. **Sweat glands** help lower body temperature as sweat (water, salts, and other waste products) evaporates at the surface. **Sebaceous glands** secrete sebum that prevents hair and skin from drying out. **Hair follicles** are present, in association with involuntary **arrector pili muscles,** which respond to emotional and thermal stimuli to cause hairs to "stand up" and goose bumps to appear. Also present are blood vessels that supply nutrients to skin cells and help maintain body temperature (when too cold, **vasoconstriction** reduces the flow of warm blood near the surface and thus reduces heat loss to the air; when too warm, **vasodilation** increases blood flow and subsequent heat loss at the surface). Various nervous system **receptors** for light touch, pressure, pain, heat, and cold are also distributed throughout the dermis.

Subcutaneous Layer

The **subcutaneous layer (hypodermis)** is primarily composed of **adipose tissue** (for storage of fat and temperature insulation) and **loose connective tissue (areolar)** to attach the entire skin to the skeletal muscles below.

B. SKELETAL SYSTEM

Functions and Divisions

The functions of the skeletal system include protection, support and posture, storage of inorganic salts and fat, blood cell production, and as a source of attachment sites for muscles, tendons, and ligaments so that movement is possible. The human skeleton has axial and appendicular divisions. The **axial skeleton** consists of the skull, hyoid bone, thoracic cage, and vertebral column. The **appendicular skeleton** is comprised of the pectoral girdle, upper limbs, pelvic girdle, and lower limbs.

Bone Tissue

Bone is primarily composed of collagen fibers and **hydroxyapatite** (a combination of calcium salts) in a mucopolysaccharide matrix. Bone exists as **compact bone,** which microscopically consists of densely packed units of concentric layers known as **osteons** or **Haversian systems,** and as **spongy bone** (cancellous bone) containing numerous air spaces that help lighten the weight and provide areas for marrow (red: blood cell formation; yellow: fat storage). **Osteocytes** are mature bone cells that maintain the health of bone tissue.

Long Bones

Long bones have a shaft or **diaphysis** between the **epiphyses** at each end that are covered with **articular cartilage** (made of hyaline cartilage) for protection within joints. The bone is covered with **periosteum**, which gives rise to **osteoblasts** (bone-making cells), provides a route for blood vessel entry, and is an attachment site for **tendons** (hold muscles to bone) and **ligaments** (hold bones to each other). Spongy bone in the diaphysis (**medullary cavity** lined with **endosteum**) is a site for fat storage, whereas the spongy bone at the epiphysis is where blood cell production occurs in young individuals. Spongy bone in flat bones is where most blood cell production occurs in adults. Long bones can continue to grow as long as a cartilaginous **epiphyseal plate** (disk) is present between the diaphysis and epiphysis. Once this last remaining strip of mitotic hyaline cartilage ossifies, growth in length can no longer occur.

Bone Development

Most bones form by **endochondral ossification** after first developing as hyaline cartilage. Only certain flat bones of the skull form from a fibrous connective tissue membrane **(intramembranous ossification).** "Soft spots" **(fontanels),** areas of this fibrous connective tissue that have not yet completely ossified, allow some compression of the bones of the skull at birth. Throughout life, bone is constantly being "remodeled" as new bone is added on the outside by **osteoblasts** and bone is eroded away from within by **osteoclasts.**

Articulations

Joints classified as **diarthrotic** (synovial) allow various amounts of relatively free movement: ball-and-socket, hinge, gliding, pivot, etc. Synovial joints contain articular cartilage at the ends of the bones, a joint capsule lined with fluid-secreting synovial membrane, and they are reinforced by ligaments. Joints with little free movement are designated as **amphiarthrotic** (symphysis), while joints that exhibit no movement are called **synarthrotic** (sutures).

A Long Bone (Femur)

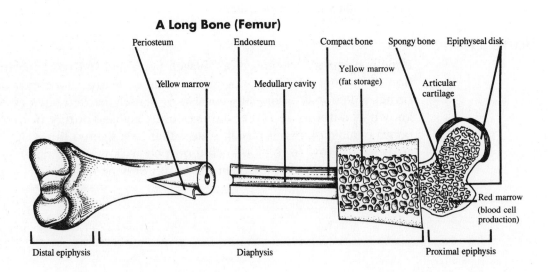

Periosteum • Endosteum • Compact bone • Spongy bone • Epiphyseal disk

Yellow marrow • Medullary cavity • Yellow marrow (fat storage) • Articular cartilage

Red marrow (blood cell production)

Distal epiphysis • Diaphysis • Proximal epiphysis

C. MUSCLE SYSTEM

Muscles move the skeletal elements and body parts to which they are attached, they move material through body parts (blood, swallowed food), and they help produce heat when they are active to maintain body temperature.

Muscle System

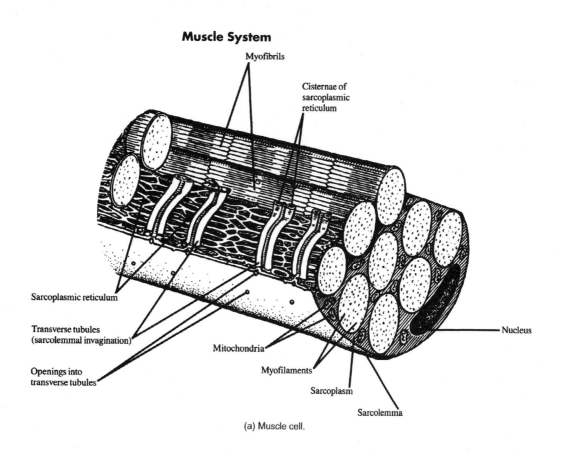

(a) Muscle cell.

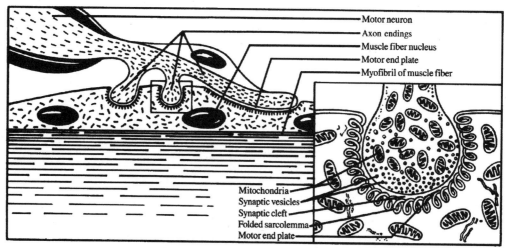

(b) Neuromuscular junction.

Skeletal Muscle Structure and Function

Skeletal muscles are attached to bones and are responsible for voluntary movement. Muscles that do most of the work for a particular action are called **agonists** or **prime movers.** Muscles that help perform the same actions are called **synergists.** Whereas, muscles that act in pairs performing opposite actions are called **antagonists.** Each muscle is attached to bones at both ends. Upon contraction, the muscle attachment site that moves is called the **insertion,** while the end that does not move is called the **origin.**

Skeletal muscle consists of bundles **(fascicles)** of muscle cells (muscle fibers), each cell consisting of **myofibrils.** Contraction occurs when a motor neuron releases a neurotransmitter (usually **acetylcholine**) at the site where neuron meets muscle cell, the **neuromuscular,** or **myoneural junction.** The neurotransmitter acts as a stimulus, causing a disturbance of the muscle cell membrane **(sarcolemma).** This allows Na+ ions to move inside and causes the sarcolemma and **t-tubules** to depolarize, subsequently leading to the release of calcium from the sarcoplasmic reticulum, and contraction of the sarcomeres within the myofibrils. **Cholinesterase** (acetylcholinesterase) is released at the neuromuscular junction to break down the acetylcholine and prevent overstimulation.

Muscle spindles inside the muscle feed back sensory information to the brain concerning the current length, position, and tension of the muscle and its tendon **(proprioception).** This helps prevent overstretching of muscle cells. Individual muscle cells respond to neural stimulation in an **all-or-none** fashion. However, graded responses of whole muscles can occur as more muscle cells within the muscle are stimulated.

Energy Sources

Energy for contraction derives from ATP produced during the normal cellular respiration of glucose. Additional sources of energy come from stored **glycogen** (which can be converted to glucose) as well as **creatine phosphate** (which, when broken down, can provide high-energy phosphates to form additional ATP molecules). During increased activity, oxygen cannot be supplied rapidly enough by the respiratory and circulatory systems. Pyruvic acid (produced during glycolysis) can temporarily be converted to **lactic acid** under these anaerobic conditions. The lactic acid that accumulates in muscle cells must be reconverted back to pyruvic acid after the activity is done. This requires additional oxygen taken in by the respiratory system and is referred to as **oxygen debt.**

Smooth and Cardiac Muscle

Smooth muscles form part of the walls of involuntary organs and blood vessels. Motor neurons from the autonomic nervous system control these muscles through the release of neurotransmitters such as acetylcholine and **norepinephrine. Cardiac muscle** makes up the major tissue of the heart. Cardiac muscles have **intercalated disks** that hold adjoining cells together in a meshed network. The networks rhythmically contract as units in response to stimulation from the autonomic nervous system. However, cardiac muscle cells can also be self-excitatory **(autorhythmicity).**

PRACTICE PROBLEMS
INTEGUMENTARY, SKELETAL, AND MUSCLE SYSTEMS

1. Which of the following responses would be expected to occur under the same temperature conditions?

    A. shivering and dilation of superficial blood vessels
    B. sweating and constriction of superficial blood vessels
    C. both A and B
    D. neither A nor B

2. Which substance produced in the skin can act to reduce the probability of skin cancer?

    A. keratin
    B. melanin
    C. sebum
    D. sweat

3. Females have a higher amount of adipose tissue in the skin. Where would this be found?

    A. epidermis
    B. dermis
    C. hypodermis
    D. stratum germinativum

4. Which of the following is (are) not protected by parts of the axial skeleton?

    A. brain
    B. heart and lungs
    C. spinal cord
    D. developing blood cells
    E. None of the above.

5. Sex hormones speed up bone production (ossification) by osteoblasts. If all other factors remain equal, which of the following predictions would have the greatest probability of being correct?

    A. Individuals who reach puberty early will stop growing early.
    B. Individuals who reach puberty early will stop growing late.
    C. Individuals who reach puberty late will stop growing early.
    D. Two of the above.

6. Which of the following is true about the development of bone?

    A. Fewer bones of the body form by intramembranous ossification than from endochondral ossification.
    B. More bones of the body form by intramembranous ossification than from endochondral ossification.
    C. Approximately the same number of bones form by intramembranous ossification and endochondral ossification.
    D. Compact bone develops by endochondral ossification, while spongy bone forms by intramembranous ossification.

7. Osteoblasts must synthesize

    A. proteins.
    B. carbohydrates.
    C. inorganic material.
    D. All of the above

8. The epiphyseal plates are considered cartilaginous joints called synchondroses. How would they be classified based on the amount of movement observed at these joints?

    A. synarthrotic
    B. amphiarthrotic
    C. diarthrotic
    D. synovial

9. The biceps brachii muscle flexes the lower arm, whereas the triceps brachii extends the lower arm. What relationship do these muscles have to each other?

    A. agonists
    B. synergists
    C. prime movers
    D. antagonists

10. Based on the information given in Question 9, which statement is correct about the biceps brachii and triceps brachii muscles?

    A. One has its origin on the lower arm.

    B. One has its insertion on the lower arm.

    C. Both have their insertions on the lower arm.

    D. Both have their origins on the lower arm.

11. What would be the expected result if cholinesterase were not released at the neuromuscular junction?

    A. The muscle would fully contract and relax once.

    B. The muscle would relax only.

    C. The muscle would continue to contract without being able to relax normally.

    D. The muscle would fully contract and relax repeatedly.

12. Which sequence of depolarization best describes the order in which a muscle contracts?

    A. sarcoplasmic reticulum, t-tubules, sarcolemma

    B. sarcoplasmic reticulum, sarcolemma, t-tubules

    C. sarcolemma, t-tubules, sarcoplasmic reticulum

    D. sarcolemma, sarcoplasmic reticulum, t-tubules

    E. t-tubules, sarcolemma, sarcoplasmic reticulum

13. When exercising, skeletal muscles can continue to carry out glycolysis and produce small amounts of ATP, even though glucose is not arriving via the blood rapidly enough. Which of the following best explains this phenomenon?

    A. Glycolysis is anaerobic and doesn't require oxygen.

    B. Extra glucose molecules can be supplied from stored glycogen within the muscle.

    C. Extra glucose molecules can be supplied from stored glycogen within the liver.

    D. All of the above.

14. When skeletal muscles grow and place extra stress on bones as a result of weight training, bones respond by increasing in thickness. This is most likely due to the action of

    A. osteoblasts.

    B. osteocytes.

    C. osteoclasts.

    D. motor neurons.

ANSWER KEY

1. D	3. C	5. A	7. D	9. D	11. C	13. B
2. B	4. E	6. A	8. A	10. C	12. C	14. A

ANSWERS AND EXPLANATIONS

1. **The correct answer is (D).** When the body is too cold, we shiver and our superficial blood vessels constrict to save heat. When the body is too warm, we sweat and our superficial blood vessels dilate to lose heat more efficiently.

2. **The correct answer is (B).** UV radiation is mutagenic and can be absorbed by DNA in skin cells. Melanin absorbs UV radiation, reducing the chances of it reaching the cells below. Keratin and sebum help conserve moisture in the skin.

3. **The correct answer is (C).** The hypodermis (subcutaneous layer) contains adipose tissue and loose connective tissue. The epidermis is stratified squamous epithelium. The stratum germinativum is the mitotic layer of epithelium in the epidermis. The dermis contains most of the complex structures of the skin (hair follicles, glands, blood vessels, receptors, etc.) and relatively few adipose cells.

4. **The correct answer is (E).** The axial skeleton includes the skull, vertebral column, and thoracic cage (sternum and ribs). Thus, all choices are protected by these bony regions. The sternum (breast bone) is one of the flat bones in which blood cells develop.

5. **The correct answer is (A).** Since growth can continue as long as the cartilaginous cells in the epiphyseal plates continue to undergo mitosis, the sooner the cartilage ossifies (due to sex hormones), the sooner growth stops.

6. **The correct answer is (A).** Only the flat bones of the skull ossify by intramembranous ossification. All other bones start off as hyaline cartilage and ossify by endochondral ossification. Choice D may sound like a good answer, but just sounding correct doesn't count!

7. **The correct answer is (D).** Osteoblasts make bone tissue which includes protein (collagen), inorganic calcium salts (hydroxyapatite), and a carbohydrate matrix (mucopolysaccharides).

8. **The correct answer is (A).** Since no movement occurs *inside* the ends of long bones, synchondroses are synarthrotic joints. Choice D (synovial) refers to the synovial membrane that lines freely movable (diarthrotic) joints.

9. **The correct answer is (D).** When muscles perform opposite actions, they are considered antagonists. The terms agonist and prime mover are synonymous for the muscle that does most of the work for a specific movement. Synergists assist the prime mover.

10. **The correct answer is (C).** Both muscles cause movement of the lower arm (flexion and extension). Therefore, the insertions of both muscles must be on the lower arm. The origin is the muscle's attachment site that does not move.

11. **The correct answer is (C).** Cholinesterase is released at the neuromuscular junction in order to break down acetylcholine and prevent this neurotransmitter from re-stimulating the muscle cell. The enzyme thus allows the muscle cell to relax. If ACh were not broken down, it would continue to allow Na+ ions across the sarcolemma, and repolarization would not be possible.

12. **The correct answer is (C).** When acetylcholine is released from the motor neuron to the neuromuscular junction, the sarcolemma depolarizes. Depolarization then spreads along the outside, through the t-tubules to the inside, and finally to the sarcoplasmic reticulum, where calcium ions are released.

13. **The correct answer is (B).** Each glycogen molecule stored in a muscle cell is made of thousands of monosaccharides (glucose) linked together. When needed, each glycogen can be broken down to supply these glucose molecules for the muscle cell to use in glycolysis. The cell does not have to wait for glucose molecules to be delivered by the blood. Glycogen stored in the liver can also be broken down to glucose, but it still would have to arrive at the muscle cells via the bloodstream. Although choice A is a true statement, it is not relevant to why glucose is still available.

14. **The correct answer is (A).** Only osteoblasts make new bone tissue. Osteoclasts break down bone tissue, while osteocytes maintain healthy bone tissue that is already present. Motor neurons stimulate muscle cells to contract and are not directly relevant to the question.

D. NERVOUS SYSTEM

General Functions

Functions of the nervous system include 1) detecting changes in the external and internal environment through **receptors** specialized to depolarize when specific changes occur, 2) integrating this sensory information as **sensory neurons** (afferent neurons) carry impulses from receptors to interneurons (association neurons) in the **central nervous system** (spinal cord and brain), and then 3) directing the appropriate responses as **motor neurons** (efferent neurons) relay impulses from interneurons of the central nervous system to the body's **effectors** (muscles and glands) which then respond accordingly. Impulses are transmitted from neuron to neuron, when a neurotransmitter is released from one depolarized neuron across a **synapse,** so that the next neuron in the circuit also depolarizes (see Section 9.2.D).

The CNS and PNS

A. Central Nervous System
   1. Brain (interneurons)
   2. Spinal Cord (interneurons)

B. Peripheral Nervous System*
   1. Somatic Nervous System
      (a) Sensory neurons carry information into the CNS from external skin receptors (touch, pressure, heat, cold, pain, etc.).
      (b) Motor neurons carry information out of the CNS to voluntary effectors (skeletal muscles).

   2. Autonomic Nervous System
      (a) Sensory neurons carry information into the CNS from internal receptors (oxygen, carbon dioxide, pH, etc.).
      (b) Motor neurons carry information out of the CNS to involuntary effectors (smooth muscles, cardiac muscle, glands).

* In the peripheral nervous system, sensory and motor neurons travel together in cranial nerves (connected directly to the brain) and spinal nerves (connected directly to the spinal cord).

Nervous System Organization: CNS and PNS

The interneurons of the brain and spinal cord are considered parts of the **central nervous system** (CNS). The receptors and sensory neurons leading to the CNS, as well as the motor neurons leading from the CNS, are considered parts of the **peripheral nervous system** (PNS). The sensory and motor neurons that enter and leave the spinal cord, respectively, travel together in structures called **spinal nerves.** Each spinal nerve services a specific segment of the body (sensory neurons "bring information in" from receptors in a particular segment, or **dermatome,** while motor neurons "carry information to" effectors in the same area). After a sensory neuron enters the spinal cord (from a spinal nerve), it **synapses** with an interneuron in the cord. This interneuron ascends the cord to the brain where other interneurons continue the circuit to the appropriate brain area for interpretation. Other interneurons of the brain then send appropriate signals that eventually descend the cord and ultimately synapse with motor neurons that relay the impulse (in a spinal nerve) to the muscle and/or gland effectors responsible for the body's specific response to the situation.

Example: An insect walking on your shoulder is detected by a touch receptor that depolarizes. The impulse travels along a sensory neuron (attached to the touch receptor) in a specific PNS spinal nerve (C4). Spinal nerve C4 enters the spinal cord (CNS), where the sensory neuron synapses with an ascending interneuron. A circuit of interneurons eventually leads to the somatic sensory area of the brain **(cerebrum),** where the touch sensation and its source location is perceived. Other interneurons lead to the primary motor area of the brain (cerebrum), where motor impulses start their descent—eventually traveling down the cord (CNS) and synapsing with motor neurons. These motor neurons leave the cord through PNS spinal nerves and form a neuromuscular junction with effector muscles that will contract and allow you to brush away the insect.

Sensory input and motor output for a particular situation need not always travel along the same spinal nerve, e.g., an insect walking on your leg may be brushed away with muscles from the arm! Above the spinal cord (head and face regions), sensory and motor neurons perform similar functions, but directly enter and leave the brain itself, respectively, via PNS structures called **cranial nerves.**

The Cranial Nerves

Nerve		Type	Function
I	Olfactory	Sensory	Sensory fibers transmit impulses associated with the sense of smell.
II	Optic	Sensory	Sensory fibers transmit impulses associated with the sense of vision.
III	Oculomotor	Primarily motor	Motor fibers transmit impulses to muscles that raise the eyelids, move the eyes, adjust the amount of light entering the eyes, and focus the lenses.
			Some sensory fibers transmit impulses associated with the condition of muscles.
IV	Trochlear	Primarily motor	Motor fibers transmit impulses to muscles that move the eyes.
			Some sensory fibers transmit impulses associated with the condition of muscles.
V	Trigeminal	Mixed	
	Ophthalmic division		Sensory fibers transmit impulses from the surface of the eyes, tear glands, scalp, forehead, and upper eyelids.
	Maxillary division		Sensory fibers transmit impulses from the upper teeth, upper gum, upper lip, lining of the palate, and skin of the face.
	Mandibular division		Sensory fibers transmit impulses from the scalp, skin of the jaw, lower teeth, lower gum, and lower lip.
			Motor fibers transmit impulses to muscles of mastication and to muscles in the floor of the mouth.
VI	Abducens	Primarily motor	Motor fibers transmit impulses to muscles that move the eyes.
			Some sensory fibers transmit impulses associated with the condition of muscles.
VII	Facial	Mixed	Sensory fibers transmit impulses associated with taste receptors of the anterior tongue.
			Motor fibers transmit impulses to muscles of facial expression, tear glands, and salivary glands.
VIII	Vestibulocochlear	Sensory	
	Vestubular branch		Sensory fibers transmit impulses associated with the sense of equilibrium.
	Cochlear branch		Sensory fibers transmit impulses associated with the sense of hearing.

The Cranial Nerves—(Continued)

Nerve		Type	Function
IX	Glossopharyngeal	Mixed	Sensory fibers transmit impulses from the pharynx, tonsils, posterior tongue, and carotid arteries.
			Motor fibers transmit impulses to salivary glands and to muscles of the pharynx used in swallowing.
X	Vagus	Mixed	Somatic motor fibers transmit impulses to muscles associated with speech and swallowing; autonomic motor fibers transmit impulses to the viscera of the thorax and abdomen.
			Sensory fibers transmit impulses from the pharynx, larynx, esophagus, and viscera of the thorax and abdomen.
XI	Accessory Cranial branch	Primarily motor	Motor fibers transmit impulses to muscles of the soft palate, pharynx, and larynx.
	Spinal branch		Motor fibers transmit impulses to muscles of the neck and back.
XII	Hypoglossal	Primarily motor	Motor fibers transmit impulses to muscles that move the tongue.

The simplest nervous system circuits, **spinal reflexes** (which do not involve the brain), are shown below

Spinal Reflexes

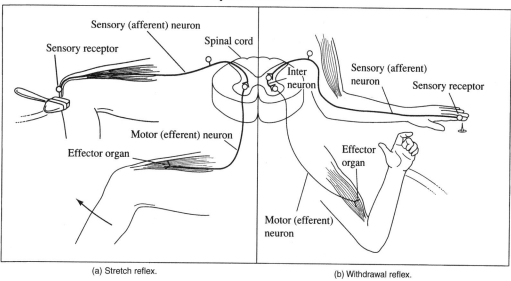

(a) Stretch reflex.　　(b) Withdrawal reflex.

PNS: Somatic and Autonomic Portions

The somatic portion of the PNS consists of neurons (in both spinal and cranial nerves) that connect the CNS with receptors in the skin and with skeletal muscles. Voluntary activity is regulated through the **somatic nervous system.** The autonomic portion of the PNS is involved with neurons (in both spinal and cranial nerves) that connect the CNS with internal receptors and with smooth muscle, cardiac muscle, and various glands. Involuntary activity is regulated through the **autonomic nervous system.** The **parasympathetic division** of the autonomic nervous system regulates involuntary effectors during normal, everyday activities through the release of the neurotransmitter acetylcholine. The **sympathetic division** of the autonomic nervous system regulates involuntary effectors during stressful situations (sometimes referred to as "fight or flight" situations) through the release of norepinephrine.

Autonomic Nervous System Effects

Effector Location	Response to Sympathetic Stimulation	Response to Parasympathetic Stimulation
Integumentary System		
Apocrine glands	Increased secretion	No action
Eccrine glands	Increased secretion (cholinergic effect)	No action
Special Senses		
Iris of eye	Dilation	Constriction
Tear gland	Slightly increased secretion	Greatly increased secretion
Endocrine System		
Adrenal cortex	Increased secretion	No action
Adrenal medulla	Increased secretion	No action
Digestive System		
Muscle of gallbladder wall	Relaxation	Contraction
Muscle of intestinal wall	Decreased peristaltic action	Increased peristaltic action
Muscle of internal anal sphincter	Contraction	Relaxation
Pancreatic glands	Reduced Secretion	Greatly increased secretion
Salivary glands	Reduced Secretion	Greatly increased secretion
Respiratory System		
Muscle walls of bronchioles	Dilation	Constriction
Cardiovascular System		
Blood vessels supplying muscles	Constriction (alpha adrenergic) Dilation (beta adrenergic) Dilation (cholinergic)	No action
Blood vessels supplying skin	Constricted	No action
Blood vessels supplying heart (coronary arteries)	Dilation (beta adrenergic) Constriction (alpha adrenergic)	Dilation
Muscles in wall of heart	Increased contraction rate	Decreased contraction rate

Autonomic Nervous System Effects—(Continued)

Effector Location	Response to Sympathetic Stimulation	Response to Parasympathetic Stimulation
Urinary System		
Muscle of bladder wall	Relaxation	Contraction
Muscle of internalurethral sphincter	Contraction	Relaxation
Reproductive System		
Blood vessels to clitoris and penis	No action	Dilation leading to erection
Muscles associated with male internal reproductive organs	Ejaculation	
Muscles of uterus	Contraction during pregnancy	
	Relaxation during non-pregnancy	

CNS: The Brain

The brain contains centers that ultimately receive, integrate, and interpret all sensory information, direct motor activity, and carry out more complex activities (thinking, learning, memory, emotions, etc.). Both the brain and spinal cord are covered with protective membranes called the **meninges.** Within the meninges, and inside the hollow regions of the CNS (**central canal** of the spinal cord and **ventricles** of the brain), **cerebrospinal fluid (CSF)** bathes the exposed surfaces of the CNS. This fluid provides a protective cushion and various transport and other supportive functions. The major parts of the brain and their functions are listed below.

The **brain stem** includes the following:

1. **Medulla Oblongata**
   The link for all ascending and descending circuits between the spinal cord and higher centers of the brain; site of cardiac (heart rate) and vasomotor (blood pressure) centers; primary respiratory centers; and coughing, swallowing, sneezing, and vomiting reflexes.

The Brain (Longitudinal Section)

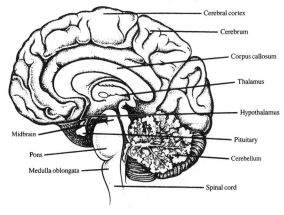

2. **Pons**

The bridge between brain stem, cerebrum, and cerebellum; site of secondary respiratory centers.

3. **Midbrain**

Contains sites associated with visual and auditory reflexes, as well as important descending motor pathways.

The **diencephalon** includes the following:

1. **Thalamus**

The central sensory relay station to the cerebrum.

2. **Hypothalamus**

The link with endocrine system via the **pituitary gland;** link with autonomic nervous system; centers involved with hunger, satiety, reproductive behavior, body temperature regulation, thirst, and water balance.

- **Reticular Formation**

Helps regulate sensory information to the cerebrum; states of sleep, arousal, and wakefulness (parts of the reticular formation extend from the brain stem into the diencephalon and cerebrum).

- **Limbic System**

Associated with emotions, and motivations (parts of the limbic system extend from the brain stem into the diencephalon and cerebrum).

Cerebellum

Coordinates voluntary motor activity; helps in maintenance of balance and equilibrium (receives input from muscles, tendons and joints, inner ear, and cerebrum).

Cerebrum

Governs higher functions such as thought, reasoning, memory, judgment, etc. (association areas); interpretation of somatic sensory input (parietal lobe); directs voluntary motor activity (frontal lobe); speech (frontal lobe); vision (occipital lobe); hearing and olfaction (temporal lobe); and taste (parietal lobe). The outer layer, the **cerebral cortex,** forms a series of ridges **(gyri)** and depressions **(sulci)** that help increase the total surface area of the cerebrum. The **corpus callosum** is a tract that connects the two cerebral hemispheres.

E. Sensory System

Receptors and Sensations

Receptors are structures of neural tissue specialized to depolarize when particular environmental changes occur. Mechanoreceptors for touch, pressure, blood pressure, hearing, etc., respond to mechanical energy forces. Chemoreceptors in blood vessel walls, in the nose, and on the tongue respond to changes in chemical concentrations (oxygen and carbon dioxide levels in the blood, airborne chemicals that dissolve on nasal receptors, and food molecules that dissolve on **taste buds** on **papillae** of the tongue). Thermoreceptors in the skin and blood vessels (hypothalamus) respond to changes in temperature. Pain receptors respond to tissue damage or excesses of temperature, pressure, and chemical concentrations. Proprioceptors respond to stretch and other tensions brought about by changes in muscle, tendon, and joint position. Visual receptors in the eye respond to changes in light intensity, color, and pattern. Hearing receptors of the inner ear respond to mechanical forces produced by sound wave vibrations. Ultimately, sensations are experienced when impulses along neuron circuits are completed from specific receptor to specific brain interpretation centers.

Vision

The eye has three layers: (1) the outer **fibrous tunic** contains the tough, protective **sclera,** and the transparent **cornea** which allows light to enter the eye, (2) the middle **vascular tunic** includes a variety of vascular, muscular, and pigmented structures, and (3) the inner **neural tunic** or **retina,** which contains the receptors for vision, the **rods** and **cones.**

The smooth muscles of the **iris** control how much light passes through the opening of the iris, the **pupil.** The **lens** is a transparent elastic structure, whose shape (flat for distant objects versus round for near objects) determines to what extent light must be bent **(refracted)** in order to focus onto the receptors of the retina **(accommodation).** The **ciliary body** and **suspensory ligaments** control the shape of the lens. Spaces between the cornea and iris, and iris and lens, are filled with **aqueous humor.** The space between the lens and retina is filled with **vitreous humor.** Both fluids help maintain the shape of the eye. The **choroid** contains vascular networks that service the retina and pigments for retaining light that enters the eye.

Cones are color-vision receptors sensitive to stimulation from different wavelengths of light (red, green, and blue), that require high light intensity to work. That is why we only see colors in bright light. Rods allow vision in dim light. A pigment in rods **(rhodopsin)** breaks down to **retinal** and **opsin** in the presence of light. This leads to a nerve impulse that travels along the optic nerve (cranial nerve II) and eventually reaches the occipital lobe of the cerebrum. In dim light or darkness, rhodopsin reforms and the rod is ready to fire again.

The Eye

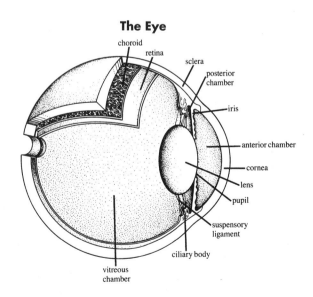

Hearing

The ear has three regions:

1. The external ear includes the outer **pinna** which collects sound waves and passes them through the **external auditory meatus** to the **tympanum** or eardrum, which separates the external ear from the middle ear.

2. The middle ear houses the **ossicles** or middle ear bones (malleus, incus, and stapes) which amplify vibrations from the tympanum. (The middle ear also contains the **eustachian tube** which leads to the pharynx and helps equalize pressure on both sides of the ear drum.)

3. Vibrations from the middle ear ossicles pass through the **oval window** into the inner ear, where hearing receptors (hair-cells) in the **cochlea** are located. The cochlea is a coiled chamber of fluid-filled compartments. The central compartment (cochlear duct) contains the **Organ of Corti** (hair-cell receptors and support cells with **basilar membrane** below and **tectorial membrane** above). As fluids of the inner ear vibrate, hair cells in the Organ of Corti are stimulated and impulses travel along the auditory nerve (cochlear branch of cranial nerve VIII), eventually reaching the temporal lobe of the cerebrum. Different hair-cell receptors respond to different sound-wave frequencies. Vibrations leave the inner ear and return to the middle ear through the **round window,** ultimately leaving the body through the eustachian tube. This prevents overstimulation of the inner ear hair-cell receptors.

The internal ear also houses the **vestibule,** which contains two structures, the **utricle** and **saccule,** responsible for maintaining balance and equilibrium when the body is stationary and during linear acceleration. The **semicircular canals** are also located in the internal ear, and are responsible for maintaining balance and equilibrium during linear and rotational acceleration. These parts of the internal ear send impulses to the cerebellum (vestibular branch of nerve VIII).

Hearing

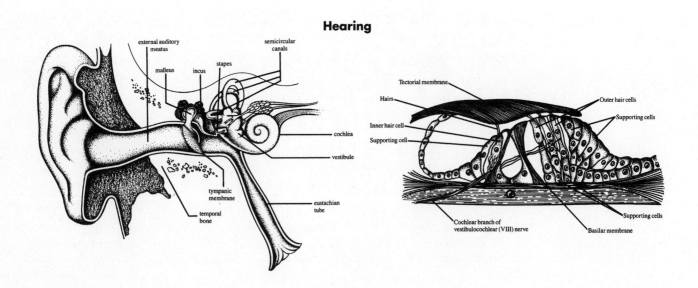

F. ENDOCRINE SYSTEM

Endocrine glands secrete **hormones** into the blood which then influence the activity of other target cells. In this way, the endocrine system has similar communicative functions to those of the nervous system. Once environmental changes are detected, appropriate homeostatic responses can be directed through these blood-borne chemical messengers (**exocrine glands** secrete substances into ducts leading directly to cavities or surfaces).

The endocrine and nervous systems are continuously interacting systems linked by the hypothalamus.

Mechanisms of Hormone Action

Hormones can affect their target cells in a number of ways.

1. Steroid hormones can enter cells and bind with receptor sites in the nucleus. The hormone-receptor complex can then bind with a chromosome, thereby regulating gene action (activating or suppressing the synthesis of particular proteins).

2. Protein and amine hormones bind to the outer membrane of target cells. This leads to the production of a second messenger molecule inside the cell such as cyclic adenosine monophosphate (**cAMP**). The second messenger then activates enzymatic processes that lead to the appropriate responses by the target cell. Such responses are often amplified because small amounts of hormone can cause the production of large amounts of second messenger molecules.

Control of Hormone Secretion

The release of many hormones is controlled by **negative feedback.** Glands are sensitive to the concentration of the substances that their hormones are designed to regulate. When the concentration of the regulated substance *goes down,* gland activity and hormone production *go up,* bringing the concentration of the substance back within its homeostatic range. If the concentration of the regulated substance *goes up* too high, gland activity and hormone production *go down,* again bringing the substance back within its homeostatic range. Such feedback loops may be activated directly by the regulated substance itself, by nerve impulses leading to the controlling gland's response, or by hormones released by other glands causing the controlling gland's response.

Major Glands and Hormones of the Endocrine System

1. **Thyroid Gland**
   The thyroid gland produces three hormones. **Thyroxine (T4)** and **triiodothyronine (T3)** increase oxygen consumption and metabolic rate in all cells. **Calcitonin** helps lower blood calcium levels.

2. **Parathyroid Glands**
   These glands produce parathyroid hormone (**parathormone**), which helps raise blood calcium levels. Target cells include osteoclasts which help break down bone material, cells of the small intestine which absorb extra calcium from foods, and kidney tubule cells which increase reabsorption of calcium.

3. **Pancreas**

   The pancreas acts as both an exocrine and endocrine gland. Exocrine functions are related to the release of digestive substances by **acinar cells** into the pancreatic duct to the small intestine. Special areas of the pancreas **(Islets of Langerhans)** produce two endocrine hormones. **Glucagon** helps raise blood glucose levels by stimulating the liver to convert glycogen into glucose, and by stimulating the breakdown of fats. **Insulin** helps decrease blood glucose levels by allowing the passage of glucose from blood to cells, by stimulating the formation of glycogen in the liver and skeletal muscles, and the formation of fat in adipose cells from excess glucose.

4. **Adrenal Glands**

   The *adrenal cortex* produces **aldosterone (mineralocorticoid)** which causes a rise in blood sodium through an increase in sodium reabsorption by kidney cells (potassium ions are secreted); **cortisol** and **cortisone (glucocorticoids)** which increase blood glucose levels by stimulating the conversion of glycogen, as well as non-carbohydrates (gluconeogenesis), and acts as an anti-inflammatory substance in response to stress; and sex hormones (mostly **androgens**) which supplement the activity of the gonads. The *adrenal medulla* secretes epinephrine and norepinephrine, which reinforce the effects of the sympathetic division of the autonomic nervous system.

5. **Ovaries**

   The ovaries secrete **estrogen** and **progesterone,** which help maintain sexual development, the menstrual cycle, and preparation for pregnancy.

6. **Testes**

   The testes produce **testosterone,** which leads to development of the male reproductive system (in the embryo), maintains male sexual characteristics and behavior, and contributes to adequate sperm production.

7. **Anterior Pituitary Gland (adenohypophysis)**

   The anterior pituitary gland produces many hormones, a number of which help regulate the activity of other glands. **Thyroid Stimulating Hormone** (TSH) controls the secretions of the thyroid gland (T3 and T4). **Adrenocorticotropic Hormone** (ACTH) controls the secretion of glucocorticoids by the adrenal cortex. **Follicle Stimulating Hormone** (FSH) stimulates estrogen production and ovum development in the ovaries and sperm production by the testes. **Luteinizing Hormone** (LH) leads to ovulation and the production of progesterone by the ovary, as well as an increase in testosterone production in the testes (**Interstitial Cell Stimulating Hormone,** ICSH). **Growth Hormone** (GH) stimulates protein synthesis, gluconeogenesis, and growth of cells in size and number. **Prolactin** (PRL) stimulates breast development and milk production.

   Due to its controlling effects on other glands, the anterior pituitary gland is often called the "master gland." However, all secretions by the anterior pituitary gland are themselves controlled by the *hypothalamus* through **releasing hormones** (prolactin inhibitory factor prevents overproduction of prolactin).

8. **Posterior Pituitary Gland (neurohypophysis)**
   Two hormones are stored and released by the posterior pituitary gland although they are produced by the hypothalamus. **Antidiuretic Hormone** (ADH or vasopressin) stimulates the reabsorption of water by kidney cells, thus regulating water balance and blood pressure. **Oxytocin** stimulates both the contraction of smooth muscle in the walls of the uterus during labor and the ejection of milk from mammary glands during nursing.

Other Endocrine Activity

The *thymus gland* secretes **thymosin,** which influences the maturation of special immune system cells (T-lymphocytes). The *pineal gland* secretes **melatonin,** which influences the body's 24-hour patterns of activity (**circadian rhythms**). The *stomach and small intestine* also have cells that secrete hormones influencing the digestive process (see Section 9.4.J). The *kidney* secretes **erythropoietin,** which stimulates red blood cell production. The *heart* releases **atrial natriuretic peptide** (ANP), which helps regulate (lower) blood pressure.

PRACTICE PROBLEMS
NERVOUS, SENSORY, AND ENDOCRINE SYSTEMS

1. A collection of neurons traveling together in the spinal cord or brain is called a tract. What kind of neurons would be found in a tract?

   A. sensory neurons
   B. motor neurons
   C. interneurons
   D. All of the above.

2. Which of the following statements is true about sensory receptors?

   A. Chemoreceptors, mechanoreceptors, and thermoreceptors detect external changes only.
   B. Chemoreceptors, mechanoreceptors, and thermoreceptors detect internal changes only.
   C. Chemoreceptors, mechanoreceptors, and thermoreceptors detect internal and external changes.
   D. Chemoreceptors and mechanoreceptors can detect internal and external changes, but thermoreceptors cannot.

3. Which statement is true about all spinal reflexes?

   A. No synapses are necessary for the response to occur.
   B. No motor neurons are necessary for the response to occur.
   C. The brain does not have to receive or send information for the response to occur.
   D. No interneurons are necessary for the response to occur.

4. Which of the following circuits would not involve one or more cranial nerves?

   A. taste
   B. vision
   C. chewing
   D. None of the above.

5. When a neurotransmitter released from one neuron (pre-synaptic neuron) makes it more difficult for the next neuron (post-synaptic neuron) to depolarize, this phenomenon is called inhibition. What might be happening at the synapse to cause inhibition?

A. The neurotransmitter causes extra Na+ to immediately enter the post-synaptic neuron.

B. The neurotransmitter causes extra K+ to immediately enter the post-synaptic neuron.

C. The neurotransmitter causes extra Na+ to immediately leave the post-synaptic neuron.

D. The neurotransmitter causes extra K+ to immediately leave the post-synaptic neuron.

6. Through which part(s) of the brain would you expect voluntary motor signals to your legs to travel?

A. cerebrum
B. cerebellum
C. midbrain
D. medulla
E. All of the above.

7. Which statement is true about the autonomic nervous system?

A. The sympathetic neurotransmitter, norepinephrine, speeds up all involuntary effectors.

B. The parasympathetic neurotransmitter, acetylcholine, slows down all involuntary effectors during "normal" activities.

C. Norepinephrine speeds up some involuntary effectors and slows down others during "fight-or-flight" activities.

D. Acetylcholine slows down some involuntary effectors and speeds up others during "normal" activities.

E. A and B
F. C and D

8. One technique previously used to reduce the effects of massive epileptic seizures in the cerebrum was to sever the corpus callosum. What result would you expect from such a procedure?

A. The seizure would be limited to one half of the cerebrum.

B. The seizure would be limited to the cerebral cortex only.

C. The patient would not feel any pain after the procedure.

D. Future seizures would involve sensory systems or motor systems but not both.

9. The type of neural cells responsible for interpreting sensory input and coordinating motor output are

A. neuroglia.
B. sensory neurons.
C. motor neurons.
D. interneurons.

10. Which cranial nerve(s) play no role in our "special senses"?

A. VII
B. VIII
C. IX
D. X

11. What is the primary difference between the various types of sensory receptors?

A. They are sensitive to different kinds of stimuli.

B. They pass signals along to different types of neurons.

C. Some pass their information into the CNS while others pass their information out of the CNS.

D. They each utilize different neurotransmitters.

E. All of the above.

12. Which of the following does not refract light as it passes through the eye?

    A. cornea
    B. aqueous humor
    C. lens
    D. retina

13. The optic disc is the site where axons from cells in the retina leave the eye and where the optic nerve originates. Since there is no room for any rods or cones at this location, what would you expect to happen when light strikes the optic disc?

    A. The visual image will not be in focus.
    B. Impulses along the optic nerve will speed up.
    C. Impulses along the optic nerve will slow down.
    D. No visual image will form.

14. An object appears red because

    A. the object absorbs wavelengths corresponding to red light.
    B. the object absorbs wavelengths other than red.
    C. "red" cones in the eye are stimulated by wavelengths corresponding to red light.
    D. "red" cones in the eye are stimulated by all wavelengths except red.
    E. B and C
    F. A and D

15. Identify the correct sequence of structures through which sound vibrations pass when hearing receptors in the cochlea are stimulated.

    A. tympanum, oval window, round window, basilar membrane
    B. tympanum, round window, oval window, basilar membrane
    C. tympanum, oval window, basilar membrane, round window
    D. tympanum, round window, basilar membrane, oval window

16. Where in the body are the receptors for detecting the kind of movement that occurs when a car suddenly accelerates?

    A. saccule and utricle
    B. semicircular canals
    C. cochlea
    D. A and B

17. Where on target cells would you expect to find receptor sites for the protein hormones, insulin and glucagon?

    A. In the nucleus of the target cells
    B. On the outer membrane of the target cells
    C. In the Islets of Langerhans of the pancreas
    D. In the acinar cells of the pancreas

18. Hormone production and release can be controlled by:

    A. hormones from other glands.
    B. signals from motor neurons.
    C. the blood concentration of the substance that the hormone regulates.
    D. All of the above.

19. Which hormone does not have hyperglycemic effects (helps raise blood glucose levels)?

    A. glucagon
    B. insulin
    C. epinephrine
    D. cortisol

20. Which organ is both the target of hormones and the producer of hormones?

    A. ovary
    B. kidney
    C. pancreas
    D. All of the above.

ANSWER KEY

1. C	3. C	5. D	7. F	9. D	11. A	13. D	15. C	17. B	19. B
2. C	4. D	6. E	8. A	10. D	12. D	14. E	16. D	18. D	20. D

ANSWERS AND EXPLANATIONS

1. **The correct answer is (C).** Since a tract is inside the brain or spinal cord (CNS), it can only contain interneurons. Collections of sensory and motor neurons are found in the peripheral nervous system and are called nerves.

2. **The correct answer is (C).**

    Chemoreceptors: *examples of internal changes:* blood oxygen, carbon dioxide, and pH levels; *examples of external changes:* olfaction and taste.

    Mechanoreceptors: *examples of internal changes:* blood pressure; *examples of external changes:* touch and pressure (skin), hearing, and balance.

    Thermoreceptors: *examples of internal changes:* body temperature; *examples of external changes:* heat and cold (skin).

3. **The correct answer is (C).** Spinal reflexes do not involve the brain. In a stretch reflex such as the patellar reflex, a sensory neuron carries information into the spinal cord from stretch receptors in the knee. The sensory neuron forms a synapse with a motor neuron that then leaves the cord to form a neuromuscular junction back in the muscle that extends the knee. Although this spinal reflex does not involve an interneuron (choice D), a withdrawal reflex (pulling the hand away from a fire) is a 3-neuron circuit (sensory n., interneuron, motor n.).

4. **The correct answer is (D).** All choices involve at least one cranial nerve. Taste: facial (VII) and glossopharyngeal (IX); vision: optic (II); chewing: trigeminal (V).

5. **The correct answer is (D).** Prior to stimulation, membranes in the polarized state are more ($-$) inside and more ($+$) outside. They have more Na+ outside and more K+ and ($-$) proteins inside. The difference in charge is approximately -70mv. For normal excitation at a synapse or neuromuscular junction to occur, the pre-synaptic neurotransmitter makes it easier for Na+ to enter the post-synaptic cell, making the inside ($+$). Inhibition usually involves the neurotransmitter allowing K+ to leave the post-synaptic cell, making the transmembrane voltage difference more than -70mv (-80mv or more), thus making it *more difficult* to cause depolarization. If extra Na+ entered (choice A), depolarization would occur more easily. The movement of K+ into the post-synaptic cell (choice B) and the movement of Na+ out of the post-synaptic cell (choice C) are not good answers since both would be against concentration gradients and would require active transport and the expenditure of ATP.

6. **The correct answer is (E).** Voluntary motor signals originate in the primary motor cortex of the cerebrum, and then pass through the midbrain (cerebral peduncles) and the medulla on their way to the spinal cord. The cerebellum coordinates these signals along the way.

7. **The correct answer is (F).** The sympathetic division of the autonomic nervous system regulates our involuntary effectors during situations such as stress and exercise (sometimes referred to as "fight-or-flight"). In such situations, norepinephrine speeds up cardiac muscle while slowing down the smooth muscle tissue of the digestive tract. In contrast, parasympathetic neurons, which release acetylcholine, will regulate these effectors as activities normalize. Thus, acetylcholine will slow down the heart back to normal, while speeding up the digestive processes back to normal.

8. **The correct answer is (A).** The corpus callosum is the tract that connects the right and left cerebral hemispheres. There is no particular pathway that could separate the entire cerebral cortex from other parts of the cerebrum (choice B). Pain (choice C) can be experienced on either side of the brain (somatic sensory area) whether or not the two cerebral hemispheres are connected. Both cerebral hemispheres contain somatic sensory and motor areas (choice D). Therefore, a seizure confined to either half could still affect both sensory and motor functions.

9. **The correct answer is (D).** The interpretation of sensory information and the coordination of motor activity take place in the neurons of the brain, which are interneurons. Neuroglia (choice A) in the CNS provide various other support functions.

10. **The correct answer is (D).** Even though the vagus nerve (X) helps regulate many of our vital systems (heart rate, blood pressure, etc.), it has no connections to our special senses. Cranial nerves VII and IX provide pathways for taste, while cranial nerve VIII provides pathways for hearing and balance.

11. **The correct answer is (A).** Different kinds of receptors respond to different forms of energy such as light (visual receptors), chemicals (chemoreceptors), mechanical (mechanoreceptors), and heat (thermoreceptors). They all directly or indirectly affect sensory neurons (choice B). All relay information *into* the CNS (choice C). Some receptors communicate with sensory neurons via electrical signals, while others release neurotransmitters onto the sensory neuron. However, each *does not* utilize a different neurotransmitter (choice D).

12. **The correct answer is (D).** The cornea, aqueous humor (between the cornea and lens), and lens each refract light as it passes through them. The result of this refraction is that the image is focused onto the receptors of the retina. The retina itself does not refract light.

13. **The correct answer is (D).** If there are no receptors, no electrical signals will be initiated and no visual image will form. Impulses along the optic nerve will not occur at all.

14. **The correct answer is (E).** Red objects basically absorb wavelengths other than red and *reflect* red light. This red light reaches our eyes from the object and stimulates our "red" cones, which are sensitive to "red" wavelengths.

15. **The correct answer is (C).** The path of sound-wave vibrations through the different parts of the ear is as follows: tympanum (eardrum) to middle ear ossicles to oval window (into the cochlea) to basilar membrane to hair-cell receptors in the Organ of Corti to round window (out of the cochlea) to eustachian tube.

16. **The correct answer is (D).** The receptors in the saccule and utricle respond primarily to gravitational forces when stationary and during *linear acceleration*. Receptors in the semicircular canals (choice B) respond to both linear and rotational acceleration, while receptors in the cochlea (choice C) respond to sound waves.

17. **The correct answer is (B).** Receptor sites for protein hormones are located on the outer membrane of target cells. Receptor sites in the nucleus (choice A) are for lipid hormones. The Islets of Langerhans (choice C) are where insulin and glucagon are made in the pancreas. Acinar cells (choice D) are where pancreatic digestive secretions are made.

18. **The correct answer is (D).** Hormones such as most of those from the anterior pituitary are produced in response to hypothalamic releasing hormones. Epinephrine and norepinephrine are released from the adrenal medulla in response to stimulation from sympathetic motor neurons. Hormones such as parathormone (parathyroid glands) and aldosterone (adrenal cortex) are regulated by negative feedback systems based on blood levels of calcium ions and sodium ions, respectively.

19. **The correct answer is (B).** Insulin *reduces* blood glucose levels by stimulating body cells (glucose uptake), liver cells (glycogen production), and adipose cells (fat formation). Thus, insulin is hypoglycemic. The other choices each help raise glucose levels by stimulating glycogenolysis, mobilization of fat, and/or gluconeogenesis.

20. **The correct answer is (D).** The ovary has target cells for hormones such as FSH and LH, and makes the hormones estrogen and progesterone. The kidney has target cells affected by aldosterone and ADH, and makes erythropoietin. The pancreas has target cells affected by the intestinal hormones, CCK, and secretin, and makes glucagon and insulin.

G. CIRCULATORY SYSTEM (CARDIOVASCULAR SYSTEM)

Functions

The circulatory system serves many functions including:

1. Transport of gases (oxygen and carbon dioxide), nutrients, wastes, and hormones.

2. Maintenance of fluid and salt balance (the blood is a source of osmotic exchange between the intracellular and extracellular fluids).

3. Defense (blood **clotting factors** play a vital role in the healing of wounds white blood cells and **antibodies** help fight invading organisms).

4. Thermoregulation (constriction of superficial blood vessels in the skin helps conserve heat, while dilation of these vessels allows heat to be lost by radiation to the environment).

5. pH balance (**buffers** transported in the blood prevent drastic changes in pH by substituting weak acids or bases when strong acids or bases are present).

Blood Composition

The blood contains **formed** (cellular) **elements** traveling in a fluid **plasma.**

1. **Formed Elements**

   (a) Red blood cells (**erythrocytes**) are primarily oxygen carriers. Oxygen combines with iron atoms that are part of the protein **hemoglobin** in RBCs. As blood is transported through the body and passes tissues low in oxygen concentration, oxygen in RBCs dissociates with hemoglobin and enters those cells by diffusion. RBCs live approximately 120 days before being destroyed by the spleen and liver.

(b) White blood cells (**leukocytes**) include granular and non-granular forms. Granular WBCs like **neutrophils** are important macrophages that phagocytize invading organisms or worn-out cellular debris. Other granular WBCs include **eosinophils** and **basophils.** Non-granular WBCs include **monocytes** (other macrophages) and **lymphocytes** (vital for antibody production and the body's cell-mediated immunity: see Section 9.4.H).

(c) **Platelets** are fragments of larger cells that play an important role in **hemostasis,** the stoppage of bleeding.

2. **Plasma**

(a) The major component of plasma is water (>90%).

(b) *Proteins*
Various plasma proteins are important for osmotic balance (albumin), clotting (fibrinogen, prothrombin), lipid transport (alpha and beta globulins), and defense (antibodies such as gamma globulins).

(c) *Nutrients*
Glucose, amino acids, and lipid molecules all play roles as sources of energy (ATP production) to be used by cells in cellular respiration and as building blocks for the synthesis of cellular components and products.

(d) *Wastes*
Metabolic byproducts such as nitrogen-containing urea and uric acid, as well as other molecules, including creatinine and ketones, are transported.

(e) *Electrolytes*
Various positive ions (sodium, potassium, calcium, hydrogen, magnesium, etc.) and negative ions (chloride, bicarbonate, phosphate, sulfate, etc.) are transported in the plasma. They are vital homeostatic components in maintaining water, salt, and pH balance, as well as in numerous other specific bodily processes.

(f) *Gases*
Approximately 3% of oxygen and 7% of carbon dioxide dissolve in the plasma.

The Heart and Blood Vessels

The human heart consists of two **atria** and two **ventricles** that help pump blood into **arteries** and then smaller branching **arterioles** carrying blood away from the heart to all major regions of the body. Materials are exchanged between the blood and body tissues across microscopic vessels called **capillaries.** Capillaries merge to form small **venules** and then larger **veins** that return blood back to the heart. Relatively thick walls of smooth muscle and elastic connective tissue in arteries and arterioles help propel blood to all regions. Valves in veins prevent its back-flow and keep it moving toward the heart.

Circulation through the Heart

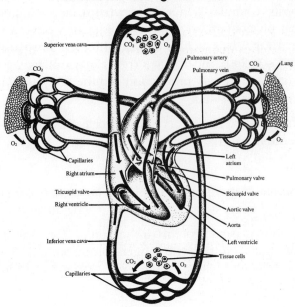

The right atrium receives blood low in oxygen and high in carbon dioxide returning in large veins (**vena cavae**) from tissues throughout the body. It then passes the blood through the right atrio-ventricular valve (**tricuspid valve**) to the right ventricle. The right ventricle pumps this deoxygenated blood to the lungs (via the **pulmonary semi-lunar valve** and **pulmonary artery**), where fresh oxygen is received and carbon dioxide is given up (both by diffusion). The newly oxygenated blood returns in **pulmonary veins** to the left atrium, passes through the left atrio-ventricular valve (**bicuspid or mitral valve**), and is then pumped (via the **aortic semi-lunar valve** and **aorta**) into the arterial system to all regions of the body. **Papillary muscles** in the ventricles and the **chordae tendinae** prevent the A-V valves from opening in the wrong direction.

Special conductile tissues in the heart receive stimuli from autonomic motor neurons that originate in the cardiac center of the brain. These special regions of the heart muscle then initiate and conduct the normal sequence of impulses that maintain a regular heart beat. These regions include the sino-atrial node (**SA node** or **pacemaker**), atrio-ventricular node (**AV node**), atrio-ventricular bundle (**AV bundle** or **Bundle of His**), and **Purkinje fibers.** Recording the electrical activity (depolarization and repolarization) through these regions of the heart represents a valuable diagnostic tool (electrocardiogram).

Blood Pressure

Normal blood pressure must be maintained to service all regions of the body efficiently. Blood pressure is the force exerted by the blood against the walls of the blood vessels. This pressure can increase due to a rise in **heart rate,** or a rise in the amount of blood pumped per beat (**stroke volume**). Together, these factors determine **cardiac output.** Blood pressure is also a function of **peripheral resistance** (friction between the blood and blood vessel walls). An increase in peripheral resistance (caused by **vasoconstriction** or increased blood **viscosity**) can also lead to an increase in blood pressure.

Systolic pressure represents the force exerted on the blood resulting from contraction **(systole)** of the ventricles. This also leads to expansion of the elastic arteries, such that when the ventricles relax **(diastole),** the recoil and the resistance of the arteries maintains the flow of blood, usually at a lesser force referred to as **diastolic pressure.** Increased peripheral resistance in the arteries due to accumulated fatty deposits (atherosclerosis) or hardening (arteriosclerosis) can lead to chronically high blood pressure.

H. LYMPHATIC SYSTEM AND IMMUNITY

Functions

The lymphatic system is closely associated with the circulatory system. Lymphatic capillaries, vessels, and accessory structures form a parallel system to the blood vessels. The functions of the lymphatic system include: a) collecting tissue fluids (water and small proteins) that normally leak out of the blood capillaries and returning them to the general circulation (via the **thoracic duct** and **right lymphatic duct**); b) absorbing digested fats (through **lacteals** in the small intestinal wall) and eventually distributing them to the adipose tissue and blood; and c) defending the body. Accessory structures include the thymus gland, spleen, and lymph nodes.

Lymph Nodes

Lymph nodes occur in groups along the pathway of lymphatic vessels. They act as screens that filter the **lymphatic fluid** (lymph). Normal constituents of lymphatic fluid pass through lymph nodes. However, macrophages are present to phagocytize trapped foreign particles, and lymphocytes that can directly act against foreign organisms or indirectly act against invaders through the production of antibodies are also found in lymph nodes.

Thymus Gland and Spleen

The **thymus gland** contains some lymphocytes that originated in bone marrow (all blood cells originate in the bone marrow). The **thymus** produces the hormone thymosin, which stimulates these lymphocytes to become **T-lymphocytes** or T-cells. The thymus gland is largest at puberty and, thereafter, decreases in size.

The **spleen** filters both lymph and blood. Its structure is somewhat similar to that of the lymph nodes (containing macrophages and lymphocytes). It helps break down worn-out RBCs and also serves as a blood reservoir.

Immunity

Two general forms of immunity are classified as **non-specific immunity** or resistance and **specific immunity** or resistance.

1. **Non-Specific Immunity/Resistance**
   Non-specific immunity/resistance includes mechanical barriers (skin and mucous membranes), enzymes (gastric enzymes and those in tears), macrophages (phagocytotic cells like neutrophils and monocytes formed in bone marrow), fever, inflammation due to **histamine** (produced by mast cells in connective tissue as well as basophils), and special anti-microbial proteins **(interferons).**

2. **Specific Immunity/Resistance**

Specific immunity/resistance includes the actions of **antibodies (antibody-mediated immunity)** that respond to the presence of foreign molecules or **antigens. Humoral antibodies** are chemicals (proteins such as gamma globulins) produced by plasma cells that have differentiated from **B-lymphocytes** or B-cells. Antibodies recognize specific antigens associated with foreign organisms such as bacteria and viruses. Such antibodies can defend in many ways. These include: combining with the antigen (sometimes called **agglutination**), covering the toxic portion of the antigen, or causing the cell on which the antigen is located to rupture. **Cell-mediated immunity** involves cells (**T-lymphocytes** or T-cells) that recognize and respond to antigens associated with foreign organisms or infected host cells. Different types of T-cells include:

(a) **cytotoxic T-cells** (killer T-cells), which attack foreign organisms or infected cells and destroy them by releasing either toxic substances that directly kill or **lymphokines** that attract other components of the immune system (macrophages and other types of T-cells).

(b) **Helper T-cells** that stimulate B-cells in their production of antibodies and work to coordinate macrophages, T-cells, and B-cells.

(c) **Suppressor T-cells** that help regulate the appropriate level of response by the immune system.

(d) **Memory T-cells** that remain dormant in the lymph nodes and circulation after being produced in response to first contact with a specific foreign antigen **(primary immune response).** When the same antigen is encountered a second time in the future, these memory T-cells, as well as **memory B-cells,** can then rapidly multiply and lead to a much faster response **(secondary immune response).**

I. RESPIRATORY SYSTEM

Function

The respiratory system consists of organs and tubes forming a passageway for air to enter and leave the body so that oxygen can be made available for cellular respiration, and carbon dioxide produced during cellular respiration can be eliminated. **Ventilation** refers to the exchange of oxygen and carbon dioxide between the outside environment and lungs. **External respiration** refers to the exchange of these gases between lungs and blood. In the blood, most oxygen (97%) travels bound to hemoglobin in RBCs, while most carbon dioxide (70%) is converted to bicarbonate ion and dissolves in the plasma (7% dissolves in the plasma as carbon dioxide, 23% binds to hemoglobin). **Internal respiration** is gas exchange between the blood and cells. Cellular respiration, where oxygen is consumed and carbon dioxide is produced, occurs within individual cells.

Respiratory Anatomy

The nose and vascular nasal mucous membranes allow air to enter, be filtered, warmed, and moistened.

The **pharynx,** behind the mouth between the nose and larynx, is a common passageway for air and food. It contains the **tonsils,** lymphatic structures that help protect against infection.

The **larynx** contains the vocal cords. The opening of this structure (the **glottis**) is associated with a strip of hyaline cartilage, the **epiglottis**, which covers the air passageway during swallowing to prevent food and liquids from entering the trachea.

The **trachea** is a tube, supported by hyaline cartilage rings, that branches into two primary **bronchi** that enter the lungs.

The **lungs** contain smaller and smaller branches of bronchi, eventually leading to **bronchioles** and clusters of grape-like air sacs called **alveoli.** Alveoli are moist, thin, highly vascular (pulmonary capillaries), and represent a huge surface area (about the size of a tennis court). As a result, they are excellent respiratory membranes for gas exchange. **Visceral pleura** cover the lungs, while **parietal pleura** line the thoracic cavity.

Mechanism of Breathing

Stimuli along motor neurons from the primary respiratory center in the medulla cause the **diaphragm** and **external intercostal muscles** to contract and, thereby, increase the volume of the thoracic cavity. As the volume of the thoracic cavity increases, the adhering parietal and visceral pleura are drawn outward so that lung volume also increases. When volume inside the lungs increases, pressure inside drops and air (now under higher pressure outside the body than inside the lungs) rushes in (inspiration). As the lungs fill with air, stretch receptors send inhibitory impulses to the respiratory centers of the brain and the diaphragm and intercostals relax. This compresses the thoracic cage and volume inside the lungs decreases. This results in an increase in pressure inside the lungs, and air (now under higher pressure inside the lungs than outside the body) rushes out (expiration). Secondary respiratory centers in the pons and various accessory muscles become involved when breathing patterns are voluntarily altered.

Respiratory Physiology

Tidal volume is the amount of air entering and leaving the lungs during normal, quiet breathing. **Inspiratory reserve** volume is the amount of air beyond tidal volume that can enter the lungs. **Expiratory reserve** volume is the amount of air beyond tidal volume that can be expelled from the lungs. **Vital capacity** is the sum of tidal volume, inspiratory reserve, and expiratory reserve volumes. **Residual volume** is that volume remaining in the lungs at all times. **Total lung capacity** is the sum of vital capacity and residual volume.

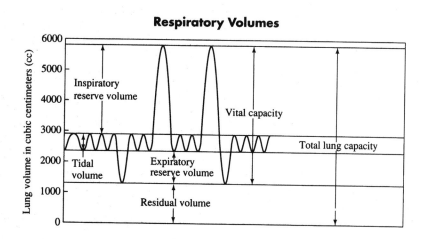

Respiratory Volumes

PRACTICE PROBLEMS
CIRCULATORY, LYMPHATIC/IMMUNE, AND RESPIRATORY SYSTEMS

1. Creatinine, a product of creatine metabolism, is transported in the plasma for removal by the kidneys. Where is creatinine most likely to have entered the blood?

   A. villi of the small intestine
   B. alveoli of the lungs
   C. skeletal muscles
   D. Bowman's capsules in the kidney nephrons

2. A deficiency of Fe in the diet can result in

   A. reduced hemoglobin concentration in erythrocytes.
   B. reduced oxygen-carrying capacity.
   C. reduced size of erythrocytes.
   D. All of the above.

3. Starling's Law states that as the volume of the blood entering the heart increases, the cardiac muscle cells in the ventricles will stretch and respond with a stronger contraction. What aspect of cardiovascular physiology will be affected?

   A. stroke volume
   B. cardiac output
   C. blood pressure
   D. All of the above.

4. The products of hemoglobin breakdown include the pigments biliverdin and bilirubin. Where are these molecules most likely produced?

   A. kidneys
   B. spleen and liver
   C. arteries and veins
   D. arteries, veins, and capillaries

5. Which blood vessels carry blood with a relatively high oxygen concentration?

   A. all arteries
   B. all arteries and the pulmonary veins
   C. pulmonary veins and all arteries except the pulmonary arteries
   D. pulmonary arteries and pulmonary veins

6. The two sounds associated with the cardiac cycle ("LUBB-dupp") are heard in sequence when the valves of the heart close during ventricular systole and ventricular diastole, respectively. Which valves produce the first sound?

   A. tricuspid valve and bicuspid valve
   B. pulmonary semi-lunar valve and aortic semi-lunar valve
   C. tricuspid valve and pulmonary semi-lunar valve
   D. bicuspid valve and aortic semi-lunar valve

7. During "normal activities," signals along parasympathetic motor neurons reach the SA node to help coordinate the contractions of the heart. Where do these signals originate?

   A. cerebrum
   B. medulla
   C. cerebellum
   D. diencephalon

8. End-diastolic volume (EDV) refers to the amount of blood present in the left ventricle after diastole (relaxation). End-systolic volume (ESV) represents the amount of blood in the left ventricle after systole (contraction). What term represents the difference between these two?

   A. cardiac output
   B. heart rate
   C. stroke volume
   D. peripheral resistance

9. The fetal heart has an opening between the two atria, called the foramen ovale, which allows blood to flow directly from the right atrium to the left atrium. What results from blood flowing through this opening?

   A. It bypasses the fetal lungs.
   B. It ensures that the fetal lungs receive extra blood.
   C. It bypasses both ventricles.
   D. It provides additional time for the blood to pick up extra oxygen.

10. One of the ways that HIV causes AIDS is by infecting those cells that coordinate the body's defenses against pathogens. Which cells of the immune system does HIV infect?

    A. cytotoxic T-cells
    B. helper T-cells
    C. plasma cells
    D. memory B-cells

11. Which cells are most important in the rapid and extensive secondary immune response when contact with a foreign antigen is made a second time?

    A. memory cells
    B. macrophages
    C. plasma cells
    D. suppressor T-cells

12. Surfactant is a secretion in the lungs that prevents alveoli from collapsing. Without this substance, what problem(s) might occur?

    A. The diameter of the bronchioles would remain constant.
    B. Inhalation would have to be more forceful.
    C. Exhalation would have to be more forceful.
    D. All of the above.

13. Antibodies are "Y-shaped" molecules consisting of four polypeptide chains: two larger (heavy) chains and two smaller (light) chains. Each chain has a constant region and a variable region that contains a unique amino acid sequence. Which region of the antibody will most likely form the binding site with the foreign antigen?

    A. constant regions
    B. variable regions
    C. both A and B
    D. neither A nor B

14. If an individual's vital capacity is 5200ml, her tidal volume is 500ml, and her inspiratory reserve volume is 3600, what is her expiratory reserve volume?

    A. 1100ml
    B. 1600ml
    C. 3100ml
    D. 4700ml

15. When carbon dioxide diffuses from tissue cells to the blood, it combines with water to form carbonic acid. Then, the enzyme carbonic anhydrase causes the ionization of carbonic acid into $H+$ and $HCO3-$. This suggests that in active tissues, pH will tend to

    A. decrease.
    B. increase.
    C. remain the same.
    D. first increase and then decrease.

16. Hemoglobin's affinity for oxygen is directly proportional to pH and is inversely proportional to temperature. Which tissue environment will receive the most oxygen from RBCs as they circulate through?

    A. cooler and more alkaline
    B. cooler and more acidic
    C. warmer and more alkaline
    D. warmer and more acidic

ANSWER KEY

1. C	3. D	5. C	7. B	9. A	11. A	13. B	15. A
2. D	4. B	6. A	8. C	10. B	12. B	14. A	16. D

ANSWERS AND EXPLANATIONS

1. **The correct answer is (C).** Creatine phosphate is an energy-storing molecule found in skeletal muscle tissue. When creatine is metabolized into creatinine, it enters the blood for removal by the kidneys. Bowman's capsule (choice D) is where creatinine will be filtered out of the blood into the kidney filtrate. Creatinine is not obtained from food (choice A) and it is obviously not taken in through the air (choice B).

2. **The correct answer is (D).** Fe is the component of heme (part of hemoglobin) to which oxygen binds in RBCs. An iron deficiency prevents normal levels of hemoglobin from being made. As a result, RBCs can be smaller and the blood's oxygen-carrying capacity will be reduced.

3. **The correct answer is (D).** When the ventricular muscle cells are stretched, they respond with a stronger contraction and more blood can be pumped with each beat (stroke volume). Anything that increases stroke volume also increases cardiac output (heart rate × stroke volume). Anything that increases cardiac output also increases blood pressure.

4. **The correct answer is (B).** The spleen and liver are primarily responsible for the breakdown of worn-out RBCs and the metabolism of the heme portion of hemoglobin. Biliverdin and bilirubin are eventually sent by the liver (via the hepatic duct) to the small intestine as part of bile. From there, these pigments leave the body as part of feces.

5. **The correct answer is (C).** The pulmonary arteries bring blood (low in oxygen and high in carbon dioxide) that has returned from the body's tissues to the lungs. They are the only arteries that are relatively oxygen-poor. In contrast, the pulmonary veins bring freshly oxygenated blood from the lungs back to the heart, and are the only veins that are relatively oxygen-rich.

6. **The correct answer is (A).** When the ventricles contract, the A-V valves (tricuspid and bicuspid) close and make the first louder sound: LUPP. This prevents the backflow of blood into the atria, and forces blood through the open semi-lunar valves into the two major arteries. When the ventricles relax, the A-V valves open, blood enters the ventricles from the atria, and blood in the aorta and pulmonary arteries backs up slightly—closing the semi-lunar valves and making the second softer sound: dupp.

7. **The correct answer is (B).** The cardiac center is in the medulla oblongata of the brain stem.

8. **The correct answer is (C).** If EDV is the volume of blood in the left ventricle after relaxation (before contraction) and ESV is the volume of blood still in the left ventricle after contraction, then the difference must be the volume that was pumped out of the left ventricle *during* contraction. This is stroke volume. Cardiac output (choice A) is stroke volume × heart rate.

9. **The correct answer is (A).** In the adult, blood leaving the right atrium enters the right ventricle, which pumps it to the lungs for gas exchange. This blood then leaves the lungs in the pulmonary veins and returns to the left atrium freshly oxygenated. Since the fetal lungs are submerged in amniotic fluid and are not yet functioning (fetal capillaries obtain oxygen by diffusion from maternal capillaries in the placenta), this temporary opening (foramen ovale) provides an efficient detour that bypasses the non-functional lungs.

10. **The correct answer is (B).** Helper T-cells (one of the primary host cells for HIV) help coordinate the complete immune response by stimulating B-cells (antibody-mediated immunity), macrophages, and T-cells (cell-mediated immunity). Although cytotoxic T-cells help battle infections, plasma cells produce antibodies, and memory cells provide long-term protection, it is the helper T-cells that bring all forces together.

11. **The correct answer is (A).** Memory B-cells and memory T-cells are cloned during first contact with the antigens of an "invading organism." Afterwards, they are found in the circulation and lymph nodes where they provide the body with long-term protection. If a second contact with the same foreign antigen is made, the response is rapid, extensive, and usually effective. Suppressor T-cells (choice D) prevent overreaction by the immune system.

12. **The correct answer is (B).** If alveolar walls collapse onto themselves (like inner walls of a balloon sticking together prior to inflation), it would take very forceful inhalation to fill them with air. Exhalation would not be as difficult, and the diameter of the bronchioles is irrelevant.

13. **The correct answer is (B).** Since the variable regions have their own unique amino acid sequences, these are the parts of antibodies that can be designed to "fit" the unique antigen structures of each invading organism. This helps account for the "specificity" of antibody-mediated immunity. The constant region is usually one of five types that help us classify antibodies with respect to where they are made and where they are found.

14. **The correct answer is (A).** Vital capacity is the maximum amount of air that can be exhaled after maximum inhalation (IRV + TV + ERV).

15. **The correct answer is (A).** If carbon dioxide contributes to H+ concentration, then the more carbon dioxide that is produced, the more acidic the tissue will become and the more pH will decrease (acids have a pH less than 7, while alkaline substances have a pH greater than 7). Active tissues carry out more cellular respiration and, therefore, produce more carbon dioxide.

16. **The correct answer is (D).** If hemoglobin's affinity for oxygen is directly proportional to pH, then it will be able to "hold on tighter" to oxygen as pH goes up (becomes more alkaline). In addition, if hemoglobin's affinity for oxygen is inversely proportional to temperature, then it will be able to "hold on tighter" as temperature goes down. Therefore, it will be able to "hold on" to oxygen in a cool, alkaline environment, but it must "let go" of oxygen in a warmer, more acidic environment.

J. DIGESTIVE SYSTEM

Functions

The major functions of the digestive system after taking in food (**ingestion**) include the chemical breakdown of large food molecules (**digestion**) into small enough sizes so that they can pass across the cells in the wall of the small intestine and enter the bloodstream (**absorption**). In addition, undigested materials must be passed along the tract for **elimination** from the body.

Digestive Anatomy and Physiology

The walls of the major hollow digestive organs have four distinct layers: an inner **mucosa**, the **submucosa**, a double layer of smooth muscles arranged in a circular and longitudinal pattern (**muscularis externa**), and an outer **serosa.** The rhythmic contraction of the smooth muscle layer (maintained at normal levels by the parasympathetic division of the autonomic nervous system, and slowed down by the sympathetic division) helps move food material through organs of the tract (**peristalsis**) and through muscular **sphincters** that surround the openings leading from one

Major Digestive Enzymes

Enzyme	Source	Digestive Action
Salivary Enzyme		
Amylase	Salivary glands	Begins carbohydrate digestion by converting starch and glycogen to disaccharides
Gastric Enzymes		
Pepsin	Gastric glands	Begins the digestion of proteins
Intestinal Enzymes		

Peptidases
  a. dipeptidase
  b. aminopeptidase
	Mucosal cells	Convert peptides into amino acids

Disaccharidases
  a. sucrase
  b. maltase
  c. lactase
	Mucosal cells	Convert disaccharides into monosaccharides

Enterokinase	Mucosal cells	Converts trypsinogen into trypsin
Pancreatic Enzymes		
Amylase	Pancreas	Converts starch and glycogen into disaccharides
Lipase	Pancreas	Converts fats into fatty acids and glycerol

Proteinases
  a. trypsin
  b. chymotrypsin
  c. carboxypolypeptidase
	Pancreas	Convert proteins or partially digested proteins into peptides

Nucleases Ribonuclease Deoxyribonuclease	Pancreas	Convert nucleic acids into nucleotides

Functions of the Liver

General Function	Specific Function
Carbohydrate metabolism	Converts glucose to glycogen (**glycogenesis**), glycogen to glucose (**glycogenolysis**), and noncarbohydrates to glucose or glucose substitutes (**gluconeogenesis**)
Lipid metabolism	Oxidizes fatty acids; synthesizes lipoproteins, phospholipids, and cholesterol; converts excess carbohydrates and proteins into fats
Protein metabolism	**Deaminates** amino acids; synthesizes urea; synthesizes blood proteins; interconverts amino acids (**transaminates**)
Storage	Stores glycogen; lipids; vitamins A, D, and B_{12}; iron; and blood
Blood filtering	Removes damaged red blood cells and foreign substances by phagocytosis
Detoxification	Alters composition of toxic substances
Secretion	Secretes bile; eliminates bilirubin and biliverdin from hemoglobin breakdown

organ to the next. The **peritoneum** is a double layer of serous membrane that lines the abdominopelvic cavity (parietal layer) and covers the organs (visceral layer: serosa). Extensions of the peritoneum that support and protect the internal organs are the mesenteries, greater omentum, and lesser omentum.

1. **Mouth**

   The tongue and teeth (**incisors:** 8, **canines:** 4, **premolars:** 8, and **molars:** 12) help manipulate food for chewing and swallowing. The **salivary glands** help moisten the food with saliva, which also contains **salivary amylase,** an enzyme that begins the chemical digestion of polysaccharide carbohydrates to disaccharides.

2. **Esophagus**

   Swallowing pushes the ball of chewed food (**bolus**) into the esophagus (the epiglottis covers the opening into the trachea), which leads into the stomach.

3. **Stomach**

   The stomach stores food until absorptive space becomes available in the small intestine. In addition, **pepsin** and **hydrochloric acid** are secreted (gastric juice) which begin the digestion of large proteins into smaller peptides. A thick, mucous lining helps protect the inner walls of the stomach from its own digestive action. Smooth muscle contractions help mix and move food along. Alcohol can be absorbed across the gastric mucosa. The mixture that finally empties into the small intestine is an acidy soup called **chyme.** The hormone **gastrin** helps regulate the stomach's activity.

4. **Pancreas**

The pancreas has both endocrine (islets of Langerhans secrete insulin and glucagon into the blood) and exocrine functions (digestive substances are secreted into the **pancreatic duct** which leads directly to the small intestine). **Pancreatic juice** contains **sodium bicarbonate** (to adjust the pH of materials arriving in the small intestine from the stomach), **pancreatic amylase** (digests polysaccharides to disaccharides), **pancreatic lipase** (digests triglycerides to glycerol and fatty acids), **trypsin, chymotrypsin,** and **carboxypolypeptidase** (needed for various stages of protein digestion), and both **ribonuclease** and **deoxyribonuclease** (digestion of nucleic acids to nucleotides). **Secretin,** a hormone secreted by the small intestine, regulates pancreatic release of sodium bicarbonate, while **cholecystokinin** or **CCK,** another intestinal hormone, controls pancreatic release of digestive enzymes, and the release of bile from the liver and gallbladder.

5. **Liver and Gallbladder**

The liver has many life-dependent functions. However, the only digestion-related function is the production of **bile.** Bile contains **bile salts** (which help emulsify fats into small droplets so that pancreatic lipase digests them more efficiently), bile pigments (biliverdin and bilirubin resulting from the breakdown of old red blood cells—another liver function), cholesterol, and various salts and electrolytes. Bile is sent to the gallbladder where it is stored and concentrated. Bile is released (also controlled by CCK) through the **common bile duct** to the small intestine as fatty substances arrive there.

6. **Small Intestine**

In the small intestine (**duodenum, jejunum,** and **ileum**), all digestion is completed (with the help of bile from the liver and gallbladder, and digestive enzymes from the pancreas and small intestinal cells themselves); absorption of digested food, water, and electrolytes occurs; and undigested material is passed further along the tract to the large intestine. Hormones produced by intestinal cells such as **intestinal gastrin** (speeds up) and **gastric inhibitory peptide** or **GIP** (slows down) regulate stomach activity, while cholecystokinin and secretin control secretions from the liver, gallbladder, and pancreas. The intestinal enzymes **lactase, sucrase,** and **maltase** complete carbohydrate digestion (disaccharides resulting from salivary and pancreatic amylase are finally broken down to monosaccharides) so that monosaccharides can be absorbed across the intestinal wall. Similarly, the intestinal enzymes **dipeptidase** and **aminopeptidase** complete the digestion of proteins (peptides to amino acids) begun by the stomach and pancreas.

The intestinal wall has its surface area multiplied many times over by the presence of folds called **villi** and their subdivisions (**microvilli**). Villi contain capillaries for the absorption of most water and water-soluble products of digestion, as well as **lacteals** for the absorption of insoluble lipids (lacteals are the endings of lymphatic vessels). Undigested materials are passed along by peristaltic waves to the large intestine. Once food is completely digested, the small molecules are absorbed and eventually transported, first to the liver (via the **hepatic portal system**) for distribution, and then to the body's cells for use in cellular respiration (ATP production) or as building blocks for the synthesis of cellular and body components.

7. **Large Intestine**
The parts of the large intestine include the **cecum, colon** (ascending, transverse, descending, and sigmoid), **rectum,** and **anal canal.** Additional water and electrolytes are absorbed through its walls. Bacteria such as *E. coli* help break down some undigested materials, help in the synthesis of certain vitamins, and regulate the normal activity. **Feces** form, are stored, and eventually are eliminated from the large intestine.

K. EXCRETORY SYSTEM

Functions

The major functions of the urinary system include the removal of various metabolic waste products and the maintenance of fluid, electrolyte, and pH balances. In addition, the kidney stimulates red blood cell production and helps maintain blood pressure.

Excretory Organs

The **kidney** is the major organ of the urinary system. Through the processes of **filtration, reabsorption,** and **urinary secretion, nephrons** (the functional units of the kidney) form a urine that contains numerous waste products and other materials not needed by the body. The kidney consists of an outer **renal cortex,** an inner **renal medulla** (with masses of tissue called **renal pyramids**), and a funnel-shaped **renal pelvis.** Urine formed in the kidney empties into extensions of the pelvis called **calyces,** which lead to tubes, the **ureters,** that carry the urine away from the kidney. The ureters lead to the **urinary bladder,** where urine can be stored before it passes out of the body through the **urethra.**

The Nephron and Urine Formation

Approximately one million nephrons are found in each human kidney. The nephron consists of a **Bowman's capsule, proximal convoluted tubule, loop of Henle, distal convoluted tubule,** and **collecting duct.** Filtration of blood takes place through the **glomerulus** (glomerular capillaries) into the hollow space of Bowman's capsule. Together, the glomerulus and Bowman's capsule are referred to as the **renal corpuscle.** The **filtrate** consists of water and small solutes, while blood cells and large molecules remain in the blood. These unfiltered materials are carried away from the glomerulus and travel through **peritubular capillaries,** which surround the nephron and eventually rejoin the venous circulation. Filtrate components include metabolic wastes such as **urea** (a nitrogenous product resulting from amino acid metabolism), **uric acid** (a nitrogenous product resulting from nucleic acid metabolism), **creatinine** (resulting from the metabolism of creatine in muscles), and **ketones** (produced during fatty acid metabolism), as well as vital nutrients (glucose, amino acids, etc.), electrolytes, and water. Much of these essential substances must be returned to the blood and are reabsorbed back into the

Urinary System

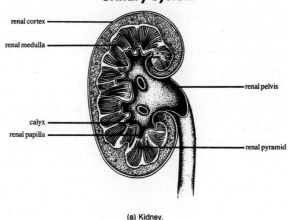

(a) Kidney.

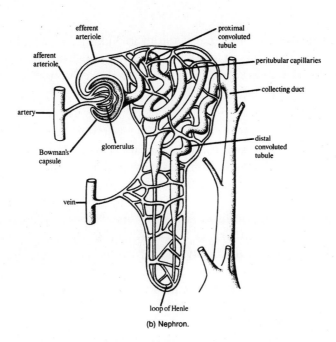

(b) Nephron.

peritubular capillaries. Most reabsorption occurs at the proximal convoluted tubules. Reabsorption mechanisms include active transport (glucose, amino acids, sodium, calcium, and potassium ions), diffusion following charge gradients (chloride, phosphate, and bicarbonate ions), and osmosis (water). At the distal convoluted tubules, additional sodium ions are reabsorbed if needed (regulated by the hormone **aldosterone**), while potassium ions are secreted from peritubular capillaries to filtrate. Other materials secreted into the filtrate include ammonia, histamine, various drugs, hydrogen ions, and other ions that help regulate blood pH. Additional water can also be reabsorbed at the distal convoluted tubules and collecting ducts (regulated by the hormone **ADH**). A **countercurrent mechanism** associated with the directional flow of salts across the loops of Henle causes the medullary tissues between the loops and collecting ducts to become extremely hypertonic and the filtrate, hypotonic. This facilitates the reabsorption of water at the distal convoluted tubule and collecting duct.

Other Kidney Functions

The kidney secretes the hormone **erythropoietin,** which stimulates red blood cell production in the bone marrow. In response to low blood pressure (detected by the nephron's **juxtaglomerular apparatus**), the kidney also produces an enzyme, **renin,** which activates the blood protein, **angiotensinogen,** to form **angiotensin.** Angiotensin then stimulates the adrenal cortex to release aldosterone, causing an increased reabsorption of sodium ions. Since water osmotically follows the sodium ions (and chloride ions) into the peritubular capillaries, blood volume rises—resulting in a higher cardiac output and increased blood pressure **(renin-angiotensin system).** With respect to pH balance, the kidney can retain alkaline buffers, while actively secreting hydrogen ions and ammonium ions when body fluid pH is too acidic, or retain more hydrogen ions while releasing bicarbonate ions and other buffers when fluids become too alkaline.

PRACTICE PROBLEMS
DIGESTIVE AND EXCRETORY SYSTEMS

1. There are 20 primary or deciduous teeth in a child's first set of teeth. These include two incisors, one canine (cuspid), and two molars on each side of the upper and lower jaw. Which types of teeth in the primary set differ in number from those in the permanent set?

   A. incisors, canines, premolars, and molars
   B. incisors, premolars, and molars
   C. premolars and molars
   D. molars only

2. Chief cells in the stomach lining produce the inactive enzyme pepsinogen, which is activated to form pepsin by HCl produced by neighboring parietal cells. In which layer of the stomach are these cells located?

   A. mucosa
   B. submucosa
   C. muscularis externa
   D. serosa

3. The hepatic portal system sends venous blood to the liver from various organs in the abdominopelvic cavity. Based on your knowledge of liver function, which of the following does not require direct venous blood flow to the liver?

   A. Transport of absorbed nutrients from the small intestine
   B. Transport of pancreatic hormones
   C. Transport of filtered blood from the kidney
   D. Transport of RBC metabolites from the spleen
   E. Transport of absorbed alcohol from the stomach

4. Which of the following can take place in the esophagus?

   A. Digestion of carbohydrates
   B. Digestion of proteins
   C. Digestion of lipids
   D. None of the above.

5. The pulp cavity is the innermost region of a tooth that lies within the mineralized dentin that makes up the bulk of each tooth. Root canals are narrow passageways in the root of each tooth that connect blood vessels and nerve branches to the pulp cavity. Which cranial nerve loses sensations when the dentist anesthetizes these nerve branches?

   A. Trigeminal (V)
   B. Facial (VII)
   C. Glossopharyngeal (IX)
   D. Hypoglossal (XII)

6. Which pancreatic secretion enables digestion of all macromolecules to take place in the duodenum of the small intestine?

   A. insulin
   B. glucagon
   C. trypsin
   D. sodium bicarbonate

7. Most of the liver's important functions occur

   A. while a meal is passing through the digestive tract.
   B. while digested food is being absorbed.
   C. at times other than during meals.
   D. All of the above.

8. Which of the following has both exocrine and endocrine functions?

   A. stomach
   B. small intestine
   C. pancreas
   D. all of the above

9. The appendix is a structure on the most proximal part of the large intestine with no apparent digestive function. Where would you find the appendix?

   A. ascending colon
   B. cecum
   C. rectum
   D. sigmoid colon

10. The afferent arteriole, which brings blood to the glomerulus, has a wider diameter than the efferent arteriole, which carries blood away from the glomerulus. How does this arrangement contribute to kidney function?

    A. It enhances filtration.
    B. It enhances reabsorption.
    C. It enhances urinary secretion.
    D. All of the above.

11. Portions of the afferent arteriole, efferent arteriole, distal convoluted tubule, and renal corpuscle make up the juxtaglomerular apparatus, which produces renin. The juxtaglomerular apparatus is involved with regulation of

    A. glucose.
    B. pH.
    C. wastes.
    D. blood pressure.
    E. All of the above.

12. From where do materials move into the filtrate by urinary secretion?

    A. afferent arteriole
    B. Bowman's capsule
    C. efferent arteriole
    D. peritubular capillaries

13. Under the microscope, numerous structures observed in the renal pyramids have a relatively "straight-line" appearance. What parts of the nephron are probably present in the renal pyramids?

    A. Bowman's capsules and proximal convoluted tubules
    B. loops of Henle
    C. distal convoluted tubules
    D. collecting ducts
    E. B and D
    F. A and C

14. Membrane carrier molecules in the cells of the proximal convoluted tubules are capable of reabsorbing normal amounts of glucose that have been filtered out of the blood at the renal corpuscle. What happens when hyperglycemic blood has excess glucose filtered at the renal corpuscle?

A. Membrane carrier molecules at the proximal convoluted tubules will increase their maximum transport rate.

B. Extra carrier molecules will be synthesized in the cells of the proximal convoluted tubules.

C. The excess glucose will continue in the filtrate and be excreted in the urine.

D. Hormones will stimulate a second round of glucose reabsorption at the distal convoluted tubules.

15. Under what conditions would you expect elevated ketone levels in the urine?

A. High carbohydrate diet.
B. Low carbohydrate diet.
C. Fasting.
D. A and C.
E. B and C.

16. The rapid reabsorption of water brought about by ADH is made easier by the "countercurrent multiplier," which involves the active transport of salts at the ascending loop of Henle. What is the result of this countercurrent multiplier effect?

A. The filtrate becomes hypotonic while the surrounding tissues become hypertonic.

B. The filtrate becomes hypertonic while the surrounding tissues become hypotonic.

C. The filtrate becomes isotonic to the surrounding tissues.

D. The tissues become isotonic to the filtrate.

ANSWER KEY

| 1. C | 3. C | 5. A | 7. C | 9. B | 11. D | 13. E | 15. E |
| 2. A | 4. A | 6. D | 8. D | 10. A | 12. D | 14. C | 16. A |

ANSWERS AND EXPLANATIONS

1. **The correct answer is (C).** The permanent set of teeth contains 32 teeth: 8 on each side of the upper and lower jaws (two incisors, one canine, two premolars, and three molars).

2. **The correct answer is (A).** The mucosa is the innermost lining of the stomach. The chief and parietal cells release their secretions directly into the lumen of the stomach, where food is being processed.

3. **The correct answer is (C).** The renal vein, carrying blood that has already had some of its wastes removed in the kidney, returns its contents directly to the inferior vena cava. All of the other choices involve subsequent functions of the liver involving the hepatic portal system.

4. **The correct answer is (A).** Although no digestion occurs as a result of direct action by esophageal cells, the pH of the esophagus is compatible with the carbohydrate digestion that began in the mouth (salivary amylase). Until the swallowed food arrives in the acidic stomach, this digestion continues. Protein digestion (choice B) begins in the stomach, while lipid digestion (choice C) begins in the small intestine.

5. **The correct answer is (A).** This question is a practical review of cranial nerve functions. The trigeminal nerve (V) carries somatic sensory information from most of the areas of the face including the teeth and gums.

6. **The correct answer is (D).** Sodium bicarbonate neutralizes the acidic chyme to a pH (slightly alkaline) compatible with all pancreatic and intestinal enzymes. Trypsin (choice C) partially digests only proteins, while insulin and glucagon (choices A and B) play a role in regulating nutrients in the blood after digestion and absorption have been completed.

7. **The correct answer is (C).** At mealtime (choices A and B) the liver's only function is to prepare fats for digestion (through the emulsifying action of bile) by pancreatic lipase. The liver's numerous other functions occur at all times.

8. **The correct answer is (D).** Gastric exocrine secretions: pepsinogen, HCl, mucous, and intrinsic factor (for vitamin B_{12} absorption); gastric endocrine secretion: gastrin. Intestinal exocrine secretions: digestive enzymes and enterokinase (for activating trypsinogen to trypsin); intestinal endocrine secretions: intestinal gastrin, GIP, secretin and CCK. Pancreatic exocrine secretions: digestive enzymes and sodium bicarbonate; pancreatic endocrine secretions: insulin and glucagon.

9. **The correct answer is (B).** The cecum is the most proximal part of the large intestine, followed by (moving distally) the ascending colon, transverse colon, descending colon, sigmoid colon, and rectum.

10. **The correct answer is (A).** By having more blood enter the glomerulus (via the efferent arteriole) than can leave at the same time (via the efferent arteriole), pressure within the glomerulus builds up so that efficient filtration can take place.

11. **The correct answer is (D).** Renin, secreted by cells of the juxtaglomerular apparatus, activates a sequence that eventually converts the blood protein angiotensinogen to angiotensin I and II. This stimulates the release of aldosterone by the adrenal cortex, so that extra Na+ ions are reabsorbed at the distal convoluted tubules. Water follows by osmosis, increasing blood volume and subsequently increasing stroke volume (Starling's law). The increased stroke volume increases cardiac output and blood pressure (renin-angiotensin system).

12. **The correct answer is (D).** Urinary secretion refers to the transport of materials from the blood (peritubular capillaries) to the filtrate at the latter parts of the nephron.

13. **The correct answer is (E).** The "straight-line" structures, the loops of Henle and the collecting ducts, are mostly found in the pyramids of the renal medulla, while the Bowman's capsules, proximal convoluted tubules, and distal convoluted tubules are mostly found in the renal cortex.

14. **The correct answer is (C).** If an individual has high blood glucose levels, extra glucose will be filtered through Bowman's capsule into the lumen of the nephron. However, since there are still only the normal number of glucose carrier molecules in the cells of the proximal convoluted tubules, only "normal" levels of glucose can be reabsorbed. The excess glucose that could not be reabsorbed stays in the filtrate through the entire nephron and ends up in the urine. This contributes to why individuals with diabetes mellitus have glucose in their urine.

15. **The correct answer is (E).** High ketone levels in the urine are most commonly a result of fatty acid metabolism. The body metabolizes fats to provide molecules (glycerol and fatty acids) that can be used as substitutes for glucose in cell respiration when glucose levels are low. This can occur during situations such as the time between meals, during exercise, during periods of low carbohydrate intake, and during fasts.

16. **The correct answer is (A).** The active transport of salt from the ascending loop makes the surrounding tissues hypertonic, while leaving the filtrate hyptonic as it continues through the distal convoluted tubules and collecting ducts.

L. REPRODUCTIVE SYSTEM

Functions

The major functions of the reproductive system include the production of sex cells or **gametes,** ensuring that gametes meet so that **fertilization** can occur, and then successfully supporting the developing offspring.

Gamete Production

Gametogenesis occurs by **meiosis** in the **gonads** (**testes** and **ovaries**). In contrast to mitosis, where two **diploid** and genetically identical products are formed, meiosis results in four **haploid** products that are each genetically different from the original cell undergoing meiosis, as well as genetically different

Meiosis

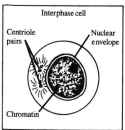

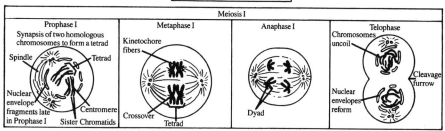

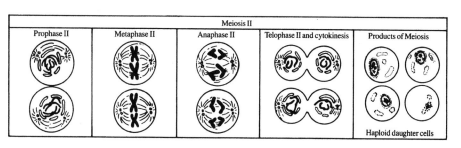

Meiosis and Mitosis Compared

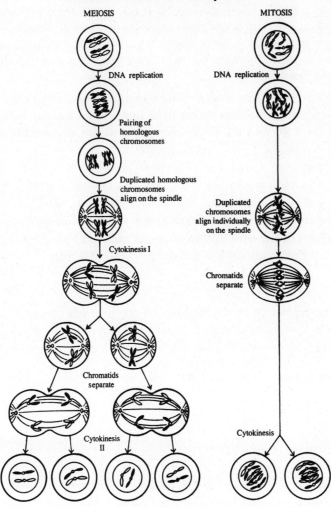

from each other. In addition, meiosis involves two cycles of division. During the metaphase of the first meiotic cycle (Metaphase I), the 46 doubled chromosomes (each consisting of two **chromatids** attached at the **centromere**) line up in such a way that **homologous pairs** of chromosomes are next to each other (in mitosis, the 46 doubled chromosomes line up randomly, i.e., homologous pairs are not next to each other). Anaphase I and Telophase I of meiosis then result in homologous pairs (still doubled) being separated into two daughter cells. Thus, each daughter cell from the first meiotic division contains 23 doubled chromosomes (in mitosis, all 46 doubled chromosomes are split as chromatids are pulled apart—resulting in 46 single chromosomes in each of the two daughter cells). Only after the second cycle of division do the chromatids separate in the first two cells. This results in four daughter cells, each containing 23 single chromosomes. Gametes contain one of each of the 23 types of chromosomes, rather than two of each (homologous pairs have been separated). The genetic uniqueness of each of the four meiotic products is due, to a great degree, to **crossing over** of genetic material between homologous chromatids during Prophase I of meiosis.

The Male System

Spermatogenesis by meiosis occurs in the **seminiferous tubules** of the testes. **Spermatogonia** (diploid) undergo meiosis: (1) all 46 chromosomes replicate forming **primary spermatocytes,** (2) the first meiotic division results in two **secondary spermatocytes,** and (3) the second meiotic division produces four **spermatids** which later mature into **spermatozoa** (in **epididymis**). A mature sperm head contains 23 chromosomes and an **acrosome** with enzymes that help penetrate the ovum. Sperm also have a neck or midpiece with mitochondria, and a flagellum. **Interstitial cells** (Leydig cells) in the testes produce **testosterone,** the primary male hormone **(androgen).**

The testes are situated in an external enclosed sac, the **scrotum.** A tightly coiled tube leading from each testis, the epididymis, stores sperm cells and is the site of their final maturation. During **ejaculation,** sperm leave the epididymis and enter the **vas deferens,** a tube that leads into the body cavity (through **inguinal canal**) as part of the **spermatic cord.** Inside the body wall, the vas deferens joins the duct from the **seminal vesicles** to form the **ejaculatory duct.** The seminal vesicles secrete an alkaline fluid containing nutrients. The **prostate** and **bulbourethral glands** (Cowper's glands) also contribute alkaline secretions to help neutralize any harmful acidity encountered in the environment during ejaculation. Sperm cells and their surrounding fluid are called **semen** (seminal fluid). Semen leaves the body through the urethra in the penis. The penis consists of a sensory head, the **glans penis,** as well as vascular erectile tissues (**corpus spongiosum** and **corpora cavernosa**), which fill with blood during erection.

Hormonal Control in the Male

Follicle Stimulating Hormone (FSH) from the anterior pituitary gland stimulates spermatogenesis, while another anterior pituitary hormone, **Interstitial Cell Stimulating Hormone** or **Luteinizing Hormone** (ICSH or LH), stimulates the production of testosterone. Testosterone itself causes the development of male structures in the embryo, secondary sex characteristics during puberty, and the maintenance of male characteristics throughout life. Both FSH and ICSH are regulated by hypothalamic releasing hormones.

The Female System

Oogenesis by meiosis occurs in **follicles** within the ovaries. **Oogonia** (diploid) undergo meiosis:

1. All 46 chromosomes replicate forming **primary oocytes** (this occurs before birth!).

2. The first meiotic division results in two structures, a large **secondary oocyte** and a much smaller **polar body** (unequal cytokinesis).

3. The second meiotic division, if it occurs, produces the functional ovum and three polar bodies. The second meiotic cycle of division usually occurs after the secondary oocyte is ovulated, and only if it has been fertilized.

After **ovulation** (the release of the secondary oocyte from the ovarian follicle), the oocyte is drawn into the **fallopian tubes** (uterine tubes) by finger-like projections called **fimbriae.** The oocyte slowly moves through the tubes (where most fertilizations take place) until it reaches the **uterus,** an organ with a thick wall of smooth muscle (**myometrium**), an inner lining (**endometrium**), part of which is shed each month during the menstrual cycle, and a narrow neck (**cervix**) leading to the vagina. The vagina receives the erect penis during intercourse and is the passageway for the menstrual flow and the fetus at birth. External genitalia include the **labia majora** and **minora,** which are folds of skin and tissue enclosing the vaginal opening, and the **clitoris,** a sensory projection equivalent (homologous) to the male glans penis. **Vestibular gland** secretions provide lubrication to the vagina and vestibular area.

Hormonal Control in the Female

Estrogen causes the development of secondary sex characteristics at puberty and helps maintain them thereafter. Starting at puberty, the monthly **menstrual cycle** results from the following cyclic hormonal changes: FSH from the anterior pituitary stimulates the development of an ovarian follicle, maturation of the oocyte, and production of estrogen by the follicle. Increased estrogen levels stimulate the growth of the endometrial lining, and lead to the secretion of LH by the anterior pituitary and inhibition of FSH (ensuring that only one follicle develops at a time). The LH causes ovulation and the formation of the **corpus luteum** (the now-empty follicle that produces high levels of estrogen and **progesterone**). Both FSH and LH are regulated by hypothalamic-releasing hormones. Progesterone is the major hormone maintaining the preparedness of the uterus to receive the embryo if fertilization takes place. LH levels decline after ovulation. If fertilization does not occur, the decrease in LH leads to degeneration of the corpus luteum. The resulting drop in estrogen and progesterone leads to the disintegration of the uterine lining and menstrual flow. The reduced estrogen levels no longer inhibit FSH and a new cycle begins. If fertilization does occur, embryonic cells produce **Human Chorionic Gonadotropin (HCG),** which acts as a "substitute" hormone that maintains the corpus luteum in spite of the decline in LH. As long as the corpus luteum is active, the uterus remains supportive of the developing embryo. Eventually, the **placenta** takes over the role of the corpus luteum as a major producer of hormones and in the maintenance of the uterus. During pregnancy, estrogen and progesterone cause the mammary glands and ducts to develop. **Prolactin** (from the anterior pituitary) stimulates the production of milk, while **oxytocin** (made in the hypothalamus and stored in the posterior pituitary gland) causes the milk to be ejected during nursing activity.

M. EMBRYOLOGY AND DEVELOPMENT

Fertilization and Cleavage

Fertilization of the haploid ovum by the haploid sperm produces the diploid first cell of the new organism, the **zygote.** The zygote undergoes many rapid mitotic divisions resulting in many small cells. No growth of these new cells occurs during this **cleavage** stage. In various vertebrates, cleavage planes of division follow a pattern relative to the **vegetal** pole (more yolk) and **animal pole** (less yolk) of the egg. In humans, the first cleavage division takes place within 24–30 hours after fertilization, and then divisions continue every 10–12 hours.

Blastulation and Gastrulation

Cleavage produces a solid ball of cells called a **morula,** which soon develops a fluid-filled space **(blastocoel).** Thereafter, the hollow ball of cells is referred to as a **blastula.** In humans, this stage is called the **blastocyst,** which has an **inner cell mass** that gives rise to the embryo, and an outer layer of cells, the **trophoblast,** which merges with the endometrium of the uterus during i**mplantation** and forms the embryonic membrane, the **chorion.** Other embryonic membranes—**allantois, amnion,** and **yolk sac**—also form later. During **gastrulation,** cells of the blastula start to push inward forming a second, and eventually a third layer of cells. These **primary germ layers** are the **ectoderm, endoderm,** and **mesoderm.**

Early Development (Amphioxus)

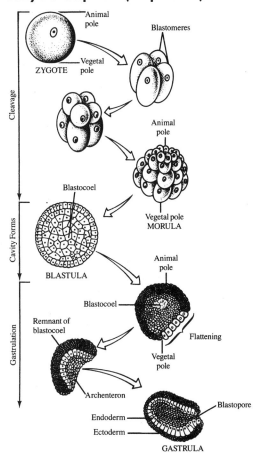

Neurulation and Organogenesis

The cells of the primary germ layers ultimately give rise to the beginnings of the organs, limbs, and other body parts **(organogenesis)**. **Neurulation** refers to the very early formation of the nervous system when dorsal cells of the ectoderm thicken, sink, and roll over to form the **neural tube,** which will later develop into the brain and spinal cord. During organogenesis, ectoderm cells will give rise to all nervous tissue, sense organs, the epidermis of the skin and its associated structures (nails, hair follicles, sweat glands, etc.), much of the pituitary gland, and parts of linings of the mouth and anal canal. Endoderm cells will develop into structures including the linings of the digestive tract, pancreas, liver, many glands, the lungs, and much of the respiratory tract, urinary bladder, and urethra. Mesoderm cells produce muscles, bones, blood and blood vessels, lymphoid tissues, kidneys, reproductive organs, and body cavity membranes. All the essential external and internal body parts of the embryo are formed by the eighth week. After this time the developing individual is called a **fetus.**

Developmental Processes and Mechanisms

The process by which cells mature and become specialized is called **differentiation. Determination** is the process by which the developmental range of options of a cell gradually becomes narrower. Each cell, at some point, becomes determined to a particular developmental pathway and will differentiate into a specific type of cell. Differentiation results from particular genes being "turned on" and "turned off" in the cell. Mechanisms by which such genes can be regulated include the actions of factors inside the cell itself **(cytoplasmic determinants),** and factors associated with other cells **(inducers). Induction** involves one group of cells influencing the development of other cells. Other general processes at work during development include **morphogenesis** (the development of form and body structures resulting from cell movement) and **pattern formation** (the shaping and positioning of body parts relative to the whole).

PRACTICE PROBLEMS:
REPRODUCTIVE SYSTEM, EMBRYOLOGY, AND DEVELOPMENT

1. Which statement is correct about homologous pairs of chromosomes?

    A. One homologous chromosome is inherited from each parent.
    B. Homologous chromosomes have genes for the same traits in the same regions (loci).
    C. Homologous chromosomes may be genetically identical for some traits but not others.
    D. All of the above.

2. Synapsis occurs between two homologous chromosomes during Prophase I of meiosis. During synapsis, one of two identical chromatids on one homologous chromosome can exchange genetic material with one of two identical chromatids on the other homologous chromosome. What will result from such an exchange?

    A. The two "genetically identical" chromatids on one of the homologous chromosomes will no longer be identical.
    B. The two "genetically identical" chromatids on both of the homologous chromosomes will no longer be identical.
    C. All four chromatids will be genetically different.
    D. A and C
    E. B and C

3. The inguinal canals are passageways connecting the scrotum with the abdominopelvic cavity. Which of the following structures would not be expected to be part of the spermatic cord passing through the inguinal canals?

    A. ejaculatory duct
    B. vas deferens
    C. blood vessels
    D. lymph vessels
    E. nerves

4. Which of the following cells has the most genetic material?

    A. spermatogonia
    B. primary spermatocytes
    C. secondary spermatocytes
    D. spermatids
    E. spermatozoa

5. Support cells in the testes called Sertoli cells (sustentacular cells) produce the hormone inhibin. One of the functions of this hormone is to inhibit FSH, which results in

    A. speeding up sperm production.
    B. slowing down sperm production.
    C. speeding up testosterone production.
    D. slowing down testosterone production.

6. Which of the following male accessory glands contributes directly to the ability of sperm to produce ATP?

    A. seminal vesicles
    B. prostate gland
    C. bulbourethral (Cowper's) glands
    D. testes

7. Which of the following statements about meiosis is true?

    A. Each sperm has approximately one-fourth (or less) of a normal cell's cytoplasm.
    B. Each sperm has approximately one-half (or less) of a normal cell's cytoplasm.
    C. Each ovum has approximately three-fourths (or more) of a normal cell's cytoplasm.
    D. A and C
    E. B and C

8. If fertilization usually occurs in the fallopian tubes, and implantation takes place 4–7 days later, what developmental stage actually implants in the endometrium?

   A. zygote
   B. solid ball of cells
   C. hollow ball of cells
   D. ball of cells with three germ layers

9. Which statement is true about ovulation?

   A. One secondary oocyte leaves the ovarian follicle, while one secondary oocyte remains behind.
   B. One secondary oocyte and one polar body leave the ovarian follicle.
   C. Two secondary oocytes leave the ovarian follicle.
   D. One ovum leaves the ovarian follicle, while three polar bodies remain behind.

10. The embryonic hormone HCG stimulates the corpus luteum to continue producing hormones. What hormone does HCG mimic?

    A. FSH
    B. LH
    C. estrogen
    D. progesterone

11. The smooth muscle wall of the uterus (myometrium) is regulated by

    A. somatic nervous system circuits.
    B. autonomic nervous system circuits.
    C. somatic nervous system circuits and hormones.
    D. autonomic nervous system circuits and hormones.

12. Which of the following is the source of hormones that initiate the female reproductive cycle?

    A. anterior pituitary gland
    B. posterior pituitary gland
    C. ovaries
    D. hypothalamus

13. Which of the following sequences is in the correct developmental order?

    A. fertilization, zygote, blastula, morula, gastrula
    B. zygote, fertilization, morula, blastula, gastrula
    C. fertilization, zygote, morula, blastula, gastrula
    D. zygote, fertilization, blastula, morula, gastrula

14. In some organisms, the first four cells of the early embryo (if isolated and grown in the laboratory) can only lead to the development of a specific quarter of the developing individual. In other organisms, however, the first four cells can each lead to the development of an entire individual. What term is associated with these phenomena?

    A. implantation
    B. neurulation
    C. determination
    D. yolk formation

15. Which embryonic membrane is most closely associated with implantation?

    A. amnion
    B. chorion
    C. allantois
    D. yolk sac

16. Which gland(s) is (are) responsible for providing the newborn with milk?

    A. anterior pituitary
    B. posterior pituitary
    C. both A and B
    D. neither A nor B

17. Which of the following sets of structures derive from the same primary germ layer?

   A. bones, muscles, kidneys, and blood
   B. stomach, lungs, urinary bladder, and liver
   C. sweat glands, brain, lining of the mouth, and eyes
   D. all of the above

18. Which of the following functions is not carried out by the placenta?

   A. Production of hormones that maintain the uterus
   B. The site at which fertilization takes place
   C. The site at which maternal and fetal circulation exchange materials
   D. The site at which the umbilical cord connects

ANSWER KEY

| 1. D | 3. A | 5. B | 7. D | 9. B | 11. D | 13. C | 15. B | 17. D |
| 2. E | 4. B | 6. A | 8. C | 10. B | 12. D | 14. C | 16. C | 18. B |

ANSWERS AND EXPLANATIONS

1. **The correct answer is (D).** Individuals receive one whole set of 23 chromosomes from each parent. Thus, we have two #1 chromosomes, two #2 chromosomes, two #3 chromosomes, etc. (one of each homologous pair from each parent). With the exception of the 23rd pair (sex chromosomes X and Y), each pair has genes for specific traits encoded at the same loci. For traits A, B, and C, the maternal chromosome may have alleles A, b, and C. For those traits, the paternal chromosome may have alleles A, B, and c. Thus, the homologous pair of chromosomes has identical genes at locus A, but they are genetically different at loci B and C.

2. **The correct answer is (E).** When a part of a paternal chromatid "crosses over" with the equivalent part of the maternal chromatid, *all 4* chromatids will be different. There will be an "original" paternal chromatid, a second paternal chromatid that now has a part of the maternal chromatid, an "original" maternal chromatid, and a second maternal chromatid that now has a part of the paternal chromatid.

3. **The correct answer is (A).** The ejaculatory duct begins where the two vas deferens meet the ducts from the seminal vesicles, dorsal to the urinary bladder. All the other structures are part of the spermatic cord.

4. **The correct answer is (B).** Spermatogonia (choice A) are normal diploid cells (2n = 46). In the primary spermatocyte, however, each chromosome has replicated to form two chromatids (92 chromatids are present). The secondary spermatocytes (choice C) are the products of the first meiotic division and contain 23 doubled chromosomes (46 chromatids). Spermatids (choice D) and spermatozoa (choice E) are haploid and have 23 chromosomes.

5. **The correct answer is (B).** In males, FSH stimulates spermatogenesis. Thus, inhibin slows down further sperm production. Since inhibin does not inhibit ICSH, the hormone that stimulates testosterone production, choices C and D are not correct.

6. **The correct answer is (A).** Only the seminal vesicles contribute sugar (fructose) to the seminal fluid, which can then be utilized by sperm cells in cellular respiration to produce ATP.

7. **The correct answer is (D).** Since cytokinesis in males produces four equal-sized products, each sperm has one-fourth (or less) of the cytoplasm that was in the original spermatogonium. In females, on the other hand, cytokinesis is unequal. The oocytes get the majority of the cytoplasm, while the polar bodies get very little.

8. **The correct answer is (C).** If the zygote forms at fertilization, there will be two cells within 24–30 hours, and additional cleavage divisions occurring every 10–12 hours thereafter. Within 4–7 days, there will be at least 64–128 cells. This stage is the hollow ball of cells called the blastula (blastocyst in humans). The 32-cell solid ball of cells (morula: choice B) would form earlier, while the gastrula (choice D) would form later.

9. **The correct answer is (B).** It is the major product of the first meiotic division, the secondary oocyte that is ovulated, along with a still-attached polar body. The second meiotic division will take place only if the secondary oocyte is fertilized by a sperm cell (usually in the fallopian tubes).

10. **The correct answer is (B).** LH is the hormone that maintains the corpus luteum. Even though LH production has decreased by the time implantation occurs, HCG acts in its place.

11. **The correct answer is (D).** Since the myometrium is primarily smooth, involuntary muscle, autonomic motor neurons are responsible for its contraction. In addition, oxytocin (made in the hypothalamus and released from the posterior pituitary gland) stimulates uterine contractions as well. Somatic motor neurons (choices A and C) only stimulate voluntary (skeletal) muscles.

12. **The correct answer is (D).** Although the anterior pituitary (choices A) produces FSH and LH which regulate the ovaries, it is the hypothalamus, through releasing hormones, that stimulates the anterior pituitary at the appropriate time.

13. **The correct answer is (C).** The zygote forms after the gametes combine during fertilization. The 32-cell morula is followed by the 64-cell blastula, and then the more complex gastrula with its three primary germ layers.

14. **The correct answer is (C).** The first example described in the question represents "determinate cleavage," whereas the second example represents "indeterminate cleavage." The other choices are terms related to different aspects of early embryology but are irrelevant to this specific question.

15. **The correct answer is (B).** In humans, the blastocyst contains an *inner cell mass* from which the embryo develops and the *trophoblast*, which forms the chorion and chorionic villi. The chorionic villi form the attachment with the endometrial lining of the uterus during implantation.

16. **The correct answer is (C).** The anterior pituitary secretes prolactin, which stimulates milk production and milk release into the ducts of the mammary glands. The posterior pituitary releases oxytocin (produced by the hypothalamus), which stimulates ejection of milk from the breast during nursing.

17. **The correct answer is (D).** Choice A includes structures that all derive from mesoderm, choice B consists of endodermal organs, and choice C contains ectodermal structures.

18. **The correct answer is (B).** Fertilization usually occurs in the fallopian tubes. Even though the corpus luteum maintains the uterus early in pregnancy, the placenta takes over completely by the end of the first trimester. Therefore, choice A is *not* the incorrect statement.

9.5 GENETICS AND EVOLUTION

A. GENETICS

Genetic Terminology and Mendelian Principles

Genes are sequences of DNA nucleotides on chromosomes that code for a specific protein (or part of that protein). The site a gene occupies on a chromosome is its **locus.** The different forms that a gene can take are called **alleles.** Each diploid organism carries two alleles for each trait because pairs of **homologous chromosomes** have corresponding loci for specific traits. An individual who carries two identical alleles (one on each homologous chromosome) for a given locus is **homozygous** for that locus or trait. If the two alleles are different, the individual is heterozygous for that locus or trait. When a trait is expressed in a **heterozygous** individual, one allele (**dominant** allele) may mask the expression of the other (**recessive** allele). Therefore, an individual's appearance for a particular trait **(phenotype)** is a function of the allelic combination **(genotype)** for that trait. Both homozygous dominant (genotype) individuals and heterozygous (genotype) individuals will express the dominant phenotype.

Mendel's *law of segregation* states that pairs of alleles for a gene locus separate during gamete formation (during meiosis, gametes receive only one of each homologous pair of chromosomes). Mendel's *law of independent assortment* states that a pair of alleles at a locus on one pair of chromosomes will separate independently of a pair of alleles at a different locus on a different pair of chromosomes (during meiosis, each pair of homologous chromosomes separates independently of all other pairs). Different traits determined by genes at loci on the same chromosome **(linked genes)** do not undergo independent assortment. However, these linked genes can be rearranged into new combinations due to **crossing over** (breaking and rejoining of homologous chromatids) during Prophase I of meiosis. As a result of crossing over, *all gametes* have different combinations of genes on their chromosomes. **Gene maps** of a chromosome can be determined by counting offspring that result from crossover events **(recombinants).**

A cross involving parents **(P generation)** homozygous for different alleles (BB × bb) at one locus is called a **monohybrid cross.** All offspring **(F1 generation)** will be heterozygous (Bb) and have the dominant phenotype. If two such heterozygotes are crossed (Bb × Bb), 3/4 of the next generation **(F2 generation)** will reflect the dominant phenotype (1BB and 2Bb: dominant, for every 1bb: recessive or 3:1 ratio). An individual with a dominant phenotype but unknown genotype (BB or Bb) can have its genotype determined with a **test cross,** in which a homozygous recessive individual (bb) is used as a partner (if BB, all offspring will be Bb and have the dominant phenotype; if Bb, one-half will be Bb and have the dominant phenotype, while one-half will be bb and have the recessive phenotype).

A cross involving parents homozygous for different alleles at two independent loci is called a **dihybrid cross** (AABB × aabb). All F1 offspring will have to be heterozygotes and show the dominant phenotype for both traits (AaBb). A cross of two such individuals (AaBb × AaBb) will produce an F2 generation that reflects a 9:3:3:1 phenotypic ratio (9A___B___ , 3A___bb, 3aaB___, and 1aabb).

Genetics

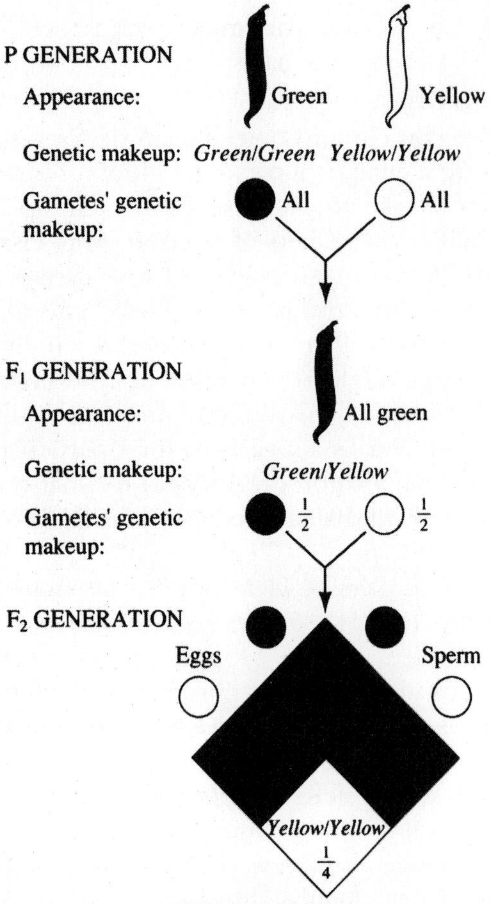

P GENERATION

Appearance: Green   Yellow

Genetic makeup: *Green/Green   Yellow/Yellow*

Gametes' genetic makeup: All   All

F₁ GENERATION

Appearance: All green

Genetic makeup: *Green/Yellow*

Gametes' genetic makeup: $\frac{1}{2}$ $\frac{1}{2}$

F₂ GENERATION

Eggs   Sperm

Yellow/Yellow $\frac{1}{4}$

(a) Monohybrid cross.

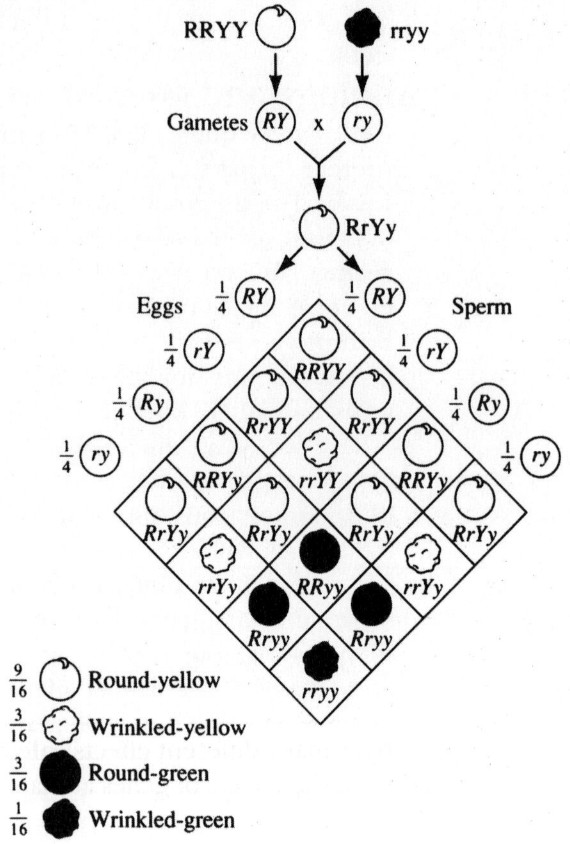

RRYY   rryy

Gametes (RY) x (ry)

RrYy

Eggs $\frac{1}{4}$(RY) $\frac{1}{4}$(RY) Sperm

$\frac{1}{4}$(rY) $\frac{1}{4}$(rY)

$\frac{1}{4}$(Ry) $\frac{1}{4}$(Ry)

$\frac{1}{4}$(ry) $\frac{1}{4}$(ry)

RRYY RrYY RrYY RrYY RRYy rrYY RRYy RrYy rrYy RrYy RrYy RRyy rrYy Rryy Rryy rryy

$\frac{9}{16}$ Round-yellow

$\frac{3}{16}$ Wrinkled-yellow

$\frac{3}{16}$ Round-green

$\frac{1}{16}$ Wrinkled-green

(b) Dihybrid cross.

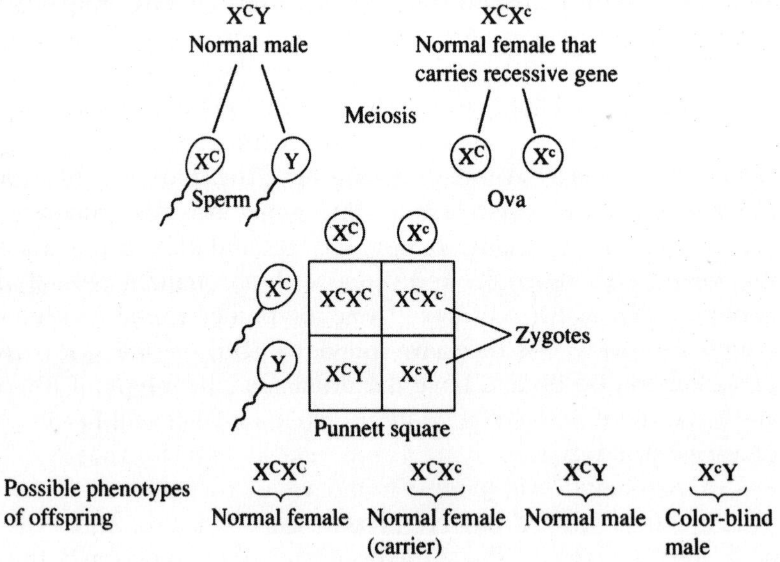

X^C Y Normal male   X^C X^c Normal female that carries recessive gene

Meiosis

X^C Y Sperm   X^C X^c Ova

Punnett square

	X^C	X^c
X^C	X^C X^C	X^C X^c
Y	X^C Y	X^c Y

Zygotes

Possible phenotypes of offspring: X^C X^C Normal female   X^C X^c Normal female (carrier)   X^C Y Normal male   X^c Y Color-blind male

(c) Sex-linked cross.

Variations on Mendelian Themes

The 23rd pair of human chromosomes are the **sex chromosomes,** which determine the sex of the individual (XX produces females; XY produces males). The Y chromosome does not carry genes for the same traits as the X chromosome. Therefore, the X and Y chromosomes (in males) are not homologous. The other 22 pairs of chromosomes are called **autosomes.** Traits that are expressions of loci on the X chromosome are called **X-linked** or **sex-linked** traits. In order for an X-linked recessive trait to be expressed in a female, the recessive allele must be present on both X-chromosomes. However, a male need only receive one recessive allele (from his mother) on his lone X chromosome. Thus, X-linked recessive traits are far more common in males then females.

For some traits, a heterozygote may reflect a phenotype in-between the dominant and recessive phenotypes (both alleles partially contribute to the final phenotype). This is referred to as **partial dominance** or **incomplete dominance.** For other traits where more than the usual two alleles may be possible **(multiple alleles),** a heterozygote may have both alleles contribute their full effects in the final phenotype **(codominance).** This can be seen with the alleles for common blood cell antigens resulting from the ABO locus. Both A and B alleles are dominant to the O allele. AB individuals have both antigens on their blood cells.

The alleles at a particular gene locus may affect the expression of a separate set of alleles at a different locus: **epistasis.** The alleles at a specific gene locus may also have many different effects: **pleiotropy.** A particular trait (like height) might result from the effects of genes at many different loci **(polygenic inheritance).**

Mutations

Genes can be considered as sequences of DNA nucleotides that determine the amino acid sequence of proteins made by cells. These proteins, in turn, contribute to the phenotype expressed for that genetic trait. Any change in the DNA nucleotide sequence is considered a **mutation,** and can lead to an incorrect final form in the protein being synthesized, a nonfunctional protein, or no protein at all. Such DNA changes can involve single nucleotide pairs **(point mutations)** or large portions of chromosomes involving many genes **(chromosomal alterations).** Point mutations include **substitutions,** in which the wrong nucleotide pair is present and only one codon is affected. In **additions** (an extra nucleotide pair is added) and **deletions** (a nucleotide pair is omitted), the entire triplet code is affected after the specific point mutation! Chromosomal alterations include various rearrangements after chromosomes break and reform incorrectly **(translocations** involve pieces of one chromosome attaching to another; **inversions** involve pieces of one chromosome reattaching in the wrong direction). Gametes may also wind up with the wrong number of chromosomes **(aneuploidy)** or extra sets of chromosomes **(polyploidy).**

B. EVOLUTION

Evolution refers to changes in gene frequencies in a population over time. Such changes can be used to help explain the vast diversity of living things.

Natural Selection

The principles of **natural selection** reflect the major mechanism by which evolution occurs over time. These include: (1) Differences exist among individuals in a population **(variation).** (2) Such differences can have a heritable component, (3) more individuals are produced than can survive and will, therefore, compete for resources, and (4) individuals whose heritable traits give them a reproductive advantage in their particular environment over other individuals (i.e., individuals more likely to survive and reproduce), will leave more offspring in the next generation. Thus, more and more individuals with those advantageous or **adaptive** traits will make up subsequent generations. **Fitness** refers to the relative reproductive success or **adaptive value** of an individual genotype in comparison to alternative genotypes. The genotype producing the most fertile individuals in the next generation is the "fittest." A strong, long-lived individual that leaves no offspring has a fitness value of zero. Natural selection is primarily assumed to act on individuals and heritable traits that benefit those individuals. Proponents of **group selection** suggest that heritable traits in individuals that benefit (reproductive advantage) the entire group or breeding population can also be maintained in this way (e.g., altruistic warning calls that potentially threaten the individual "caller" are maintained by selection because they benefit other individuals in the group and improve the chances of survival for the group itself). When other group members are genetically related to the "altruist," this kind of group selection is referred to as **kin selection.**

Hardy-Weinberg Equilibrium and Population Genetics

The Hardy-Weinberg law or theorem states that gene frequencies in a breeding population **(gene pool)** will remain the same (constant) from generation to generation (even with crossing over and sexual reproduction taking place) unless other factors are operating. In other words, evolution will not occur without one or more other factors at work. However, one or more of these other factors are always at work:

1. **Mutation**
   Spontaneous changes in DNA producing new alleles or changing one allele to another.

2. **Natural Selection**
   Some alleles provide individuals bearing them with a reproductive advantage over others.

3. **Migration**
   Individuals with particular alleles can enter or leave the population.

4. **Non-Random Mating**
   Certain individuals are more likely to mate than others in a population that is not infinitely large.

5. **Genetic Drift**
   Random events can affect the frequency of alleles in a population that is not infinitely large.

Since most of these factors are always operating, evolution does occur. The Hardy-Weinberg Equilibrium only exists under hypothetical conditions that are never met!

Speciation

Individuals are considered to belong to the same biological **species** if they can mate and produce fertile offspring. Various **reproductive isolating mechanisms** may be at work leading to "splitting" of gene pools so that successful breeding can no longer occur and **speciation** eventually takes place. **Pre-zygotic isolating mechanisms** include geographic, ecological, or temporal isolation (individuals do not meet and eventually become adapted to different environments), behavioral isolation (courtship or mating behavior are not compatible), and mechanical isolation (reproductive body parts are incompatible). **Post-zygotic isolating mechanisms** include hybrid inviability (successful development of offspring does not occur), hybrid sterility (offspring are born sterile), and hybrid breakdown (offspring are fertile but weak and unable to ultimately maintain reproductive success). Speciation is one of the processes contributing to the vast diversity observed in the living world.

Vertebrate Diversity

Vertebrates (fish, amphibians, reptiles, birds, and mammals) belong to the phylum **Chordata (Chordates),** a group of animals with a supporting **notochord, a dorsal tubular nerve cord,** and **pharyngeal gill slits** at some stage in the life cycle. Vertebrates share the following characteristics: a vertebral column that forms the main skeletal axis inside the body **(endoskeleton)**; a pronounced head region **(cephalization)** that is part of the endoskeleton enclosing a highly developed brain; two pairs of appendages; muscles attached to the endoskeleton for movement; a chambered heart and closed circulatory system; a vascular respiratory system for gas exchange (gills, lungs, and/or skin); a digestive tract; an excretory system for waste removal with paired kidneys; and separate sexes. Vertebrates, like members of some other phyla (arthropods, mollusks, annelids, etc.) have an inner body cavity called a **coelom** which reflects a "tube-within-a-tube" body plan (hollow digestive tract with two openings inside the body wall).

Origin of Life

Speculation about the origin of life suggests that chemical evolution required the absence of oxygen, the presence of fundamental chemical building blocks (water, carbon dioxide, hydrogen, nitrogen, carbon monoxide, methane, etc.), energy, and large periods of time. The events of chemical evolution include: the origin of small organic molecules or monomers (amino acids, monosaccharides, fatty acids, and nucleotides); the combination of monomers into macromolecules (primitive proteins and nucleic acids); assemblages or aggregates of macromolecules **(microspheres, coacervates, liposomes)**; and the formation of primitive cells (probably anaerobic, heterotrophic, and prokaryotic) with hereditary capabilities. The first autotrophs probably appeared later, and with the production of oxygen resulting from photosynthesis, the evolution of aerobic, eukaryotic organisms followed. This possible sequence is part of the **heterotroph hypothesis.**

PRACTICE PROBLEMS
GENETICS AND EVOLUTION

1. Fruit flies of the genotype AaBb were crossed with individuals of the genotype aabb. The first 1000 offspring included 470 AaBb, 485 aabb, 24 Aabb, and 21 aaBb. What can be inferred from this cross?

   A. It is a dihybrid cross.
   B. It involves independent assortment.
   C. Both A and B
   D. Neither A nor B

2. A test cross of a black guinea pig male produced six black male offspring and two brown female offspring. If black is dominant to brown, what is the genotype of the male parent?

   A. $X_B Y$
   B. $X_b Y$
   C. Bb
   D. BB

3. The gene A leads to the production of a blue plant pigment, while the gene B leads to the *deposition* of that blue pigment in the petals of the flower. If a dihybrid cross of two heterozygotes (AaBb × AaBb) produces some offspring with blue petals and others with white petals in a phenotypic ratio of 9:7, what genetic phenomenon is the most likely explanation?

   A. pleiotropy
   B. linkage
   C. epistasis
   D. polygenic inheritance

4. If, in one of two secondary spermatocytes, one of the 23 replicated chromosomes does not separate properly (nondisjunction) during Telophase II of meiosis, how many chromosomes will be present in the four spermatids produced at the end of the second meiotic division?

   A. 23, 23, 22, 24
   B. 23, 23, 23, 23
   C. 22, 22, 24, 24
   D. 0, 0, 46, 46

5. If a substitution occurs in a sequence of 15 nucleotides at the 7th nucleotide, what can we be sure will happen when this sequence is translated?

   A. Only the first amino acid will be correct.
   B. The first two amino acids will be correct.
   C. The first three amino acids will be correct.
   D. The first two amino acids and the last two amino acids will be correct.

6. The probability of parents having a daughter is 50% $\left(\dfrac{1}{2}\right)$. What is the probability of parents having three daughters in a row?

   A. $\dfrac{1}{2}$

   B. $\dfrac{1}{4}$

   C. $\dfrac{1}{8}$

   D. $\dfrac{1}{16}$

7. What blood type is not possible in a child produced by a Type A father and a Type B mother?

   A. A
   B. B
   C. AB
   D. O
   E. All are possible.

8. If a polygenic trait in plants involves genes at three different loci, which determine fruit weight, and each dominant allele contributes 0.5 lb, while each recessive allele contributes .25 lb, what would fruits weigh in individuals that are heterozygous at all three loci?

   A. 2 lb
   B. 2.25 lb
   C. 2.5 lb
   D. 2.75 lb
   E. 3.0 lb

9. A hemophiliac woman and her husband whose blood clots normally, have a son. What is the probability that this child will have hemophilia? Hemophilia is a sex-linked recessive trait.

   A. 0%
   B. 25%
   C. 50%
   D. 75%
   E. 100%

10. If one of the abnormal sperm cells described in Question 4 successfully fertilizes a normal ovum, how many chromosomes will the zygote contain?

   A. 22 or 44
   B. 23 or 46
   C. 24 or 47
   D. 45 or 47

11. Which male elephant would be the fittest?

   A. An individual that fathered five offspring each breeding season and lived through six breeding seasons
   B. An individual that fathered three offspring each breeding season and lived through ten breeding seasons
   C. An individual that fathered one offspring each breeding season and lived through thirty breeding seasons
   D. All of the above

12. According to the Hardy-Weinberg theorem, which of the following conditions would not contribute to gene frequencies in a population remaining in equilibrium?

   A. absence of natural selection
   B. absence of a large breeding population
   C. absence of migration
   D. absence of mutation
   E. random mating

13. In certain bluejay species, the siblings of parent birds help incubate their eggs and guard their young after hatching. This is an example of

   A. classical natural selection.
   B. genetic drift.
   C. kin selection.
   D. post-zygotic reproductive isolation.

14. Which of the following is not representative of the vertebrate body plan?

   A. open circulatory system
   B. coelom
   C. two sets of paired appendages
   D. separate sexes

15. Which sequence is correct according to the heterotroph hypothesis?

- A. organic molecules, coacervates, inorganic molecules, heterotrophs, autotrophs
- B. inorganic molecules, organic molecules, coacervates, autotrophs, heterotrophs
- C. coacervates, inorganic molecules, organic molecules, autotrophs, heterotrophs
- D. inorganic molecules, organic molecules, coacervates, heterotrophs, autotrophs

16. A mating between a female horse (mare) and a male donkey produces a mule. All mules are sterile. This is an example of

- A. mutation.
- B. post-zygotic reproductive isolation.
- C. pre-zygotic reproductive isolation.
- D. speciation.

ANSWER KEY

| 1. A | 3. C | 5. B | 7. E | 9. E | 11. D | 13. C | 15. D |
| 2. C | 4. A | 6. C | 8. B | 10. D | 12. B | 14. A | 16. B |

ANSWERS AND EXPLANATIONS

1. **The correct answer is (A).** This is definitely a dihybrid cross, as reflected by the alleles for the A trait and B trait. However, if these traits assorted independently (which happens when traits are on independent chromosomes), one would expect 25% of each genotype produced. The results suggest that the two traits are linked. The heterozygous parent (AaBb) has one chromosome with AB and the other with ab. Thus, most of the offspring are AaBb and aabb. The genotypes Aabb and aaBb are "recombinants" resulting from crossing over in the heterozygous parent.

2. **The correct answer is (C).** A test cross is performed to determine the genotype of an individual using a double recessive partner. Since both black and brown offspring were produced, the black male guinea pig parent must have been Bb. If he had been BB (choice D), all offspring would have been black. If coat color was a sex-linked trait, no black male offspring could be produced by a brown mother and black father (choice A). Choice B (X^b) is incorrect because that is the genotype of a brown guinea pig father.

3. **The correct answer is (C).** Epistasis refers to a kind of gene interaction in which alleles at one locus can influence the effects of alleles at a separate locus. In this case, all AB individuals can make and deposit the blue pigment in their petals and will be blue (9), all aa individuals would not be able to produce the pigment and would be white (3), all A_bb individuals would be unable to deposit the pigment in their petals and would be white (3), and all aabb individuals would neither be able to make nor deposit the pigment and would be white (1).

4. **The correct answer is (A).** Because one secondary spermatocyte (containing 23 replicated chromosomes or 46 chromatids) proceeds normally, it will produce two normal spermatids (23 chromosomes each) after the second meiotic division. The other secondary spermatocyte will have nondisjunction occur in one (2 chromatids) of the 23 replicated chromosomes, while the other 22 replicated chromosomes (44 chromatids) will separate normally. Therefore, one of these two spermatids will contain 22 chromosomes (it received neither of the still-attached chromatids) while the other will have 24 chromosomes (it received both of the still-attached chromatids).

5. **The correct answer is (B).** Since the substitution is at the seventh nucleotide, the first six nucleotides remain unchanged and will code for the original two amino acids. The substitution is part of the third codon. However, we cannot be sure that the last two amino acids will also be correct (choice D) because the substitution in the third codon may produce early termination.

6. **The correct answer is (C).** The chance of having a daughter is $\frac{1}{2}$, but the chance of having two daughters in a row as independent events is $\frac{1}{2} \times \frac{1}{2} = \frac{1}{4}$. Similarly, the chance of having three daughters in a row would be $\frac{1}{2} \times \frac{1}{2} \times \frac{1}{2} = \frac{1}{8}$.

7. **The correct answer is (E).** All are possible because the question does not specify the exact genotype of either parent. If the father (Type A) had the $I^A i$ genotype and the mother (Type B) had the $I^B i$ genotype, all combinations can be produced: $I^A i$ (Type A), $I^B i$ (Type B), $I^A I^B$ (Type AB), and ii (Type O).

8. **The correct answer is (B).** If the plant was heterozygous at all three loci (AaBbCc), and each dominant allele contributes 0.5 lb while each recessive allele contributes 0.25 lb, the fruit would weigh 2.25 lb.

9. **The correct answer is (E).** If mom has hemophilia, her genotype is $X^h X^h$. She can only contribute an X chromosome with the recessive allele for hemophilia to all her sons. (They must receive the Y chromosome from dad in order to be sons in the first place!) Therefore, all sons produced by this couple will have the genotype $X^h Y$, and will have hemophilia.

10. **The correct answer is (D).** The normal female gamete will have 23 chromosomes. If the abnormal sperm from Question 4 with 22 chromosomes fertilized this ovum, the result would be a zygote with 45 chromosomes. However, if the sperm with 24 chromosomes fertilized the ovum, the zygote would contain 47 chromosomes. Each would represent a different example of aneuploidy.

11. **The correct answer is (D).** Reproductive fitness is based on an individual's ability to successfully pass its genes on to future generations, relative to the success of other individuals. Even though choice A produced the most offspring each season and choicer C lived the longest, all three elephants produced thirty offspring and thus were equally "fit."

12. **The correct answer is (B).** When a breeding population is relatively small, chance events can lead to changes in gene frequencies (genetic drift). Thus, the population would not remain at equilibrium and would "evolve." The other choices all reflect conditions that lead to gene frequencies remaining *unchanged*.

13. **The correct answer is (C).** When apparently altruistic behavior is performed to benefit one's relatives, this is known as kin selection. Since the individuals that benefit from such behavior share genes with the "altruist," the altruist is actually increasing his/her own "fitness."

14. **The correct answer is (A).** All vertebrates have a closed circulatory system in which the blood flows continuously through the heart and blood vessels, without bathing the tissues directly.

15. **The correct answer is (D).** Organic molecules (amino acids, nucleotides, etc.) are thought to have formed from inorganic precursors, coacervates (enclosed collections of macromolecules) preceded the evolution of cells, and heterotrophic cells are believed to have evolved before photosynthetic cells.

16. **The correct answer is (B).** Pre-zygotic isolation refers to any conditions that prevent fertilization from taking place (breeding at different times, breeding in different geographic regions, reproductive structures are incompatible, etc.). Since the horse and donkey have successfully mated and produced an offspring, this is an example of a post-zygotic isolating mechanism (hybrid sterility). A new species (mules) would not arise in such a situation (choice D) because the mules themselves cannot produce offspring.

CHAPTER 10

Organic Chemistry

10.1 MOLECULAR STRUCTURE OF ORGANIC MOLECULES

A. SIGMA AND PI BONDS

Bonding occurs in organic molecules (as well as others) when pairs of electrons are concentrated between the centers of atoms in such a way as to maximize the distance between different bonding pairs.

Many bonds can be described by first identifying **hybrid orbitals** on individual atoms, most commonly carbon and nitrogen. As an example of why hybrid bonding is a useful concept, consider methane, CH_4. In order to form a molecule in which the electron pairs in the bonds are at maximal distance from each other, the molecule should have tetrahedral geometry. Yet of the available valence orbitals on the carbon, the three $2p$ orbitals are at 90° angles to one another, not 109.5°, and the $2s$ orbitals have no particular directionality at all.

To create orbitals pointing in the correct direction, assume that a $2s$ is promoted into $2p$ orbital, and then assume that the four orbitals are combined so that each points to a different corner of a tetrahedron. The resulting hybrid is called "sp^3."

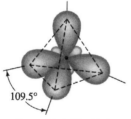

109.5°

Four sp^3 hybrid orbitals

Not all carbon compounds require 109.5° angles. In benzene, each carbon makes three bonds, at 120°, by using its $2s$ and two of its $2p$ orbitals to form an "sp^2" hybrid. Where two bonds at 180° are needed, "sp" hybrids are formed.

The bonds formed when the hybrid orbitals overlap with orbitals from an adjacent atom toward which they point are called **sigma orbitals.** The characteristic feature of a sigma orbital is **cylindrical symmetry**: When rotated around the axis between the bonded atoms, the shape of the orbital is unchanged.

In contrast, a "pi" orbital is formed by the overlap of two atomic orbitals, usually unhybridized p orbitals, which are parallel and adjacent to each other.

A common example occurs in double-bonded $\overset{\diagdown}{\underset{\diagup}{C}}=\overset{\diagup}{\underset{\diagdown}{C}}$ where one of the bonds,

the **sigma bond,** is formed by the overlap of sp^2 hybrid orbitals; while the second bond is a **pi bond** formed by the overlap of the remaining p orbitals on each carbon. The latter are parallel and are close enough for effective overlap.

Application of Sigma (σ) and Pi (π) Bonds to Structural Formulas

In describing organic structure, we need to keep several principles in mind:

1. Identify the location of all bonds in the molecule, including multiple bonds (correct Lewis structure).

2. Locate the nonbonding pairs of electrons.

3. Determine the sigma framework by deciding on the appropriate angles between bonds and between nonbonding pairs. Assign appropriate hybridization to central atoms, particularly carbons and nitrogens. The central atom must have one hybrid orbital for each bonding pair and each nonbonding pair.

4. After the sigma framework is accounted for, add a pi bond to a sigma base to describe a **double bond**; add two pi bonds to describe a **triple bond.**

Examples

CH_2CClF:

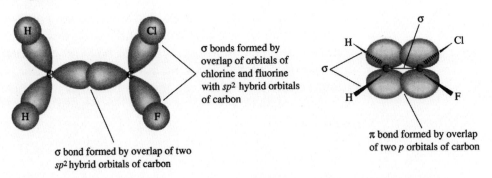

σ bonds formed by overlap of orbitals of chlorine and fluorine with sp^2 hybrid orbitals of carbon

σ bond formed by overlap of two sp^2 hybrid orbitals of carbon

π bond formed by overlap of two p orbitals of carbon

Note that there are no **lone pairs.** To generalize from this example, had the molecule been SiH_2ClF—note that silicon is directly below carbon in the Periodic Table—the structure would have been identical, with silicon the central atom in place of carbon, and with hybrids deriving from the $3s$ and $3p$ atomic orbitals of the central atom.

NH_3:

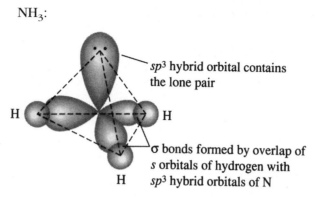

sp³ hybrid orbital contains
the lone pair

σ bonds formed by overlap of
s orbitals of hydrogen with
sp³ hybrid orbitals of N

Here we see an example of the need to leave room for the lone pair on the nitrogen. Were the molecule PH_3, we would have had to construct the central hybrid from the valence 3*s* and 3*p* orbitals on the phosphorus.

Formaldehyde, HCHO:

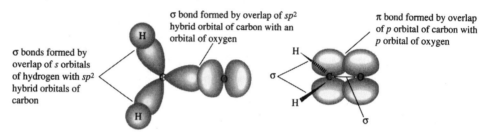

σ bond formed by overlap of *sp²* hybrid orbital of carbon with an orbital of oxygen

π bond formed by overlap of *p* orbital of carbon with *p* orbital of oxygen

σ bonds formed by overlap of *s* orbitals of hydrogen with *sp²* hybrid orbitals of carbon

The sigma structure of the molecule is formed from an sp^2 hybrid on the carbon atom. (The oxygen may be sp^2 hybridized as well, although the fact that it forms only one bond makes this conjecture impossible to verify through measurement of bond angles.) The C═O pi bond is formed by the overlap of out-of-plane 2*p* orbitals on each of the carbon and the oxygen atoms.

Delocalized Electrons and Resonance in Ions and Molecules

Benzene is said to have two **resonance forms**:

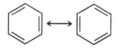

This pair of formulas is *not* meant to imply that there is equilibrium between the two forms written. Rather, each bond in the benzene molecule has the *same* bond lengths and electron density (roughly $1\frac{1}{2}$ bonds). Twelve electrons occupy the sigma framework. The additional electrons arising from the out-of-plane 2*p* orbitals are delocalized—they travel throughout the ring in pi molecular orbitals.

B. MULTIPLE BONDING

Effect on Bond Length and Bond Energies

Organic molecules display single bonds based on sigma overlap, plus double and triple bonds, which have both a sigma bond and either one or two pi bonds. Bond dissociation energies increase as the number of bonds increases; e.g., the energies of the carbon-carbon bond in ethane (single bond), ethylene (double bond), and acetylene (triple bond) are 347, 523, and 962 kJ/mol, respectively.

The length of a double bond is less than that of a single bond, and a triple bond has the shortest length of all three. Taking the same examples as above, we find bond lengths of 1.54 Å for ethane, 1.35 Å for ethylene, and 1.21 Å for acetylene.

Rigidity in Molecular Structure

Since a sigma bond has, by definition, symmetry about the internuclear axis, the degree of overlap of the atomic orbitals that constitute it is unchanged by rotation of one of the atoms. This is not so with double bonds, since the p-orbital overlap that is the basis of a pi bond is maximal when the p orbitals are parallel, and it falls to zero as one of the p orbitals is rotated to a 90° orientation relative to its neighbor. For this reason, single bonds allow rotation (unless bulky substituents interfere), while double and triple bonds prevent rotation. The implication of this rigidity for stereoisomerism is discussed below.

C. STEREOCHEMISTRY OF COVALENTLY BONDED MOLECULES

Isomers

Isomers are distinct compounds that have the same molecular formulas, but different molecular structures. The major categories of isomers are discussed in the sections that follow.

Structural Isomers

Structural isomers share a common molecular formula but their atoms are connected in different ways. Examples are n-pentane

$$CH_3—CH_2—CH_2—CH_2—CH_3$$

and 2-methylbutane.

$$CH_3—\overset{\overset{\displaystyle H}{|}}{C}—\overset{\overset{\displaystyle H}{|}}{\underset{\underset{\displaystyle H}{|}}{C}}—CH_3$$
$$\underset{\displaystyle CH_3}{}$$

No amount of rotation of atoms around their bond axes will interconvert these isomers; we would have to break and then reconnect bonds to change one to the other.

Stereoisomers

In contrast to structural isomers, stereoisomers share the same order of atoms, but differ in the orientation of those atoms.

Enantiomers

Enantiomers are pairs of compounds that are mirror images of each other and cannot be superimposed on each other. Below we see examples of compounds that are (or are not) enantiomers:

Not Enantiomers:

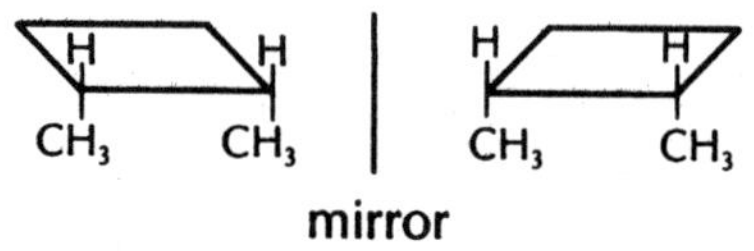

mirror

The two drawings are of the same molecule.

Enantiomers:

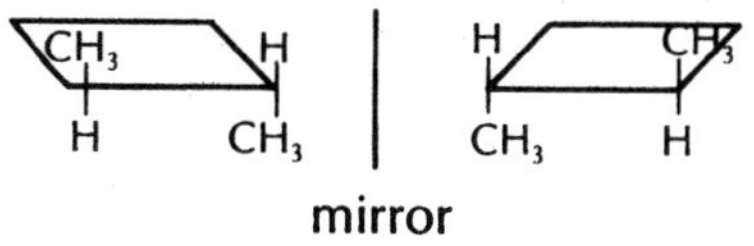

mirror

Chiral Compounds; Chiral Carbon Atoms

The term *chiral* refers to a compound that has an enantiomer. Applied to a carbon atom, it indicates that the carbon has four different substituents. Such a carbon is also called **asymmetric.** If a compound has only one chiral carbon, it is chiral; the presence of several chiral carbons may or may not indicate that the compound is chiral.

Here are examples of chiral and non-chiral carbon atoms:

Chiral carbon:

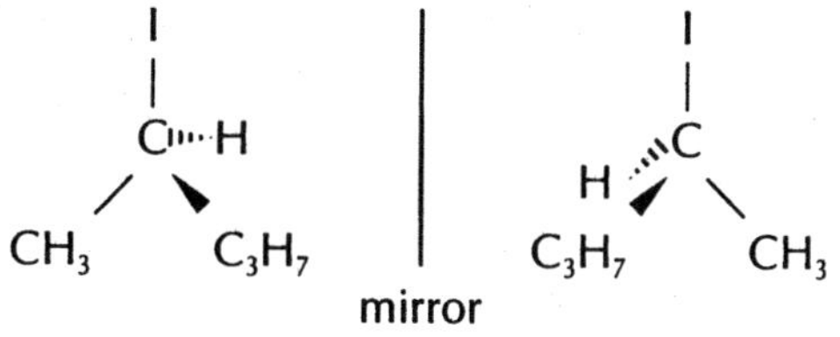

mirror

Non-chiral carbon:

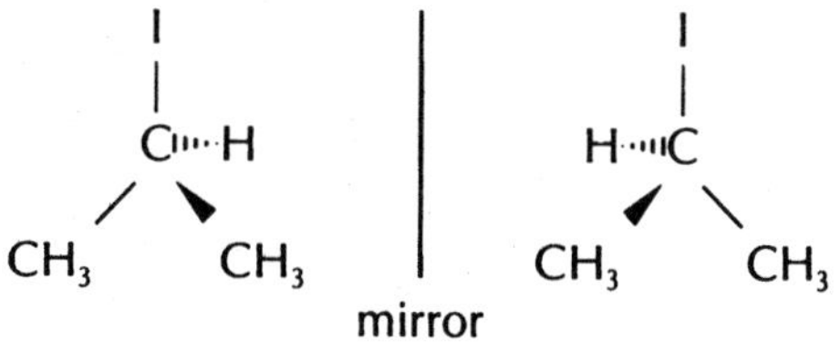

mirror

Diastereomers

Diastereomers are a class of stereoisomers that are *not* mirror images of each other. They include geometrical isomers, conformational isomers, and molecules with multiple chiral carbons.

Geometric (cis/trans) Isomers

As we have seen, double bonds prevent rotation. For this reason, we may have **cis** or **trans** forms (generalized as "geometric isomers") of alkenes such as 1,2-dichloroethylene:

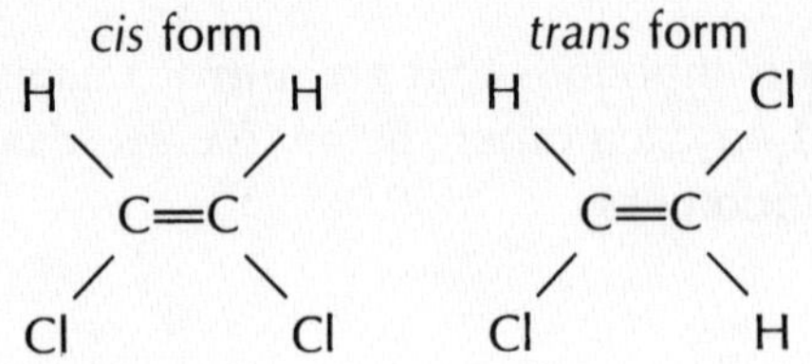

Conformational Isomers ("Conformers")

In biphenyl,

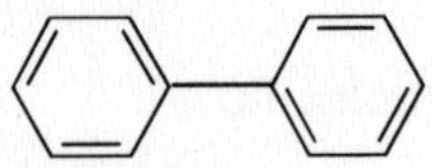

there is relatively free rotation about the C—C bond connecting the two benzene rings, and no distinct isomers result. But rotation is hindered in the following substituted biphenyls:

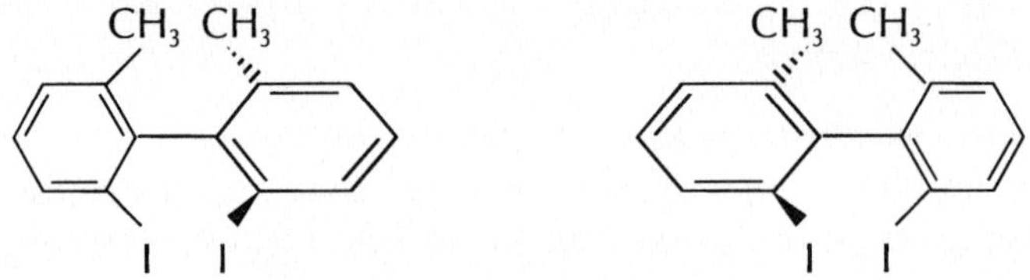

Such a pair of enantiomers are called **conformational isomers.** Note that if rotation were less hindered, so that the forms could interconvert, then there would be no enantiomers.

Diastereomers Having Two or More Chiral Carbons

In the following pair of compounds, each has two chiral carbons and each has the same ordering of atoms in its structure. Yet the two forms are not mirror images (thus, they are diastereomers) and they cannot be superimposed.

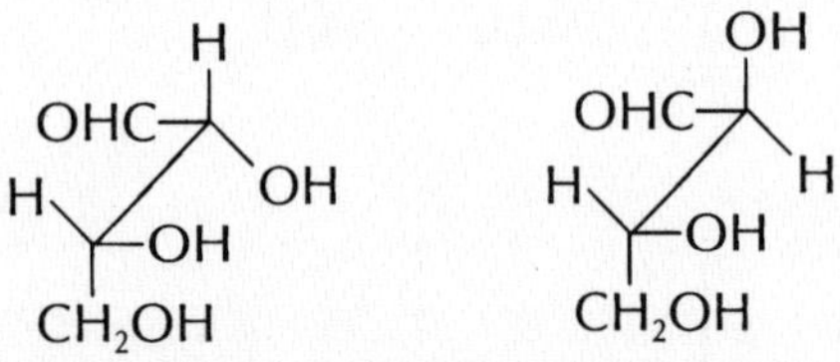

Polarization of Light: Specific Rotation

Enantiomers have a remarkable property that allows them to be studied and distinguished by physical measurements. To explain this property, we must first discuss polarized light.

Polarized Light

Normal light sources produce light that is said to be "unpolarized." This means that the electric field vector of the light wave points in all directions in the plane perpendicular to the direction that the light beam travels. A polarizing filter selects out light whose electric field vector points in only one direction; the light is then said to be linearly polarized.

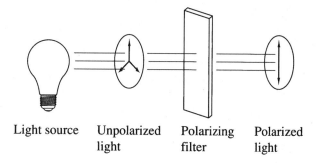

Light source   Unpolarized   Polarizing   Polarized
light   filter   light

Optical Activity of Chiral Compounds

When linearly polarized light is passed through a solution containing one enantiomer of a pair, *its direction of polarization is rotated*. If light is passed through a solution containing the second enantiomer of the pair (with the same concentration and optical path length), then the polarization will again be rotated, by an angle equal in magnitude but opposite in direction to the initial rotation. This property of chiral compounds is termed **optical activity.**

Optical Activity

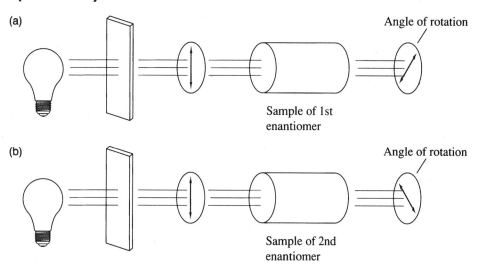

(a)

Angle of rotation

Sample of 1st enantiomer

(b)

Angle of rotation

Sample of 2nd enantiomer

Specific Rotation

For consistency in reporting the direction and magnitude of optical activity of various compounds, chemists report a substance's **specific rotation,** alpha, defined as

$$[\alpha]_D^{25^\circ} = \alpha_{obs}/c \, l$$

Here $[\alpha]_D^{25^\circ}$ is the specific rotation at 25°C using the intense *"D"* spectral line of a sodium lamp; $\alpha_{(obs)}$ is the observed angle of rotation (given a "+" designation for clockwise, or **dextrorotatory rotation** and a "−" designation for counterclockwise, or **levorotatory rotation**); c is the concentration of the compound in g/mL of solution, and l is the cell length in decimeters, where 1 decimeter = 10 cm.

Absolute and Relative Configuration

The **absolute configuration** of a molecule is the complete stereochemical description of its structure, either through a three-dimensional diagram or a two-dimensional depiction plus the "R/S" configuration (described below) at each chiral carbon. By contrast, **relative configuration** refers to an experimentally determined configuration of two molecules in the absence of complete structural information. As an example of determination of relative configuration, polarimetry can indicate that a compound having a (+) optical rotation has been converted to a product that also has (+) rotation ("retention of configuration") or to a product that has (−) rotation ("inversion").

R/S Convention

By use of the **Cahn-Ingold-Prelog convention,** we can assign each chiral carbon atom the prefix R or S, thus allowing anyone familiar with the R/S system and with the compound's two-dimensional structural diagram to draw the correct three-dimensional structure.

Steps in Assigning R/S Values

1. Identify the chiral carbon atoms to be characterized.

2. Assign a priority to each group attached to the chiral carbon. In assigning priority, look at the atom on each substituent which is attached to the chiral carbon.

    (a) Highest priority is given to the substituent whose joining atom is of the highest atomic number.

    (b) If the first atoms of two or more groups are identical, look at the second atom on each and prioritize using the highest atomic number.

    (c) Double and triple bonds are treated as in the following example: Imagine each pi bond to be broken and the atoms at both ends duplicated. (Added atoms have a square around them.)

    Example

    (d) Draw the chiral carbon and its four substituents in the following way, where the numbers refer to the previously determined priorities. Place the fourth priority substituent at the rear position and draw in the others in a way consistent with the known structure. Then draw an arrow from group 1 through group 2 to group 3. If the arrow describes a clockwise circle, then the configuration is "R." If the circle is counterclockwise, the configuration is "S."

Example
"S" Configuration.

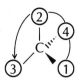

Example
"R" Configuration.

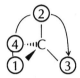

Racemic Mixture

A racemic mixture consists of equal amounts of (+) and (−) isomers of a given compound. Many reactions are not stereoselective and yield a racemic mixture.

10.2 HYDROCARBONS

A. SATURATED HYDROCARBONS (ALKANES)

Properties

Alkanes are compounds of hydrogen and carbon that contain only single bonds. Relatively unreactive, their physical properties depend largely on the number of carbons they contain, with the degree of branching being important as well. The table below gives the names of the first eight "normal" (i.e., straight-chain) alkanes, as well as the chain length, boiling point, and melting point for each.

Number of C Atoms	Name	b.p., (°C)	m.p., (°C)
1	methane	−161.5	−183
2	ethane	−88.6	−172
3	propane	−42.1	−188
4	butane	−.5	−135
5	pentane	36.1	−130
6	hexane	68.7	−95
7	heptane	98.4	−91
8	octane	125.7	−57

Compared to the straight-chain compounds, *branched* alkanes have lower boiling points because of their smaller surface area, which leads to decreased intermolecular forces. Alkanes are nonpolar, so they are soluble in non-polar solvents like benzene and chloroform but insoluble in water.

Important Reactions

1. **Combustion**

   Combustion—i.e., rapid reaction with oxygen—occurs with all alkanes. For the example of ethane, the overall reaction is

   $$C_2H_6 + 7/2\ O_2 \rightarrow 2\ CO_2 + 3\ H_2O$$

   Combustion of alkanes gives CO_2 and H_2O.

2. **Halogenation**

   Alkanes react with Cl_2 and Br_2 to form substituted alkanes such as CH_2Cl_2, CH_2Br_2, etc. The usual result is a mixture of substitution products. The reaction requires either light or heat to drive it; a curious feature is that each photon of light that is incident may lead to the formation of many molecules of products. The mechanism, a **chain reaction,** is described below.

   Chain reaction in halogenation:
   (light)
   $Cl_2 \rightarrow 2Cl\bullet$ (initiation)
   $Cl\bullet + CH_4 \rightarrow HCl + CH_3\bullet$ (propagation)
   $CH_3\bullet + Cl_2 \rightarrow CH_3Cl + Cl\bullet$ (propagation)
   $Cl\bullet + CH_3\bullet \rightarrow CH_3Cl$ (termination)
   $2\ Cl\bullet \rightarrow Cl_2$ "
   $2CH_3\bullet \rightarrow CH_3CH_3$ "

Once initiated by light, the propagation steps continue to generate additional chlorine radicals, continuing the "chain" for hundreds or thousands of cycles until the termination process halts the reaction.

Inhibition

A chain reaction is "inhibited" by substances that trap the **free radicals** essential to its continuation. In the reaction above, oxygen molecules may act as inhibitors by reacting with the methyl radical to form the relatively unreactive CH_3OO radical.

Ring Strain in Cyclic Compounds

Cycloalkanes resemble normal alkanes (n-alkanes) but their ends are joined. The most commonly occurring rings have five or six carbons, and the explanation for this lies in the tendency (described in Section 10.6) for carbon to form tetrahedral bond angles of 109.5°. In rings of three or four carbons, the bond angles must be considerably less than 109.5° (e.g., 90° for planar cyclobutane), with the result that the bonds will not have optimal overlap. Thus, the ring will be less stable; this drop in stability is termed **ring strain.**

Ring strain is conveniently measured by comparing the **heat of combustion** of the cyclic compound with that of the straight-chain compound. The following chart shows values of ring strain per CH_2 group:

Number of Carbons in Ring	Ring Strain per CH_2 (kJ/mol)
3	38.3
4	28
5	5
6	0
7	4
8	5

B. UNSATURATED COMPOUNDS (ALKENES)

Description

Alkenes are hydrocarbons with one or more double bonds. The reactivity of the double bond, as well as the fact that the resistance to free rotation of the double bond leads to isomerism, causes marked differences in chemical behavior between alkanes and alkenes.

1. **Structure and Isomerization**
   The two geometrical isomers of 2-butene are shown below. The **"trans" isomer** has the CH_3 groups on opposite sides of the double bond, while in the **"cis" isomer,** the CH_3's are on the same side:

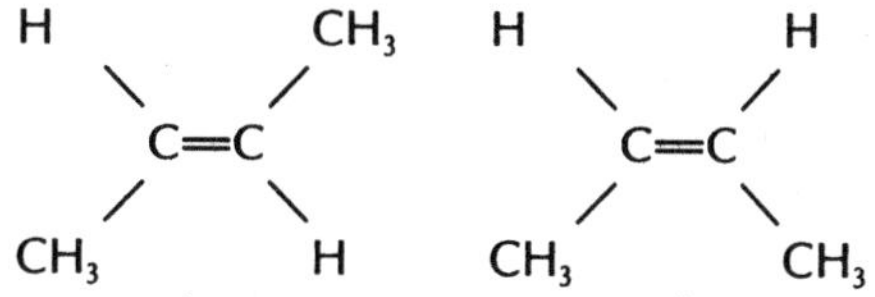

Steric hindrance causes the *cis* isomer to be less stable than the *trans*, by about 4 kJ/mol.

2. **Physical Properties**
   The melting and boiling points of the alkenes are similar to those of the alkanes; as with the alkanes, both melting and boiling points increase with chain length. Alkenes are only slightly more polar than the alkanes so that they are also insoluble in water but soluble in nonpolar solvents.

Electrophilic Addition

An electrophile is a species that is attracted to an electron-rich group; the double bond in an alkene is such a group. An example of electrophilic addition is shown in the following reaction sequence, in which HBr is the **electrophile**:

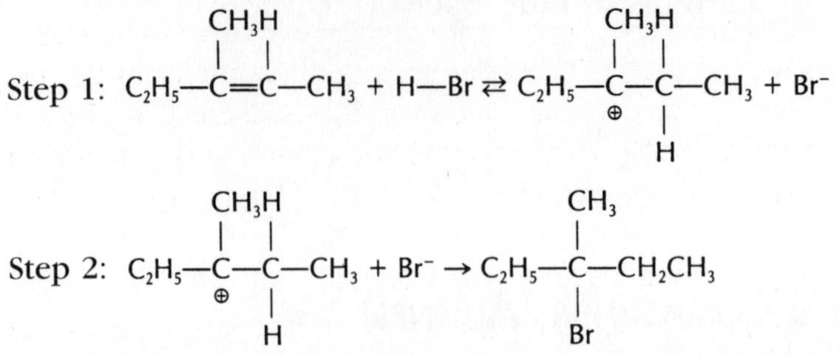

Step 1: $C_2H_5\!-\!\overset{\overset{\displaystyle CH_3}{|}}{C}\!=\!\overset{\overset{\displaystyle H}{|}}{C}\!-\!CH_3 + H\!-\!Br \rightleftarrows C_2H_5\!-\!\overset{\overset{\displaystyle CH_3}{|}}{\underset{\oplus}{C}}\!-\!\overset{\overset{\displaystyle H}{|}}{\underset{\underset{\displaystyle H}{|}}{C}}\!-\!CH_3 + Br^-$

Step 2: $C_2H_5\!-\!\overset{\overset{\displaystyle CH_3}{|}}{\underset{\oplus}{C}}\!-\!\overset{\overset{\displaystyle H}{|}}{\underset{\underset{\displaystyle H}{|}}{C}}\!-\!CH_3 + Br^- \rightarrow C_2H_5\!-\!\overset{\overset{\displaystyle CH_3}{|}}{\underset{\underset{\displaystyle Br}{|}}{C}}\!-\!CH_2CH_3$

In the first step, H^+ attaches to the carbon on one side of the original double bond, while in the second step, Br^- attaches to the adjacent carbon.

Is it simply by chance that the hydrogen ion adds to the left side, as pictured above? The answer is no—the positively-charged **carbocation** shown above is favored greatly over the alternative ion which would have the H^+ add to the other side of the double bond:

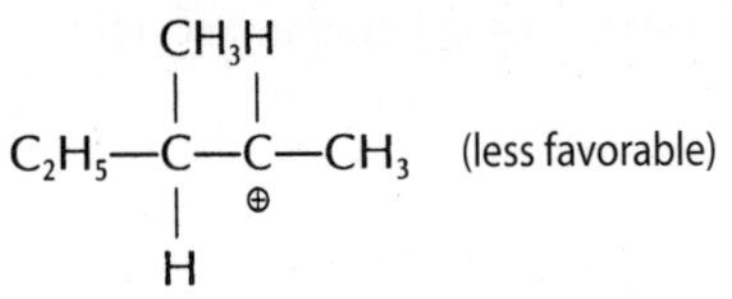

$C_2H_5\!-\!\overset{\overset{\displaystyle CH_3}{|}}{\underset{\underset{\displaystyle H}{|}}{C}}\!-\!\overset{\overset{\displaystyle H}{|}}{\underset{\oplus}{C}}\!-\!CH_3$ (less favorable)

This is so because the first reaction gives a *tertiary* carbocation, which is more stable than a secondary one. As a result, we find that the hydrogen of an acid that adds to a double bond in an alkene goes to the carbon that already has the greater number of hydrogens attached to it. More generally, electrophilic addition to an alkene double bond proceeds via the most stable intermediate carbocation. These (compatible) statements are summarized as **Markovnikov's Rule.**

Water can also act as an electrophile in an acidic solution, where hydrogen ions exist as H_3O^+:

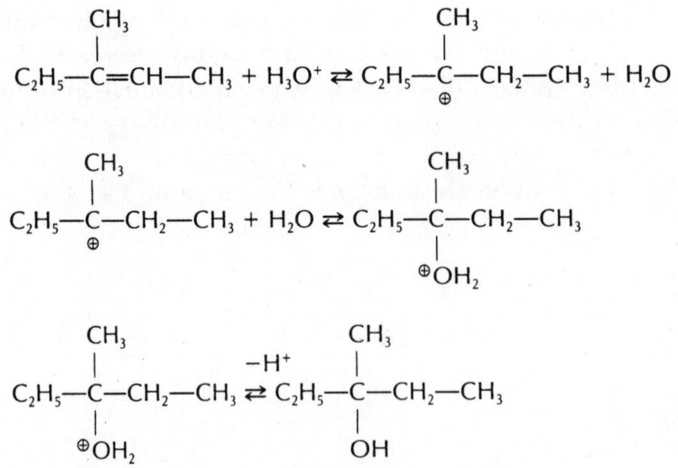

$C_2H_5\!-\!\overset{\overset{\displaystyle CH_3}{|}}{C}\!=\!CH\!-\!CH_3 + H_3O^+ \rightleftarrows C_2H_5\!-\!\overset{\overset{\displaystyle CH_3}{|}}{\underset{\oplus}{C}}\!-\!CH_2\!-\!CH_3 + H_2O$

$C_2H_5\!-\!\overset{\overset{\displaystyle CH_3}{|}}{\underset{\oplus}{C}}\!-\!CH_2\!-\!CH_3 + H_2O \rightleftarrows C_2H_5\!-\!\overset{\overset{\displaystyle CH_3}{|}}{\underset{\underset{\displaystyle \oplus OH_2}{|}}{C}}\!-\!CH_2\!-\!CH_3$

$C_2H_5\!-\!\overset{\overset{\displaystyle CH_3}{|}}{\underset{\underset{\displaystyle \oplus OH_2}{|}}{C}}\!-\!CH_2\!-\!CH_3 \overset{-H^+}{\rightleftarrows} C_2H_5\!-\!\overset{\overset{\displaystyle CH_3}{|}}{\underset{\underset{\displaystyle OH}{|}}{C}}\!-\!CH_2\!-\!CH_3$

C. Aromatic Compounds

Description

An aromatic compound, of which benzene is the most familiar example, is planar, contains one or more rings, and has delocalized π electrons numbering $4n + 2$ (**Hückel Rule**). The π cloud gives rise to an extra stability described below. Benzene itself is insoluble in water, although substituted benzenes containing polar groups can dissolve in water. Benzene and other aromatics have higher melting points than nonaromatic compounds of similar atomic weights, a fact explained by their ability to pack efficiently into crystals.

Resonance Energy and Delocalization

An early description of benzene utilized two equivalent resonance structures:

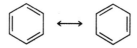

Rather than implying a rapid equilibrium, this resonance model is meant to suggest that each bond is equivalent and has properties midway between those of a single and a double bond. Yet benzene does not react as an alkene—e.g., it fails to react with Br_2. When H_2 is added to it, it will react to form cyclohexane, just as the 6-membered alkene cyclohexene does. Because the enthalpy of hydrogenation of cyclohexene, with its one double bond, is 120 kJ/mol, we might expect that benzene, which according to the resonance structures above has three double bonds, would release 360 kJ/mol on hydrogenation. Instead, the measured value is only 208 kJ/mol; thus, benzene is far more stable, by 152 kJ/mol, than an alkene having three double bonds. This increased stability is referred to as **resonance energy.**

The molecular orbital description of benzene shows it to be planar, with a sigma framework of overlapping sp^2 orbitals on each carbon atom. Each atom has one unused p orbital, which points in and out of the plane of the molecule. These orbitals overlap to form a continuous pi-bonded system that encircles the molecule above and below the plane. The six pi electrons are said to be **delocalized** since they no longer are restricted to motion in the vicinity of individual carbon atoms.

By use of pi molecular orbitals constructed from linear combinations of the original atomic p orbitals, we can calculate energy levels for the benzene molecule. All six of the pi electrons are found to be in bonding orbitals, a result consistent with benzene's high resonance energy. Similar delocalization of electrons, with consequent stability, is found for other aromatic molecules.

PRACTICE PROBLEMS
SECTIONS 10.1 AND 10.2

1. Hybrid orbitals form

   A. sigma bonds only.
   B. pi bonds only.
   C. sigma and pi bonds.
   D. lone-pair orbitals and sigma bonds.

2. As the multiplicity of bonds increase, the

   A. bond energies increase and bond lengths decrease.
   B. bond energies and lengths both decrease.
   C. bond energies and lengths both increase.
   D. bond energies decrease and bond lengths increase.

3. Which of the following statements is untrue about enantiomers?

   A. Enantiomers are pairs of compounds that are mirror images of each other.
   B. Enantiomers are also structural isomers.
   C. Enantiomers have one or more chiral atoms.
   D. Enantiomers are optically active.

4. Which of the following statements is untrue about diastereomers?

   A. Diastereomers are not mirror images.
   B. Diastereomers are not structural isomers.
   C. Diastereomers include geometric isomers and conformational isomers.
   D. Diastereomers can never have chiral carbon atoms.

5. A racemic mixture of 2-bromobutane contains

   A. the R enantiomer only.
   B. the S enantiomer only.
   C. equal amounts of the (+) and (−) optical isomers.
   D. only diastereomers.

6. Alkenes differ from alkanes in that

   A. they are more reactive.
   B. they can have geometrical isomers and alkanes cannot.
   C. they undergo halogenation and alkanes do not.
   D. None of the above.

7. 1-butene undergoes electrophilic addition with HCl. The main product is

   A. 1-chlorobutane.
   B. 2-chlorobutane.
   C. 1,1-chlorobutane.
   D. 1-butyne.

8. What is always true about an aromatic compound?

   A. It contains only carbon and hydrogen atoms.
   B. It undergoes addition reactions at room temperature.
   C. It has delocalized electrons.
   D. It has cis and trans isomers.

ANSWER KEY

1. D 2. A 3. B 4. D 5. C 6. A 7. B 8. C

ANSWERS AND EXPLANATIONS

1. **The correct answer is (D).** Hybrid orbitals around central atoms overlap with orbitals of bonding atoms along the internuclear axis to form sigma bonds. Non-bonding or lone-pair electrons occupy hybrid orbitals of the central atom.

2. **The correct answer is (A).** Single bonds contain one sigma bond while double and triple bonds have one and two pi bonds, respectively, in addition to the sigma bond. The energy required to break these bonds, i.e., the bond dissociation energy, increases as the number of bonds increases. As the number of bonds between atoms increases, the atoms are pulled closer together and the bond length decreases.

3. **The correct answer is (B).** Structural isomers have the same formula but the atoms are bonded to each other in a different sequence. Enantiomers are stereoisomers that have the same order of atoms.

4. **The correct answer is (D).** Diastereomers are stereoisomers that are not mirror images. They can have more than one chiral atom and have superimposable mirror images, as in meso compounds. 2,3-dichlorobutane, for example, has a meso structure (diastereomer) along with a pair of optically active enantiomers.

5. **The correct answer is (C).** A racemic mixture does not rotate the plane of polarized light because it contains equal amounts of enantiomers. One enantiomer rotates polarized light clockwise (dextrorotary), while its nonsuperimposable mirror image rotates the plane of polarized light in the opposite direction (levorotary) by the same angle.

6. **The correct answer is (A).** Alkenes contain one or more pi bonds, which makes them more reactive than saturated compounds. They typically undergo electrophilic addition reactions because of the electron-rich pi bond.

7. **The correct answer is (B).** Markovnikov's Rule indicates that the H of the electrophile will bond to the carbon atom already attached to most hydrogen atoms. Thus, the chloro group will bond to carbon-2 in the compound, the atom connected to the least number of hydrogen atoms.

8. **The correct answer is (C).** Aromatic compounds have $4n+2$ delocalized electrons. Nitrogen atoms, for example, can also participate in the ring, as in pyridine. Because the ring or rings are flat, cis and trans isomers do not exist. Aromatic compounds tend to undergo substitution reactions so as to maintain the stable aromatic character of the rings.

10.3 OXYGEN-CONTAINING COMPOUNDS

A. ALCOHOLS

General Principles

The general formula of an alcohol is ROH where R is an alkyl group (or substituted alkyl group). Alcohols are categorized as primary (1°), secondary (2°), or tertiary (3°). Some examples are:

$CH_3CH_2CH_2OH$ —OH bound to a carbon, which is attached to only one other carbon

propanol (1°)
(n-propyl alcohol)

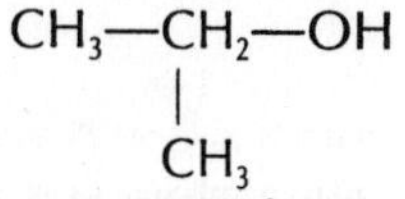

CH_3—CH_2—OH   —OH bound to a C, which is attached to two C's
|
CH_3

isopropanol (2°)
(isopropyl alcohol)

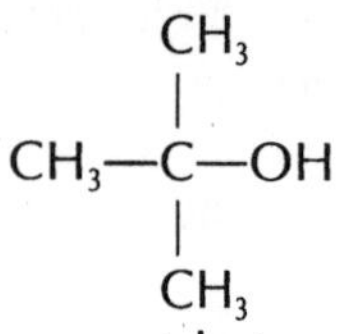

CH_3
|
CH_3—C—OH   —OH bound to a C, which is attached to three C's
|
CH_3

t-butanol (3°)
(t-butyl alcohol)

The basic properties of alcohols are due to the —OH functional group. These properties can vary, however, depending on the nature of R.

Physical Properties

The —OH group in alcohols is hydrophilic mostly due to its tendency to hydrogen bond with water:

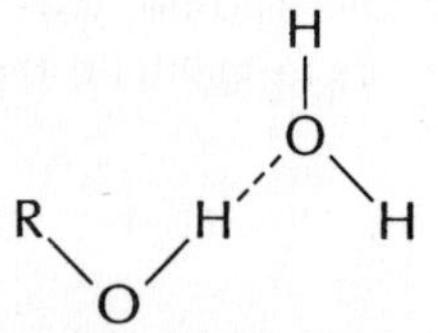

Thus, light alcohols in particular have high solubilities (miscible with water) in aqueous solution. As the R group increases, the hydrophobic (lipophilic) moiety grows in size and the solubility in water of the alcohol decreases.

Boiling points of alcohols increase with increasing molecular weights and decrease with increased branching. Alcohols, however, have markedly higher boiling points than hydrocarbons, ethers, or addehydes of the same molecular weight because of intermolecular hydrogen-bonding:

$$R-O\underset{H}{\overset{H-O^{\diagup R}}{\diagup}}$$

Some Chemical Properties

Alcohols as Bases

Like water, alcohols contain O with unshared electrons, which make them able to accept protons from acids:

$$\underset{\text{base}}{R-\overset{..}{\underset{..}{O}}-H} + \underset{\text{acid}}{H^+} \rightleftharpoons R-\overset{\overset{\displaystyle H}{|}}{\underset{\underset{\oplus}{..}}{O}}-H$$

Alcohols are about as basic as water. They also accept protons from carbocations, bringing about elimination reactions.

Alcohols as Acids

Alcohols are weaker acids than water

$$RO^\ominus + \underset{\substack{\text{stronger}\\\text{acid}}}{H-O-H} \rightarrow OH^- + \underset{\substack{\text{weaker}\\\text{acid}}}{ROH}$$

but they're stronger than NH_3.

$$NH_2^- + \underset{\substack{\text{stronger}\\\text{acid}}}{R-O-H} \rightarrow NH_3 + \underset{\substack{\text{weaker}\\\text{acid}}}{RO^-}$$

Relative Acidities
$$H_2O > ROH > NH_3 > RH$$

Alcohols as Nucleophiles

Alcohols are nucleophilic due to their unshared electrons and can thus participate in substitution reactions (S_N2 and S_N1).

Important Reactions

Dehydration of Alcohols

An alcohol loses a molecule of water to form an alkene in dehydration reactions:

$$\underset{\substack{|\ \ |\\H\ \ OH\\\text{alcohol}}}{-C-C-} \underset{\text{heat}}{\overset{\text{acid}}{\rightarrow}} \underset{\text{alkene}}{-C=C-} + H_2O$$

Tertiary alcohols undergo dehydration readily. For 3° and 2° alcohols, the mechanism is:

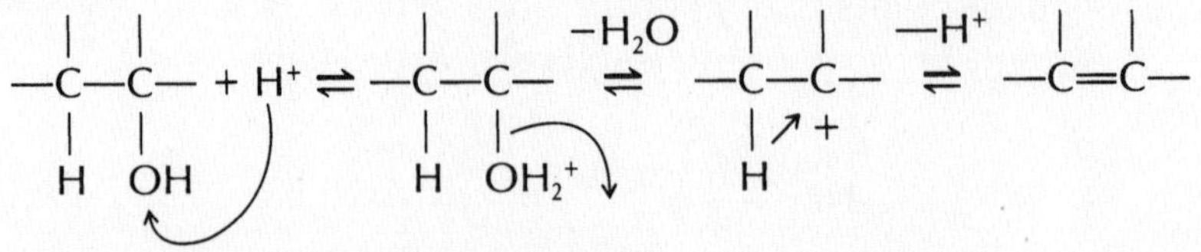

The acid converts —OH into a good leaving group so that a carbocation is formed giving rise to an E1 elimination reaction. (E1 elimination involves a carbocation intermediate, and its rate depends only on the concentration of the substrate.)

Where more than one alkene can be formed, the preferred product is the more stable one (the one with the most alkyl groups attached to the $\text{C}{=}\text{C}$).

For example,

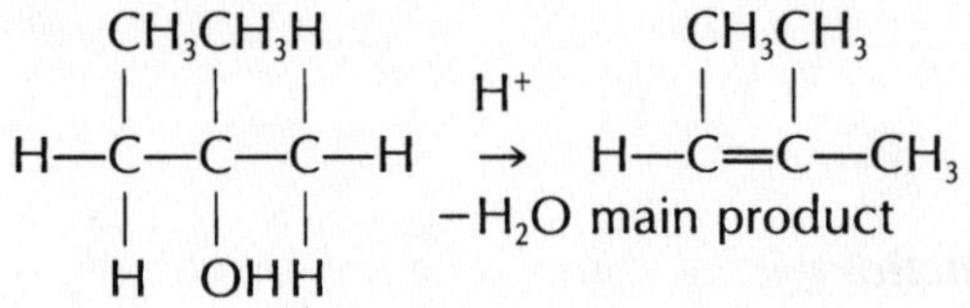

A phenyl group is preferred over one or two alkyl groups:

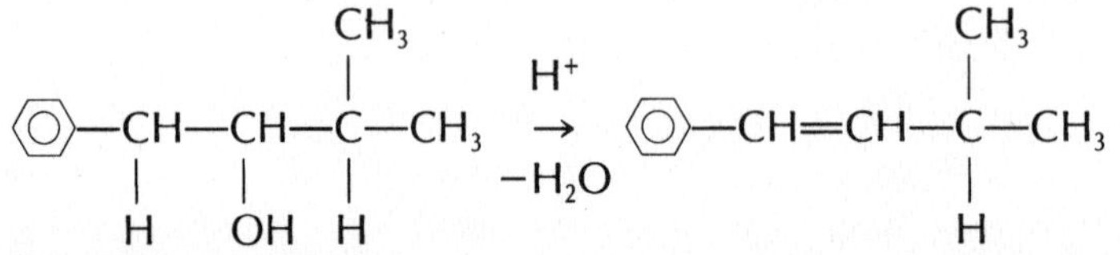

Substitution Reactions

Reactions of an alcohol can involve the cleavage of the C—OH bond in which another nucleophile joins with the carbon. This is a substitution reaction. Note that the —OH is a poor leaving group so that protonation usually occurs first. Substitution reactions can follow two paths: S_N1—Nucleophilic Substitution of 1st order, or S_N2—Nucleophilic Substitution of 2nd order.

S_N1 Substitution Reaction

The S_N1 substitution reaction is characterized by the following:

- first-order kinetics (rate depends only on concentration of substrate, not the concentration of the attacking nucleophile)

- the reactivity is very dependent on the nature of the R group:

  $3° > 2° > 1° > CH_3L$ (L = leaving group)

- racemization (enantiomers formed in equal concentration) because a carbocation is planar around the positively charged site so that attack by a nucleophile is equally probable from either side, giving rise to equal concentrations of enantiomers

- rearrangement can occur, giving rise to the most stable carbocation intermediate

Examples of S_N1 reactions where alcohols are the substrate include

$$
\begin{array}{ccc}
& CH_3 & & CH_3 \\
& | & HCl & | \\
CH_3-C-CH_3 & \rightarrow & CH_3-C-CH_3 \\
& | & room & | \\
& OH & temperature & Cl
\end{array}
$$

where the mechanism involves a carbocation intermediate.

$$ROH + HX \rightleftharpoons ROH_2^+ + X^-$$

$$ROH_2^+ \rightleftharpoons R^+ + H_2O$$

$$R^+ + X^- \rightarrow RX$$

$$
\begin{array}{ccc}
CH_3H & & CH_3H \\
| \ | & HCl & | \ | \\
CH_3-C-C-CH_3 & \rightarrow & CH_3-C-C-CH_3 \\
| \ | & & | \ | \\
CH_3OH & & Cl \ CH_3
\end{array}
$$

(Note the rearrangement.)

S_N2 Substitution Reactions

The S_N2 substitution reaction has the following characteristics:

- second-order kinetics (the rate of reaction is dependent on the concentration of both the substrate and the nucleophile)

- the reactivity is also dependent on the nature of R but with the less substituted R groups being most favored by this mechanism:

    $$CH_3L > 1° > 2° > 3°$$

- an inversion of configuration occurs if the reacting alcohol is optically active

- rearrangement does not occur: the attacking nucleophile joins the carbon once bonded to the leaving group

Examples of S_N2 reactions are

$$CH_3OH + H^+ \rightleftharpoons CH_3OH_2^+$$

$$CH_3OH_2^+ + Cl^- \rightarrow [^{\delta-}Cl\text{---}CH_3\text{---}OH_2^{\delta+}] \rightarrow ClCH_3 + H_2O$$
$$\text{transition state}$$

The mechanism can be shown as

$$CH_3OH + H^+ \rightleftharpoons CH_3OH_2^+$$

$$CH_3OH_2^+ + Cl^- \rightarrow [^{\delta-}Cl\text{--}CH_3\text{---}OH_2^{\delta+}] \rightarrow ClCH_3 + H_2O$$
$$\text{transition state}$$

B. Aldehydes and Ketones

Aldehydes and ketones contain the carbonyl C=O group that, for the most part, determines their general properties. Their general formulas are:

aldehyde ketone

R and R′ can be aliphatic or aromatic groups. Some examples are:

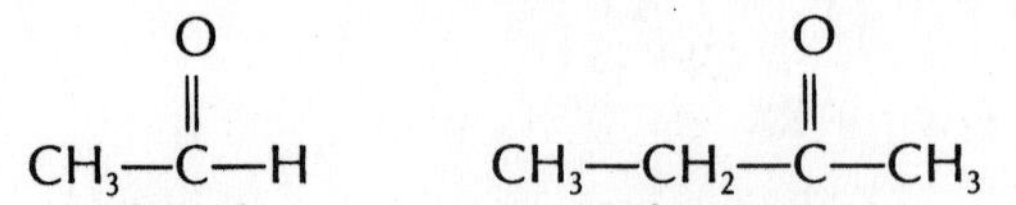

ethanal (acetaldehyde) 2-butanone (methyl ethyl ketone)

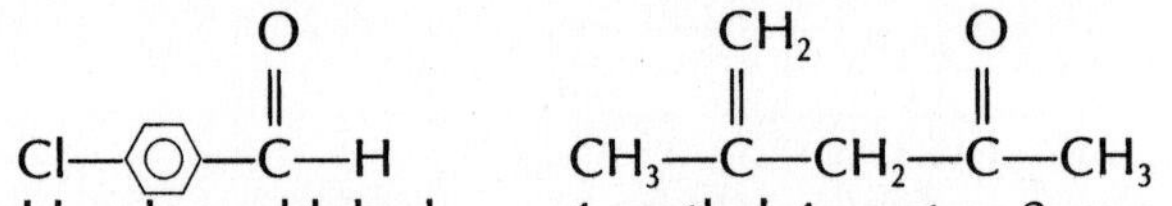

p-chlorobenzaldehyde 4-methyl-4-penten-2-one

The IUPAC system of naming ketones replaces the e of the corresponding alkane by one for ketones and by al for aldehydes.

General Principles

The carbonyl group is the site of *nucleophilic addition* and also serves to increase the acidity of a hydrogen. The mechanism is

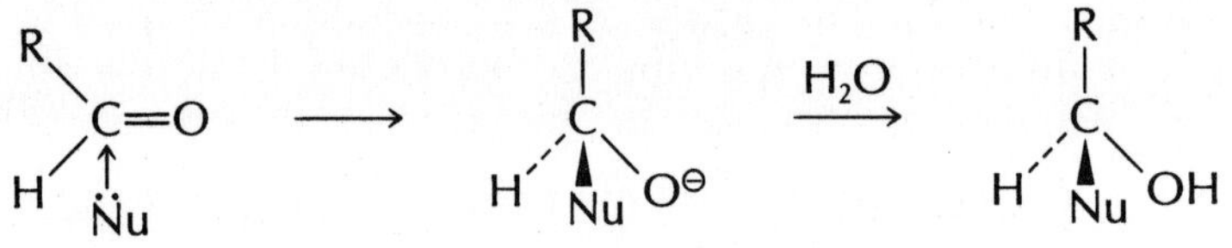

Trigonal planar Tetrahedral

Note that the nucleophilic additions are catalyzed by H^+ because the protonated aldehyde or ketone undergoes nucleophilic attack more readily.

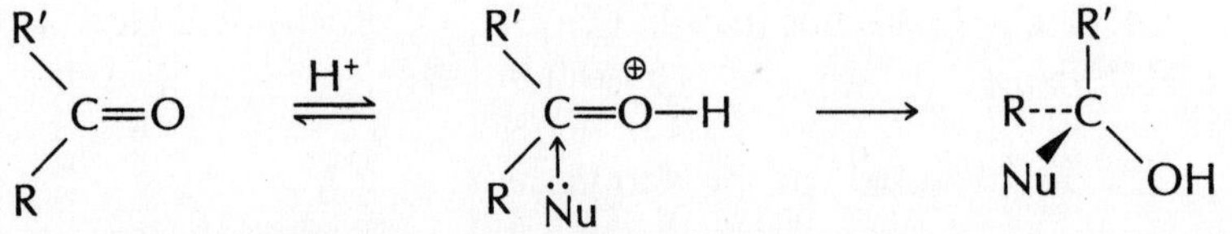

Effect of Substituents on Reactivity

Aldehydes generally undergo nucleophilic addition more readily than ketones due to both steric and electronic effects. The additional R group in the ketone increases crowding in the transition state as well as intensifies the negative charge on the oxygen. As a rule, larger R groups decrease reactivity to nucleophilic addition.

Aryl groups tend to deactivate aldehydes and ketones due to resonance stabilization of the reactant:

$$\text{\large\textcircled{+}} \; \bigotimes - = \overset{\overset{\displaystyle H}{|}}{C} - O^{\ominus}$$

Note: There are two other structures.

Acidity of α-Hydrogen Atoms

The carbonyl moiety makes the α-hydrogens acidic so that they can be abstracted by bases to form carbanions:

$$CH_3 - \underset{\underset{\displaystyle H}{|}}{\overset{\overset{\displaystyle \alpha}{|}}{C}H} - \overset{\overset{\displaystyle O}{\|}}{C} - H \; \underset{}{\overset{OH^-}{\rightleftharpoons}} \; [CH_3 - CH - CHO]^-$$

carbanion

The carbanion forms because it is resonance stabilized.

$$CH_3 - \underset{\underset{\displaystyle \ominus}{..}}{CH} - \overset{\overset{\displaystyle O}{\|}}{C} - H \leftrightarrow CH_3 - CH = \overset{\overset{\displaystyle O^{\ominus}}{|}}{C} - H$$

α-Hydrogen atoms located between two carbonyl groups show greater acidity due to greater resonance stabilization (more resonance structures can be drawn).

Reactivity of α-β Unsaturated Carbonyls

The β position of $\overset{\overset{\displaystyle O}{\|}}{\underset{\underset{\displaystyle \beta \quad \alpha}{}}{-CH=CH-C-}}$ is the site of attack by a nucleophile in addition reactions because of resonance stabilization of the resulting carbanion.

$$\overset{Nu:}{\underset{\underset{\displaystyle |}{}}{-\overset{\downarrow}{C}=CH-}}\overset{\overset{\displaystyle O}{\|}}{C-} \rightarrow \left[\overset{\overset{\displaystyle Nu}{|}}{\underset{\underset{\displaystyle |}{}}{-C-}}\underset{\underset{\displaystyle ..}{\overset{\displaystyle \ominus}{}}}{CH}\overset{\overset{\displaystyle O}{\|}}{C-} \leftrightarrow \overset{\overset{\displaystyle Nu}{|}}{\underset{\underset{\displaystyle |}{}}{-C-}}CH=\overset{\overset{\displaystyle O^{\ominus}}{|}}{C-} \right]$$

Important Reactions: Nucleophilic Addition

Nucleophiles that add to aldehydes and ketones include alcohols to form acetals and ketals, carbanions in aldol condensations, and derivatives of ammonia to form imines.

Addition of ROH

$$\underset{/}{\overset{\backslash}{}}C=O + ROH \rightleftharpoons \overset{\overset{\displaystyle OH}{|}}{\underset{\underset{\displaystyle |}{}}{-C-}}OR \underset{H^+}{\overset{ROH}{\rightleftharpoons}} \overset{\overset{\displaystyle OH}{|}}{\underset{\underset{\displaystyle |}{}}{-C-}}OR$$

hemiacetal or hemiketal   acetal or ketal

Note that the product is formed through nucleophilic addition to $-\overset{\overset{\displaystyle O}{\|}}{C}-$ and then ether formation through a carbocation (S_N1).

Aldol Condensation: Addition of Carbanions

In the presence of a base, two molecules of aldehyde or ketone can combine to form a β-hydroxyaldehyde or β-hydroxyketone. The aldehyde or ketone must, however, contain an α-H because a carbanion is the attacking nucleophile.

$$R—CH_2—\overset{\overset{\displaystyle O}{\|}}{C}—H + OH^- \rightleftharpoons R—\overset{\overset{\displaystyle O}{\|}}{\underset{\underset{\ominus}{..}}{C}H}—C—H + H_2O$$

carbanion

$$R—CH_2—\overset{\overset{\displaystyle O}{\|}}{C}—H \rightleftharpoons R—CH_2—\overset{\overset{\displaystyle O^\ominus}{|}}{\underset{\underset{R—CH—CHO}{|}}{C}}—H \overset{H_2O}{\rightleftharpoons} R—CH_2—\overset{\overset{\displaystyle OH}{|}}{CH}—\overset{\overset{\displaystyle}{|}}{\underset{\underset{R}{|}}{CH}}—\overset{\overset{\displaystyle O}{\|}}{C}—H$$

$$\underset{R—\overset{\underset{\ominus}{\underset{..}{}}}{C}H—\overset{\overset{\displaystyle O}{\|}}{C}—H}{}$$

Addition of Ammonia Derivatives

Some ammonia derivatives add to the carbonyl group to form products that are used to identify the aldehyde or ketone. A carbon-nitrogen double bond is formed from the elimination of water.

$$\overset{\diagdown}{\underset{\diagup}{C}}=O + H_2N—X \rightarrow \left[—\overset{\overset{\displaystyle |}{}}{\underset{\underset{OH}{|}}{C}}—NH—X \right] \rightarrow \overset{\diagdown}{\underset{\diagup}{C}}=N—X + H_2O$$

imine

Amines can be formed from aldehydes and ketones by a reduction in the presence of ammonia.

$$R—\overset{\overset{\displaystyle R'}{|}}{C}=O + NH_3 \rightarrow \left[R—\overset{\overset{\displaystyle R'}{|}}{C}=NH \right] \overset{H_2/Ni}{\rightarrow} R—\overset{\overset{\displaystyle R'}{|}}{C}—NH_2$$

amine

Primary amines react with carbonyl compounds to form N-substituted imines.

$$R—\overset{\overset{\displaystyle H}{|}}{C}=O + H_2NR' \rightarrow R—\overset{\overset{\displaystyle H}{|}}{\underset{\underset{OH}{|}}{C}}—NHR' \rightarrow R—\overset{\overset{\displaystyle H}{|}}{C}=NR'$$

imine

Note that dehydration occurs to give the imine product.

With a secondary amine R'_2NH, a similar addition product is formed.

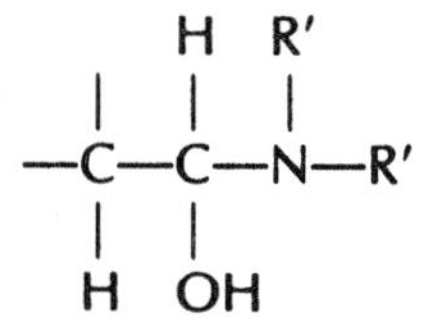

$$-\overset{\overset{\displaystyle H}{|}}{\underset{\underset{\displaystyle H}{|}}{C}}-\overset{\overset{\displaystyle R'}{|}}{\underset{\underset{\displaystyle OH}{|}}{C}}-N-R'$$

However, because there are no H's on N to permit elimination of water, an enamine is formed.

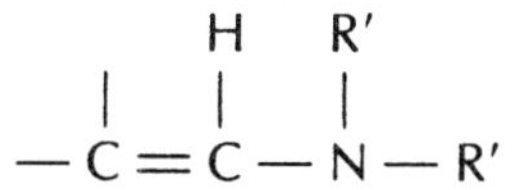

$$-C=\overset{\overset{\displaystyle H}{|}}{C}-\overset{\overset{\displaystyle R'}{|}}{N}-R'$$
enamine

Tautomers

Tautomers are compounds that are in rapid equilibrium and differ in their arrangement of atoms. The tautomers discussed below differ in the position of a hydrogen.

Keto-enol Tautomerism

When —OH is joined to —C=C—, an enol is formed that exists in equilibrium with a more stable keto structure:

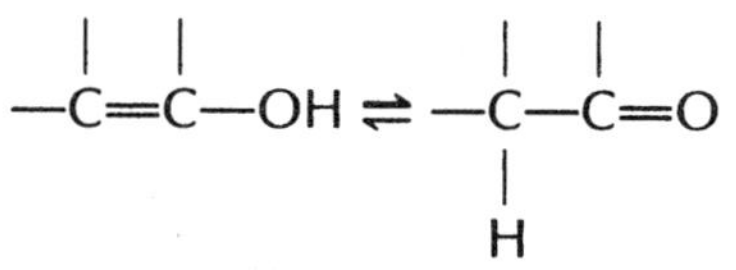

$$-\overset{|}{C}=\overset{|}{C}-OH \rightleftharpoons -\overset{|}{C}-\overset{|}{\underset{\underset{\displaystyle H}{|}}{C}}=O$$

enol   keto

Phenol is an exception: the enol form is more stable.

Enamine—imine tautomers

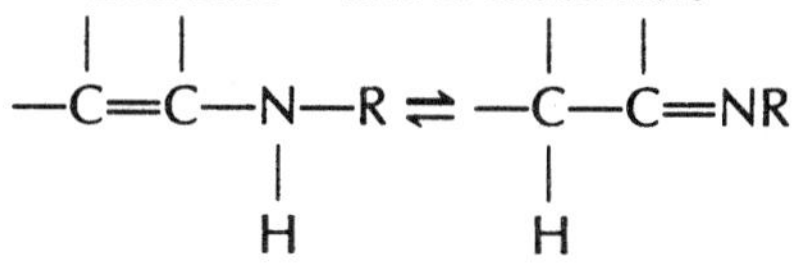

$$-\overset{|}{C}=\overset{|}{C}-\overset{|}{\underset{\underset{\displaystyle H}{|}}{N}}-R \rightleftharpoons -\overset{|}{C}-\overset{|}{\underset{\underset{\displaystyle H}{|}}{C}}=NR$$

enamine   imine

C. CARBOXYLIC ACIDS

Carboxylic acids are organic acids (weak acids) containing the carboxyl group

$$-\overset{\overset{\text{O}}{\|}}{\text{C}}-\text{O}-\text{H}.$$ Their general formula is $R-\overset{\overset{\text{O}}{\|}}{\text{C}}-\text{OH}$ where R can be an aliphatic or an aryl group. Some examples are:

$$\text{H}_3\text{C}-\overset{\overset{\text{CH}_3}{|}}{\text{CH}}-\text{CH}_2-\overset{\overset{\text{O}}{\|}}{\text{C}_4}-\text{OH}$$

3-methyl butanoic acid
(β-methylbutyric acid)

m-chlorobenzoic acid (with Cl and —COOH on ring)

$$\text{CH}_3-\overset{\overset{\text{Cl}}{|}}{\text{CH}}-\text{CH}_2-\text{CH}_2-\overset{\overset{\text{O}}{\|}}{\text{C}}-\text{OH}$$
4-chloropentanoic acid
(δ-chlorovaleric acid)

The IUPAC system replaces the -e of the root name of the alkane with -oic acid.

General Principles

The carboxyl group gives rise to the following properties.

Physical Properties

Boiling points are higher than expected based on molecular weight due to intermolecular H-bonding:

$$R-C\overset{\text{O}\cdots\text{H}-\text{O}}{\underset{\text{O}-\text{H}\cdots\text{O}}{}}C-R$$

They tend to be even higher than boiling points of alcohols. Low-molecular-weight carboxyl acids are very soluble in water due to H-bonding with water. As R gets larger, solubility decreases.

Chemical Properties of the Carboxyl Group

Acidity
The most characteristic property of carboxylic acids is their acidity

$$R-\overset{\overset{\text{O}}{\|}}{\text{C}}-\text{OH} \overset{\text{H}_2\text{O}}{\rightleftharpoons} R-\overset{\overset{\text{O}}{\|}}{\text{C}}-\text{O}^\ominus + \text{H}_3\text{O}^+$$
carboxylate anion

The reason for the acidic behavior of the hydrogen of the —OH in COOH is resonance stabilization of the anion.

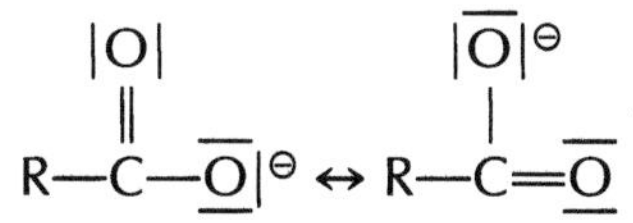

$$\underset{\substack{\| \\ R-C-\overline{O}|^{\ominus}}}{|O|} \leftrightarrow \underset{\substack{| \\ R-C=\overline{O}}}{|\overline{O}|^{\ominus}}$$

In an alcohol where an —OH is also present, there is no appreciable resonance stabilization of the conjugate base.

The nature of the R group affects the acidity of the carboxylic acid. Any substituent that stabilizes the anion of the carboxylic acid, i.e., electron-withdrawing, increases acidity; any substituent that destabilizes, i.e., intensifies charge or electron-donating, decreases acidity. Hence, halogens increase acidity through inductive effects. Their effect decreases the farther they are located from the carboxyl group. The following acids are listed in order of increasing acidity (increasing K_a's).

$$CH_3CH_2COOH < CH_3COOH < ClCH_2COOH < Cl_2CHCOOH < Cl_3CCOOH$$

Similar effects are seen with aromatic acids. Electron-withdrawing groups such as —Cl and —NO_2 strengthen benzoic acid while electron-releasing groups such as —CH_3, —OH, —OCH_3, and —NH_2 weaken the acid.

Nucleophilic Substitution
Carboxylic acids tend to undergo nucleophilic substitution reactions in which a

nucleophile replaces the $-\overset{\overset{\displaystyle O}{\|}}{C}-OH$. When these nucleophiles contain —Cl, —OR′, or —NH_2, they form acid chlorides, esters, and amides, respectively. Note that all

of the carboxylic acid derivatives contain the acyl group $R-\overset{\overset{\displaystyle O}{\|}}{C}-$.

Important Reactions

Conversion into Acid Derivatives

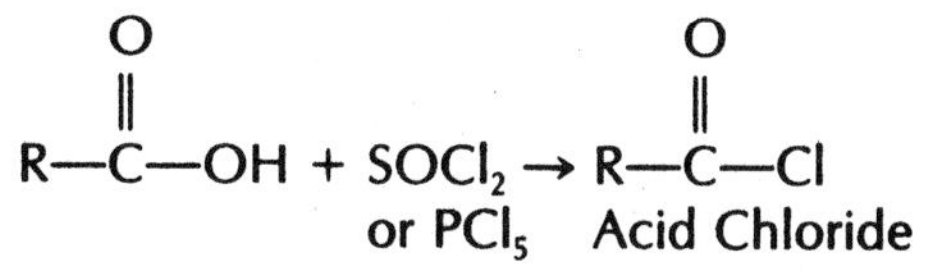

$$R-\overset{\overset{\displaystyle O}{\|}}{C}-OH + SOCl_2 \rightarrow R-\overset{\overset{\displaystyle O}{\|}}{C}-Cl$$
$$\text{or } PCl_5 \quad \text{Acid Chloride}$$

Acid chlorides are very reactive and are often used to synthesize the other acid derivatives.

Conversion into Esters

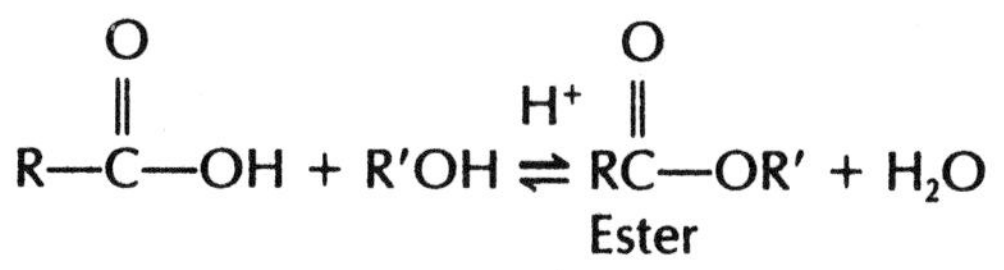

$$R-\overset{\overset{\displaystyle O}{\|}}{C}-OH + R'OH \underset{}{\overset{H^+}{\rightleftharpoons}} RC-OR' + H_2O$$
$$\text{Ester}$$

Note the above reaction is catalyzed by H^+.

Bulky groups present near the site of the reaction either on the acid or alcohol slow the rate of esterification.

Conversion to Amides

Amides are usually formed from the acid chloride.

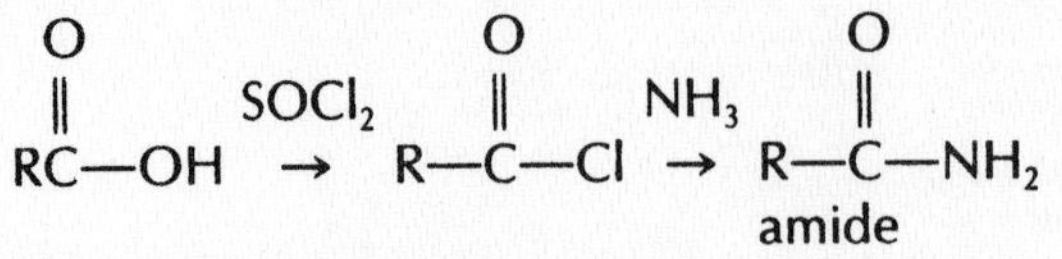

$$\underset{RC-OH}{\overset{\overset{\displaystyle O}{\|}}{}} \quad \xrightarrow{SOCl_2} \quad \underset{R-C-Cl}{\overset{\overset{\displaystyle O}{\|}}{}} \quad \xrightarrow{NH_3} \quad \underset{\underset{amide}{R-C-NH_2}}{\overset{\overset{\displaystyle O}{\|}}{}}$$

Reduction to Alcohols

$LiAlH_4$ can reduce R-COOH to RCH_2OH. Aldehydes, RCHO, are also reduced to RCH_2OH and are also easily oxidized to the carboxylic acid.

Decarboxylation Reactions

Decarboxylation reactions often involve β-diacids or β-ketoacids.

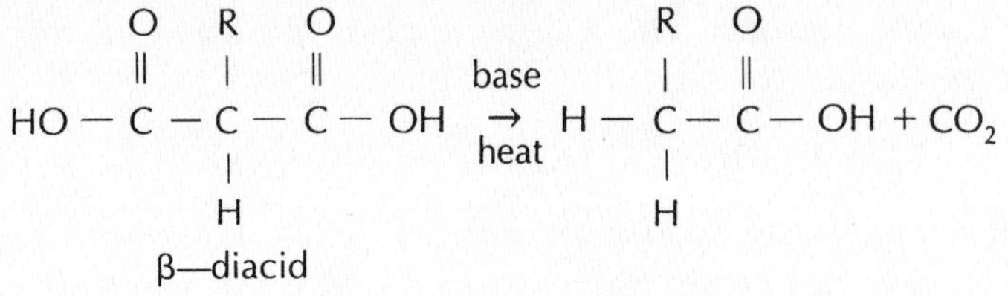

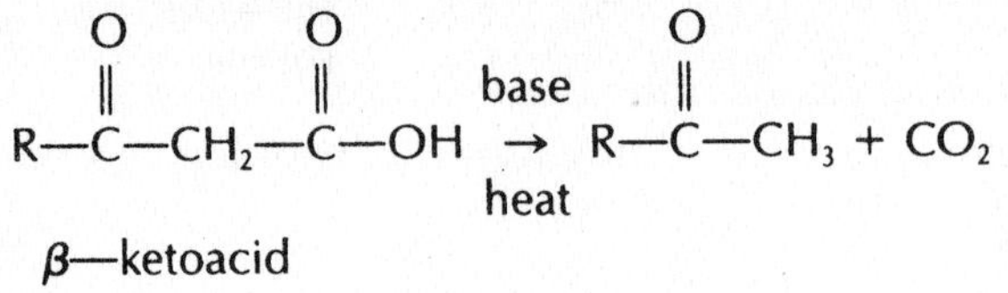

$$\underset{\text{β—diacid}}{HO-\overset{\overset{\displaystyle O}{\|}}{C}-\underset{\underset{\displaystyle H}{|}}{\overset{\overset{\displaystyle R}{|}}{C}}-\overset{\overset{\displaystyle O}{\|}}{C}-OH} \quad \xrightarrow[heat]{base} \quad H-\underset{\underset{\displaystyle H}{|}}{\overset{\overset{\displaystyle R}{|}}{C}}-\overset{\overset{\displaystyle O}{\|}}{C}-OH + CO_2$$

$$\underset{\text{β—ketoacid}}{R-\overset{\overset{\displaystyle O}{\|}}{C}-CH_2-\overset{\overset{\displaystyle O}{\|}}{C}-OH} \quad \xrightarrow[heat]{base} \quad R-\overset{\overset{\displaystyle O}{\|}}{C}-CH_3 + CO_2$$

D. COMMON ACID DERIVATIVES

These are acid chlorides, amides, esters, and anhydrides. The formula for acetic anhydride, the most common anhydride, is

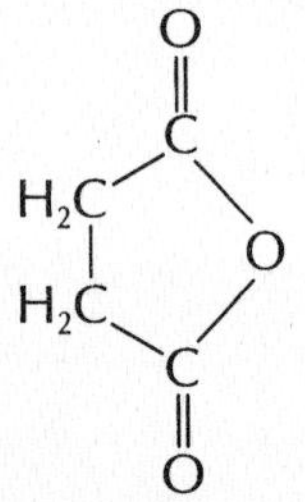

$$\underset{H_2C}{\overset{}{}}\underset{H_2C}{\overset{C=O}{}}\underset{C}{\overset{}{}}\underset{\displaystyle O}{\overset{}{}}$$

Important Reactions

Esters

Conversion into acids

Hydrolysis

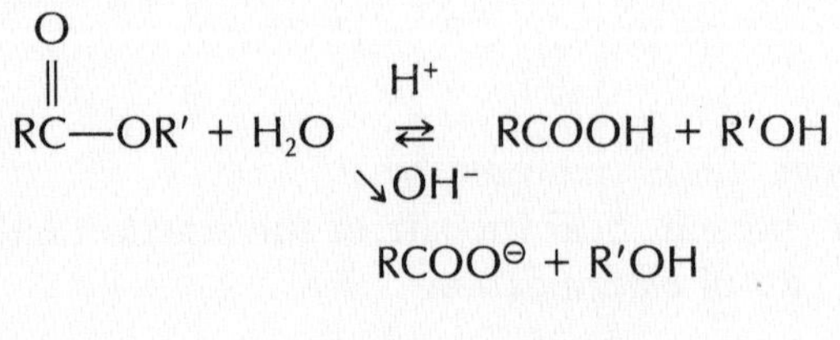

$$\underset{RC-OR' + H_2O}{\overset{\overset{\displaystyle O}{\|}}{}} \quad \underset{\searrow OH^-}{\overset{H^+}{\rightleftarrows}} \quad RCOOH + R'OH$$

$$RCOO^{\ominus} + R'OH$$

In the basic hydrolysis, the hydroxide ion attacks the carbonyl carbon forming

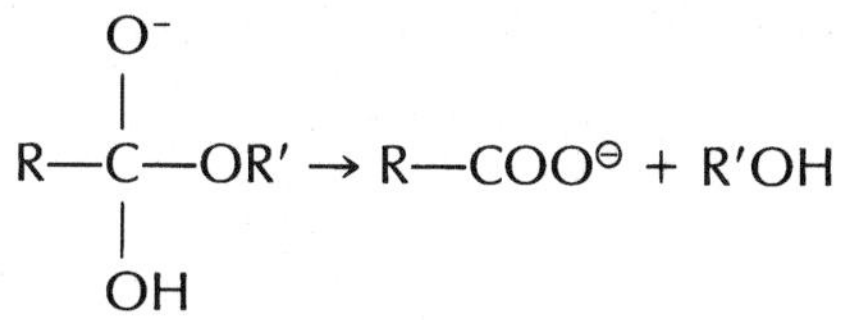

$$\underset{\underset{\displaystyle OH}{|}}{\overset{\overset{\displaystyle O^-}{|}}{R-C-OR'}} \rightarrow R-COO^{\ominus} + R'OH$$

In the above reaction, cleavage occurs between oxygen and the acyl group.

In acidic hydrolysis, the H^+ attaches to the carbonyl oxygen making the carbonyl more susceptible to nucleophilic attack ($H-O-H$) because the oxygen can absorb the π electrons without accepting a negative charge.

Saponification is the base catalyzed hydrolysis of esters such as fats. Fats are esters of fatty acids.

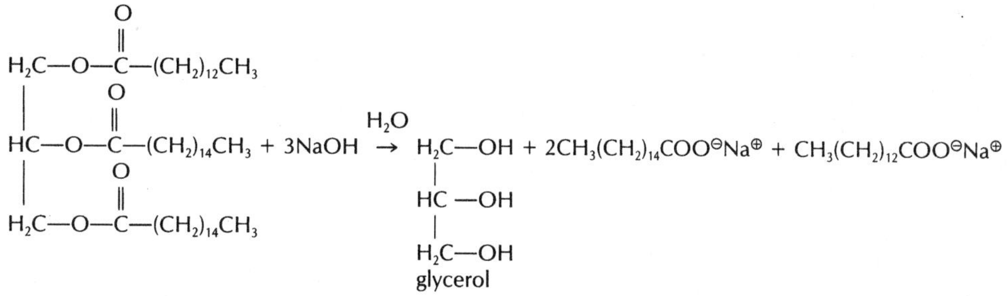

$$\begin{array}{l} H_2C-O-\overset{\overset{\displaystyle O}{\|}}{C}-(CH_2)_{12}CH_3 \\ | \qquad\qquad \overset{\displaystyle O}{\|} \\ HC-O-\overset{}{C}-(CH_2)_{14}CH_3 + 3NaOH \xrightarrow{H_2O} H_2C-OH + 2CH_3(CH_2)_{14}COO^{\ominus}Na^{\oplus} + CH_3(CH_2)_{12}COO^{\ominus}Na^{\oplus} \\ | \qquad\qquad \overset{\displaystyle O}{\|} \qquad\qquad\qquad\qquad\qquad | \\ H_2C-O-\overset{}{C}-(CH_2)_{14}CH_3 \qquad\qquad\qquad\qquad HC-OH \\ \qquad\qquad\qquad\qquad\qquad\qquad\qquad\qquad | \\ \qquad\qquad\qquad\qquad\qquad\qquad\qquad\qquad H_2C-OH \\ \qquad\qquad\qquad\qquad\qquad\qquad\qquad\qquad glycerol \end{array}$$

The sodium salts of fatty acids produced by saponification of fats or oils are soap. The above triester is called a triglyceride because all three —OH groups of glycerol are esterified.

Ammonolysis of Esters

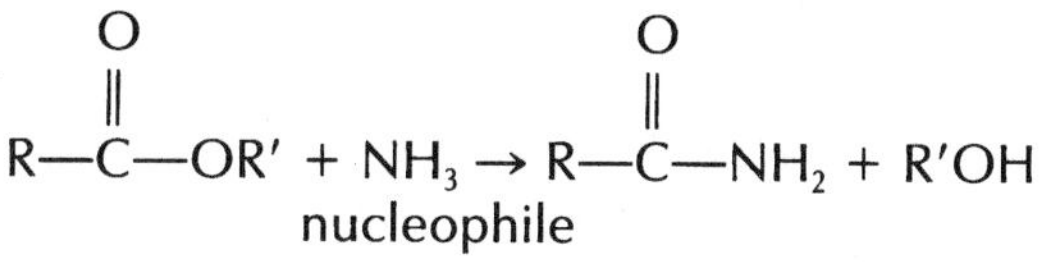

$$\underset{\displaystyle nucleophile}{\overset{\overset{\displaystyle O}{\|}}{R-C-OR'} + NH_3} \rightarrow \overset{\overset{\displaystyle O}{\|}}{R-C-NH_2} + R'OH$$

Transesterification

$$\underset{\displaystyle nucleophile}{\overset{\overset{\displaystyle O}{\|}}{R-C-OR'} + R''OH} \overset{H^+ \text{ or } R''O^{\ominus}}{\rightleftharpoons} RCOOR'' + R'OH$$

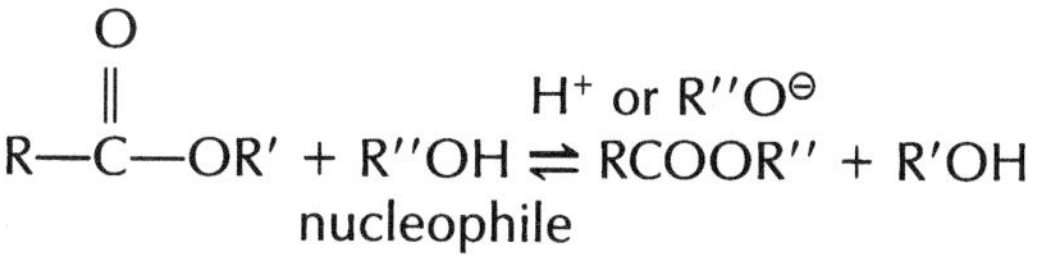

The above reaction is also called alcoholysis of an ester.

Amides

Hydrolysis

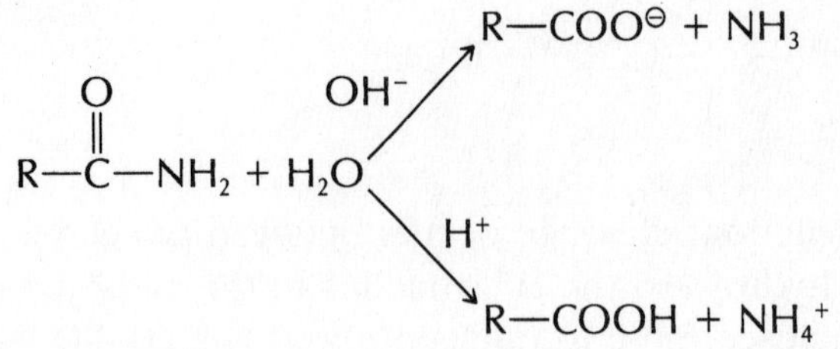

$$R-COO^{\ominus} + NH_3$$

$$R-\overset{\overset{\displaystyle O}{\|}}{C}-NH_2 + H_2O \underset{\underset{\displaystyle H^+}{\nearrow}}{\overset{\overset{\displaystyle OH^-}{\searrow}}{}}$$

$$R-COOH + NH_4^+$$

Again in basic hydrolysis, OH^- is the nucleophile while H_2O is the nucleophile in acidic hydrolysis.

Anhydrides

Hydrolysis

$$(CH_3CO)_2O + H_2O \rightarrow 2CH_3COOH$$

Ammonolysis: Conversion into Amides

$$(CH_3CO)_2O + 2NH_3 \rightarrow CH_3CONH_2 + CH_3COO^{\ominus}NH_4^{\oplus}$$
$$\text{acetamide}$$

Alcoholysis: Conversion into Esters

$$(CH_3CO)_2O + CH_3OH \rightarrow CH_3-\overset{\overset{\displaystyle O}{\|}}{C}-OCH_3 + CH_3COOH$$
$$\text{methyl acetate}$$

E. ETHERS

The general formula for an ether is

R—O—R′

where R or R′ (or both) can be an aliphatic or an aromatic group. Some examples are:

$CH_3CH_2OCH_2CH_3$
Diethyl ether

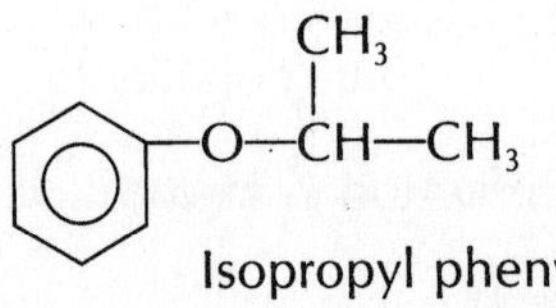

Isopropyl phenyl ether

Ethers are named by following the names of each group with ether.

Physical Properties

The C—O—C bond angle is about 110°

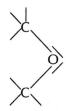

so that the ether molecule is weakly polar.

Hydrogen bonding between ether molecules is not possible (H bonded only to C), so that the boiling points of ethers are comparable to alkanes of similar molecular weights. Solubilities of ethers in water, however, are comparable to solubilities of alcohols because of H-bonding between H_2O and R—O—R′:

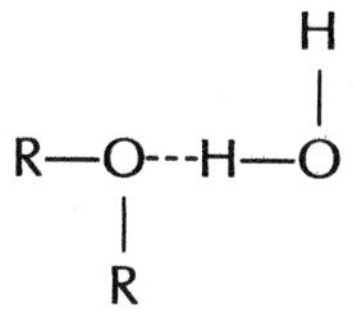

$$R—O\cdots H—O\overset{\displaystyle H}{\underset{\displaystyle R}{|}}$$

Chemical Properties: Cleavage by Acids

Ethers are fairly unreactive. The ether linkage, C—O—C, is resistant to attack by bases, oxidizing, and reducing agents. Ethers, however, undergo cleavage by acids.

The reaction is

$$R—O—R' \overset{HX}{\rightarrow} RX + R'OH \overset{HX}{\rightarrow} R'—X$$

Reactivity increases according to HCl < HBr < HI.

Note that the above reaction generally occurs only under rigorous conditions: concentrated acids and high temperatures.

The mechanism involves the initial protonation of the ether followed by nucleophilic attack of X^- in an S_N1 or S_N2 substitution reaction:

$$R—O—R' + HX \rightleftarrows R—\overset{\displaystyle H}{\underset{\displaystyle \oplus}{O}}—R' + X^- \overset{S_N1 \text{ or}}{\underset{S_N2}{\rightarrow}} RX + R'OH$$

A tertiary alkyl group (R) tends to undergo an S_N1 reaction while a primary alkyl group tends to undergo an S_N2 substitution reaction.

F. PHENOLS

The general formula of phenols is ArOH where Ar can be phenyl, a substituted phenyl group, or one of the other aromatic groups. Phenols differ from alcohols because the —OH group is joined directly to an aromatic ring. As a result, many of the properties of phenols differ markedly from those of alcohols.

Physical Properties

H-bonding is thought to account for the high boiling points of the *simple* phenols, which are liquids or solids. H-bonding between water and phenol itself accounts for its solubility. However, most other phenols are insoluble in water. O-Nitrophenol exhibits a low boiling point and solubility in water due to intramolecular H-bonding.

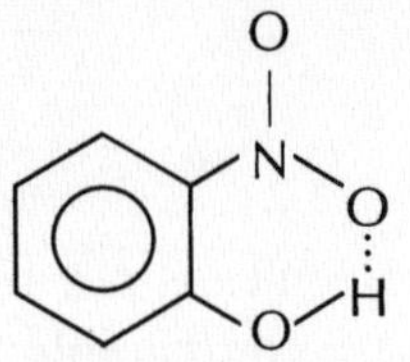

Chemical Properties: Acidity of Phenols

Phenols are stronger acids than water and alcohols but weaker than carboxylic acids. Their K_a values are about 10^{-10}. They undergo the following reactions:

$$ArOH + OH^- \rightarrow ArO^- + H_2O$$
stronger acid   weaker acid

$$ArO^- + RCOOH \rightarrow ArOH + RCOO^-$$
        stronger acid

Resonance stabilization of the phenoxide anion accounts for the acidity of phenol relative to an alcohol.

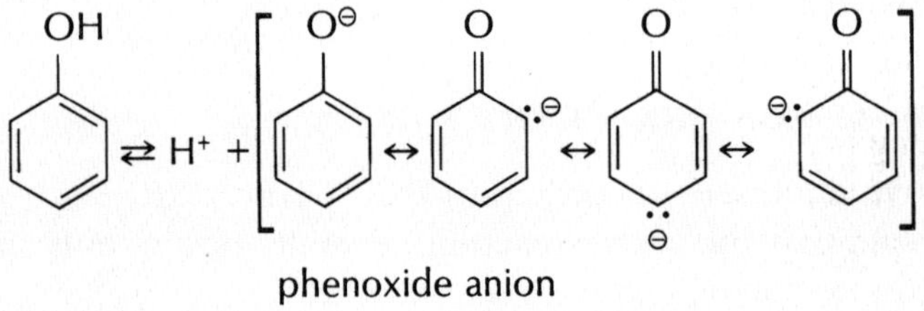

phenoxide anion

These structures show how the negative charge on the O is delocalized onto the ring.

Substituents affect the acidity of phenols as they do the acidity of carboxylic acids. Electron-attracting groups disperse the negative charge of the phenoxide anion, increasing acidity. These groups include $-NO_2$ and $-X$. Electron-releasing groups such as $-CH_3$ intensify the negative charge of the ion, decreasing acidity.

10.4 AMINES

A. DESCRIPTION

Amines are alkyl or aryl derivatives of NH_3. The general formulas of amines are $RNH_2(1°)$, $R_2NH(2°)$, or $R_3N(3°)$ where R is any alkyl or aryl group. Amines are classified as primary (1°), secondary (2°), or tertiary (3°) according to the number of groups attached to N. Some examples are:

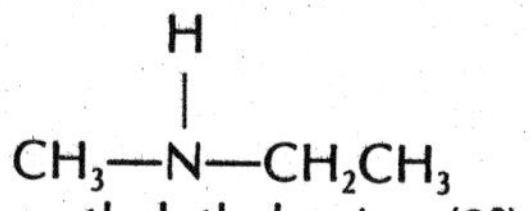

methylethylamine (2°)

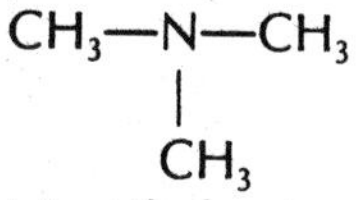

trimethylamine (3°)

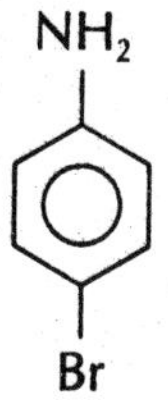

p-bromoaniline (1°)

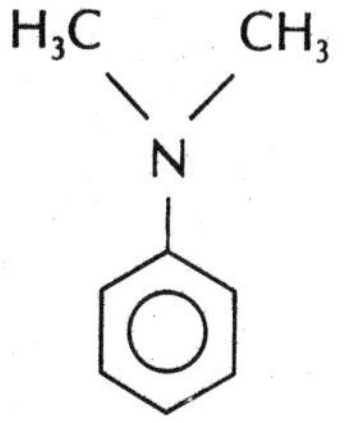

N, N-dimethylaniline (3°)

Replacing the 4H's of NH_4^+ with R gives a quaternary salt (4°) such as:

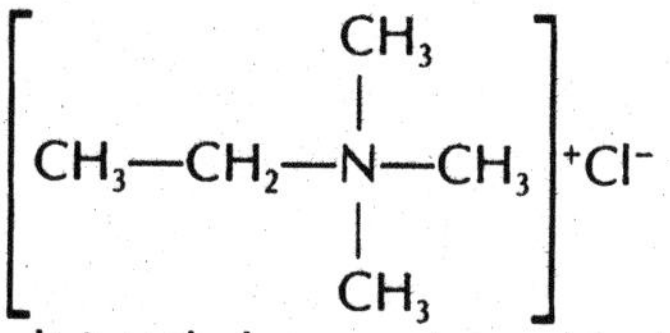

ethyltrimethylammonium chloride

Stereochemistry

Amines have pyramidal shapes like NH_3:

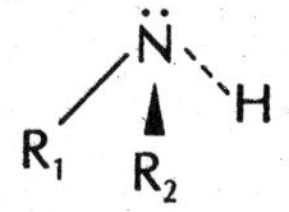

Nitrogen uses three sp^3 hybrid orbitals for bonding with carbon or hydrogen. These sp^3 orbitals are pointed toward the corners of a tetrahedron. The fourth sp^3 orbital contains an unshared pair of electrons. Models indicate that when N is bonded to three different groups, it is chiral and that two enantiomers should exist. However, because the energy barrier between the two pyramidal arrangements is so low, they are readily interconverted and consequently enantiomers of simple amines have not been isolated:

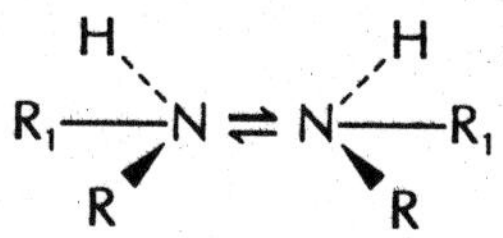

Physical Properties

Amines are polar compounds and can form intermolecular H-bonds (except for 3° amines). These bonds account for the lower boiling points of nonpolar compounds of the same molecular weight. Note, however, that boiling points of amines are lower than those of comparable molecular weight alcohols or carboxylic acids where H-bonding is stronger due to the more electronegative oxygen atom.

Amines of all three classes can form hydrogen bonds, with water accounting for the high solubility of small amines. As the hydrocarbon chain grows larger, solubility in water decreases with minimal solubility at about six carbons.

B. GENERAL PRINCIPLES

The chemical properties of the three classes of amines are similar to NH_3 due to the tendency of N to share its lone pair of electrons. This tendency accounts for the basicity of NH_3 and its derivatives, for their behavior as nucleophiles, as well as for the high reactivity of aromatic rings attached to amino or substituted amino groups.

Basicity

Like NH_3, amines form basic solutions in water

$$RNH_2 + H_2O \rightleftharpoons RNH_3^+ + OH^- \qquad K_b$$

and react with mineral acids to form their salts.

$$RNH_2 + H_3O^+ \rightarrow RNH_3^+ + H_2O$$

Aliphatic amines are stronger than NH_3 ($K_b = 10^{-5}$) with K_b's that are one or two magnitudes greater. This difference in basicity can be attributed to the electron-releasing ability of alkyl groups that disperse the positive charge on the substituted ammonium cation, increasing its stability relative to the amine. As with carbocations, electron-releasing groups increase stability.

The increase in basicity can also be explained by the increased availability of the unshared electrons due to the electron-releasing effects of the alkyl groups pushing negative charge onto N.

Aromatic amines exhibit very low K_b's (10^{-10}). This low basicity can be accounted for by the resonance structures that stabilize aniline relative to its conjugate acid.

One could also explain the lower basicity of aromatic amines relative to NH_3 as being due to the partial withdrawal of the unshared electron pair by the ring, making the unshared electrons less available to an attacking proton. Note that the resonance structures show increased electron density on the ortho and para positions, accounting for the increased reactivity of the aromatic ring toward electrophilic attack as well as the preferential attack on these positions by electrophiles.

Effect of Substitutents on Basicity of Aromatic Amines

Electron-releasing groups such as $-NH_2$, $-OCH_3$, $-OH$, and $-CH_3$ tend to increase basicity of aromatic amines because they push electrons toward N, making the unshared pair of electrons more vulnerable to attack by H^+. These groups also increase reactivity of the ring toward electrophilic attack because of the increase in negative charge on the ring.

$$CH_3-\overset{\oplus}{\ddot{O}} = \overset{\ominus}{\overset{\cdot\cdot}{\bigcirc}} -\ddot{N}H_2$$

On the other hand, electron-withdrawing groups, such as $-NH_3^+$, $-NO_2$, $-SO_3$, $-COOH$, $-Br$, and $-Cl$, pull electrons away from N, making the unshared electron pair less available. The ring is also deactivated toward electrophilic attack due to the withdrawal of negative charge from the ring.

Note that *both* electron-withdrawing and electron-donating groups weaken basicity of aromatic amines when they are in the ortho positions (ortho effect).

C. MAJOR REACTIONS

Amide Formation

Ammonia and primary and secondary amines react with acid chlorides to form amides and substituted amides.

$$\underset{\underset{\text{nucleophile}}{\uparrow}}{NH_3} + R-\overset{O}{\overset{\|}{C}}-Cl \rightarrow R-\overset{O}{\overset{\|}{C}}-NH_2 + HCl$$

$$\underset{\downarrow}{RNH_2} + R'-\overset{O}{\overset{\|}{\underset{\underset{\text{leaving group}}{\nwarrow}}{C}}}-Cl \rightarrow R'-\overset{O}{\overset{\|}{C}}-NHR + HCl$$

Amide formation occurs in peptide formation or protein synthesis.

$$\underset{\text{amino acid}}{H_2N-CHR-\overset{O}{\overset{\|}{C}}-OH} + \underset{\text{amino acid}}{H_2N-CHR'-\overset{O}{\overset{\|}{C}}-OH} \rightarrow \underset{\text{peptide}}{H_2N-CHR-\overset{O}{\overset{\|}{C}}-\overset{H}{\overset{|}{N}}-CHR'-\overset{O}{\overset{\|}{C}}-OH}$$

Tertiary amines do not react most likely because they cannot lose a hydrogen to stabilize the product after they join to the carboxyl carbon.

Ring Substitution in Aromatic Amines

As already indicated under General Principles, amino and substituted amino groups release electrons into the ring, activating the ring toward electrophilic attack. Resonance structures of the intermediate formed after attack by an electrophile, E, show the stabilizing effect of the amino group on the carbocation when the attack is on the ortho or para positions.

These structures are particularly stable due to the completed octet around all atoms other than H. Hence, they account for the ortho, para-directing properties of amino and substituted amino groups.

Alkylation of Amines

Amines are alkylated by alkyl halides according to

$$RNH_2 \xrightarrow{RX} R_2NH \xrightarrow{RX} R_3N \xrightarrow{RX} R_4N^{\oplus}X^{\ominus}$$

The reaction is a nucleophilic substitution with the amine replacing X.

Alkylation of 1° and 2° amines is a method of synthesis for 2° and 3° amines.

Alkylation of a tertiary amine produces a quaternary ammonium salt.

$$R_3N + RX \rightarrow R_4N + X^-$$

D. QUATERNARY AMMONIUM SALTS

As indicated above, the complete alkylation of an amine leads to a quaternary ammonium salt in which four organic groups are bound to N, producing a positive charge on the N. An anion must be present to balance the charge.

Properties

The quaternary ammonium salts tend to be soluble in water. Drugs that are high-molecular-weight amines are often made soluble in body fluids by introducing them as chloride, or sulfate ammonium salts. Note that unlike other amine salts (RNH_3^+, $R_2NH_2^+$+, R_3NH^+), quaternary ammonium salts have the same structure in aqueous solution regardless of the pH.

PRACTICE PROBLEMS
SECTIONS 10.3 AND 10.4

1. Alcohols boil at much higher temperatures than hydrocarbons of the same molecular weight due to

   A. hydrogen bonding.
   B. branching.
   C. polarity.
   D. tertiary structures.

2. In both dehydration and substitution reactions of alcohols,

   A. heating is required.
   B. only tertiary alcohols react.
   C. —OH is the leaving group.
   D. protonation usually occurs first because —OH is a poor leaving group.

3. Which statement is false about S_N1 reactions of alcohols?

   A. It follows first-order kinetics.
   B. Racemization occurs.
   C. Tertiary alcohols are more reactive than secondary or primary alcohols.
   D. Rearrangement never occurs.

4. The typical reaction of aldehydes and ketones is

   A. electrophilic addition.
   B. nucleophilic addition.
   C. nucleophilic substitution.
   D. electrophilic substitution.

5. The carbonyl group increases the acidity of the hydrogen atoms attached to the alpha carbon. The best explanation is which of the following?

   A. The oxygen in the carbonyl group can accommodate a negative charge.
   B. The carbonyl group is flat.
   C. The carbonyl carbon has sp^2 hybridization.
   D. The carbonyl group has a pi bond.

6. When acetaldehyde reacts with ethanol in the presence of acid, the product is

   A. an acetal.
   B. a hemiacetal.
   C. a ketal.
   D. a hemiketal.

7. The formation of a β-hydroxyaldehyde results from

   A. an aldol condensation.
   B. the reaction of two molecules of an aldehyde in the presence of dilute base.
   C. the reaction of two molecules of aldehyde in the presence of dilute acid.
   D. All of the above.

8. Tautomers are

   A. different resonance structures of the same compound.
   B. mirror images of each other.
   C. in rapid equilibrium.
   D. always keto and enol forms.

9. The carboxyl group gives rise to which properties?

   A. acidic, undergoes electrophilic addition, hydrophilic
   B. basic, undergoes nucleophilic substitution, hydrophobic
   C. acidic, undergoes nucleophilic substitution, hydrophilic
   D. acidic, undergoes nucleophilic addition, hydrophilic

10. Which of the following statements is false?

    A. Basic hydrolysis of fats produces glycerol and salts of fatty acids.
    B. $LiAlH_4$ can reduce carboxylic acids to alcohols.
    C. β diacids and β ketoacids in the presence of base and heat undergo decarboxylation.
    D. Water is the nucleophilic agent in the basic hydrolysis of esters.

11. The resonance structures of aniline account for

    A. the lower basicity compared with aliphatic amines.

    B. the increase in reactivity of the aromatic ring toward electrophilic attack.

    C. the increase in negative charge on the ortho and para positions.

    D. All of the above.

12. The base-strengthening substituents on aromatic amines

    A. activate the ring toward electrophilic substitution.

    B. activate the ring toward nucleophilic substitution.

    C. activate the ring toward meta substitution.

    D. deactivate the ring toward electrophilic substitution.

ANSWER KEY

1. A   2. D   3. D   4. B   5. A   6. A   7. D   8. C   9. C   10. D   11. D   12. A

ANSWERS AND EXPLANATIONS

1. **The correct answer is (A).** Abnormally high boiling points are due to the greater energy needed to break H-bonds that tightly hold molecules together. Light alcohols are miscible also because of H-bonds that link the alcohol molecules to water molecules.

2. **The correct answer is (D).** —OH is a poor leaving group. Protonation allows H_2O to leave so that dehydration and substitution can occur.

3. **The correct answer is (D).** S_N1 reactions involve a carbocation intermediate. Rearrangement often occurs to increase the number of alkyl groups around the positively charged carbon and thus stabilize the intermediate.

4. **The correct answer is (B).** The carbonyl group is the site of nucleophilic addition that is catalyzed by acid. The protonated oxygen of the aldehyde or ketone removes charge from the carbonyl carbon, making it more susceptible to attack by a nucleophile.

5. **The correct answer is (A).** The negative charge of the resulting carbanion is stabilized by the carbonyl oxygen.

6. **The correct answer is (A).** Two ethanol molecules will bond to the carbonyl carbon in the presence of acid.

7. **The correct answer is (D).** Aldol condensation reactions occur whenever aldehydes or ketones are in the presence of a dilute acid or base. The product results from the addition of the alpha carbon of one molecule of aldehyde or ketone to the carbonyl carbon of the other molecule of aldehyde or ketone. For example,

8. **The correct answer is (C).** An example is

The acidic H jumps from the —OH group over to the double bond. Another example of tautomers are enamine-imine tautomers. An example is

9. **The correct answer is (C).** The carboxylate anion is resonance stabilized, giving the carboxyl group its acidic properties.

Carboxylic acids and their derivatives typically undergo nucleophilic substitution in which —Cl, —OH, —NH$_2$, —OOCR, or OR is replaced by some other basic group. For an aldehyde or ketone to undergo nucleophilic substitution, a hydride (H$^-$) or alkide (R$^-$), the strongest bases of all, would have to leave. Thus, they undergo addition as opposed to substitution.

10. **The correct answer is (D).** OH$^-$ ion attacks the carbonyl carbon.

11. **The correct answer is (D).** Resonance structures show how the lone-pair electrons are distributed around the aromatic ring. The increased negative charge on the ortho and para positions accounts for the increased reactivity of the molecule to electrophilic attack as well as the preferred attack at these positions.

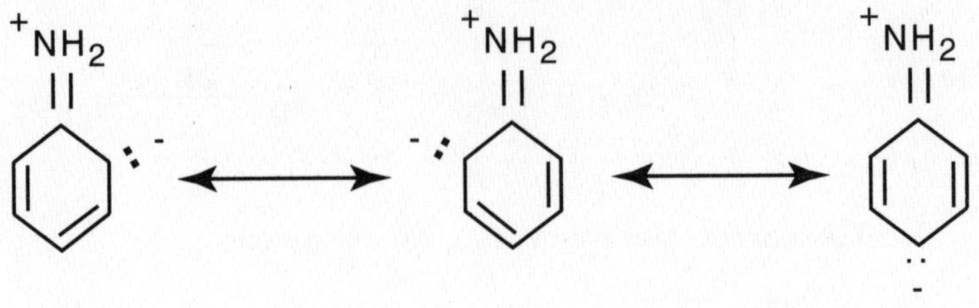

12. **The correct answer is (A).** Base-strengthening substituents send electrons into the ring, thus activating it to electrophilic attack as well as localizing the lone-pair electrons on nitrogen and increasing its basicity.

10.5   BIOLOGICAL MOLECULES

A.   AMINO ACIDS AND PROTEINS

Proteins are polyamides; their monomers are α-amino carboxylic acids (amino acids), that are more than twenty in number. The general formula for an amino acid is

$$\overset{\oplus}{H_3N}-CH-COO^{\ominus}$$
$$\underset{R}{|}$$

(Note that in proline and hydroxyproline, the amino group is part of a pyrrolidine ring.) If the R group of the amino acid contains a carboxyl group as in aspartic acid or glutamic acid, or a carboxamide as in asparagine, the amino acid is classified as *acidic*. *Basic amino acids* contain a second basic group; lysine, for example, contains another amino group; arginine, a guanidino group; and histidine, an imidazole ring.

Amino Acids as Dipolar Ions

Amino acids have high melting points (at which they decompose), solubilities in water, and K_a and K_b values that are very low for —COOH and —NH_2 groups. These properties are consistent with a dipolar structure as shown above. The acidic and basic equilibrium reactions for glycine are

$$\overset{\oplus}{H_3N}-CH-COO^- + H_2O \rightleftharpoons H_2N-CH-COO^{\ominus} \qquad K_a$$
$$\underset{H}{|} \qquad\qquad\qquad \underset{H}{|}$$
$$\textit{dibasic form}$$

and

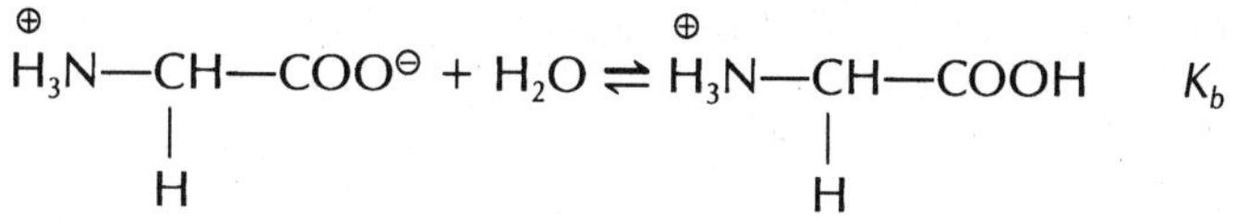

$$\overset{\oplus}{H_3N}—\underset{\underset{H}{|}}{CH}—COO^{\ominus} + H_2O \rightleftharpoons \overset{\oplus}{H_3N}—\underset{\underset{H}{|}}{CH}—COOH \qquad K_b$$

protonated form

which accounts for the unusually low values of K_a and K_b.
In acidic and basic solution, the reactions are

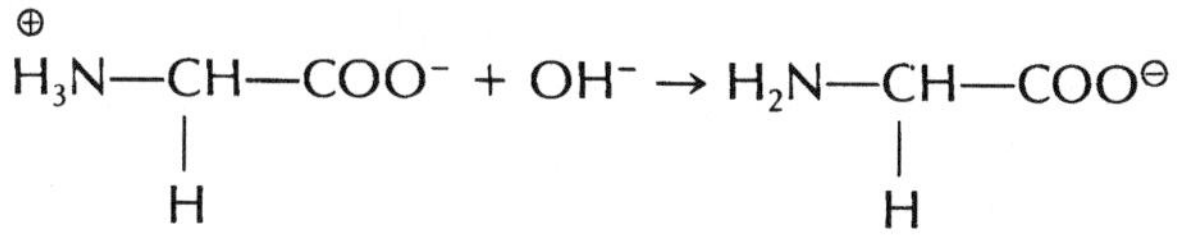

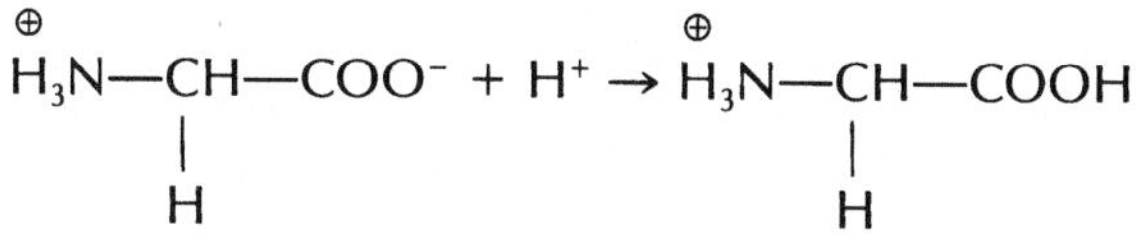

$$\overset{\oplus}{H_3N}—\underset{\underset{H}{|}}{CH}—COO^- + OH^- \rightarrow H_2N—\underset{\underset{H}{|}}{CH}—COO^{\ominus}$$

$$\overset{\oplus}{H_3N}—\underset{\underset{H}{|}}{CH}—COO^- + H^+ \rightarrow \overset{\oplus}{H_3N}—\underset{\underset{H}{|}}{CH}—COOH$$

In basic solution, the dibasic form (two basic groups on amino acid) predominate, while the fully protonated form predominates in acid solution.

The pH at which the concentration of these two forms are equal is called the *isoelectric point:* There is no net migration by the amino acid in the presence of an electric field at this pH. For glycine it is 6.1. The highest concentration of the dipolar ion is at the isoelectric point.

Configuration of Amino Acids

From the table titled "Natural Amino Acids," it is clear that in all of the amino acids except for glycine (R = H), there is a chiral carbon, so they are optically active. *Naturally occurring amino acids almost all have the S-configuration:*

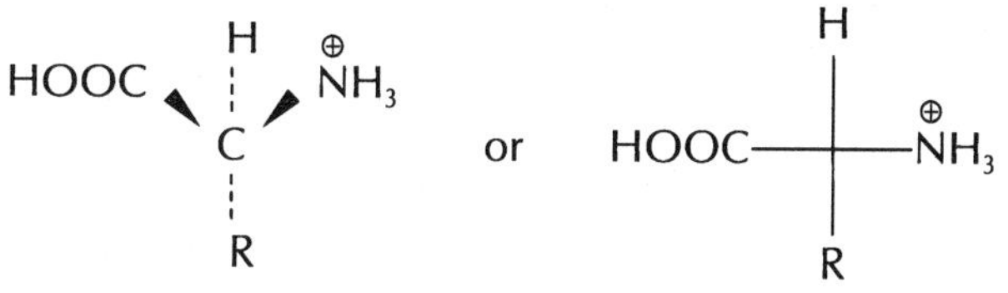

Fischer Projection

Natural Amino Acids

Name	Abbreviation	Formula
(+)-Alanine	Ala A	CH_3CHCOO^- with $^+NH_3$
(+)-Arginine[e]	Arg R	$H_2NCNHCH_2CH_2CH_2CHCOO$ with $^+NH_2$ and NH_2
(−)-Asparagine	Asn N	$H_2NCOCH_2CHCOO^-$ with $^+NH_3$
(+)-Aspartic acid	Asp D	$HOOCCH_2CHCOO^-$ with $^+NH_3$
(−)-Cysteine	Cys C	$HSCH_2CHCOO^-$ with $^+NH_3$
(−)-Cystine	Cys—Cys	$^-OOCCHCH_2S-SCH_2CHCOO$ with $^+NH_3$ and $^+NH_3$
(+)-Glutamic acid	Glu E	$HOOCCH_2CH_2CHCOO^-$ with $^+NH_3$
(+)-Glutamine	Gln Q	$H_2NCOCH_2CH_2CHCOO^-$ with $^+NH_3$
Glycine	Gly G	$H_3\overset{\oplus}{N}-CH_2-COO^-$
(−)-Histidine[e]	His H	imidazole ring CH_2CHCOO^- with $^+NH_3$
(−)-Hydroxylysine	Hyl	$^+H_3NCH_2CHCH_2CH_2CHCOO^-$ with OH and NH_2
(−)-Hydroxyproline	Hyp	HO-pyrrolidine ring $-COO^-$

Natural Amino Acids—*Continued*

Name	Abbreviation	Formula
(+)-Isoleucine[e]	Ile I	$CH_3CH_2CH(CH_3)CHCOO^-$ $\mid$ $^+NH_3$
(−)-Leucine[e]	Leu L	$(CH_3)_2CHCH_2CHCOO^-$ $\mid$ $^+NH_3$
(+)-Lysine[e]	Lys K	$^+H_3NCH_2CH_2CH_2CH_2CHCOO^-$ $\mid$ NH_2
(−)-Methionine[e]	Met M	$CH_3SCH_2CH_2CHCOO^-$ $\mid$ $^+NH_3$
(−)-Phenylalanine[e]	Phe F	CH_2CHCOO^- $\mid$ $^+NH_3$
(−)-Proline	Pro P	
(−)-Serine	Ser S	$HOCH_2CHCOO^-$ $\mid$ $^+NH_3$
(−)-Threonine[e]	Thr T	$CH_3CHOHCHCOO^-$ $\mid$ $^+NH_3$
(−)-Tryptophane[e]	Trp W	
(−)-Tyrosine	Tyr Y	$HO$$CH_2CHCOO^-$ $\mid$ $^+NH_3$
(+)-Valine[e]	Val V	$(CH_3)_2CHCHCOO^-$ $\mid$ $^+NH_3$

[e]Essential amino acid

Peptides and Proteins

Amino acids undergo the same reactions as other organic molecules containing a —NH_2 and —COOH and any other group present (R). Hence, an amide can form from the interaction of the carboxyl group on one amino acid and the amino group on another. For example:

$$\overset{\oplus}{H_3N}-CH-COO^\ominus + \overset{\oplus}{H_3N}-CH-COO^\ominus \rightarrow$$

|
H
Glycine

|
CH_3
Alanine

$$\overset{\oplus}{H_3N}-CH-\overset{\overset{O}{\parallel}}{C}-\overset{\overset{H}{|}}{N}-CH-COO^\ominus + H_2O$$

|
H

|
CH_3

Glycylalanine (Gly-Ala)

The peptide linkage (—NHCO—) gives rise to dipeptides (as above), tripeptides, etc. Proteins are polypeptides. The convention for writing the structures of peptides is to put the N-terminal amino acid residue (free amino group) on the left and the C-terminal acid residue (free carboxyl group) on the right.

1. **Hydrolysis**

   Like other amides, the peptide linkage can be cleaved during basic or acidic hydrolysis to form the amino acids back again. The tripeptide Gly-Ala-Phe yields glycine, alanine, and phenylalanine amino acids upon hydrolysis.

2. **Isoelectric Point and Side Chains**

   As with amino acids, at the *isoelectric* point the protein shows no net migration in an electric field. This means that the positive and negative charges are exactly balanced. At pH values less than the isoelectric point, positive charges prevail (protein moves to cathode); while at pH values greater than the isoelectric point, negative charges prevail (protein moves to anode). Different proteins have different isoelectric points because they contain different quantities of acidic and basic side chains associated with their amino acid residues. These side chains have marked effects on the behavior of proteins by their chemical properties (such as acid-base properties) as well as by their sizes and shapes.

3. **Sulfur Linkages**

   The R groups of the amino acids cysteine and cystine contain S. Hence, sulfur linkages between proteins containing these amino acids occur (disulfide bridges).

B. CARBOHYDRATES

Carbohydrates are polyhydroxy aldehydes or ketones or compounds that form from their hydrolysis. A *monosaccharide* is a carbohydrate that cannot be hydrolyzed to form a simpler compound. Upon hydrolysis, a *disaccharide* forms two monosaccharides while a *polysaccharide* forms many monosaccharide units.

A monosaccharide is an aldose if it contains an aldehyde group; ketose if it contains a keto group. Also, the number of carbon atoms is included in the name so that an aldotriose contains three carbons and an aldehyde group. A ketohexose is a monosaccharide that contains six carbon atoms and a keto group.

Some common sugars are

```
        CHO                  CH₂OH
         |                     |
        CHOH                  C=O
         |                     |
        CHOH                  CHOH
         |                     |
        CHOH                  CHOH
         |                     |
        CHOH                  CHOH
         |                     |
        CH₂OH                 CH₂OH
  Glucose (aldohexose)   Fructose (2-ketohexose)
```

Sucrose is a disaccharide consisting of (+)-glucose and (−)-fructose. Cellulose, starch, and glycogen are all polysaccharides containing the (+)-glucose monomer.

Stereochemistry of Sugars

Aldohexoses contain four chiral carbons:

$$H-\overset{\overset{\textstyle O}{\|}}{C}-(CHOH)_4-CH_2OH$$

Consequently, 2^4 or 16 stereoisomers (eight pairs of enantiomers) exist. Only three are common: (+)-glucose, (+)-mannose, and (+)-galactose.

```
        CHO                  CHO                  CHO
   H———————OH           HO———————H           H———————OH
  HO———————H           HO———————H           HO———————H
   H———————OH           H———————OH           HO———————H
   H———————OH           H———————OH           H———————OH
       CH₂OH                CH₂OH                CH₂OH
    (+)-glucose          (+)-mannose         (+)-galactose
```

Sugars are given a relative configuration based on glyceraldehyde, $CH_2OHCHOHCHO$, an aldotriose.

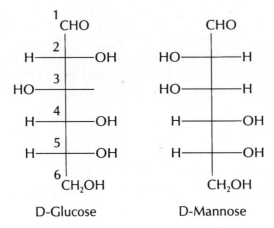

The orientation of the next to last —OH in a sugar is compared to D-glyceraldehyde.

D-Glucose   D-Mannose

Epimers are a pair of aldose diastereomers that differ only in configuration about carbon-2.

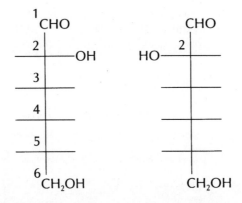

D-glucose and D-mannose shown above are examples of epimers.

Cyclic Structure of D-(+)-Glucose

In aqueous solution, D-(+)-glucose exists as an equilibrium mixture of two cyclic structures that undergo mutorotation.

α-D-(+)-Glucose   β-D-(+)-Glucose

Note that the α and β forms (called *anomers*) differ only by the orientation of —OH on carbon-1. Because they are hemiacetals, they are hydrolyzed by water so that either anomer is converted through an open chain structure into the other anomer.

Reactions of Sugars

Oxidation of Monosaccharides

Aldoses undergo oxidation readily. However, the product depends on the oxidizing agent and the conditions of the reaction.

Formation and Hydrolysis of Disaccharides

Monosaccharides bond together through glycosidic linkages between the hemiacetal carbon and a hydroxyl group of the other sugar. For example,

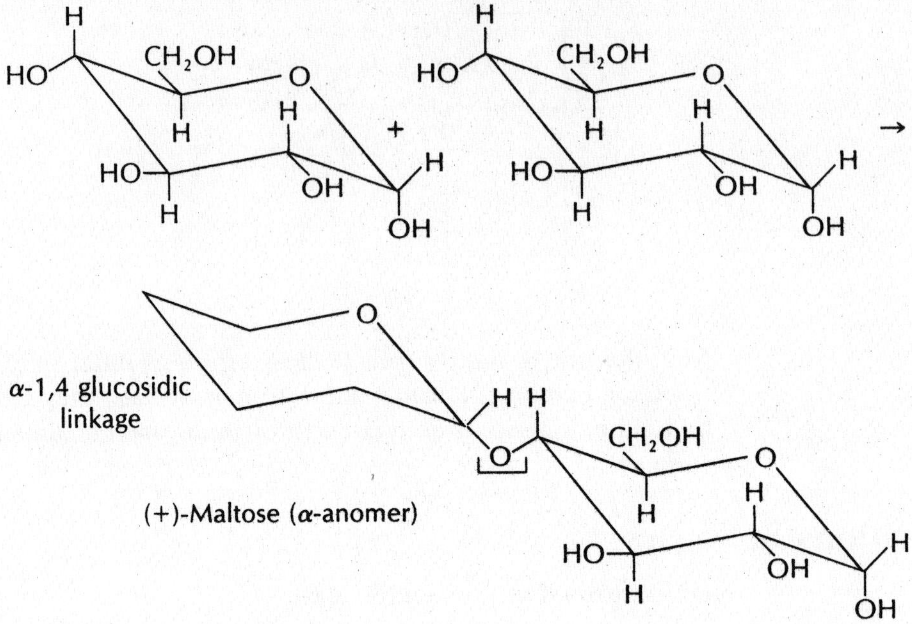

α-1,4 glucosidic linkage

(+)-Maltose (α-anomer)

Hydrolysis of maltose will yield the two glucose molecules back again, while sucrose will form glucose and fructose.

Polysaccharides consist of many monosaccharide units joined by glycosidic bonds. Cellulose, for example, has β-1,4 glycosidic bonds that do not occur in starch and glycogen.

C. LIPIDS

Lipids consist of many different kinds of biomolecules including fats, oils, steroids, and terpenes. They are insoluble in water and can be extracted from cells by organic solvents such as chloroform.

Fats

Fats are esters of fatty acids and glycerol and are called glycerides or more specifically triacylglycerols.

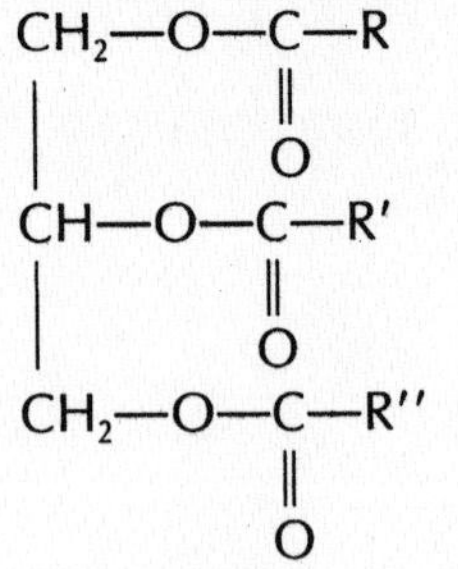

fat
(triacylglycerol)

Fatty acids (RCOOH, R′COOH, R″COOH) contain from 3 to 18 C's, but only an even number of C atoms occur in substantial amounts due to biosynthesis. The composition of fats varies, but each fat tends to have a characteristic composition. For example, in butter saturated acids contain 18 C's and represent 8–13% by weight, while in soybean oil these same fatty acids represent 2–5%. (Oils are liquid fats.) Unsaturated fatty acids that contain one or more double bonds per molecule are also present in fats. The most common of these are oleic (cis-isomer) and linoleic (cis, cis-isomer) acids:

$$CH_3(CH_2)_7CH=CH(CH_2)_7COOH$$
oleic acid

$$CH_3(CH_2)_4C=C-CH_2C=C(CH_2)_7COOH$$
| | | |
H   H   H   H
linoleic acid

The presence of cis-unsaturated fatty acids in fats lowers melting points because those fatty acids do not fit well with the saturated chains of other fatty acids. Consequently, cis-unsaturated fatty acids are more abundant in oils. Hydrogenation of some of these double bonds converts fats like corn oil and cottonseed oil into solids. This process is called hardening of oils and produces cooking fats.

Fatty acids can be made from the hydrolysis of glycerides or fats.

$$CH_2-O-C-R$$
‖
O
$$CH-O-C-R'$$ NaOH/H_2O
‖   → CH_2OH + $RCOO^-Na^+$
O
$$CH_2-O-C-R''$$ CHOH $R'COO^-Na^+$
‖
O CH_2OH $R''COO^-Na^+$
Glyceride   Glycerol   Soap
(Fat)

The above saponification reaction forms sodium salts of fatty acids or soap. Acid hydrolysis produces a mixture of the free carboxylic acids.

Soaps clean because they possess both a hydrophilic (water-soluble) and hydrophobic or lipophilic (water-insoluble) end. The hydrocarbon chain or hydrophobic part of the fatty acid dissolves in the grease or oil, while the negatively charged carboxyl group is dissolved in water. When the water is removed, the grease or oil follows.

Steroids
Steroids have four fused rings of carbon atoms with functional groups attached.

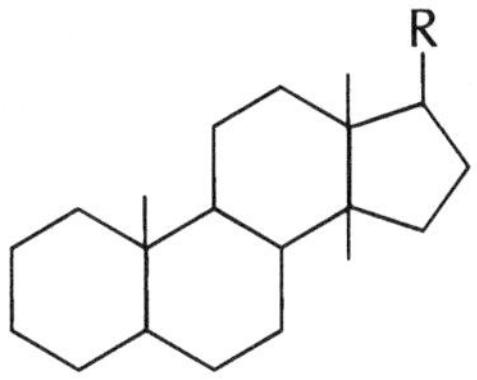

Steroid

Steroids include cholesterol (the predominant component of gallstones), sex hormones, and adrenal cortical hormones.

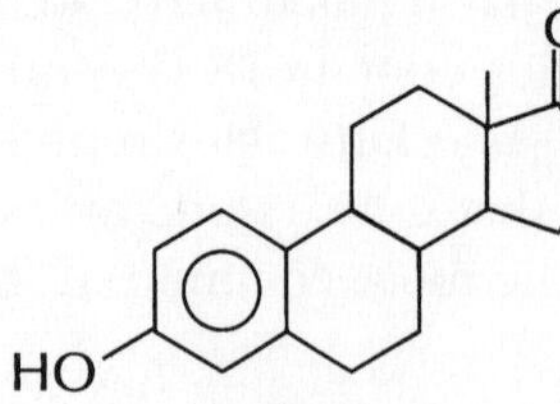

Estrone
(an estrogen)

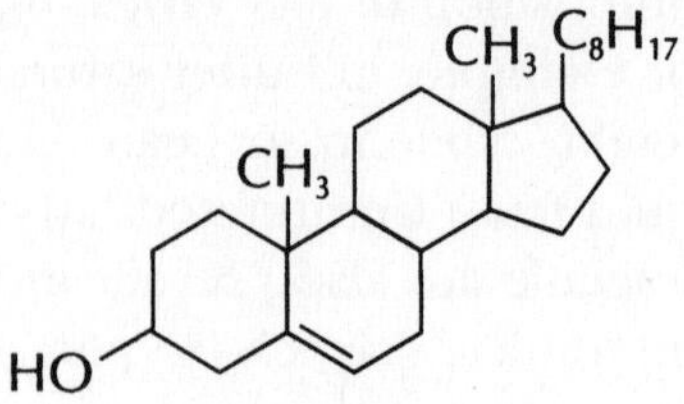

Cholesterol

D. PHOSPHOROUS COMPOUNDS

Phosphate esters are important biomolecules. They include phosphoglycerides.

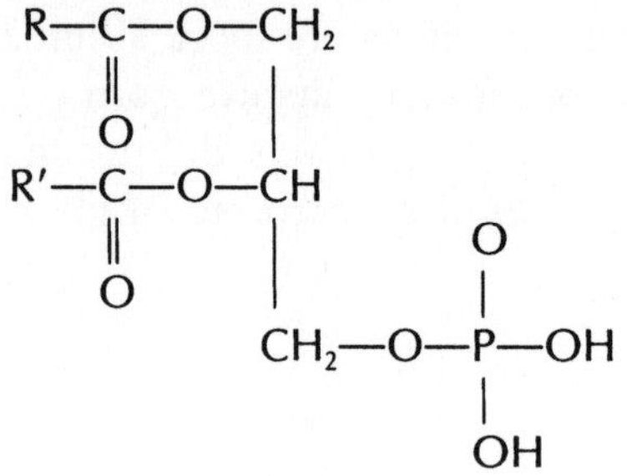

Phosphatidic Acid
(phosphoglyceride)

Note that in the above phospholipid there are two acyl groups (as opposed to three in a fat) and a phosphate group. Other important phosphorous-containing biomolecules include adenosine triphosphate, which transfers energy by converting molecules to phosphate esters and nucleic acids, which control heredity. Nucleic acids are polyesters of phosphoric acid.

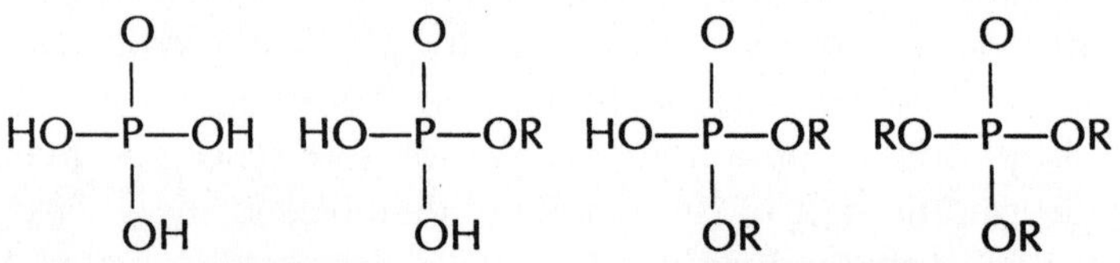

Phosphoric
acid

Phosphate esters

Acid-Base Behavior of Phosphoric Acid and Derivatives

Phosphoric acid as well as its monoalkyl and dialkyl esters are very acidic and exist predominantly as anions in aqueous solution.

In acidic solution, phosphate esters hydrolyze to form phosphoric acid as a result of C—O cleavage.

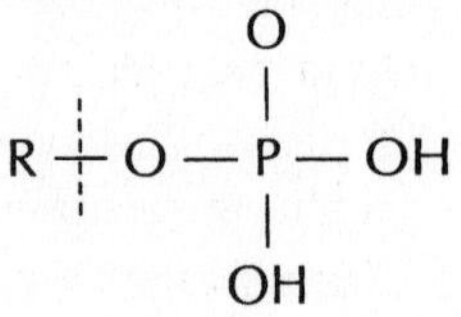

Phosphate acts as a leaving group. In basic solution only trialkyl phosphate esters hydrolyze, losing one alkoxy group due to P—O cleavage.

$$R-O-\!\!\!\!|-P-OR$$

(structure: R—O ⫶ P—OR, with P double-bonded to O above, bonded to OR and OH⁻ below)

The OH⁻ attacks the phosphorous in the ester. Mono- and dialkyl phosphate esters do not hydrolyze in alkaline solution because the OH⁻ ion is repelled by the ester, which exists as the anion in basic solution.

Phospholipids mostly exist as

(structure: G—O—P—OH, with P double-bonded to O above, bonded to OR below)

where G is the glyceryl group and R is often ethanolamine $HOCH_2CH_2NH_2$ or choline $HOCH_2CH_2N(CH_3)_3{}^+$.

(structure of phospholipid:
R'—C—O—CH₂ (C double bonded to O)
R''—C—O—CH (C double bonded to O)
CH₂—O—P—O⁻ (P double bonded to O)
OCH₂CH₂NH₃⁺)

Note that this phospholipid is a dipolar ion. It tends to undergo hydrolysis by cleavage at the P—OR bond.

10.6 USE OF SPECTROSCOPY IN STRUCTURAL IDENTIFICATION

A. NUCLEAR MAGNETIC RESONANCE

Nuclear magnetic resonance (NMR) is a powerful tool for the determination of molecular structure. As its name implies, it utilizes the *magnetic* properties of atomic *nuclei* (most commonly using hydrogen nuclei) to infer structural information by measuring the energies at which "resonances," or absorptions of radio frequency energy, take place.

The nucleus of a hydrogen atom is simply a proton. Like an electron, it can have two **spin states,** each one generating a magnetic moment. When no external magnetic field is present, these states have equal energies, but in the presence of an external field, alignment of the magnetic moment against the field corresponds to a slightly higher energy. The difference between the two states is

Acetaldehyde Spectrum.

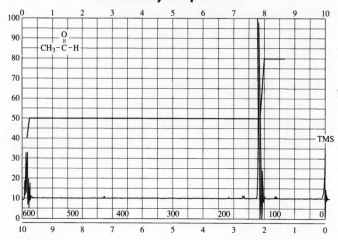

proportional to the strength of the external field. The commonly used magnetic field strength of 14,092 gauss produces an energy gap corresponding to radio frequency photons having a frequency of 60 MHz ($60 \times 10^6 \text{sec}^{-1}$).

Different hydrogen nuclei within the same molecule will require slightly different energies to promote them to the excited state. These differences arise because of **shielding** by the electrons surrounding the nuclei. A highly shielded hydrogen nucleus—e.g., one bonded to an electron-donating group—will require a photon of greater energy for promotion than will a less shielded nucleus. These differences are slight, on the order of parts per million, but they can be accurately measured.

As an example of an nmr spectrum, consider acetaldehyde, CH_3CHO. The three methyl hydrogens all experience an equivalent magnetic environment fairly well-shielded, since the carbon is not highly electron-withdrawing, while the hydrogen on the CHO is less shielded owing to the electronegative oxygen nearby.

The "Acetaldehyde Spectrum" shows it displayed in the conventional way. To generate the spectrum, the spectrometer varies the applied magnetic field, which increases to the right on the *x*-axis, while holding the photon energy of the radio frequency source constant. (Some spectrometers obtain an identical spectrum by varying the photon frequency at constant magnetic field.)

Note the following features of the spectrum:

- Each signal corresponds to each kind of proton.

- The step-shaped curves above the signals show the integrated areas beneath each of those signals; the height of each step is proportional to the area under the corresponding signal.

- The peak marked **TMS** gives the radio frequency absorption of a small amount of the reference compound **tetramethylsilane,** which is added to the acetaldehyde. TMS is used because its hydrogens are all equivalent and are extremely well-shielded.

- As anticipated, the absorption of the methyl hydrogens, which were predicted to be well-shielded, is closer to the absorption of TMS than is the absorption of the CHO hydrogen. The difference between the absorption of a given hydrogen and that of the reference TMS hydrogens is called the **chemical shift,** which is customarily measured in units of "delta," where each delta unit is a part per million shift from TMS. The hydrogen on the CHO is found at 9.9 ppm, while the methyl hydrogens are found at 2.2 ppm.

The table below lists typical values of the chemical shift for common hydrogen-containing groups. Note that many of the values are variable, depending upon other atoms or groups in the molecule.

Proton environment	Approximate chemical shift (ppm)
$R—CH_3$	0.9
$R_2—CH_2$	1.3
$R_3—CH$	1.4
$\overset{\displaystyle O}{\overset{\displaystyle \|}{—C—CH_3}}$	2.1
Ar—H	6–8.5
Ar—C—H	2.2–3
R—CHO	9–10
R—COOH	10–12
R—OH	2–5
Ar—OH	4–7
$R—NH_2$	1.5–4

Spin-Spin Coupling

We have so far omitted an important characteristic of nmr spectra, that of "splitting" of peaks due to interaction of neighboring hydrogens. The acetaldehyde spectrum provides an excellent example of such splitting.

First, consider the effect of the methyl hydrogens on the NMR absorption by the CHO hydrogen. If all of the methyl hydrogen nuclei were exactly the same, there might be a shift in this absorption, but there would be no splitting; however, since the CH_3 hydrogens can be aligned either with or against the external field, the CHO hydrogen can "feel" either an increase in the total magnetic field or a slight decrease. The result is a splitting into N + 1 peaks, where N is the number of adjacent interacting hydrogens. Here N is 3 (i.e., from the three methyl hyrogens), resulting in four peaks in the absorption of the CHO hydrogen.

Note that the peak for the CHO hydrogen is split because it has multiple near-neighbors (and not because there are multiple CHO hydrogens). Note also that splitting is reciprocal, so that if one group of hydrogens causes a splitting in the absorption spectrum of a second group, then the converse will also occur.

The NMR signals from —OH groups and —NH groups may be broadened owing to exchange of protons between different molecules and, in the case of —NH, owing to the magnetic moment of the nitrogen nucleus. Thus, any broad peaks may be diagnostic for these functional groups.

B. INFRARED SPECTROSCOPY

Important structural information about a molecule is revealed by its infrared spectrum. Absorption of light of the correct infrared frequencies excites molecular vibrations; e.g., a vibration in which a singly bonded carbon and hydrogen move back and forth as if their bond were a spring.

Vibrational frequencies measured by infrared spectroscopy are usually reported in **wave numbers,** with units of cm^{-1}. The frequency in wave number units is determined by taking the reciprocal of the wavelength (expressed in cm) of the exciting photon. Since wavelength is inversely proportional to photon energy, the frequency in wave numbers is directly proportional to the photon energy.

A second common means of reporting infrared data is through wavelength measured in **microns** (μ), where 1 micron = 10^{-6} m. The two systems are related through the expression

$$\text{frequency (wave numbers)} = 10^4/\text{wavelength in microns}$$

The table below gives some common **infrared absorption** frequencies. The exact position of the absorption depends on details of the molecule. In general, frequencies decrease as the atoms participating in the vibration become more massive, and increase as the bond order (i.e., single, double) increases.

Functional group	Approximate frequency (cm^{-1})
O—H, N—H, ≡C—H	3300
\—C—H /	3000 or slightly less
=C—H \	3000 or slightly more
—C≡C— \	2200 or slightly less
C=O /	1710 for ketones, aldehydes, acids 1735 for esters 1650 for amides
\ / C=C / \	1660

An example of an infrared spectrum, that for 1-butene, is shown in the figure below with some of the absorptions labeled:

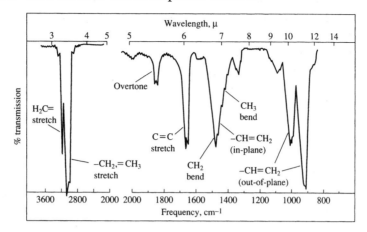

Not all vibrations will appear in an infrared spectrum. Those that are found, which are termed **infrared active,** are those that alter the dipole moment of the molecule.

Thus, of the two substituted alkenes,

(a) $H_2C{=}CH_2$

(b) $(C_2H_5{-}HC{=}CH_2)$

the $C{=}C$ stretching frequency will be evident in the spectrum of the less symmetrical molecule (b), but not (a).

PRACTICE PROBLEMS
SECTIONS 10.5 AND 10.6

1. Amino acids

   A. have one amino and one carboxylic acid group.
   B. have low melting points.
   C. exist as dipolar ions only.
   D. have different ionic forms depending on the pH.

2. Naturally occurring amino acids

   A. have mostly the S configuration.
   B. react with each other to form peptide linkages.
   C. are soluble in water.
   D. All of the above.

3. Which statement is true about the structures of carbohydrates?

   A. Carbohydrates are polyhydroxy aldehydes or ketones or compounds that can be hydrolyzed to form them.
   B. Carbohydrates include glucose, starch, and glycogen only.
   C. Carbohydrates are all aldohexoses.
   D. All carbohydrates are epimers.

4. Glucose anomers differ only

   A. by their glycosidic linkages.
   B. in their number of carbon atoms.
   C. in their configuration about carbon-1.
   D. in the number of chiral carbons.

5. Oils are liquids because they

    A.   contain cis-unsaturated acid chains that do not fit well together.

    B.   contain saturated acid chains that fit together well due to tetrahedral bond angles.

    C.   undergo hydrogenation.

    D.   have high melting points.

6. Phosphoglycerides are

    A.   carboxylate esters.

    B.   phosphate esters.

    C.   carboxylate esters and phosphate esters.

    D.   triacylglycerols.

7. Infrared spectroscopy can generally be used to distinguish between

    A.   alcohols and ketones.

    B.   enantiomers.

    C.   cis-trans isomers.

    D.   conformers.

8. The number of signals in the NMR spectrum of 2-bromopropene is

    A.   2

    B.   3

    C.   cannot be determined

    D.   0

9. The NMR spectrum of $CH_2Br\text{-}CHBr_2$ shows

    A.   a triplet downfield and a doublet.

    B.   two triplets.

    C.   two doublets.

    D.   a doublet downfield and a triplet.

ANSWER KEY

1. D	2. D	3. A	4. C	5. A	6. C	7. A	8. B	9. A

ANSWERS AND EXPLANATIONS

1. **The correct answer is (D).** Some amino acids contain a second acidic group (e.g., aspartic acid) or a second basic group (e.g., lysine). Glycine is not optically active. In basic solution the dibasic form of amino acids predominates, while in acidic solution the protonated form is in highest concentration.

2. **The correct answer is (D).** Except for glycine, naturally occurring amino acids are optically active. Stereochemical studies show that all have the S configuration about the carbon atom bonded to the alpha amino group. Amides are formed by the reaction between amino groups and carboxyl groups to form peptides. In fact, the —NHCO— group is called a peptide linkage. Amino acids are nonvolatile crystalline solids with high melting points and are water soluble. These properties are explained by a dipolar structure, $+H_3N$—CHR—COO$^-$.

3. **The correct answer is (A).** Although glucose, starch, and glycogen are vital biochemical compounds, there are numerous other carbohydrates. Cellulose, which we use for paper, clothing, and shelter, is just an example of another carbohydrate. Monosaccharides are aldoses or ketoses and are usually also pentoses or hexoses. Disaccharides and polysaccharides can be hydrolyzed to monosaccharides.

4. **The correct answer is (C).** Aldoses and their glycosides have cyclic structures that can differ in the configuration about C-1. The C-1—OH is on the right in the α anomer and on the left in the β glucose anomer.

5. **The correct answer is (A).** Fats are all glycerides, composed of glycerol and carboxylic acids. These fatty acids are both saturated and unsaturated, the latter exhibiting mostly cis configurations about the double bonds. Fats with mostly saturated fatty acids have higher melting points because the tetrahedral carbons fit more tightly together than the cis fatty acid chains, making for stronger intermolecular forces. Oils or liquid fats have high numbers of unsaturated fatty acid chains that conversely cause lower melting points.

6. **The correct answer is (C).** Phosphoglycerides are lipids that are similar to fats but contain only two acyl groups (R—C═O) and a phosphate group in place of the third. The parent molecule is called diacylglycerol phosphate or phosphatidic acid.

7. **The correct answer is (A).** The infrared spectrum of an organic molecule gives the most information about its structure. Each functional group generally has a range of characteristic absorption frequencies: Carbonyl bonds in aldehydes and ketones absorb at about $1700 \ cm^{-1}$, while —OH groups absorb at much higher energies of approximately $3300 \ cm^{-1}$.

8. **The correct answer is (B).**

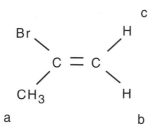

a,b, and c indicate the three different kinds of protons. a and (b,c) are clearly chemically inequivalent protons, that is, protons with different environments. b and c, however, are stereochemically inequivalent, and therefore their environments differ as well. Consequently, one would expect three NMR signals to match with three different protons.

9. **The correct answer is (A).** The NMR spectrum has a doublet associated with —CH_2^- protons because they are split by the —CH^- proton, and a triplet for the —CH^- proton, split by the two —CH_2^- protons.

10.7 SEPARATIONS AND PURIFICATIONS

Organic compounds do not usually occur either in the natural state or in a reaction mixture from a laboratory synthesis in a pure form. Consequently, separation and purification procedures are necessary to obtain organic chemicals in a pure form. Distillation, crystallization, and extraction are the most frequently used lab procedures to separate and purify organic compounds.

A. DISTILLATION

Distillation consists of boiling a liquid and then condensing the vapor into a separate container. The goal is to separate a mixture of two or more compounds that differ in their volatilities.

Distillation of a Pure Compound

At constant pressure, the temperature of the distilling vapor of a pure substance will remain constant as long as heat is supplied at a uniform rate and superheating does not occur. The temperature of the distilling vapor represents the boiling point of that fraction of the distillate. The temperature is the boiling point of the liquid in the flask only if the composition of the liquid is the same as the composition of the distilling vapor.

A constant temperature is therefore associated with a pure liquid and is used as a criterion of purity of a liquid. There are, however, mixtures (azeotropes) that boil at a constant temperature because the composition of the solution in the distilling flask is the same as the composition of their vapor. The components of an azeotropic mixture cannot therefore be separated by ordinary distillation.

Fractional Distillation

Fractional distillation is a multistep process in which receivers are changed during the distillation of a mixture. Two or more fractions are collected during different boiling temperature ranges. The first fraction is enriched in the lower boiling point component, while subsequent fractions are enriched in higher boiling point compounds. By repeating the process for each fraction, a much better separation of the mixture into its components is realized. The more times the process is repeated, the more complete the separation.

Fractional distillation is often carried out with fractionating columns. Each plate in the column ideally does the separation equivalent of one distillation procedure.

The effectiveness of a column to separate a mixture is measured by an enrichment factor (α), which is the ratio of the mole fraction of the components in the vapor to the ratio of their mole fractions in the liquid. For a two-component solution

$$\alpha = \frac{X_A / X_B \text{ (vapor)}}{X_A / X_B \text{ (liquid)}}$$

The above formula gives the enrichment factor for each plate. The number of plates theoretically required for a separation that gives 95% purity of the lower boiling point component is

$$\frac{2.85}{\log \alpha} = \text{number of theoretical plates for 95\% purity}$$

A more useful equation is

$$\frac{250}{T_B - T_A}$$

T_B = boiling point of component B

T_A = boiling point of component A

The above equation indicates that the closer the boiling temperatures of the components of the liquid, the more plates (or distillations) are required to achieve a standard separation.

B. CRYSTALLIZATION

When a crystalline solid forms in a reaction mixture, it is generally contaminated and must be purified. Often, purification is achieved by dissolving the solid in an appropriate solvent at the boiling point and then recrystallizing the material at a low temperature. A good solvent will dissolve an appreciable amount of the compound at high temperatures and very little at low temperatures. It will also dissolve impurities readily at both low and high temperatures. To recover most of the sample from the solvent, it is critical to use as little of the solvent as possible. In practice, only slightly more hot solvent is used to dissolve the solid so that the solution will not be quite saturated. To collect a pure product, the solvent must be separated from the sample after crystallization has occurred. Suction filtration followed by several washings with the cold solvent and evaporation of the solvent is generally sufficient. A melting point should not be taken until all of the solvent is removed.

Fractional Crystallization

Fractional crystallization may be used to separate two or more components from a reaction mixture. One procedure separates the hot solution (components dissolved in a selected solvent) into fractions by slowly cooling to a selected temperature so that the first crop of crystals form. The solution is then filtered and cooled to another selected temperature so that a second fraction of crystals form, and so on.

C. EXTRACTION

Solvent extraction can be used to

1. separate and isolate substances from naturally occurring mixtures

2. isolate dissolved compounds from solutions

3. remove soluble impurities from mixtures

An immiscible solvent is often used to isolate dissolved organic compounds from solution. For example, an organic solvent like ether or chloroform can be used to extract organic substances from aqueous solution. An organic compound Y, for example, distributes itself between the two solvents A and B according to its distribution coefficient or partition coefficient K given by

$$K \text{ (at constant temperature)} = \frac{[Y]_A}{[Y]_B}$$

The distribution coefficient can be approximated by finding the solubility of the solute in each pure solvent. In addition to a favorable distribution coefficient, other factors that should be considered in selecting a solvent include:

1. Solvent should not extract other dissolved substances.

2. Solvent should be easily separated from solute after extraction (usually by distillation).

3. Solvent should not react with the solute of interest.

Multiple Extractions

The most efficient extraction procedure is one that involves several successive extractions using a fixed quantity of solvent as opposed to a simple extraction with that same total quantity of solvent. The following formula gives the fraction of compound Y left in solvent A after n extractions with solvent B, using a volume of V_B/n.

Multiple extractions are also used to remove soluble impurities. An organic substance mixed with an impurity is treated with an immiscible solvent. The impurity distributes itself between the organic substance and the solvent according to its distribution coefficient. The same formulas apply.

D. CHROMATOGRAPHY

Chromatography refers to many purification procedures, all of which distribute a sample between a stationary phase and a mobile one. As with extractions (liquid-liquid), the success of separation depends on the distribution coefficients. These procedures include liquid-solid, ion-exchange, liquid-liquid, and gas-liquid chromatography.

Liquid-Solid Chromatography

Surfaces of solids adsorb molecules of liquids and gases. Generally, the more polar the surface of the solid, the more it selectively adsorbs polar molecules from liquid or gases. The adsorption coefficient of solute A (K_A) adsorbed onto a solid surface is given by

$$K = \frac{\text{Amount of solute A adsorbed/Unit Surface Area}}{\text{Concentration of solute A in Solution}}$$

Solutes having different adsorption coefficients toward a solid surface can be separated by liquid-solid chromatography. One method uses a thin film of solid covering a sheet of glass or some other material that serves as the stationary phase. The solution or mobile phase containing the solutes to be separated is introduced to the bottom of the plate, usually as a spot. The plate is dropped vertically into a small amount of solvent, which then ascends by capillary action carrying the solutes with it. The solutes with the higher adsorption coefficients will adsorb onto the plate first, forming bands closer to the spot. The less tightly held solutes will appear farther up the plate.

Gas-Liquid Chromatography

In this chromatographic technique, a film of nonvolatile liquid adsorbed on a solid support serves as the stationary phase while the moving phase consists of a mixture of the vaporized sample with a carrier gas such as N_2 or He. The components of the vaporized sample distribute themselves between the carrier gas as a vapor and liquid as a solute. As in fractional distillation, the degree of separation depends on differences in the vapor pressure of the components of the mixture. The number of theoretical plates required for a 95% pure sample with 80% recovery from a 50:50 mixture is given by

$$\text{number of plates needed} = \frac{2.0}{(\log \alpha)^2}$$

The above expression differs from the analogous expression for fractional distillation by the exponent of the log α term. Because α (the relative volatility of the components in the mixture) is most likely to be close to unity for mixtures that are being fractionally distilled or chromatographed, log α approaches zero. Consequently, gas-liquid chromotography requires significantly more theoretical plates than fractional distillation to achieve the same separation. This can be attained by using long columns coiled into a small volume. It is important to note that with gas-liquid chromatography, you can choose from a long list of liquid phases to maximize the value of α.

CHAPTER 11

Biological Sciences Sample Exam

TIME: 100 MINUTES   77 QUESTIONS

Directions: This test includes 10 sets of questions related to specific passages (62 questions) and 15 shorter, independent questions. The passages represent all four format styles (Information Presentation, Problem Solving, Research Study, and Persuasive Argument that you may see on the MCAT exam). Explanatory answers immediately follow the test.

Passage I (Questions 1–6)

In red blood cells, oxygen forms a relatively unstable bond with hemoglobin. Whether oxygen remains bound to hemoglobin (hemoglobin saturation) or whether it dissociates from hemoglobin is a function involving many variables, including the concentration of oxygen in the blood and surrounding tissues (measured as PO_2 in mm of mercury), the concentration of carbon dioxide in the blood and surrounding tissues (measured as PCO_2 in mm of mercury), and the temperature and pH of the blood. The experiments described below were carried out to determine the effects of some of these variables.

Experiment 1

Samples of mouse blood were tested for hemoglobin saturation levels at different conditions of PO_2 in a controlled experimental chamber. The temperature (36°C), pH (7.4), and PCO_2 (40mm) of the blood were all kept constant. Table 1 shows the results of the experiment.

Experiment 2

PO_2 conditions identical to those in Experiment 1 were used to measure hemoglobin saturation at different PCO_2 levels (20mm and 80mm). The temperature and pH of the blood samples were

Table 1.

Hemoglobin Saturation at Different PO_2 Levels (36°C; pH = 7.4; PCO_2 = 40mm).

PO_2 Levels	% Hemoglobin Saturation
20	40
30	60
40	80

held constant at levels identical to those in Experiment 1. Table 2 shows the results.

Experiment 3

Table 3 shows the results of the third experiment, in which hemoglobin saturation was measured under varying conditions of blood pH (7.2 and 7.6). All other experimental conditions

Table 2.

Hemoglobin Saturation at Different PCO_2 Levels (36°C; pH = 7.4).

PO_2 Levels	% Hemoglobin Saturation	
	PCO_2 = 20mm	PCO_2 = 80mm
20	50	20
30	70	40
40	90	60

(PO_2, PCO_2, and temperature) were identical to those used in Experiment 1.

Table 3.

Hemoglobin Saturation at Different pH Levels (36°C; PCO_2 = 40mm).

	% Hemoglobin Saturation	
PO_2 Levels	pH = 7.2	pH = 7.6
20	20	50
30	40	70
40	60	90

1. Based on the results of Experiments 2 and 3, which of the following statements is most appropriate?

   A. Changes in pH have less of an effect than changes in PCO_2.
   B. Changes in pH have more of an effect than changes in PCO_2.
   C. An increase in pH will have a similar effect to a decrease in PCO_2.
   D. An increase in pH will have a similar effect to an increase in PCO_2.

2. Experiment 1 suggests that hemoglobin saturation will be highest

   A. in the brain.
   B. in the lungs.
   C. in the vena cavae.
   D. in body tissues farthest from the lungs.

3. The variable not tested by this set of experiments is

   A. PO_2.
   B. alkalinity level.
   C. PCO_2.
   D. temperature.

4. Under acidic conditions, hemoglobin saturation levels at PO_2 = 30mm would be expected to

   A. increase above 70%.
   B. decrease below 40%.
   C. increase above 90%.
   D. decrease below 20%.

5. Carbon monoxide is toxic because it combines with hemoglobin more readily than oxygen does, and because it does not dissociate from hemoglobin as readily as oxygen does. Treating the effects of carbon monoxide poisoning can include administering air that is high in oxygen concentration, and administering carbon dioxide to stimulate rapid breathing. Which statement is most appropriate with regard to this pattern of treatment?

   A. The rationale for the treatments is supported by the results in Experiments 1 and 2.
   B. The rationale for the treatments is contradicted by the results in Experiment 1 and supported by the results in Experiment 2.
   C. The rationale for the treatments is contradicted by the results in Experiments 1 and 2.
   D. The rationale for the treatments is supported by the results in Experiment 1 and contradicted by the results in Experiment 2.

6. An increase in blood PCO_2 also increases the acidity of blood. Do the trends in hemoglobin saturation levels shown in Tables 2 and 3 support this idea?

   A. Yes
   B. No
   C. Only at the lowest PO_2
   D. Only at the highest PO_2

Passage II (Questions 7–13)

The electrocardiogram (ECG) is a record of the electrical changes that take place in the myocardium during a cardiac cycle. Since body fluids, with their various electrolytes, can conduct an electrical current, depolarizations and repolarizations that occur in muscle cells can be detected from the surface of the body. By placing metal electrodes at specific locations on the skin, the electrical sequences associated with the contraction and relaxation of the atria and ventricles can be viewed pictorially using an instrument that monitors and records these events.

As impulses move through the cardiac conduction system—i.e., the S-A node or *pacemaker* (in the right atrium with fibers extending across to the left atrium), the A-V node (also in the right atrium), the A-V bundle or bundle of His (in the interventricular septum), and the Purkinje fibers (in the walls of the ventricles)—the following precise sequence of representations can be seen in the normal ECG:

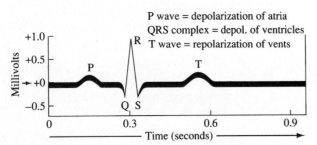

P wave = depolarization of atria
QRS complex = depol. of ventricles
T wave = repolarization of vents

7. The P wave is most closely associated with the electrical events between the

    A.   S-A node and A-V node.
    B.   S-A node and Purkinje fibers.
    C.   A-V node and A-V bundle.
    D.   A-V bundle and Purkinje fibers.

8. According to the figure, the largest net change in voltage associated with a specific event during the cardiac cycle is closest to

    A.   0.5 millivolts.
    B.   −0.5 millivolts.
    C.   1.0 millivolts.
    D.   1.5 millivolts.

9. The time interval required for the cardiac impulse to travel from the pacemaker into the ventricular walls can be estimated by measuring the

    A.   height of the P wave.
    B.   combined heights of the P wave and the QRS complex.
    C.   distance between the P wave and the QRS complex.
    D.   distance between the P wave and the T wave.

10. With respect to the figure above, which statement best explains the absence of a wave depicting repolarization of the atria?

    A.   The atria do not have to repolarize at every cardiac cycle.
    B.   Atrial repolarization occurs at a point beyond the T wave.
    C.   Atrial repolarization occurs at about the same time as ventricular depolarization.
    D.   Atrial repolarization distinctly occurs between the P wave and the QRS complex, but the electrical change is so slight that the normal instruments used are not sensitive enough to detect it.

11. If damaged heart tissue prolongs depolarization of the ventricles, what change might be detected in the patient's ECG?

    A.   A higher QRS complex.
    B.   A wider QRS complex.
    C.   A second QRS complex will be present.
    D.   The QRS complex will be absent.

12. Innervation of the S-A node and the A-V node to maintain the normal heart rate comes from

    A. motor neurons of the somatic nervous system.
    B. motor neurons of the sympathetic autonomic nervous system.
    C. motor neurons of the parasympathetic autonomic nervous system.
    D. none of these types of motor neurons, since the heart is self-excitable.

13. Which of the following should have no effect on the normal ECG?

    A. potassium ion concentrations
    B. sodium ion concentrations
    C. calcium ion concentrations
    D. none of these

Passage III (Questions 14–20)

Many of the events that occur during early human development are very similar to those developmental events described for other vertebrates. Within three days after fertilization (zygote formation), a 16–32-cell structure called a morula has formed as a result of mitosis during the cleavage stage. By the end of the first week, this structure has continued to grow in cell number; has developed a hollow, fluid-filled cavity; and is referred to as a blastocyst. The blastocyst has an outer layer of cells (trophoblast) that forms tiny finger-like projections (microvilli) that grow into the endometrial lining of the uterus, thereby facilitating implantation at this time (later, trophoblast cells will give rise to the embryonic membrane, the chorion). Inside, the blastocyst is made up of other cells that form an inner-cell mass that eventually gives rise to the embryo.

The embryonic stage includes the second through the eighth weeks. During this time, (a) gastrulation occurs among the cells of the inner cell mass, forming the primary germ layers: ectoderm, endoderm, and mesoderm; (b) neurulation takes place among ectodermal cells; and (c) components of the other major organ systems form (organogenesis) from all three germ layers (e.g., ectoderm: special sense organs, epidermal structures; endoderm: linings of the digestive and respiratory tracts; mesoderm: bone and all muscle tissues).

After the eighth week, the developing individual enters the fetal stage, during which time body parts continue to grow and mature but relatively few new structures are formed.

14. Teratogens are agents that can cause congenital defects in developing offspring due to their effects on differentiating cells. During which time would you expect these factors to have the severest effects?

    A. prior to fertilization
    B. during cleavage and implantation
    C. during gastrulation and organogenesis
    D. in the fetus

15. According to the passage, the inner cell mass forms

    A. between fertilization and the end of day 3.
    B. between days 3 and 7.
    C. just after implantation.
    D. during the embryonic stage.

16. Which statement is supported by information in the passage?

    A. The spinal cord forms from ectoderm.
    B. Parts of the eye are formed from ectoderm.
    C. Both A and B are supported.
    D. Neither A nor B is supported.

17. If a woman requiring *in vitro fertilization* has 50–72-hr cells (her own ovum had been removed, fertilized, and then incubated 50–72 hours in a special medium outside the body) transferred to her uterus, at which developmental stage should the cells be in order to most closely simulate the natural sequence of events described in the passage?

   A. zygote
   B. morula
   C. blastocyst
   D. embryo

18. If two cells of the blastocyst were chosen randomly and compared, would they be genetically identical?

   A. yes
   B. no
   C. only if the two cells were both part of the trophoblast or both part of the inner cell mass
   D. only if they were from different parts of the blastocyst (one from trophoblast, one from inner cell mass)

19. According to the passage, myocardial cells are derived from

   A. ectoderm.
   B. endoderm.
   C. mesoderm.
   D. It cannot be determined.

20. The placenta is an organ that develops from cells of the chorion and endometrium. Therefore, it is comprised of

   A. maternal tissue.
   B. embryonic tissue.
   C. both maternal and embryonic tissues.
   D. It is an independent organ consisting of tissues considered neither maternal nor embryonic.

Passage IV (Questions 21–26)

Conflicts can arise in modern evolutionary discussions concerning the "target" or "unit" of natural selection. Although it has long been accepted that if a heritable "trait" (physiological, behavioral, structural, etc.) reproductively benefits an individual with that trait, he/she will leave more offspring in the following generation than competitors who do not possess that trait. This will result in more and more individuals present in each new generation possessing the gene(s) underlying the trait. By contrast, those individuals without this "adaptive" trait will leave fewer offspring in each generation and future populations will gradually have less and less of the types who lack the advantageous gene(s). Such an increase or decrease in the frequency of the gene(s) underlying the trait in question can typically be explained on the basis of natural selection acting on the *individual* as the unit of selection.

However, certain traits have been observed that do not, at first glance, seem to provide a reproductive advantage to the individual possessing the trait. For example, a member of a group (herd, flock, etc.) that sounds an alarm call when danger is sighted often draws the danger source to itself. This can be disadvantageous to the alarm caller's reproductive potential, but may be of great advantage to other members of the group who heed the warning and escape (altruism). Possessing the gene(s) underlying such altruistic alarm calling may lead to an early death for the individual, but may benefit the longevity and reproductive potential of the group itself. Thus, such genes (and traits) may be maintained and actually increase in subsequent generations if natural selection can act on the *group* as the unit of selection (group selection).

21. "Since alarm calling is detrimental to the caller, the genes underlying such behavior should have been eliminated from the population long ago. Yet, we continue to observe such behavior." Which point of view does this statement support?

    A. The unit of selection for this behavior is the individual.
    B. The unit of selection for this behavior is the group.
    C. Evolution is a gradual, long-term process.
    D. Altruistic behavior is expected to occur only rarely in animal groups.

22. Some theorists propose that "kin selection" is a way that genes for altruistic behavior can be maintained in a population; i.e., if the group consists of genetically related individuals, the altruist (alarm caller) may be preserving many copies of its own altruistic genes by saving other members of the group. Which of the following statements is correct?

    A. Kin selection requires no special unit of selection beyond the individual.
    B. The individual as the unit of selection cannot account for kin selection.
    C. Kin selection demonstrates that both the individual and the group are units of selection.
    D. Group selection occurs in groups of related individuals.

23. Which observation can be used as evidence against the idea of group selection?

    A. An alarm call causes a flock of birds to scatter, confusing the predator and making it difficult to capture any one individual.
    B. A young baboon's alarm call immediately brings the strong, large males of the troop to protect against a leopard.
    C. Both A and B.
    D. Neither A nor B.

24. Supporters of the *reciprocal altruism* concept suggest that even if an alarm caller has immediate risks (costs) when warning others, the sum benefits of all future warnings given to him by the other group members will outweigh such costs by far. Reciprocal altruism

    A. provides an advantage to an alarm caller.
    B. demonstrates that the evolutionary "costs and benefits" of a trait come into play immediately.
    C. Both A and B.
    D. Neither A nor B.

25. Honeybee society utilizes thousands of sterile workers that contribute greatly to the maintenance and survival of the fertile queen and the entire colony, yet they never produce offspring of their own. This observation

    A. supports the view that individuals are the sole units of selection.
    B. is irrelevant to the question of whether the individual or the group is the unit of natural selection.
    C. can be addressed using a group selection explanation.
    D. suggests that gene frequencies in honeybee colonies can only change if mutations occur.

26. According to the Hardy-Weinberg Law (Equilibrium), gene frequencies in a population do not change from generation to generation (no evolution takes place) *unless* one or more of the following factors is at work: non-random mating, mutation, selection, migration, and genetic drift. If, in a natural population, individuals possessing the gene(s) underlying alarm calling have their survival and reproductive potential directly affected by this behavior, which viewpoint would be most important in showing that evolution *is* taking place (Hardy-Weinberg Equilibrium is *not* being maintained)?

A. The individual is the unit of selection.
B. The group is the unit of selection.
C. Evidence that both *units* are targets of selection should be shown to indicate that evolution is taking place.
D. The *unit* of selection is irrelevant to showing that evolution is taking place.

Passage V (Questions 27–32)

Hormones are chemical messengers synthesized by one type of cell that can affect the activity of another type of cell. Hormones are usually produced by endocrine glands and released directly into the blood, by which they are transported throughout the body. The target sites of a particular hormone may be *specific* (Thyroid Stimulating Hormone, produced by the anterior pituitary gland, primarily increases the activity of cells in the thyroid gland), or quite *general* (insulin, produced by the pancreas, affects the ability of all cells to utilize glucose).

Experimental studies often attempt to identify the endocrine tissues responsible for a research organism's response or lack of response, and then try to determine which specific hormone is at work. In some species of mammals, it has been hypothesized that testosterone influences male courtship behavior toward females and aggressive behavior toward competing males.

27. Which of the following observations would suggest that the hypothesis may be valid?

A. When males see females approaching their territories, they begin to perform courtship behaviors.
B. After males have set up their territories, they are extremely aggressive toward any other males in the area.
C. When males are injected with high levels of testosterone, courtship behavior to females and aggressive behavior toward males increases.
D. All of the above.

28. One way of testing the hypothesis would be to remove the gonads of male individuals in an experimental group of subjects. Based on the hypothesis, what prediction can be made?

A. Courtship and aggressive behavior should not be affected.
B. Courtship and aggressive behavior should decrease.
C. Courtship and aggressive behavior should increase.
D. Courtship and aggressive behavior should vary in opposite directions.

29. If, after removal of the gonads, both behaviors remain as before, should the experimenter eliminate testosterone from his/her hypothesis as the hormonal influence on courtship and aggression?

   A. Yes, because it is known that the testes are the primary sites of testosterone production.
   B. Yes, because even if testosterone is synthesized at other glandular sites as well, concentrations would not be high enough to maintain the behaviors.
   C. No, because testosterone may be made elsewhere at high enough concentrations to maintain the behaviors.
   D. No, because an experimental group does not represent what happens in nature.

30. If, after removal of the gonads, both behaviors in question disappear, how might the experimenter provide additional evidence to support the hypothesis?

   A. Inject testosterone and see if the behaviors return.
   B. Repeat the experiment with another experimental group.
   C. Both A and B.
   D. Neither A nor B.

31. According to information in the passage, it would be possible to conclude that testosterone has *specific* target sites in the experimental organism if it could be shown that it affected

   A. only the two particular behaviors in question.
   B. all cells in very specific ways.
   C. only male individuals.
   D. only particular cells in the brain that influence the behaviors in question.

32. If testosterone concentrations stimulate courtship and aggression in the same way, which hypothesis seems most appropriate if it becomes known that testosterone levels decrease in subordinate males after each defeat in aggressive encounters with dominant males?

   A. Courtship behavior should not be affected in subordinate males.
   B. Courtship behavior should be less vigorous in subordinate males.
   C. Courtship behavior should be more vigorous in subordinate males.
   D. Courtship behavior should be less vigorous in dominant males.

Passage VI (Questions 33–39)

A set of experiments was carried out to isolate unusual mutants of the bacterium *E. coli*. It is known that normal *E. coli* cells grow well on a minimal nutrient medium containing agar and a solution of glucose, salts, and ammonia. *E. coli* can also grow on a medium containing more complex sugars like lactose, because they normally have the enzymes needed to convert complex sugars to glucose. Overnight, a single bacterial cell can grow into a culture of millions of cells that appears as a raised colony on the medium.

Experiment 1

A test-tube suspension of normal *E. coli* was treated with x-rays in order to produce mutations among the bacterial cells. The bacteria were then spread across a dish containing a minimal nutrient medium. The medium also contained the antibiotic streptomycin, which kills normal bacteria. The culture was incubated overnight and examined. No bacterial cultures were found growing in the dish.

Experiment 2

The experiment was repeated exactly as before, using the same test-tube suspension. This time, when the culture was examined after incubation, two colonies of bacteria (Colony A and Colony B) were found growing on the medium.

Experiment 3

Samples from both colonies grown in Experiment 2 were spread across two different streptomycin-containing media. Medium X was the typical minimal medium. Medium Y contained the same ingredients, with the exception that instead of glucose, lactose was the only nutrient sugar present. After incubation, the four dishes were examined and the results are shown in the following table.

	Medium X	Medium Y
Colony A	growth	growth
Colony B	growth	no growth

33. What conclusion can be drawn from Experiment 1?

A. No mutations were produced.

B. Mutations were produced, but none that were streptomycin-resistant.

C. No streptomycin-resistant mutations were produced.

D. All bacterial cells became streptomycin-resistant.

34. What conclusion can be drawn from Experiment 2?

A. At least two bacterial cells were mutated and became streptomycin-resistant colonies.

B. All bacterial cells *except two* became streptomycin-resistant.

C. A variety of mutants were produced with the second dose of x-rays.

D. Colony A and Colony B can grow without glucose in the medium.

35. What do the results of Experiment 3 suggest about how Colony A and Colony B are similar to each other?

A. Both can grow on glucose, lactose, and streptomycin.

B. Both can grow on glucose and lactose.

C. Both can grow on lactose and streptomycin.

D. Both can grow on glucose and streptomycin.

36. What might be a reasonable hypothesis for explaining why Colony B is unable to grow on Medium Y?

A. Lactose is not nutritious when mixed with streptomycin.

B. The mutagenic x-rays affected the lactose in the medium.

C. The gene for the enzyme that converts lactose to glucose had mutated.

D. A gene in the cells that made up Colony A had mutated, enabling them to out-compete the cells of Colony B in the lactose medium.

37. If streptomycin-resistance arose by mutation in Experiment 2, when did the mutation that prevented Colony B from growing in the lactose medium arise?

A. in Experiment 1

B. in Experiment 2

C. in Experiment 1 or Experiment 2

D. in Experiment 3

38. If a culture taken from the original x-rayed suspension in Experiment 1 were spread across a fresh dish of minimal medium *without* streptomycin, what would you expect to observe after incubation?

    A. Colonies would be growing everywhere on the medium.

    B. One or two colonies would be growing on the medium.

    C. Only cells that produced Colony A in Experiment 2 would be able to grow.

    D. The cells that produced Colony A and Colony B in Experiment 2 would die on the medium.

39. How might streptomycin-resistance from the cells in Colony A be conveyed to other normal *E. coli* cells?

    A. by conjugation
    B. by transformation
    C. by transduction
    D. all of the above

Passage VII (Questions 40–45)

Vertebrate organisms respond in many different ways to changes in environmental temperature. *Poikilotherms* (fish, amphibians, and reptiles) have a body temperature that fluctuates with that of the environment. They lack metabolic mechanisms for regulating their temperature. However, they are able to maintain homeostatic temperature levels primarily through behavioral adaptations. Warm-blooded animals or *homeotherms* (birds, mammals) derive most of their heat from their own metabolic activities and can conserve or dissipate heat when necessary through a variety of physiological methods. The appropriate response in homeotherms is dependent on whether their body temperature is above or below their brain's normal "thermostat" setting. The figure here compares the effects of changing environmental temperatures on poikilothermic and homeothermic vertebrates.

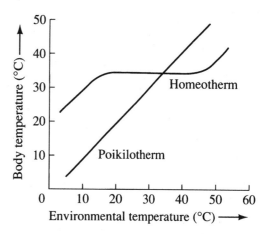

40. According to the information in the figure, at approximately what environmental temperature will the average homeotherm and poikilotherm have the same body temperature?

    A. 5–10°C
    B. 15–20°C
    C. 30–35°C
    D. 45–50°C

41. The figure indicates that the average warm-blooded animal's metabolic and physiological mechanisms, which help maintain normal body temperature, start to lose their effectiveness

    A. between 20°C and 45°C.
    B. below 35°C and above 50°C.
    C. between 5°C and 20°C.
    D. below 20°C and above 45°C.

42. At 15°C, a poikilothermic lizard would most likely

    A. take refuge in a cool burrow.
    B. bask on a sunny rock.
    C. hunt for food.
    D. vasoconstrict superficial blood vessels to conserve heat.

43. The human "thermostat" is in the hypothalamus. When body temperature "strays" from homeostatic levels, neurons from the hypothalamus send stimuli along circuits that eventually activate the appropriate responses for returning body temperature back to the homeostatic range. According to the figure, to which effectors would neuronal circuits be active when environmental temperature is approximately 40°C?

A. sweat glands and superficial blood vessels (for vasoconstriction)

B. skeletal muscles (for shivering) and superficial blood vessels (for vasodilation)

C. sweat glands and superficial blood vessels (for vasodilation)

D. skeletal muscles (for shivering) and superficial blood vessels (for vasoconstriction)

44. According to the figure, which statement best describes the difference in response options between a homeotherm (A) and poikilotherm (B) when environmental temperatures rise from 25°C to 40°C, if we assume that normal body temperature is approximately 35°C for both animals?

A. Animal A could rest in the sun the entire time, while animal B could rest in the sun for a while and then seek the shade.

B. Animal B could rest in the sun the entire time, while animal A could rest in the sun for a while and then seek the shade.

C. Animal A could rest in the sun the entire time, while animal B could first rest in the shade and then seek the sun.

D. Animal B could rest in the sun the entire time, while animal A could first rest in the shade and then seek the sun.

45. Substances produced by cells of the immune system in response to infectious microorganisms often act as *pyrogens* on the human body. That is, they cause an adjustment in the brain's thermostat so that it becomes set at a higher than normal temperature (102°F instead of 98.6°F). What symptoms might be exhibited by a patient infected by one of these pathogens?

A. sweating at 101°F
B. shivering at 101°F
C. shivering at 103°F
D. none of these

Passage VIII (Questions 46–51)

A student found that when she reacted 2-methyl-1-butanol with H_2SO_4, two low-boiling liquids formed (Solution A). She then performed the following experiments.

Experiment 1

The liquids were reacted with Cl_2 in CCl_4 and the resulting mixture distilled. Two dichloro products were identified as mostly 2,3-dichloro-2-methylbutane and some 1,2-dichloro-2-methylbutane.

Experiment 2

The liquids in Solution A were then reacted with HCl(aq) to form mostly 2-chloro-2-methylbutane.

The student concluded that the liquids were 2-methyl-1-butene and 2-methyl-2-butene. She performed Experiments 3 and 4 to elucidate the mechanism of the reaction.

Experiment 3

A kinetic study showed that the initial reaction is a first-order reaction whose rate depends only on the concentration of 2-methyl-1-butanol.

Experiment 4

The initial reaction was repeated using 2-deutero-2-methyl-1-butanol as a starting material. The rate of the reaction decreased as a result.

46. What are the intermediates that could account for the two liquid products?

A.
$$CH_3-\overset{\oplus}{CH}-\overset{\overset{\displaystyle CH_3}{|}}{CH}-CH_3, \ ^{\oplus}CH_2-CH_2-\overset{\overset{\displaystyle CH_3}{|}}{CH}-CH_3$$

B.
$$^{\oplus}CH_2-CH_2-\overset{\overset{\displaystyle CH_3}{|}}{CH}-CH_3, \ CH_3-CH_2-\overset{\overset{\displaystyle CH_3}{|}}{\underset{\oplus}{C}}-CH_3$$

C.
$$CH_3-CH_2-\overset{\overset{\displaystyle CH_3}{|}}{\underset{\oplus}{CH}}-CH_2, \ CH_3-CH_2-\overset{\overset{\displaystyle CH_3}{|}}{\underset{\oplus}{C}}-CH_3$$

D.
$$CH_3-\overset{\overset{\displaystyle CH_3}{|}}{\underset{\underset{\displaystyle CH_3}{|}}{C}}-\overset{\oplus}{CH_2}, \ CH_3-\overset{\overset{\displaystyle CH_3}{|}}{\underset{\oplus}{C}}-CH_2-CH_3$$

47. Which mechanism of the initial reaction is most consistent with the results of the experiments?

A. S_N1
B. S_N2
C. E1
D. E2

48. Chlorination of the liquids showed that Solution A consisted mostly of

A. 2-methyl-2-butene.
B. 2-methyl-1-butene.
C. 1-chloro-2-methyl-2-butene.
D. 1-chloro-2-methyl-1-butene.

49. The results of the experiments are consistent with a carbocation undergoing a

A. 1,2 methyl shift.
B. 1,2 hydride shift.
C. 1,3 methyl shift.
D. 1,3 hydride shift.

50. Based on the results of Experiments 1–4, what is most likely the chief product of the dehydrohalogenation of 2-methyl-1-bromo-pentane?

A. 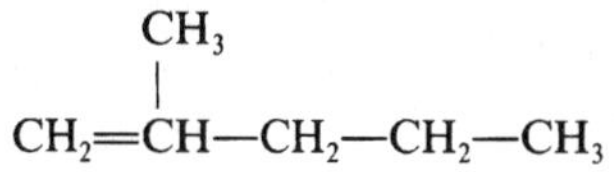
$$CH_2{=}CH-CH_2-\overset{\overset{\displaystyle CH_3}{|}}{C}H_2-CH_3$$

A.
$$\overset{\overset{\displaystyle CH_3}{|}}{CH_2{=}CH-CH_2-CH_2-CH_3}$$

B.
$$CH_3-\overset{\overset{\displaystyle CH_3}{|}}{C}{=}CH-CH_2-CH_3$$

C.
$$CH_3-\overset{\overset{\displaystyle CH_3}{|}}{CH}-CH{=}CH-CH_3$$

D.
$$CH_3-\overset{\overset{\displaystyle CH_3}{|}}{CH}-CH_2-CH{=}CH_2$$

51. Which of the following general statements applies to the mechanism of the reaction?

A. An S_N2 reaction occurs with inversion of configuration.
B. Rearrangement of H^{θ} or an alkyl group will occur if it produces a more stable carbocation.
C. Electron-withdrawing groups stabilize carbocations.
D. Only cis isomers are formed in elimination reactions.

Passage IX (Questions 52–59)

Two mechanisms are postulated for the addition of Br_2 to cis-2-butene.

Mechanism A

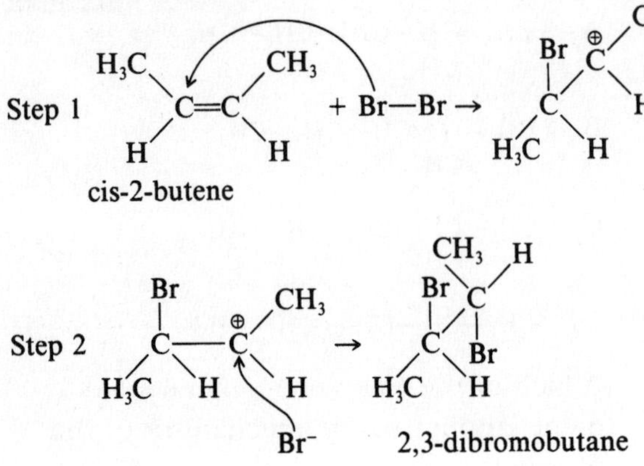

Step 1

cis-2-butene

Step 2

2,3-dibromobutane

Mechanism B

Step 1

Step 2

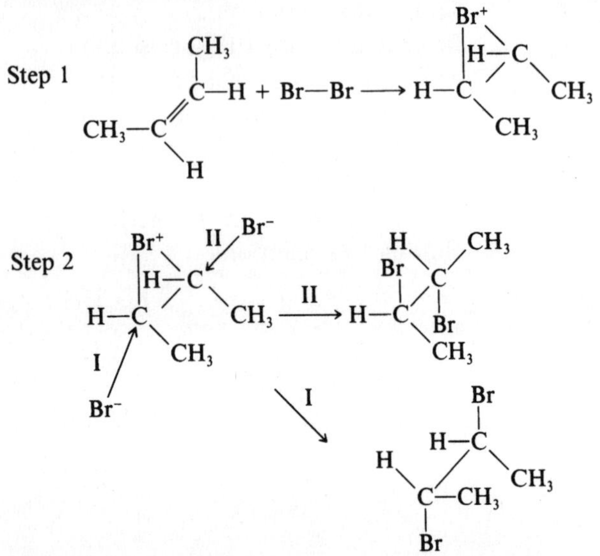

Bromination of cis-2-butene yields a racemic mixture of 2,3-dibromobutane while bromination of trans-2-butene gives meso-2,3-dibromobutane.

52. Step 2 of Mechanism A as shown yields only

A. (R,R)-2,3-dibromobutane.
B. (S,S)-2,3-dibromobutane.
C. (R,S)-2,3-dibromobutane.
D. meso-2,3-dibromobutane.

53. Step 2 of Mechanism A shows attack of Br from the bottom of the carbocation.

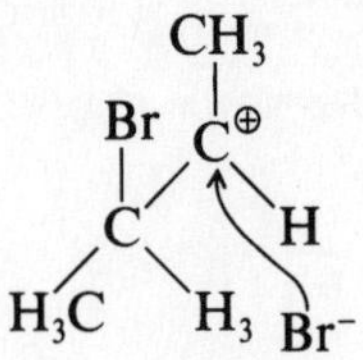

If the rotation about the CC bond occurs so that the carbocation in Step 2 of Mechanism A becomes

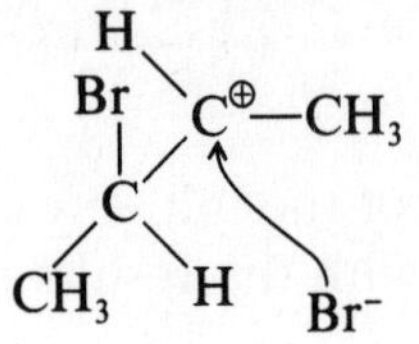

the product would be

A. meso-2,3-dibromobutane.
B. the same product.
C. (S,S)-2,3-dibromobutane.
D. (R,R)-2,3-dibromobutane.

54. The observed stereochemistry

A. supports both Mechanism A and Mechanism B.
B. does not support either mechanism.
C. supports Mechanism A only.
D. supports Mechanism B only.

55. The advantage of a bromonium ion over a carbocation as an intermediate is

A. that in a carbocation, all atoms have an octet.
B. that in a bromonium ion, all atoms have an octet.
C. that a halogen can better accommodate the positive charge.
D. There is no advantage.

56. Bromination of 2-phenyl-2-butene occurs via Mechanism A. What is the most likely explanation?

A. Phenyl groups undergo addition more readily.
B. The bromonium ion is sterically hindered.
C. The phenyl group stabilizes the carbocation.
D. The phenyl group destabilizes the bromonium ion.

57. Halogenation of both cis and trans-2-butene occurs by

A. syn addition.
B. anti addition.
C. syn addition for cis-2-butene and anti for trans.
D. anti addition for cis-2-butene and syn for trans.

58. Halohydrins contain halogen and hydroxyl groups on adjacent carbon atoms. They can be formed by the addition of chlorine or bromine to an alkene in the presence of water. There is evidence that a halonium ion is formed as an intermediate, which is then attacked by H_2O. Predict the major product(s) when cis-2-butene forms a chlorohydrin.

A.
```
     CH3                    CH3
Cl——|——H              H——|——Cl
 H——|——OH            HO——|——H
     CH3                    CH3
```

B.
```
     CH3                    CH3
 H——|——Cl             Cl——|——H
 H——|——OH            HO——|——H
     CH3                    CH3
```

C.
```
     CH2CH3                 CH2CH3
 H——|——OH            HO——|——H
     CH2Cl                  CH2Cl
```

D.
```
     CH3                    CH3
 H——|——OH            HO——|——H
     CH2CH2Cl             CH2CH2Cl
```

59. Hydroxylation of cis-2-butene with peroxy acids forms a racemic mixture of 2,3-butanediol. Which intermediate is most consistent with the stereochemical evidence?

A. a carbocation

B. an epoxide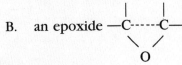

C. a carbanion
D. a halonium ion

Questions 60–77 are independent of any passage and independent of each other.

60. Which of the statements below is false regarding the following structure?

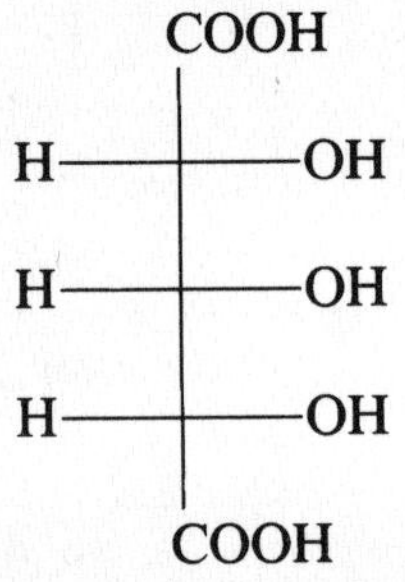

```
        COOH
         |
  H——————OH
         |
  H——————OH
         |
  H——————OH
         |
        COOH
```

A. It is optically inactive.
B. It is a meso acid.
C. It can be formed by using HNO_3 to treat

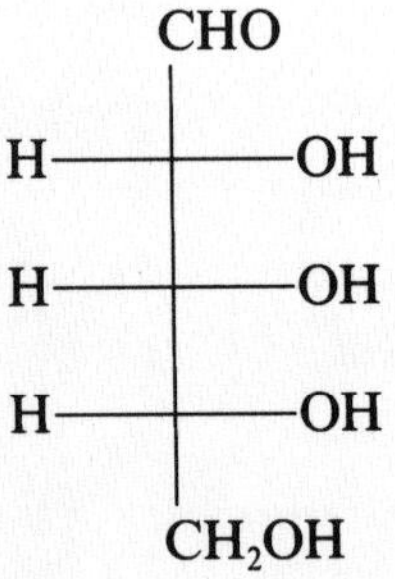

```
        CHO
         |
  H——————OH
         |
  H——————OH
         |
  H——————OH
         |
       CH_2OH
```

D. It is nonsuperimposible on its mirror image.

61. The dipolar ion of alanine is

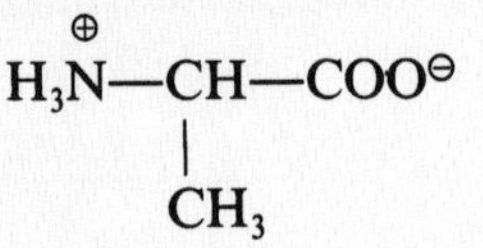

$$\overset{\oplus}{H_3N}-CH-COO^{\ominus}$$
$$|$$
$$CH_3$$

What is the predominant form in basic solution?

A. 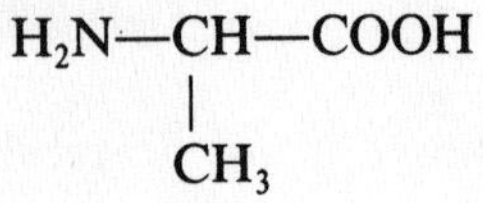 $H_2N-CH-COOH$
$\quad\quad |$
$\quad\quad CH_3$

B. 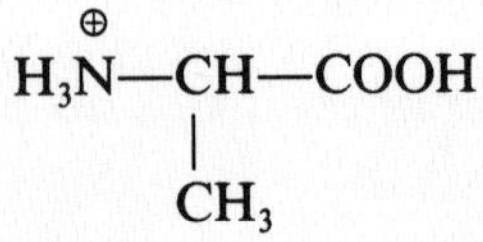 $\overset{\oplus}{H_3N}-CH-COOH$
$\quad\quad |$
$\quad\quad CH_3$

C. 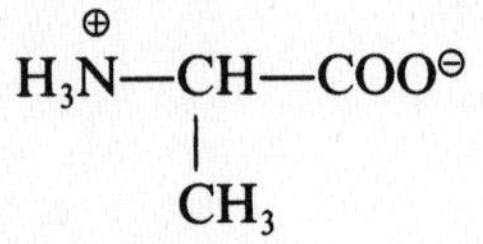 $\overset{\oplus}{H_3N}-CH-COO^{\ominus}$
$\quad\quad |$
$\quad\quad CH_3$

D. 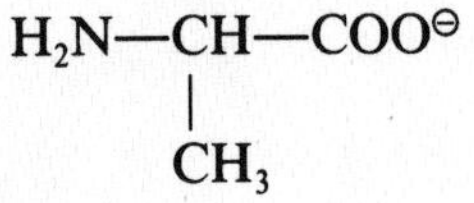 $H_2N-CH-COO^{\ominus}$
$\quad\quad |$
$\quad\quad CH_3$

62. Acetic acid reacts more rapidly with methanol than with ethanol to form the ester. Most likely this is due to

A. an inductive electronic effect.
B. a resonance effect.
C. steric hindrance.
D. an ortho effect.

63. In the kidney, the distal convoluted tubules of the nephron contain a filtrate in which the sodium concentration is lower than in the surrounding peritubular capillaries. If sodium ions move from filtrate to blood, what process is at work?

A. diffusion
B. osmosis
C. facilitated transport (facilitated diffusion)
D. active transport

64. If a cell is treated with a substance that inhibits DNA polymerase activity, what stage of the cell cycle is most likely to be affected?

A. Interphase
B. Prophase
C. Anaphase
D. Telophase

65. The following reaction must take place in all human cells:

$$\text{adenosine triphosphate} \xrightarrow{\text{ATPase}}$$
$$\text{adenosine diphosphate} + \text{phosphate}$$

For what purpose does this reaction most often occur?

A. It is needed to carry out the electron transport chain.
B. It is carried out to maintain the passage of oxygen from lungs to blood.
C. It is needed to carry out most energy-requiring cellular work.
D. It is carried out to regulate the movement of water across membranes.

66. Mouse cells are grown in culture dishes with nutrient medium containing radioactive forms of adenine and uracil. Which molecules synthesized by the cells would you expect to be radioactively labeled?

A. Adenine and uracil in DNA, RNA, and ATP
B. Adenine and uracil in DNA and ATP uracil in RNA
C. Adenine in DNA and RNA; uracil in RNA; neither in ATP
D. Adenine in DNA, RNA, and ATP; uracil in RNA

67. Cyanide is a poison that interferes with cytochrome activity. In what part of a human cell does cyanide have its effects?

A. Cytosol
B. Mitochondria
C. Ribosomes
D. All of the above

68. Colorblindness is a relatively common sex-linked trait in humans. If a woman is born colorblind, which statement is most accurate about colorblind individuals in her ancestry?

A. Both of her parents were colorblind.
B. Both of her parents were carriers of colorblindness.
C. Both of her parents, at least one of her mother's parents, and at least one of her father's parents had the gene.
D. Both of her parents, both of her mother's parents, and at least one of her father's parents had the gene.

69. Multicellular organisms are always composed of many small cells rather than fewer large cells. As a cell's surface area increases by the square of its linear dimension, its volume increases by the cube of its linear dimension. Which statement is true about how cellular function(s) would be *directly* affected in a cell that grew too large?

A. The rate of membrane transport could not keep up with the needs of the cell.
B. The distances to be traveled by molecules within the cell would make metabolic functions inefficient.
C. Both A and B.
D. Neither A nor B.

70. Nondisjunction is a phenomenon in which an error in the distribution of chromosomes occurs during meiosis. If it occurs in meiosis I, homologous chromosomes do not move apart; whereas if it happens in meiosis II, sister chromatids do not separate. In a cell in which the diploid number is six $(2N = 6)$, how many chromosomes will be in each of the four meiotic products if one pair of homologous chromosomes exhibits nondisjunction during meiosis I?

   A. Two cells will have 6 chromosomes; two cells will have none.
   B. Two cells will have 4 chromosomes; two cells will have 2 chromosomes.
   C. Two cells will have 5 chromosomes; two cells will have 1 chromosome.
   D. All four cells will have 3 chromosomes.

71. If prevention of the initial enzymatic breakdown of polysaccharides is desired, where in the body should the release of such enzymes be blocked?

   A. In the mouth, stomach, pancreas, and small intestine
   B. In the mouth, stomach, and pancreas
   C. In the mouth, pancreas, and small intestine
   D. In the mouth and pancreas

72. Parathormone (PTH) is a peptide hormone produced in the parathyroid gland. It plays a major role in increasing blood calcium (Ca) levels, primarily through a negative feedback-loop control mechanism. Which of the following statements best describes how this feedback loop works?

   A. As Ca levels go up, PTH rises. This lowers Ca levels, leading to a drop in PTH.
   B. As Ca levels go down, PTH drops. This raises Ca levels, leading to a rise in PTH.
   C. As Ca levels go down, PTH rises. This raises Ca levels, leading to a drop in PTH.
   D. None of the above is a negative feedback loop.

73. The maximum number of different tetrapeptides that can be formed from two alanine and two phenylalanine amino acid residues is

   A. 4
   B. 3
   C. 2
   D. 6

74. Infrared spectroscopy is often used to determine the presence of a carbonyl group in a compound. It is a strong band appearing at about 1700 cm^{-1} in aldehydes, ketones, and carboxylic acids and their derivatives. A carboxylic acid will show another carbon oxygen stretching band at

   A. a higher frequency.
   B. a lower frequency.
   C. the same frequency.
   D. a frequency in the ultraviolet region of the electromagnetic spectrum.

75. The anomers of D-(+)-glucose differ in their configuration around which of the following?

    A. C-1
    B. C-5
    C. C-6
    D. C-2

76. Reaction of alcohols with nucleophiles often requires the presence of acid because

    A. alcohols only react with hydrogen halides.
    B. —OH is a poor leaving group and therefore must be protonated to form a better leaving group, $\overset{\oplus}{\text{OH}}_2$.
    C. acids prevent rearrangement of the carbocation.
    D. acids prevent bond cleavage.

77. The benzene ring typically undergoes

    A. nucleophilic addition.
    B. nucleophilic substitution.
    C. electrophilic addition.
    D. electrophilic substitution.

ANSWER KEY

1. C	11. B	21. B	31. D	41. D	51. B	61. D	71. D
2. B	12. C	22. A	32. B	42. B	52. B	62. C	72. C
3. D	13. D	23. C	33. C	43. C	53. A	63. D	73. D
4. B	14. C	24. C	34. A	44. A	54. D	64. A	74. B
5. D	15. B	25. C	35. D	45. B	55. B	65. C	75. A
6. A	16. C	26. D	36. C	46. C	56. C	66. D	76. B
7. A	17. B	27. C	37. C	47. C	57. B	67. B	77. D
8. D	18. A	28. B	38. A	48. A	58. A	68. C	
9. C	19. C	29. C	39. D	49. B	59. B	69. C	
10. C	20. C	30. C	40. C	50. B	60. D	70. B	

ANSWERS AND EXPLANATIONS

1. **The correct answer is (C).** A close examination of Tables 2 and 3 reveals that hemoglobin saturation levels change in the same direction and in the same amounts when PCO_2 increases and when blood pH decreases. This should not be unexpected since carbon dioxide combines with water to form carbonic acid. Thus, as carbon dioxide levels go up, more carbonic acid will form and pH will become more acidic.

2. **The correct answer is (B).** There should be a general understanding that oxygen levels are highest in the lungs. Based on results, it should become clear that as blood passes through the lungs, hemoglobin will easily pick up and bind to oxygen for transport throughout the body. As blood passes through oxygen-poor tissues, hemoglobin is less able to remain bound to oxygen, and the gas enters the tissues where it is most needed.

3. **The correct answer is (D).** Hemoglobin saturation was examined at different oxygen, carbon dioxide, and pH levels. All experiments were carried out at 36°C.

4. **The correct answer is (B).** Table 3 shows that hemoglobin saturation decreases as pH goes down. As pH declines further (into the acidic range), hemoglobin saturation should continue to decrease. At pH: 7.6 (70%); at pH: 7.2 (40%); below 7.0, saturation should drop below 40%.

5. **The correct answer is (D).** Experiment 1 does show that as oxygen concentration increases, hemoglobin's ability to remain bound to oxygen also increases. However, the results of Experiment 2 indicate that if carbon dioxide levels increase, hemoglobin will be less able to remain bound to oxygen. Apparently, the rapid breathing stimulated by administrating carbon dioxide provides the added benefit of helping to eliminate carbon monoxide from the alveoli.

6. **The correct answer is (A).** As stated above (Question 1), increases in blood carbon dioxide levels lead to the formation of additional carbonic acid, resulting in the lowering of blood pH.
$$CO_2 + H_2O \rightarrow H_2CO_3 \rightarrow H^+ + HCO_3^-$$

7. **The correct answer is (A).** The depolarization of the atria (P wave) takes place as electrical changes initiated at the S-A node pass across the right atrium to the A-V node. Areas in the ventricles are not yet involved.

8. **The correct answer is (D).** Interpreting each peak in the figure indicates that the height of R extends above +1.0 millivolts, while S extends well below the 0.0 mark and approaches −0.5 millivolts. Thus, the net change is closest to 1.5 millivolts.

9. **The correct answer is (C).** One should immediately be able to see that time is on the horizontal axis. The P wave is initiated by depolarization at the S-A node (see Question 1), whereas depolarization of the ventricles is associated with the QRS complex. The distance between these points represents the time needed for the impulse to reach the Bundle of His and Purkinje fibers in the ventricular walls (the T wave represents a later point in time when the ventricles repolarize).

10. **The correct answer is (C).** Knowledge about the sequence of the cardiac cycle should immediately help eliminate choices A and B. Repolarization of the atria coincides with ventricular depolarization. A moment's thought should make choice D improbable. It is unlikely that an instrument designed to pick up the electrical changes in an organ as vital as the heart would not be sensitive enough to detect each event in the sequence.

11. **The correct answer is (B).** Since the QRS complex represents depolarization of the ventricles, a prolonged depolarization would make this part of the ECG wider. A higher QRS complex would indicate a stronger depolarization (contraction).

12. **The correct answer is (C).** It should be understood that regulation of heart rate is under autonomic control. The sympathetic division is responsible during stressful situations ("fight or flight"), whereas the parasympathetic division controls the heart during normal activity.

13. **The correct answer is (D).** Each of the electrolytes is vital to membrane function and muscle contraction (resting potential, depolarization, repolarization, sliding of protein filaments, etc.).

14. **The correct answer is (C).** Differentiation is the process by which cells become specialized. Clearly, major periods of specialization occur as cells within the primary germ layers begin forming the major organs and organ systems. The fetal stage is more a time for growth and maturation of structures than a period for the formation of new structures.

15. **The correct answer is (B).** The inner cell mass is the part of the blastocyst from which the embryo develops. According to the passage, the blastocyst develops from the morula by the end of the first week after fertilization.

16. **The correct answer is (C).** It should be recognized that spinal cord formation results from neurulation. The passage states that neurulation takes place among ectodermal cells and that ectodermal cells also give rise to the special sense organs.

17. **The correct answer is (B).** 50-72 hours after fertilization correspond to the 16-cell morula stage.

18. **The correct answer is (A).** The question requires you to recognize that *all somatic cells* are genetically identical. Each cell of the body forms by mitosis of previous cells, going back to the zygote. All body cells have the exact same genetic material as the zygote.

19. **The correct answer is (C).** Realizing that myocardial cells are muscle cells is the key to this question. The passage states that bone and muscle tissue derive from mesoderm.

20. **The correct answer is (C).** The chorion forms from cells of the trophoblast, clearly an embryonic tissue. The endometrium is the inner lining of the uterus, clearly a maternal tissue. Therefore, the placenta consists of tissues derived from both.

21. **The correct answer is (B).** If the individual were the only unit of selection, traits detrimental to the reproductive fitness of the individual would be eliminated. Thus, the maintenance and observance of such traits suggest other possible units of selection; i.e., the trait is maintained because it increases the reproductive fitness of the group. Choices C and D are irrelevant to the question.

22. **The correct answer is (A).** Natural selection acting on the individual maintains genes present in the individual that contribute to his/her reproductive fitness. The result is that more offspring (more copies of those genes!) with those traits will be represented in the next generation. Kin selection is a special case of individual selection, in that a behavior like alarm calling, if performed in the presence of close relatives, is a trait that enables more copies of the individual's shared genes to be maintained and represented in the next generation. No group selection hypothesis is necessary. Alarm calling is not detrimental (to the individual's genes) after all!

23. **The correct answer is (C).** It should immediately be recognized that both choices A and B indicate that alarm calling is not detrimental to the individual (it benefits the individual by increasing the chances of survival). If this is the case, then individual selection by itself can maintain such a trait.

24. **The correct answer is (C).** In evolutionary terms, the "future" benefits of a trait on an individual's fitness must be "entered into the equation immediately." If such future reproductive benefits were not part of natural selection's "formula," the "current risks" to individual fitness would outweigh the "current benefits" and such traits would be eliminated.

25. **The correct answer is (C).** The observation that individuals behave in a way that results in increased fitness for a different individual, at first glance, contradicts the view of the individual being the sole unit of selection. The *observation itself* can be addressed using the group selection approach. However, we now know that kin selection can just as easily explain such behavior.

26. **The correct answer is (D).** An understanding is required, that the only evidence necessary to show that evolution is occurring is the observation that changes in gene frequencies within a breeding population have taken place—regardless of *how* they have taken place. The unit of selection is a side issue. In fact, for a particular case, the gene frequency changes may have less to do with selection than for some other factor (emigration of individuals out of the population, non-random mating, etc.).

27. **The correct answer is (C).** The hypothesis predicts that testosterone influences courtship and aggressive behavior. The only way to test the hypothesis is to observe these behaviors as testosterone levels vary. Only choice C attempts to examine behavior as a function of testosterone level. Simply observing the expected behavior does not implicate the role of the hormone at all.

28. **The correct answer is (B).** Basic knowledge that the testes are the primary source of testosterone production in males is required. Removal of the testes (gonads) should lower testosterone levels and subsequently decrease both courtship and aggressive behavior (especially if injecting high levels of testosterone led to increases in both behaviors; see Question 27).

29. **The correct answer is (C).** Knowledge that testosterone is also produced by the adrenal cortex is helpful, but not essential. In any experimental program that attempts to demonstrate the *role* of a hormone *and its source,* all potential sources should be investigated. Before the hypothesis that testosterone influences these behaviors is rejected, other tests should be conducted to make sure there is no other source of the hormone (at least blood tests of hormone levels should be conducted before and after removal of each gland).

30. **The correct answer is (C).** "Replacement" therapy is often used to confirm the influence of a hormone. However, a large enough sample of experimental organisms (with controls) should always be part of an experimental program (this can also be "built-in" to the original experimental design).

31. **The correct answer is (D).** It should be understood from the passage that the term "specific target site" refers to particular cells/tissues in the organism (not specific behaviors or specific individuals).

32. **The correct answer is (B).** The ability to make predictions from the observed change in hormone level is important for this question. If losses in aggressive encounters cause a drop in testosterone level in subordinate males, the decreased hormone level should also be reflected in a less vigorous courtship by these individuals (since previous observations showed that testosterone stimulates courtship).

33. **The correct answer is (C).** The only clear result from Experiment 1 is that following irradiation, no cultures were able to grow on medium with streptomycin. This observation should not eliminate the possibility that other mutations may have occurred in the tube. The medium used in the dish was only designed to test for streptomycin-resistance among the normally sensitive cells.

34. **The correct answer is (A).** The passage reveals that single cells can grow into colonies after incubation. Therefore, the two colonies that grew in Experiment 2 were derived from at least one cell each. The observation that they grew on a medium with streptomycin indicates that the cells became streptomycin-resistant after the second irradiation.

35. **The correct answer is (D).** Medium Y contains lactose instead of glucose. Cells from Colony B were unable to grow on this lactose medium. Both colonies were able to grow on a minimal medium (Medium X, containing glucose), as well as on streptomycin.

36. **The correct answer is (C).** The passage states that normal cells can grow on a lactose medium because they have the enzymes needed to convert it to glucose. If cells from Colony B can no longer grow on lactose, the irradiation may have affected the gene coding for this enzyme (or one of the enzymes). Lactose is still nutritious for Colony A (we reject choice A), and the lactose medium was not irradiated—only the test-tube suspension was irradiated (we reject choice B). Finally, the colonies were placed on separate dishes—no competition was involved (we also reject choice D).

37. **The correct answer is (C).** As stated earlier (in Question 33), we cannot eliminate the possibility that the mutation at the lactose enzyme locus could have occurred in Experiment 1. Experiment 1 was simply not designed to isolate such a mutant. It is also possible (slightly) that two mutants arose in the same cell with the same dose of radiation in Experiment 2.

38. **The correct answer is (A).** The original suspension of bacteria contained normal cells that can grow on a minimal medium. Regardless of how many cells mutated, there would be innumerable cells still able to grow on this medium (cells that gave rise to Colony A and Colony B should also be able to grow on a streptomycin-free medium!).

39. **The correct answer is (D).** Basic knowledge of how bacteria can transfer genetic material is required. All three methods are means of sexual reproduction in bacteria.

40. **The correct answer is (C).** A simple reading of the graph indicates that the two lines cross at 30°C–35°C. The homeotherm will be able to maintain this body temperature at a broad range of environmental temperatures, whereas the poikilotherm's body temperature can vary as environmental temperature changes.

41. **The correct answer is (D).** The plateau representing physiological and metabolic maintenance of body temperature in homeotherms can no longer be sustained below 20°C (approximately) and above 45°C (approximately).

42. **The correct answer is (B).** The passage indicates that behavioral responses help poikilotherms maintain appropriate body temperature. At 15°C, a definite "warming" pattern of response is in order. Basking in the sun sounds about right (hunting for food would be extremely difficult because normal functioning of the body is significantly slowed by the cold temperature).

43. **The correct answer is (C).** Cooling mechanisms include the production of sweat (evaporation of sweat at the body surface is a heat-losing process) and the dilation of superficial blood vessels (in order to increase heat loss by radiation).

44. **The correct answer is (A).** The homeothermic animal (A) can physiologically maintain normal body temperature throughout this range of environmental temperatures. However, the poikilotherm (B) must first warm up (bask?), and will eventually have to seek a cooler environment (as its body temperature increases too much).

45. **The correct answer is (B).** Normally, when body temperature falls below the "thermostat setting" in the hypothalamus, heating or heat-conservation mechanisms are put into effect (shivering and vasoconstriction of superficial blood vessels). When body temperature rises above the setting, cooling mechanisms are activated (sweating and vasodilation). If the "pyrogen" has caused adjustment of the thermostat to 102°F, then a body temperature of 101°F can be accompanied by shivering. Even though the body feels warm to the touch (because body temperature is warmer than normal), the body is colder than the thermostat setting, and, as a result, the heating mechanism is activated.

46. **The correct answer is (C).**

$$CH_3-CH_2-\underset{\underset{CH_3}{|}}{CH}-CH_2^{\oplus} \xrightarrow{-H^+} CH_3-CH_2-\underset{\underset{CH_3}{|}}{C}=CH_2$$

$$CH_3-CH_2-\underset{\underset{\oplus}{\overset{\overset{CH_3}{|}}{C}}}{}-CH_3 \xrightarrow{-H^+} CH_3-CH=\underset{\underset{CH_3}{|}}{C}-CH_3$$

47. **The correct answer is (C).** Loss of water or dehydration to form an alkane indicates an elimination reaction. The first order kinetics indicates an E1 elimination with the rate of the reaction dependent on the rate of formation of the carbocation intermediate.

48. **The correct answer is (A).**

$$CH_3-CH=CH-CH_3 \xrightarrow{Cl_2} CH_3-\underset{\underset{Cl}{|}}{CH}-\underset{\underset{Cl}{|}}{\overset{\overset{CH_3}{|}}{C}}-CH_3$$

49. **The correct answer is (B).** The $CH_3-CH_2-\underset{\underset{CH_3}{|}}{CH}-CH_2^{\oplus}$ carbocation rearranges by a 1,2 hydride shift to from the more stable $CH_3-CH_2-\underset{\underset{\oplus}{\overset{\overset{CH_3}{|}}{C}}}{}-CH_3$, a tertiary carbocation. This rearrangement accounts for the chief product, $CH_3-CH=\underset{\underset{CH_3}{|}}{C}-CH_3$ which gives mostly 2,3-dichloro-2-methylbutane upon chlorination (Experiment 1). Experiment 4 shows a decrease in formation of the carbocation due to deuterium being substituted for hydrogen. The C—D bond will break more slowly, hindering the 1,2 hydride shift.

50. **The correct answer is (B).**

$$CH_3-CH_2-CH_2-\underset{\underset{CH_3}{|}}{CH}-CH_2Br \rightarrow CH_3-CH_2-CH_2-\underset{\underset{\oplus}{\overset{\overset{CH_3}{|}}{C}}}{}-CH_3 \rightarrow CH_3-CH_2-CH=\underset{\underset{CH_3}{|}}{C}-CH_3$$
$$\text{chief carbocation}$$

51. **The correct answer is (B).**

52. **The correct answer is (B).** (S,S)-2,3-dibromobutane

53. **The correct answer is (A).** meso-2,3-dibromobutane

54. **The correct answer is (D).** Mechanism A as shown produces (S,S)-2,3-dibromobutane. Rotation about the C—C bond produces the meso compound. Bromination of cis-2-butene, however, yields a racemic mixture, so Mechanism A is incorrect. Mechanism B showing a bromonium intermediate produces equal concentrations of the enantiomers.

55. **The correct answer is (B).** The carbon carrying the positive charge of the carbocation has only six electrons.

56. **The correct answer is (C).** Mechanism A produces a very stable carbocation in which the positive charge is delocalized into the ring.

57. **The correct answer is (B).** As already indicated, only Mechanism B accounts for the stereochemistry of the bromination of the cis isomer. This is an anti addition since bromine attacks from opposite sides of the molecule. Anti addition must also occur in the bromination of the trans isomer in order to produce the meso product.

58. **The correct answer is (A).** Using Mechanism B

59. **The correct answer is (B).**

60. **The correct answer is (D).** The structure represents a meso structure because a plane of symmetry can be drawn through carbon-3 and, therefore, is *superimposable* on its mirror image and optically inactive.

61. **The correct answer is (D).** The dibasic form predominates in basic solution.

62. **The correct answer is (C).** Bulky groups on either the acid or alcohol slow the reaction due to steric hindrance.

63. **The correct answer is (D).** This question requires a basic understanding of membrane transport mechanisms. When a substance moves against a concentration gradient (from low concentration to high), energy is required. Active transport is the only mechanism capable of moving sodium in the direction described.

64. **The correct answer is (A).** General knowledge of the events associated with mitosis is required. DNA polymerase is the enzyme involved with bringing DNA nucleotides into place during DNA replication. In the cell cycle, this occurs during the S phase of interphase.

65. **The correct answer is (C).** The breakdown of ATP to ADP releases energy for cellular work. Water movement across membranes (osmosis) and oxygen passing from lungs to blood (diffusion) require no cellular energy. During the electron transport chain, ATP is synthesized from ADP.

66. **The correct answer is (D).** Basic knowledge of the components of nucleic acids and related molecules is required. Adenine is one of the four nucleotide bases found in DNA and RNA, as well as in the adenosine triphosphate (ATP) molecules found in all cells. Uracil is one of the four nucleotide bases found in RNA.

67. **The correct answer is (B).** This question involves a basic understanding of the stages of cellular respiration and the role of the cytochromes in the electron transport chain. Only glycolysis takes place in the cytosol. Both the Krebs cycle and transport chain occur in the mitochondria (ribosomes are the site of protein synthesis).

68. **The correct answer is (C).** This question requires an understanding of Mendelian genetics, and sex-linked inheritance patterns in particular. If a woman is colorblind (a sex-linked recessive trait: X^cX^c), she must have had a colorblind father (X^cY) and a mother who, at least, was a carrier (X^cX^c). The subject's father received the colorblindness allele from his mother. The subject's mother must have had at least one parent with the colorblindness allele.

69. **The correct answer is (C).** A large cell would have an outer surface area (cell membrane) that would not be large enough to service the even larger cell volume inside. Similarly, the various organelles and assorted components of the cytoplasm would be too far apart for proper coupling of reactions, and for other interdependent functions to take place efficiently.

70. **The correct answer is (B).** Answering this question requires a general knowledge of the events of meiosis. Normally, in an organism with a diploid number of 6 (2N = 6), each of the four meiotic products will have three chromosomes. However, if nondisjunction occurs in the first meiotic division, one daughter cell will have four doubled chromosomes and the other daughter cell will have two doubled chromosomes (one pair of homologous chromosomes did not separate). After the second division, all chromatids will separate, resulting in four single chromosomes in two of the products and two single chromosomes in the other two products.

71. **The correct answer is (D).** A basic knowledge of the organs of digestion, their enzymes, and the functions of those enzymes is required. The initial breakdown of polysaccharide carbohydrates to disaccharides is carried out by salivary amylase (released by the salivary glands into the mouth) and pancreatic amylase (released by the pancreas into the small intestine). The question asks where the release of these enzymes *should be blocked.*

72. **The correct answer is (C).** An understanding of negative feedback control mechanisms typically at work in the endocrine system is required. Hormone concentration usually changes in the *opposite* direction (negative feedback) of the substance it regulates. When they change in the same direction, a positive feedback mechanism is at work.

73. **The correct answer is (D).**

    Ala-Ala-Phe-Phe
    Phe-Phe-Ala-Ala
    Ala-Phe-Ala-Phe
    Phe-Ala-Phe-Ala
    Phe-Ala-Ala-Phe
    Ala-Phe-Phe-Ala

    Note the N-terminal amino acid residue (having the free amino group) is written on the left, and the C-terminal amino acid residue (having the free carboxyl group) appears at the right end.

74. **The correct answer is (B).** A C—O single bond is weaker than a double bond. Therefore, less energy (or lower frequency) is needed to induce the stretching vibration. Remember, reciprocal centimeters (cm^{-1}) is a measure of frequency and energy is directly proportional to the frequency.

75. **The correct answer is (A).** Glucose anomers.

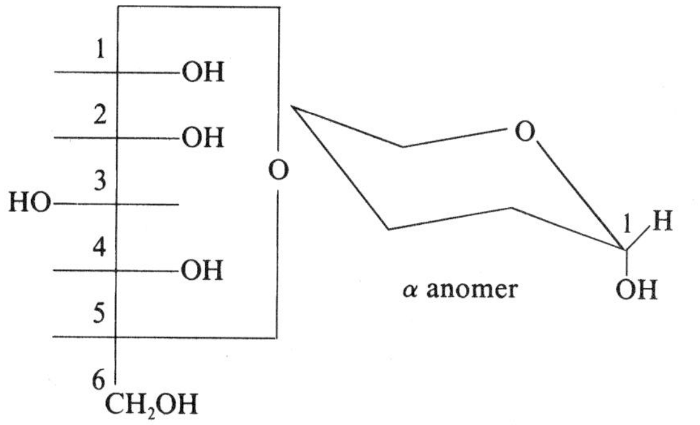

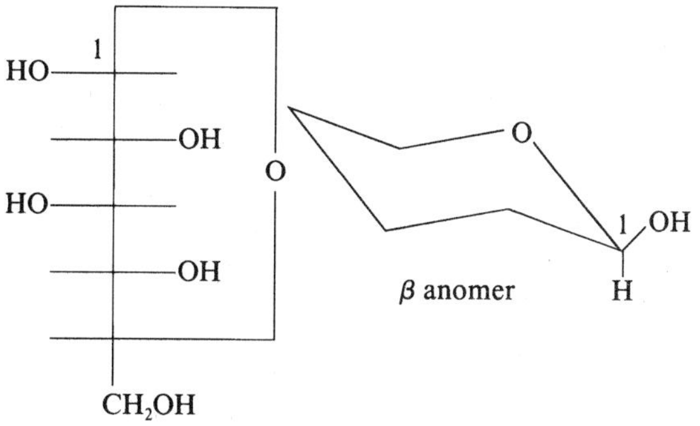

76. **The correct answer is (B).** The hydroxide group is a strong base and therefore a poor leaving group. It must be protonated to form the weak base, H_2O, so that it can leave the molecule.

77. **The correct answer is (D).** Substitution reactions are preferred because they preserve the very stable aromatic structure. Electrophiles can join the ring because of the resonance stabilization of the intermediate ion

Unit Five

THREE PRACTICE
MCAT EXAMS

PERIODIC TABLE OF ELEMENTS

1 1A Alkali metals	2 2A Alkaline earth metals	3	4	5	6	7 Transition Metals	8	9	10	11	12	13 3A	14 4A	15 5A	16 6A Halogens	17 7A	18 8A Noble gases
1 H 1.008																	2 He 4.003
3 Li 6.941	4 Be 9.012											5 B 10.81	6 C 12.01	7 N 14.01	8 O 16.00	9 F 19.00	10 Ne 20.18
11 Na 22.99	12 Mg 24.31											13 Al 26.98	14 Si 28.09	15 P 30.97	16 S 32.06	17 Cl 35.45	18 Ar 39.95
19 K 39.10	20 Ca 40.08	21 Sc 44.96	22 Ti 47.90	23 V 50.94	24 Cr 52.00	25 Mn 54.94	26 Fe 55.85	27 Co 58.93	28 Ni 58.70	29 Cu 63.55	30 Zn 65.38	31 Ga 69.72	32 Ge 72.59	33 As 74.92	34 Se 78.96	35 Br 79.90	36 Kr 83.80
37 Rb 85.47	38 Sr 87.62	39 Y 88.91	40 Zr 91.22	41 Nb 92.91	42 Mo 95.94	43 Tc (98)	44 Ru 101.1	45 Rh 102.9	46 Pd 106.4	47 Ag 107.9	48 Cd 112.4	49 In 114.8	50 Sn 118.7	51 Sb 121.8	52 Te 127.6	53 I 126.9	54 Xe 131.3
55 Cs 132.9	56 Ba 137.3	57 La* 138.9	72 Hf 178.5	73 Ta 180.9	74 W 183.9	75 Re 186.2	76 Os 190.2	77 Ir 192.2	78 Pt 195.1	79 Au 197.0	80 Hg 200.6	81 Tl 204.4	82 Pb 207.2	83 Bi 209.0	84 Po (209)	85 At (210)	86 Rn (222)
87 Fr (223)	88 Ra 226.0	89 Ac** (227)	104 Rf	105 Db	106 Sg	107 Bh	108 Hs	109 Mt	110 Uun	111 Uuu	112 Uub						

Nonmetals
Metals

*Lanthanides (Rare Earths)

58 Ce 140.1	59 Pr 140.9	60 Nd 144.2	61 Pm (145)	62 Sm 150.4	63 Eu 152.0	64 Gd 157.3	65 Tb 158.9	66 Dy (251)	67 Ho 1.008	68 Er 1.008	69 Tm 1.008	70 Yb 1.008	71 Lu 1.008

**Actinides (Transuranium)

90 Th 232.0	91 Pa (231)	92 U 238.0	93 Np (237)	94 Pu (244)	95 Am (243)	96 Cm (247)	97 Bk (247)	98 Cf (251)	99 Es (252)	100 Fm (257)	101 Md (258)	102 No (259)	103 Lr (260)

Practice Exam I

TEST	QUESTIONS	MINUTES
Physical Sciences	1–77	100 minutes
Verbal Reasoning	78–142	85 minutes
Writing Sample	2 Essays	60 minutes
Biological Sciences	143–219	100 minutes

ANSWER SHEET

PRACTICE EXAM I

Physical Sciences		Verbal Reasoning		Biological Sciences	
1. Ⓐ Ⓑ Ⓒ Ⓓ	40. Ⓐ Ⓑ Ⓒ Ⓓ	78. Ⓐ Ⓑ Ⓒ Ⓓ	111. Ⓐ Ⓑ Ⓒ Ⓓ	143. Ⓐ Ⓑ Ⓒ Ⓓ	182. Ⓐ Ⓑ Ⓒ Ⓓ
2. Ⓐ Ⓑ Ⓒ Ⓓ	41. Ⓐ Ⓑ Ⓒ Ⓓ	79. Ⓐ Ⓑ Ⓒ Ⓓ	112. Ⓐ Ⓑ Ⓒ Ⓓ	144. Ⓐ Ⓑ Ⓒ Ⓓ	183. Ⓐ Ⓑ Ⓒ Ⓓ
3. Ⓐ Ⓑ Ⓒ Ⓓ	42. Ⓐ Ⓑ Ⓒ Ⓓ	80. Ⓐ Ⓑ Ⓒ Ⓓ	113. Ⓐ Ⓑ Ⓒ Ⓓ	145. Ⓐ Ⓑ Ⓒ Ⓓ	184. Ⓐ Ⓑ Ⓒ Ⓓ
4. Ⓐ Ⓑ Ⓒ Ⓓ	43. Ⓐ Ⓑ Ⓒ Ⓓ	81. Ⓐ Ⓑ Ⓒ Ⓓ	114. Ⓐ Ⓑ Ⓒ Ⓓ	146. Ⓐ Ⓑ Ⓒ Ⓓ	185. Ⓐ Ⓑ Ⓒ Ⓓ
5. Ⓐ Ⓑ Ⓒ Ⓓ	44. Ⓐ Ⓑ Ⓒ Ⓓ	82. Ⓐ Ⓑ Ⓒ Ⓓ	115. Ⓐ Ⓑ Ⓒ Ⓓ	147. Ⓐ Ⓑ Ⓒ Ⓓ	186. Ⓐ Ⓑ Ⓒ Ⓓ
6. Ⓐ Ⓑ Ⓒ Ⓓ	45. Ⓐ Ⓑ Ⓒ Ⓓ	83. Ⓐ Ⓑ Ⓒ Ⓓ	116. Ⓐ Ⓑ Ⓒ Ⓓ	148. Ⓐ Ⓑ Ⓒ Ⓓ	187. Ⓐ Ⓑ Ⓒ Ⓓ
7. Ⓐ Ⓑ Ⓒ Ⓓ	46. Ⓐ Ⓑ Ⓒ Ⓓ	84. Ⓐ Ⓑ Ⓒ Ⓓ	117. Ⓐ Ⓑ Ⓒ Ⓓ	149. Ⓐ Ⓑ Ⓒ Ⓓ	188. Ⓐ Ⓑ Ⓒ Ⓓ
8. Ⓐ Ⓑ Ⓒ Ⓓ	47. Ⓐ Ⓑ Ⓒ Ⓓ	85. Ⓐ Ⓑ Ⓒ Ⓓ	118. Ⓐ Ⓑ Ⓒ Ⓓ	150. Ⓐ Ⓑ Ⓒ Ⓓ	189. Ⓐ Ⓑ Ⓒ Ⓓ
9. Ⓐ Ⓑ Ⓒ Ⓓ	48. Ⓐ Ⓑ Ⓒ Ⓓ	86. Ⓐ Ⓑ Ⓒ Ⓓ	119. Ⓐ Ⓑ Ⓒ Ⓓ	151. Ⓐ Ⓑ Ⓒ Ⓓ	190. Ⓐ Ⓑ Ⓒ Ⓓ
10. Ⓐ Ⓑ Ⓒ Ⓓ	49. Ⓐ Ⓑ Ⓒ Ⓓ	87. Ⓐ Ⓑ Ⓒ Ⓓ	120. Ⓐ Ⓑ Ⓒ Ⓓ	152. Ⓐ Ⓑ Ⓒ Ⓓ	191. Ⓐ Ⓑ Ⓒ Ⓓ
11. Ⓐ Ⓑ Ⓒ Ⓓ	50. Ⓐ Ⓑ Ⓒ Ⓓ	88. Ⓐ Ⓑ Ⓒ Ⓓ	121. Ⓐ Ⓑ Ⓒ Ⓓ	153. Ⓐ Ⓑ Ⓒ Ⓓ	192. Ⓐ Ⓑ Ⓒ Ⓓ
12. Ⓐ Ⓑ Ⓒ Ⓓ	51. Ⓐ Ⓑ Ⓒ Ⓓ	89. Ⓐ Ⓑ Ⓒ Ⓓ	122. Ⓐ Ⓑ Ⓒ Ⓓ	154. Ⓐ Ⓑ Ⓒ Ⓓ	193. Ⓐ Ⓑ Ⓒ Ⓓ
13. Ⓐ Ⓑ Ⓒ Ⓓ	52. Ⓐ Ⓑ Ⓒ Ⓓ	90. Ⓐ Ⓑ Ⓒ Ⓓ	123. Ⓐ Ⓑ Ⓒ Ⓓ	155. Ⓐ Ⓑ Ⓒ Ⓓ	194. Ⓐ Ⓑ Ⓒ Ⓓ
14. Ⓐ Ⓑ Ⓒ Ⓓ	53. Ⓐ Ⓑ Ⓒ Ⓓ	91. Ⓐ Ⓑ Ⓒ Ⓓ	124. Ⓐ Ⓑ Ⓒ Ⓓ	156. Ⓐ Ⓑ Ⓒ Ⓓ	195. Ⓐ Ⓑ Ⓒ Ⓓ
15. Ⓐ Ⓑ Ⓒ Ⓓ	54. Ⓐ Ⓑ Ⓒ Ⓓ	92. Ⓐ Ⓑ Ⓒ Ⓓ	125. Ⓐ Ⓑ Ⓒ Ⓓ	157. Ⓐ Ⓑ Ⓒ Ⓓ	196. Ⓐ Ⓑ Ⓒ Ⓓ
16. Ⓐ Ⓑ Ⓒ Ⓓ	55. Ⓐ Ⓑ Ⓒ Ⓓ	93. Ⓐ Ⓑ Ⓒ Ⓓ	126. Ⓐ Ⓑ Ⓒ Ⓓ	158. Ⓐ Ⓑ Ⓒ Ⓓ	197. Ⓐ Ⓑ Ⓒ Ⓓ
17. Ⓐ Ⓑ Ⓒ Ⓓ	56. Ⓐ Ⓑ Ⓒ Ⓓ	94. Ⓐ Ⓑ Ⓒ Ⓓ	127. Ⓐ Ⓑ Ⓒ Ⓓ	159. Ⓐ Ⓑ Ⓒ Ⓓ	198. Ⓐ Ⓑ Ⓒ Ⓓ
18. Ⓐ Ⓑ Ⓒ Ⓓ	57. Ⓐ Ⓑ Ⓒ Ⓓ	95. Ⓐ Ⓑ Ⓒ Ⓓ	128. Ⓐ Ⓑ Ⓒ Ⓓ	160. Ⓐ Ⓑ Ⓒ Ⓓ	199. Ⓐ Ⓑ Ⓒ Ⓓ
19. Ⓐ Ⓑ Ⓒ Ⓓ	58. Ⓐ Ⓑ Ⓒ Ⓓ	96. Ⓐ Ⓑ Ⓒ Ⓓ	129. Ⓐ Ⓑ Ⓒ Ⓓ	161. Ⓐ Ⓑ Ⓒ Ⓓ	200. Ⓐ Ⓑ Ⓒ Ⓓ
20. Ⓐ Ⓑ Ⓒ Ⓓ	59. Ⓐ Ⓑ Ⓒ Ⓓ	97. Ⓐ Ⓑ Ⓒ Ⓓ	130. Ⓐ Ⓑ Ⓒ Ⓓ	162. Ⓐ Ⓑ Ⓒ Ⓓ	201. Ⓐ Ⓑ Ⓒ Ⓓ
21. Ⓐ Ⓑ Ⓒ Ⓓ	60. Ⓐ Ⓑ Ⓒ Ⓓ	98. Ⓐ Ⓑ Ⓒ Ⓓ	131. Ⓐ Ⓑ Ⓒ Ⓓ	163. Ⓐ Ⓑ Ⓒ Ⓓ	202. Ⓐ Ⓑ Ⓒ Ⓓ
22. Ⓐ Ⓑ Ⓒ Ⓓ	61. Ⓐ Ⓑ Ⓒ Ⓓ	99. Ⓐ Ⓑ Ⓒ Ⓓ	132. Ⓐ Ⓑ Ⓒ Ⓓ	164. Ⓐ Ⓑ Ⓒ Ⓓ	203. Ⓐ Ⓑ Ⓒ Ⓓ
23. Ⓐ Ⓑ Ⓒ Ⓓ	62. Ⓐ Ⓑ Ⓒ Ⓓ	100. Ⓐ Ⓑ Ⓒ Ⓓ	133. Ⓐ Ⓑ Ⓒ Ⓓ	165. Ⓐ Ⓑ Ⓒ Ⓓ	204. Ⓐ Ⓑ Ⓒ Ⓓ
24. Ⓐ Ⓑ Ⓒ Ⓓ	63. Ⓐ Ⓑ Ⓒ Ⓓ	101. Ⓐ Ⓑ Ⓒ Ⓓ	134. Ⓐ Ⓑ Ⓒ Ⓓ	166. Ⓐ Ⓑ Ⓒ Ⓓ	205. Ⓐ Ⓑ Ⓒ Ⓓ
25. Ⓐ Ⓑ Ⓒ Ⓓ	64. Ⓐ Ⓑ Ⓒ Ⓓ	102. Ⓐ Ⓑ Ⓒ Ⓓ	135. Ⓐ Ⓑ Ⓒ Ⓓ	167. Ⓐ Ⓑ Ⓒ Ⓓ	206. Ⓐ Ⓑ Ⓒ Ⓓ
26. Ⓐ Ⓑ Ⓒ Ⓓ	65. Ⓐ Ⓑ Ⓒ Ⓓ	103. Ⓐ Ⓑ Ⓒ Ⓓ	136. Ⓐ Ⓑ Ⓒ Ⓓ	168. Ⓐ Ⓑ Ⓒ Ⓓ	207. Ⓐ Ⓑ Ⓒ Ⓓ
27. Ⓐ Ⓑ Ⓒ Ⓓ	66. Ⓐ Ⓑ Ⓒ Ⓓ	104. Ⓐ Ⓑ Ⓒ Ⓓ	137. Ⓐ Ⓑ Ⓒ Ⓓ	169. Ⓐ Ⓑ Ⓒ Ⓓ	208. Ⓐ Ⓑ Ⓒ Ⓓ
28. Ⓐ Ⓑ Ⓒ Ⓓ	67. Ⓐ Ⓑ Ⓒ Ⓓ	105. Ⓐ Ⓑ Ⓒ Ⓓ	138. Ⓐ Ⓑ Ⓒ Ⓓ	170. Ⓐ Ⓑ Ⓒ Ⓓ	209. Ⓐ Ⓑ Ⓒ Ⓓ
29. Ⓐ Ⓑ Ⓒ Ⓓ	68. Ⓐ Ⓑ Ⓒ Ⓓ	106. Ⓐ Ⓑ Ⓒ Ⓓ	139. Ⓐ Ⓑ Ⓒ Ⓓ	171. Ⓐ Ⓑ Ⓒ Ⓓ	210. Ⓐ Ⓑ Ⓒ Ⓓ
30. Ⓐ Ⓑ Ⓒ Ⓓ	69. Ⓐ Ⓑ Ⓒ Ⓓ	107. Ⓐ Ⓑ Ⓒ Ⓓ	140. Ⓐ Ⓑ Ⓒ Ⓓ	172. Ⓐ Ⓑ Ⓒ Ⓓ	211. Ⓐ Ⓑ Ⓒ Ⓓ
31. Ⓐ Ⓑ Ⓒ Ⓓ	70. Ⓐ Ⓑ Ⓒ Ⓓ	108. Ⓐ Ⓑ Ⓒ Ⓓ	141. Ⓐ Ⓑ Ⓒ Ⓓ	173. Ⓐ Ⓑ Ⓒ Ⓓ	212. Ⓐ Ⓑ Ⓒ Ⓓ
32. Ⓐ Ⓑ Ⓒ Ⓓ	71. Ⓐ Ⓑ Ⓒ Ⓓ	109. Ⓐ Ⓑ Ⓒ Ⓓ	142. Ⓐ Ⓑ Ⓒ Ⓓ	174. Ⓐ Ⓑ Ⓒ Ⓓ	213. Ⓐ Ⓑ Ⓒ Ⓓ
33. Ⓐ Ⓑ Ⓒ Ⓓ	72. Ⓐ Ⓑ Ⓒ Ⓓ	110. Ⓐ Ⓑ Ⓒ Ⓓ		175. Ⓐ Ⓑ Ⓒ Ⓓ	214. Ⓐ Ⓑ Ⓒ Ⓓ
34. Ⓐ Ⓑ Ⓒ Ⓓ	73. Ⓐ Ⓑ Ⓒ Ⓓ			176. Ⓐ Ⓑ Ⓒ Ⓓ	215. Ⓐ Ⓑ Ⓒ Ⓓ
35. Ⓐ Ⓑ Ⓒ Ⓓ	74. Ⓐ Ⓑ Ⓒ Ⓓ			177. Ⓐ Ⓑ Ⓒ Ⓓ	216. Ⓐ Ⓑ Ⓒ Ⓓ
36. Ⓐ Ⓑ Ⓒ Ⓓ	75. Ⓐ Ⓑ Ⓒ Ⓓ			178. Ⓐ Ⓑ Ⓒ Ⓓ	217. Ⓐ Ⓑ Ⓒ Ⓓ
37. Ⓐ Ⓑ Ⓒ Ⓓ	76. Ⓐ Ⓑ Ⓒ Ⓓ			179. Ⓐ Ⓑ Ⓒ Ⓓ	218. Ⓐ Ⓑ Ⓒ Ⓓ
38. Ⓐ Ⓑ Ⓒ Ⓓ	77. Ⓐ Ⓑ Ⓒ Ⓓ			180. Ⓐ Ⓑ Ⓒ Ⓓ	219. Ⓐ Ⓑ Ⓒ Ⓓ
39. Ⓐ Ⓑ Ⓒ Ⓓ				181. Ⓐ Ⓑ Ⓒ Ⓓ	

WRITING SAMPLE

Part 1

TURN PAGE FOR ADDITIONAL SPACE

_____
_____
_____
_____
_____
_____
_____
_____
_____
_____
_____
_____
_____
_____
_____
_____
_____
_____
_____
_____
_____
_____
_____

END OF PART 1

WRITING SAMPLE

Part 2

TURN PAGE FOR ADDITIONAL SPACE

END OF PART 2

PHYSICAL SCIENCES

> **Directions:** This test contains 77 questions. Most of the questions consist of a descriptive passage followed by a group of questions related to the passage. For these questions, study the passage carefully and then choose the best answer to each question in the group. Some questions in this test stand alone. These questions are independent of any passage and independent of each other. For these questions, too, you must select the one best answer. Indicate all your answers by blackening the corresponding circles on your answer sheet.
>
> A Periodic Table is provided at the beginning of this unit (page 564). You may consult it whenever you wish.

Passage I (Questions 1–8)

The figure below shows a photograph obtained when light from a low-pressure hydrogen lamp is passed through a spectrometer.

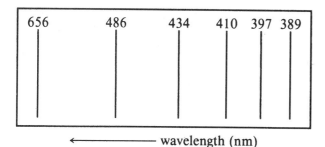

Two scientists offer their views on the interpretation of these lines.

Scientist 1: These "spectral lines" point to the existence of quantized energy levels in the hydrogen atom. The lines at different wavelengths represent photons after an electron has been promoted to a higher level in the atom, and then relaxed down to either the ground state or a low-lying excited state.

By converting the wavelengths to energies, we can construct the following diagram showing the energy levels that must exist in the atom:

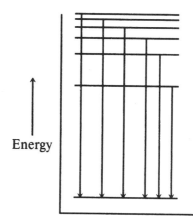

Scientist 2: My colleague has missed an important alternative explanation, which I am certain is the correct one. Hydrogen does not have discrete energy levels; rather, the glass in the spectrometer used to measure the wavelength has *peculiar gaps in its transmission properties—it allows only certain colors through.*

GO ON TO THE NEXT PAGE

1. What is the approximate ratio of the longest to the shortest wavelength shown?

   A. -0.5
   B. .5
   C. 1.2
   D. 1.7

2. The wavelengths shown are given in nanometers (nm), where 1 nm $= 10^{-9}$m. Which of the following represents the shortest-wavelength spectral line shown in meters?

   A. 3.89×10^{-11}m
   B. 3.89×10^{-9}m
   C. 3.89×10^{-7}m
   D. 3.89×10^{-6}m

3. In Scientist 1's view, the shortest wavelength transition represents the

   A. transition of lowest energy difference.
   B. transition of highest energy difference.
   C. most intense transition.
   D. transition most likely to occur.

4. Which relation would Scientist 1 use to convert wavelength to energy *most directly?*

   A. $E = hv$
   B. $E = hc/\lambda$
   C. $c = v\lambda$
   D. $En = -k/n^2$

5. For Scientist 1, a transition in hydrogen having $\lambda = 610$ nm would be

   A. impossible.
   B. obscured by the transitions around it.
   C. found between the transitions at 656 nm and 486 nm.
   D. found to represent higher energy transitions than those for 656 nm.

6. Scientist 2 views the transition at 434 nm as

   A. the only one possible in the region between 420 and 480 nm.
   B. not accurately determined.
   C. originating in the glass in the spectrometer.
   D. made visible by the glass in the spectrometer.

7. Scientist 2's views would be reinforced by which of the following?

   I. The finding that other atoms gave similar emission spectra in the same spectrometer.
   II. The finding that other atoms gave different emission spectra in the same spectrometer.
   III. Evidence that the spectrometer contained hydrogen atoms.

   A. I only
   B. II only
   C. III only
   D. I and II only

8. Another researcher analyzes the light from a tungsten filament lamp using the same spectrometer, and finds that a broad spectrum of wavelengths are present in the region from 400 to 650 nm, with no sharp lines. These findings support

   A. Scientist 1's position.
   B. Scientist 2's position.
   C. both positions.
   D. neither position.

Passage II (Questions 9–14)

A chemist wishes to separate a mixture containing 0.1 M Zn^{2+} ions and 0.1 M Pb^{2+} ions. She decides to use the difference in K_{sp}'s (see Table 1) to effect the separation.

Table 1

Salt	K_{sp}
ZnS	1×10^{-21}
PbS	8×10^{-28}

The chemist predicts the following results (Table 2).

Table 2

ion	$[S^{2-}]$ needed to precipitate
Zn^{2+}	1×10^{-20} M
Pb^{2+}	8×10^{-27} M

In preparing sulfide solutions, the chemist makes use of the following relation for the H_2S system:

$$[H^+]^2[S^{2-}] = 1 \times 10^{-23}$$

9. If a small quantity of sulfide ion is introduced into the mixture of Zn^{2+} and Pb^{2+}, what will precipitate first?

   A. ZnS
   B. PbS
   C. Both ZnS and PbS
   D. Neither will precipitate

10. Which of the following expressions should the chemist use to calculate the concentration of sulfide at which PbS will precipitate?

   A. $[S^{2-}] = (8 \times 10^{-28})^{\frac{1}{2}}$
   B. $[S^{2-}] = (8 \times 10^{-28})/(0.1)$
   C. $[S^{2-}] = (8 \times 10^{-28})^2/(0.1)$
   D. $[S^{2-}] = (8 \times 10^{-28})/(0.1)^2$

11. The chemist wonders how difficult it will be to prepare the dilute solutions of sulfide indicated in Table 2. How many S^{2-} ions per cubic centimeter are represented in the solution indicated in the first row of the table?

   A. 1×10^{-20}
   B. 6×10^{-20}
   C. 6
   D. 6000

12. The chemist must now determine a means of preparing a highly dilute solution of sulfide, and she decides to use the H_2S system. The relation already given for H_2S implies that

   A. high pH leads to low $[S^{2-}]$.
   B. low pH leads to low $[S^{2-}]$.
   C. pH is not necessarily related to $[S^{2-}]$.
   D. none of the above

13. What is the value of $[S^{2-}]$ when pH is 2.0?

   A. 1×10^{-19} M
   B. 5×10^{-24} M
   C. 2.5×10^{-23} M
   D. 2.0 M

14. At what value of $[H^+]$ will ZnS precipitate?

   A. 0.0032 M
   B. 0.032 M
   C. 0.32 M
   D. 3.2 M

GO ON TO THE NEXT PAGE

Passage III (Questions 15–20)

A student wishes to determine the solubility of $Mg(OH)_2$ under various conditions.

Experiment 1

The student dissolves some of the compound in water and finds $[Mg^{2+}]$ in the saturated solution to be 1.65×10^{-4}.

Experiment 2

The student dissolves enough $Mg(OH)_2$ in 0.1 M NaOH to make a saturated solution.

Experiment 3

The student prepares a saturated solution of $Mg(OH)_2$ in 1.0 M HCl.

15. From Experiment 1, the student concludes that the solubility of the salt is

    A. 1.65×10^{-4}
    B. 3.3×10^{-4}
    C. $(1.65 \times 10^{-4})^2$
    D. $(1.65 \times 10^{-4})^3$

16. Based on LeChatelier's Principle, how will the solubility of the compound in 0.1 M NaOH compare to the solubility of the compound in water?

    A. It will be less.
    B. It will be the same.
    C. It will be greater.
    D. It cannot be determined.

17. Which of the following expressions would allow the student to solve for the approximate concentration of Mg^{2+} in the alkaline solution?

    A. $[Mg^{2+}](.1) = K_{sp}$
    B. $[Mg^{2+}]^2(.1) = K_{sp}$
    C. $[Mg^{2+}](.1)^2 = K_{sp}$
    D. $[Mg^{2+}](.2)^2 = K_{sp}$

18. The student decides to measure the solubility of the salt in strong acid solution, as in Experiment 3. How would the solubility in acid compare to the solubility in the basic solution?

    A. It would be less.
    B. It would be about the same.
    C. It would be greater.
    D. It cannot be determined.

19. Which of the following expressions could be used to calculate the solubility of the solution prepared in Experiment 3?

    A. $[Mg^{2+}](1.0) = K_{sp}$
    B. $[Mg^{2+}](1.0)^2 = K_{sp}$
    C. $[Mg^{2+}](1.0 \times 10^{-14}) = K_{sp}$
    D. $[Mg^{2+}](1.0 \times 10^{-14})^2 = K_{sp}$

20. Which of the following can the student conclude?

    I. K_{sp} is pH-dependent.
    II. The solubility of $Mg(OH)_2$ is pH-dependent.
    III. The pH-dependence of this solubility serves as a model for all other magnesium salts.

    A. I only
    B. II only
    C. III only
    D. I and II only

Passage IV (Questions 21–26)

A student wants to know the molecular weight of a substance that is liquid at room temperature but a gas at 100°C.

She heats the substance until it vaporizes, then fills an open 400-mL flask with the gas and maintains the temperature at 100°C. She then cools the flask to room temperature. After the vapor in the flask condenses, she finds that this sample weighs 0.900 g. The barometric pressure is 750 torr.

The student then calculates that the number of moles of gas in the sample is 0.0129. She further calculates that the molecular weight of the sample must be 72.1 g/mol.

However, her instructor tells her that the molecular weight of the sample should *in fact* be 24.0 g/mol.

21. Once the substance in the flask is vaporized, how do changes in temperature affect the number of moles of gas in the flask (assuming the flask to be open and the pressure and volume to be constant)?

    A. The number increases as T increases.
    B. The number decreases as T increases.
    C. The number has no relation to T.
    D. It depends on the substance.

22. Which of the following did the student use to calculate the number of moles of gas in the flask at 100°C?

    A. (750)(.400)/(.0821)(100)
    B. (750/760)(.400)/(.0821)(100)
    C. (750/760)(.400)/(.0821)(373)
    D. (750/760)(.400)/(.0821)(273)

23. Which of the following did the student use to calculate the molecular weight of the gas in the flask?

    A. (.900)/(.0129)
    B. (.0129)(.900)
    C. (.0129)/(.90)
    D. (.900) + (.0129)

24. Which of the following errors might explain the difference between the molecular weight calculated by the student and the figure given by the instructor?

    A. Instead of being completely filled with gas, the flask contained some air.
    B. The temperature of the sample was actually higher than 100°C.
    C. The temperature of the sample was actually lower than 100°C.
    D. The volume of the flask was actually less than 400 mL.

25. The student decides to investigate whether the discrepancy in molecular weight measurements is due to molecules that bind together to form aggregates in the gas phase. If such aggregated molecules occurred in the gas sample, which of the following would be affected?

    I. The number of molecules
    II. The total weight of the gas
    III. The average speed of the molecules

    A. I only
    B. II only
    C. III only
    D. I and III only

26. If aggregation were the cause of the discrepancy in molecular weight, how many molecules must bind together on average to result in the molecular weight of 72.1 g/mol?

    A. 2
    B. 3
    C. 4
    D. 5

GO ON TO THE NEXT PAGE

Passage V (Questions 27–31)

Two theories for predicting the rate of a chemical reaction are given below. As you read them, look for both their similarities and their differences. Then answer the questions that follow.

Theory 1

The rate of a chemical reaction is defined to be the number of moles of a specified reactant that is consumed per unit of time. Because reactants must collide in order for a reaction to occur, it might seem that reaction rates would depend upon the concentration of reactants—since the more reactants are present, the greater the likelihood of a reaction. This is, in fact, the case, as the following example shows.

For the reaction

$$N_2O_5 \rightarrow 2NO_2 + 1/2\ O_2$$

the rate is proportional to the amount of N_2O_5 present. We may express this fact as a "rate law":

$$rate = k\ [N_2O_5]$$

where k is the rate constant.

A more complicated reaction will have a more complicated rate law. For the reaction

$$2NO + O_2 \rightarrow 2NO_2$$

the rate law will be

$$rate = k\ [NO]^2[O_2]^1$$

where the powers in the rate law reflect the coefficients of the reactants in the chemical equation. This relationship between numbers of reactant molecules and exponents in the rate law is a general one.

Theory 2

Theory 1 is very often true, for it expresses the reasonable insight that the greater the concentration of reactants, the greater the likelihood of a reaction. It has a great shortcoming, however, in its assumption that all reactions proceed in one fell swoop rather than in several steps. Let us take an example, using the letters A, B, and C, to represent molecules. In the reaction

$$A + 2B \rightarrow C$$

Theory 1 predicts a rate law of

$$rate = k[A][B]^2$$

But suppose the reaction actually proceeds in two stages, with the first one being

$$A + B \rightarrow AB$$

followed by

$$AB + B \rightarrow C$$

Let us also suppose that the first stage is much slower than the second, perhaps taking thousands of times as long. Then the rate of the overall process will essentially be the same as the rate of the first stage, which is given by

$$rate = k\ [A][B]$$

in contrast to Theory 1's prediction. Theory 2 implies, then, that we must understand the details of the reaction, including the relative speed of the various subreactions, in order to predict a rate law. Theory 1 is not totally wrong, it's just incomplete.

27. Theory 1 relates the

   A. rate of a reaction to the concentration of products.
   B. rate of a reaction to the concentration of reactants.
   C. relative amounts of reactants to each other.
   D. rate of a reaction to the individual rates of various stages of that reaction.

578

28. According to Theory 1, which of the following expresses the rate of this reaction?

$$3M + 2N \rightarrow 4P$$

A. $k\,[M][N]$
B. $k\,[M]^3[N]^2$
C. $k\,[M]^3[N]^2[P]^4$
D. $k\,([M]^3 + [N]^2)$

29. According to a proponent of Theory 2,

A. Theory 1 can never give a correct prediction for a rate law.
B. Theory 1 will give a correct result if the reactant coefficients are all equal to 1.
C. Theory 1 will give a correct result for a single-stage reaction.
D. Theory 1 is in error because it claims that collisions are necessary for reactions to take place.

30. A chemist studies the rate of the reaction

$$2NO_2 + F_2 \rightarrow 2NO_2F$$

According to Theory 1, the rate of this reaction is proportional to the

A. first power of NO_2 and the first power of F_2.
B. second power of NO_2 and the second power of NO_2F.
C. second power of NO_2 and the second power of F_2.
D. second power of NO_2 and the first power of F_2.

31. The chemist suspects that the reaction given in Question 30 proceeds in two stages:

$$NO_2 + F_2 \rightarrow NO_2F + F \text{ (Stage 1)}$$

$$F + NO_2 \rightarrow NO_2F \text{ (Stage 2)}$$

According to Theory 2, if Stage 1 is much slower than Stage 2, then the overall reaction rate

A. will be determined by the rate of Stage 1.
B. will be determined by the rate of Stage 2.
C. will be determined by the rate of Stage 1 minus that of Stage 2.
D. cannot be determined unless the rate law is measured experimentally.

GO ON TO THE NEXT PAGE

Salt	K_{sp}	Solubility (pure H$_2$O)	Solubility (0.1 M cation)
BaSO$_4$	1.1×10^{-10}	1.0×10^{-5}	1.1×10^{-9}
BaCO$_3$	1.6×10^{-9}	4.0×10^{-5}	1.6×10^{-8}
CaSO$_4$	2.4×10^{-5}	4.9×10^{-3}	2.4×10^{-4}
CaF$_2$	1.7×10^{-6}	3.5×10^{-4}	1.7×10^{-5}
PbS	7×10^{-29}	8.4×10^{-15}	7×10^{-28}
PbSO$_4$	1.3×10^{-8}	1.1×10^{-4}	1.3×10^{-7}
BaF$_2$	1.7×10^{-6}	7.5×10^{-3}	1.7×10^{-5}
Pb(OH)$_2$	2.8×10^{-16}	4.1×10^{-6}	2.8×10^{-15}
Fe(OH)$_2$	1.6×10^{-15}	7.4×10^{-6}	1.6×10^{-14}
Cu(IO$_3$)$_3$	1.3×10^{-7}	5.1×10^{-3}	1.3×10^{-6}

Passage VI (Questions 32–39)

We have seen that when a salt dissolves in pure water, the expression for K_{sp} can be used to solve for the concentration of the ions. For example, for AgCl,

$$K_{sp} = [Ag^+][Cl^-]$$

Since in pure water, every silver or chloride ion results from a dissociation, either concentration may be used to calculate the solubility.

The situation is different if there is another source of either ion. The table above gives solubility data for various salts in pure water (column 3) and for a solution containing 0.1 mol/L of the cation in the original salt. For example, for BaSO$_4$, the last column refers to solubility in 0.1 M Ba^{2+}.

32. The pair of salts with the least and greatest solubility in pure water, respectively, are

A. PbS and CaSO$_4$.
B. PbS and BaF$_2$.
C. BaF$_2$ and PbS.
D. CaSO$_4$ and PbS.

33. The solubility of Pb(OH)$_2$ in the presence of 0.1 M cation is

A. greater than the K_{sp} by a factor of 10.
B. less than the K_{sp} by a factor of 10.
C. less than the solubility in pure water by a factor of 10.
D. greater than the solubility in pure water by a factor of 10.

34. The solubility of a given salt in pure water is

A. less than in the 0.1 M solution of the cation.
B. greater than in the 0.1 M solution of the cation.
C. sometimes less, sometimes greater, than in the 0.1 M solution of the cation.
D. equal to the solubility in the solution of the cation.

35. The solubility of a given salt in the 0.1 M cation solution can be calculated as which of the following?

A. $(K_{sp})^{\frac{1}{2}}$
B. $(0.10)K_{sp}$
C. $K_{sp}/(0.10)$
D. The square root of the solubility in pure water

36. Which of the following is closest to the ratio of the smallest K_{sp} shown in the chart to the largest?

A. 10^{24}
B. 10^{-24}
C. 10^{12}
D. 10^{-12}

37. Which of the lead salts listed produces the greatest concentration of Pb^{2+} when added in excess to pure water?

    A. PbS
    B. $PbSO_4$
    C. $Pb(OH)_2$
    D. All the salts produce the same concentration.

38. Excess BaF_2 is added to pure water; then $Ba(NO_3)_2$ is added until the solution is 0.1 M in Ba^{2+}. Which of the following is true?

    A. BaF_2 dissolves after the addition of barium nitrate.
    B. The solubility product of BaF_2 drops as the barium nitrate is added.
    C. BaF_2 precipitates as the barium nitrate is added.
    D. $Ba(NO_3)$ precipitates at the last step.

39. Solution A is 0.1 M in both $Ba(NO_3)_2$ and $Ca(NO_3)_2$. To 100 mL of solution A, a student adds 1.0 mL of 0.1 M Na_2SO_4. What will be the result?

    A. Precipitation of $BaSO_4$
    B. Precipitation of $CaSO_4$
    C. Precipitation of both $BaSO_4$ and $CaSO_4$
    D. None of the above

Passage VII (Questions 40–44)

A worker on the third floor of a building under construction needs to remove a 100-kg block of steel. The worker, whose body mass is 70 kg, pushes the block along the level floor at a constant velocity covering 8 m in 4 s. The force applied on the block is 200 N. When the block reaches the edge of the building, it falls off. It tumbles 8 meters, accidentally strikes a stake partially embedded in the ground, and drives the stake completely into the ground.

40. What is the weight of the steel block?

    A. 9.8×10^{-2} N
    B. 4.9×10^{-2} N
    C. 4.9×10^2 N
    D. 9.8×10^2 N

41. Which statement is most accurate about the force of friction exerted while the block is pushed along the floor?

    A. $F_{friction}$ is greater than 200 N.
    B. $F_{friction}$ is less than 200 N.
    C. $F_{friction}$ is exactly equal to 200 N.
    D. $F_{friction}$ cannot be determined from the data given.

42. What is the work done by the man in pushing the block?

    A. 1600 J
    B. 400 J
    C. 50 J
    D. 25 J

43. What is the approximate velocity of the block just before striking the stake?

    A. 9.80 m/s
    B. 2.00 m/s
    C. 12.5 m/s
    D. 16.0 m/s

44. What is the approximate kinetic energy of the block just before striking the stake?

    A. 3263 J
    B. 7840 J
    C. 8500 J
    D. 12,000 J

GO ON TO THE NEXT PAGE

Passage VIII (Questions 45–49)

An electrical technician constructs a circuit that consists of three resistors, R_1, R_2, and R_3 of 30 Ω, 60 Ω, and 40 Ω, respectively, and a voltage source, V. The circuit diagram for the set up is:

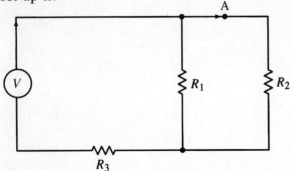

With an ammeter the technician measures the amount of current at point A.

45. If the amount of current measured at point A is 2.0 amperes, what is the rate at which R_2 uses electrical energy?

    A. 30 W
    B. 60 W
    C. 240 W
    D. 180 W

46. What is the amount of heat developed in R_2 in 3 seconds?

    A. 720 J
    B. 120 J
    C. 360 J
    D. 40 J

47. What is the voltage drop across the 30 Ω resistor, R_1?

    A. 60 V
    B. 120 V
    C. 180 V
    D. 240 V

48. What is the voltage of the potential difference source V?

    A. 60 V
    B. 120 V
    C. 240 V
    D. 360 V

49. The voltage source, V, has an internal resistance of 4 Ω. What is its electromotive force (emf)?

    A. 384 V
    B. 336 V
    C. 356 V
    D. 364 V

Passage IX (Questions 50–53)

In order to compare the refractive properties of various liquid substances, a researcher constructs the apparatus illustrated below. It consists of two adjacent chambers, 1 and 2, with walls and partitions made from very thin glass so that the effects of the glass on the refraction of light passing through the chambers is negligible. One chamber is filled with a reference liquid for which the refractive index is known. Water is a typical reference liquid. The refractive index for water is $n_{H_2O} = 1.33$. The liquid to be tested is then placed in the second chamber. The apparatus is surrounded by the air in the laboratory.

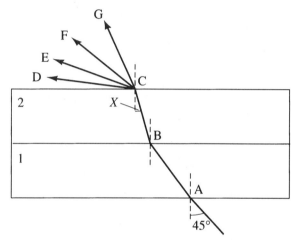

The researcher then shines a beam of light through the two liquids and traces its path. The angle of incidence of the beam on the first wall of the apparatus (chamber 1) is 45°. (Sin 45° = 0.707. Sin 30° = 0.500.)

50. In the diagram, several possible rays for the light beam exiting from chamber 2 into the air are indicated. Which ray best represents the actual exit path of the beam?

  A. D
  B. E
  C. F
  D. G

51. What is the speed of light in water?

  A. 1.13×10^3 m/s
  B. 2.26×10^8 m/s
  C. 3.00×10^8 m/s
  D. 3.99×10^8 m/s

52. If the refractive index of the unknown liquid in chamber 2 is 2.00, which of the statements below most accurately describes the angle of incidence, X, of the beam on the wall between the unknown liquid in chamber 2 and the air?

  A. It is less than 30°.
  B. It is exactly 30°.
  C. It is greater than 30° but less than 45°.
  D. It is exactly 45°.

53. What is the sine of the critical angle between the unknown liquid in chamber 2 and the air?

  A. 0.500
  B. 0.707
  C. 1.00
  D. 2.00

Passage X (Questions 54–58)

A Nebraska telephone company lineman needs to determine the size of copper wire that can best withstand the typical buildup of ice on the wires during the winter. He takes a sample that is 240 meters long and 2.0 mm in diameter. He simulates the net effect of the ice by applying a 628-N force to one of the wires so that the line of action of the force coincides with the axis of the wire. The length after stretching the wire is 240.24 m. When the force is removed, the wire returns to its original length.

54. What is the stress on the wire?

   A. 2.00×10^8 N/m^2
   B. 2.00×10^8 J
   C. 314 N/m^2
   D. 314

55. What is the strain on the wire?

   A. 0.24 m
   B. 1.0×10^{-3} N/m^2
   C. 0.24
   D. 1.0×10^{-3}

56. What is the estimated elastic modulus for copper?

   A. 2.0×10^{11} N/m^2
   B. 314 N/m^2
   C. 480 N/m^2
   D. 2.0×10^5 N/m^2

57. The elastic modulus for copper is called the

   A. Shear modulus.
   B. Bulk modulus.
   C. Young's modulus.
   D. Unit modulus.

58. The reaction of the wire to the removal of the force is called the

   A. elastic limit.
   B. breaking point.
   C. elasticity.
   D. tensile strength.

Questions 59–77 are independent of any passage and independent of each other.

59. The speed of sound in air at a given temperature is 360 m/s. What is the shortest closed-end pipe that will produce an air column length that can resonate at a frequency of 450 Hz?

   A. 20 cm
   B. 80 cm
   C. 90 cm
   D. 125 cm

60. What is the acceleration of a falling stone whose velocity increases from 80 m/s to 100 m/s in 2 seconds?

   A. 0.10 m/s^2
   B. 10 m/s^2
   C. 10 m/s
   D. 90 m/s^2

61. A ball is thrown vertically upward with an initial velocity of 40.0 meters per second. What will be its velocity after 2.00 seconds?

   A. 20.4 m/s
   B. 9.80 m/s
   C. 49.0 m/s
   D. 80.0 m/s

62. A 2.0-kg body is acted on by a 10-N force. If the body is initially at rest, what will be its velocity after 5 seconds?

   A. 5.0 m/s
   B. 10 m/s
   C. 20 m/s
   D. 25 m/s

63. If 22.5 g of $NiCl_2$ reacts completely with a sufficient amount of NH_3 and NaBr to form $Ni(NH_3)_2Br_2Cl_2$, which of the following expressions gives the number of moles of product that are formed? (at. wt. of Ni = 58.7, of Cl = 35.5, of Br = 79.9)

   A. 22.5/79.9
   B. 13/[79.9 + 2(35.5)]
   C. (2)(22.5/79.9)
   D. 22.5/[58.7 + 2(14) + 6 + 2(35.5)]

64. Which is the correct electron-dot formula for H_2O_2?

A.   H:Ö::Ö:H

B.   H:O::O:H
         ..

C.   H:O::Ö:H

D.   H:Ö : Ö:H
         ..   ..

65. Which of the following is closest to the pH of a mixture containing 1.0 mole each of formic acid (whose K_a is 1.8×10^{-4}) and potassium formate?

A.   0.1
B.   2
C.   4
D.   7

66. If 1.0 mole each of graphite at 350K (C_p = 8.63 J/mol deg) and water at 273K (C_p = 4.18 J/mol deg) are put together in an insulated container, which of the following gives the final temperature (T) of the water in degrees C?

A. $(8.63)(350 + T) = (4.18)(273 + T)$
B. $(8.63)(350 - T) = (4.18)(273 + T)$
C. $(4.18)(350 - T) = (8.63)(273 + T)$
D. $T = (8.63 - 4.18)/(350 - 273)$

67. A 0th-order reaction requires 5 minutes for the original concentration of its reactant to drop from 0.180 M to 0.090 M. How much additional time, in minutes, will be required for the reactant concentration to decline to 0.045 M?

A.   2.5
B.   5
C.   7.5
D.   10

68. A "3-minute egg" cooked in Boston might require extra cooking time in

A.   Denver, because of the higher boiling point of the water at Denver's higher altitude.
B.   Death Valley, because of the higher boiling point of the water at Death Valley's lower altitude.
C.   Denver, because of the lower boiling point of the water at high altitude.
D.   Death Valley, because of the lower boiling point of the water at low altitude.

69. An electron in a hydrogen atom is excited to a state where $l = 2$ and $n = 4$. This state is referred to as

A. $2p$.
B. $4s$.
C. $2d$.
D. $4d$.

70. The solubility of AgCl in water can be increased by

A.   adding NaCl.
B.   adding $AgNO_3$.
C.   adding AgCl.
D.   none of the above.

71. What is the force between two 10μC charges separated by a distance of 10 cm?

A. 1.0×10^{-8} N
B.   90 N
C.   30 N
D. -30 N

72. A heating device requires 1200 watts of power when supplied by a 120-volt source. What is the resistance of this device?

A.   12 Ω
B.   10 Ω
C.   6 Ω
D.   0.10 Ω

GO ON TO THE NEXT PAGE

73. The light emitted from an incandescent source follows the inverse square law of intensity. By what factor does the brightness change if the source is moved from 6 ft away from an observer to 3 ft away from the observer?

   A.   The brightness doubles.
   B.   The brightness quadruples.
   C.   The brightness is halved.
   D.   The brightness is quartered.

74. What radiation is emitted during the following decay process?

$$^{226}_{88}\text{Ra} \rightarrow {}^{222}_{86}\text{Rn} + x$$

   A. α decay
   B. β decay
   C.   Neutron emission
   D.   Positron emission

75. A 20 Ω and a 40 Ω resistor are connected in series with a voltage source as shown below.

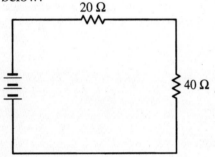

If the current through the 20 Ω resistor is 2.0 A, what is the voltage drop across the 40 Ω resistor?

   A.   40 V
   B.   80 V
   C.   120 V
   D.   400 V

76. How many neutrons are produced in the following nuclear reaction?

$$^{235}_{92}\text{U} + {}^{1}_{0}n \rightarrow {}^{144}_{56}\text{Ba} + {}^{89}_{36}\text{Kr} + X{}^{1}_{0}n$$

   A.   1
   B.   2
   C.   3
   D.   4

77. A 6-N and an 8-N force act on the same point of a body, but at right angles to each other. What is the resultant force?

   A.   2 N
   B.   7 N
   C.   10 N
   D.   14 N

END OF TEST 1.

IF YOU FINISH BEFORE THE TIME IS UP,
YOU MAY CHECK YOUR WORK ON THIS TEST ONLY.

VERBAL REASONING

TIME: 85 MINUTES   **QUESTIONS 78–142**

> **Directions:** There are nine passages in this test. Each passage is followed by questions based on its content. After reading a passage, choose the one best answer to each question and indicate your selection by blackening the corresponding circle on your answer sheet.

Passage I (Questions 78–85)

The deliberate violation of constituted law (civil disobedience) is never morally justified if the law being violated is not the prime target or focal point of the protest. Although our government maintains the principle of the Constitution by providing methods for and protection of those engaged in individual or group dissent, the violation of law simply as a technique of demonstration constitutes rebellion.

Civil disobedience is, by definition, a violation of the law. The theory of civil disobedience recognizes that its actions, regardless of their justification, must be punished. However, disobedience of laws not the subject of dissent, but merely used to dramatize dissent, is regarded as morally, as well as legally, unacceptable. It is only with respect to those laws that offend the fundamental values of human life that moral defense of civil disobedience can be rationally supported.

The assumption that a law is a valid target of civil disobedience is filled with moral and legal responsibility that cannot be taken lightly. To be morally justified in such a stance, one must be prepared to submit to legal prosecution for violation of the law and accept the punishment if the attack is unsuccessful. One should even demand that the law be enforced and then be willing to acquiesce in the ultimate judgment of the courts. As members of an organized society, we benefit from our government and our Constitution. If we challenge the law and our challenge is not vindicated, our implied duty is to accept the verdict.

For a just society to exist, the principle of tolerance must be accepted, both by the government in regard to properly expressed individual dissent and by the individual toward legally established majority verdicts. No individual has a monopoly on freedom, and all must tolerate opposition. Dissenters must accept dissent from their dissent, giving it all the respect they claim for themselves. To disregard this principle is to make civil disobedience not only legally wrong but also morally unjustifiable.

78. It can be inferred from the article that the author's attitude toward civil disobedience when properly conducted is one of

- A. contempt.
- B. respect.
- C. shock.
- D. enthusiasm.

79. The author regards the violation of law simply as a technique to dramatize dissent as

- A. unlawful.
- B. morally wrong.
- C. acceptable if changing the Constitution.
- D. an act of rebellion.

80. According to the author of the article, the violation of constituted law (civil disobedience) is never morally justified unless

  A. a greater good is being fought for.

  B. the law being broken is the law that the people involved want changed.

  C. the act of civil disobedience has taken over an important moral issue.

  D. the saving of human life is involved.

81. The author says that in order to be morally responsible for an act of civil disobedience, an individual must

  I. completely understand the law he or she is breaking.

  II. realize the law that he or she is trying to change may not be changed by the act of civil disobedience.

  III. be willing to be arrested and be prosecuted for his or her act of civil disobedience.

  A. I only

  B. III only

  C. I and II only

  D. II and III only

82. According to the article, in order for society to exist

  A. people must be tolerant of government and not break laws.

  B. government must have enormous power to control people.

  C. government must be tolerant of people and people must be tolerant of government.

  D. the relationship between the governed and the government must be balanced.

83. According to the author, civil disobedience is justifiable only when

  A. other methods to change a law have been tried and have failed.

  B. the law that people are trying to change offends fundamental values of human life.

  C. the law that people are trying to change is a violation of the Constitution.

  D. a group has decided that rebellion is the only course open to them.

84. The use of individual or group dissent in our society is interpreted by the author as a

  A. privilege.

  B. right.

  C. violation of the law.

  D. means to test governmental control.

85. The article points out that in accordance with the theory of civil disobedience, one who supports civil disobedience should be prepared to

  A. be punished.

  B. accept praise.

  C. be reviled.

  D. become ostracized.

Passage II (Questions 86–93)

Contemporary astronomy is ordinarily at least as much of an observational as a theoretical science. Sooner or later on the basis of observation and analysis, what astronomers detect finds its way into theory, or the theory is modified to accept it.

Neutrino astronomy doesn't fit this pattern. Its highly developed body of theory grew for 30 years without any possibility of verification. Despite the construction of a string of elaborate observatories, some buried in the earth from southern India to Utah to South Africa, the last five years as well have produced not a single, validated observation of an extraterrestrial neutrino.

It is a testament to the persistence of the neutrino astronomers and the strength of their theoretical base that their intensive search for these ghost particles goes on.

The neutrino is a particle with a vanishingly small mass and no charge. Having no charge, it does not interact with the fields around which most particle detection experiments are built; it can be detected only inferentially, by identifying the debris left from its rare interaction with matter.

Even such indirect observations need elaborate and highly sensitive equipment that wasn't in place until about five years ago. The goal is worth the effort; however, once detected, extraterrestrial neutrinos will provide solid, firsthand information on the sources and conditions that spawned them.

Scientists are sure of this in light of results of sophisticated experiments already conducted on neutrino reactions in particle accelerators and other earthbound apparatus. These experiments have been refined rigorously over the years and are the basis of neutrino theory, which is an integral part of modern physics.

The existence of neutrinos was first postulated in the early 1930s, to explain a form of radioactive decay in which a beta particle—an electron—is emitted. Certain quantities that physicists insist should be the same after an interaction as before—momentum, energy, and angular momentum—could be conserved only if another particle of zero charge and negligible mass were emitted.

86. The normal pattern of research in astronomy according to the article is to

   A. develop theories through the process of analytical reasoning and then make observations to see if the theories work.
   B. observe and then, after many observations, try to develop a theory that explains the observations.
   C. develop a theory and then use observations to prove the theory.
   D. conduct experimental research to validate unproven theories.

87. According to the article, equipment for studying extraterrestrial neutrinos has been available

   A. since the 1930s.
   B. for 25 years.
   C. for the last five years.
   D. for the last 15 years.

88. It can be inferred from the article that neutrino theory was first developed as a result of which one of the following laws?

   A. Magnetism
   B. Conservation
   C. Inertial
   D. Motion

89. One reason neutrinos are hard to find, according to the article, is that they are

   I. positively charged.
   II. negatively charged.
   III. neither positively nor negatively charged.

   A. I only
   B. II only
   C. I and II only
   D. III only

GO ON TO THE NEXT PAGE

90. According to the article, the theory of extraterrestrial neutrinos is based on

   A. a great number of observations.
   B. the use of earthbound equipment to neutrinos.
   C. a theory that was first developed in the 1930s based on astronomical observations made at that time.
   D. a theory that has been sustained even though no extraterrestrial neutrino has ever been observed.

91. Observing neutrinos is worth the effort according to the article because

   A. this discovery will prove that developing a theory about something before we observe it is a valid idea.
   B. observing neutrinos will give us considerable knowledge of what spawned them.
   C. if we can observe neutrinos, we will be able to build better telescopes.
   D. we will better understand neutrons.

92. Three quantities that physicists say should be the same after an interaction as before are

   A. electrons, protons, and neutrons.
   B. magnetism, force, and energy.
   C. neutrinos, atoms, and molecules.
   D. momentum, energy, and angular motion.

93. According to the article, neutrino theory is a basic part of

   A. physics.
   B. physical chemistry.
   C. astronomy.
   D. molecular biology.

Passage III (Questions 94–101)

Many persons who appreciate and admire Mr. Swinburne's genius cannot help regretting that he should ever have descended from the serene heights of poetry into the arena of criticism. Creation and analysis are two very different things; and poetic inspiration is often divorced from the sanity of judgment. It is very easy to pardon the excess of a poet's imagination; but we cannot overlook the absence of common sense and impartiality in a writer who claims to be regarded as a literary critic.

Mr. Swinburne's criticism is characterized by an utter want of proportion and an aggressive dogmatism that finds vent in offensive and vituperative language quite unsuited to the dignity of literature. . . .

A careful comparison of *Essays and Studies* with another volume published about eleven years later, under the title of *Miscellanies*, shows that their author has either deliberately or unconsciously contradicted many of the opinions he had previously expressed. . . .

No doubt Mr. Swinburne has read the best portion of modern literature. He is filled with apparently genuine admiration for lesser-known Elizabethan dramatists, and he has done a service by pointing out some of their praiseworthy characteristics. But even in this work of utility, there is an element of false criticism, for some of the weakest plays of Ford and Webster are lauded by him as great and immortal dramas. Mr. Swinburne, when he writes about Victor Hugo, cannot be taken seriously; he is a Hugomaniac, and when he refers to either *L'Homme qui Rit* or *L'Annee Terrible*, he can only express himself in the superlative degree. Indeed, nearly all that he has written about this rather overrated representative of the French romanticist school is little better than hysterical declamation.

True poet though he be, Mr. Swinburne has none of the faculties that are properly termed judicial. In his entire estimates of the merits and demerits of other men of genius (for undoubtedly he is himself a man of genius), he is too one-sided, too extravagant, too unrestrained. Literature is, perhaps, with him a consuming passion, and for that very reason he may not be able to discuss it with calmness or moderation. This fact, however, remains: His judgments upon books and their authors are the very reverse of impartial, and it is manifest that Nature never intended him for a critic.

94. It can be inferred that the author of this article believes that two characteristics of a good critic are

   A. imagination and the ability to use vituperative language.
   B. dogmatism and passion.
   C. love of romantic literature and love of poetry.
   D. common sense and impartiality.

95. According to the author, Mr. Swinburne is a good

   I. poet.
   II. playwright.
   III. critic.

   A. I only
   B. I and II only
   C. II and III only
   D. III only

96. The author states that a comparison between Mr. Swinburne's *Essays and Studies* and *Miscellanies* shows the two volumes to be

   A. consistent with each other.
   B. well connected with each other.
   C. inconsistent with each other in many respects.
   D. complementary to each other.

97. According to the author, Mr. Swinburne's criticisms can be described as all of the following except

   A. unrestrained.
   B. calm and detached.
   C. one-sided.
   D. offensive.

98. The author states that Mr. Swinburne's criticisms are very

   A. impartial.
   B. knowledgeable.
   C. poetic.
   D. partial.

99. It can be inferred from the article that the author does not think highly of

   A. Elizabethan writers.
   B. French romanticism.
   C. Mr. Swinburne's knowledge of literature.
   D. neoclassical writers.

100. It may be inferred from the passage that the author considers Mr. Swinburne's literary talents as a critic to be

   A. praiseworthy.
   B. an ideal difficult to aspire to.
   C. biased and censorious.
   D. a model for future literary critics.

101. The example of Mr. Swinburne as a biased literary critic implies that

   A. his creative literary talents were squandered on writing only criticism.
   B. his literary reviews were taken seriously by the public at the time.
   C. most of the literature he reviewed tended to be mediocre and dull.
   D. he mistakenly assumed his writing talents could also extend to literary criticism.

GO ON TO THE NEXT PAGE

Passage IV (Questions 102–108)

A proper, English-born minister, George Wharton James seemed out of his element when he arrived in the still-wild West in 1881. But James became fascinated by the endangered Native American culture he saw in California and neighboring Arizona.

Before his death in 1923, James wrote more than forty books chronicling the region and its Mojavi, Yavapai, and Havasupai tribes. A prolific photographer, he also took thousands of photographs documenting the daily lives and customs of the peoples he saw. After his death, James's unique pictorial history of the region was donated to the Southwest Museum in Los Angeles, a nonprofit educational institution founded in 1907 to preserve and interpret the art, artifacts, and documentary material of the prehistoric and historic cultures of the Americas.

But many of James's best pictures—just like the vanishing society he photographed—now are in danger. They and thousands of other pictures could literally turn to dust without quick action to preserve them. With help from the National Endowment for the Humanities, the Southwest Museum is trying to protect the visual memory of the region and make the pictures more accessible to historians and researchers.

"There is very little documentation of that period remaining," says Daniela P. Moneta, the museum's head librarian and director of its film preservation project. "Much of it has already been destroyed."

Moneta explains that James and many other photographers of the early 1900s often used a nitrate-based film to capture the culture of Native Americans facing the onslaught of American settlers. Within decades, however, the nitrate-based film begins to deteriorate. Ultimately, it can crumble into powder. The early photographers, notes Moneta, "just didn't realize it would deteriorate so quickly."

The threatened degeneration poses a major problem for historians of the period. The museum's extensive collection contains thousands of fragile negatives, taken between 1900 and 1940, of important enthnographic and archaeological documentation of California, the Southwest, and Meso-america. The photo library is a treasure house for researchers—particularly those living in the West—since it contains vintage prints that show the crafts, costume, dances, ceremonies, dwellings, and daily life of the native Americans. "The library includes unique images not contained in other photo archives," notes Moneta.

In addition to the George Wharton James collection, the museum's photo treasure chest includes such rare items as negatives of the dress and culture of the Cupeno and Luiseno Indians of Southern California in the early 1900s; scenes of the Seminole and Choctaw tribes in the Southeastern United States; pictures of daily life among the Pueblo and other tribes in Arizona and New Mexico; documentation of the Mayan ruins in Yucatan; and photos taken by the Southwest Museum staff during archaeological excavations in California, Nevada, and Colorado.

The more than eleven thousand nitrate-based negatives in the museum's collection "are still in good condition," says Moneta, but experts have already detected early warning signals of deterioration. "The negatives could turn to powder before we know it," she notes, adding the museum's anxiety over the film has increased greatly in the past five years.

For several decades, the negatives were kept in a cool storage area within the museum. But in 1981, a nitrate film expert with the San Diego Historical Society recommended that the deteriorating negatives be moved out of the museum because they could soon begin to emit destructive gaseous fumes and could even explode.

In 1983, the negatives were shipped out to a remote storage warehouse approved by the Los Angeles Fire Department. Now, the negatives are not only relatively inaccessible to researchers, but are threatened with even more rapid deterioration because the storage facility lacks temperature and humidity controls.

With help from the National Endowment for the Humanities, the museum plans to save the film by converting it into "interpositives" on safety-based film, which then can be stored in the museum for easy access by researchers. The interpositives will be similar to a positive print of the negative on paper, but it will be of finer quality, and less detail will be lost in the copying process. "Having a positive image of the negatives available will make the collection more usable and therefore more valuable to researchers," says Moneta.

102. According to the article, George Wharton James was important because he was

    I.   one of the first settlers in the Southwest.
    II. an expert in film preservation.
    III. an important photographer of Native American cultures of the Southwest.

    A.   I and III only
    B.   II only
    C.   III only
    D.   II and III only

103. The Southwestern Museum has

    A.   the only visual documentation of Native American culture of the early 1900s.
    B.   very little experience with film preservation.
    C.   converted all its nitrate negatives to interpositives.
    D.   eleven thousand nitrate negatives that are threatened with deterioration.

104. The article states that many of James's best photographs are in danger because:

    A.   the kind of film he used deteriorates over time.
    B.   they are not in the possession of the Southwestern Museum.
    C.   visitors to the museum have been careless with the photographs and have damaged them.
    D.   the museum lacks space to care for the photos and is forced to store them at facilities far from the museum.

105. George Wharton James came to the United States in

    A.   1804.
    B.   1826.
    C.   1874.
    D.   1881.

106. The article implies that the Southwestern Museum was unable to save many of the nitrate negatives because

    A.   the negatives were deteriorating so rapidly that it was virtually impossible to save them.
    B.   loss of funding from various sources had forced the museum to abandon its search for alternative methods.
    C.   a San Diego Historical Society expert on nitrate film was criticial of the museum's method of handling the negatives.
    D.   the costs of preserving nitrate negatives were so exorbitant.

107. Which of the following is the best explanation of the value of James's pictures to be drawn from the article?

    A.   They preserve a unique pictorial history of a number of Native American tribes of the Southwest.
    B.   The deterioration of the negatives proves the inefficiency of early photographic film despite the value of their cultural contribution.
    C.   They are interesting artifacts of a forgotten culture.
    D.   James was an important, leading religious authority whose influence is remembered.

GO ON TO THE NEXT PAGE

108. According to the article, which of the following statements is true about photography in the period from the 1880s to the 1920s?

    A. So many photographs were taken during this time that it is not crucial to save all of the negatives.

    B. So few photographs were taken during this time that it is essential that all of James's photographs be saved.

    C. Although few photographs were taken during this period, James's photos were of such poor quality that they are not worth the expense of saving them.

    D. No effective method for saving nitrate negatives was available then and none has yet been developed.

Passage V (Questions 109–114)

It would grieve me to seem unjust toward a writer to whom I have long felt very specially attracted—and this by no means only because of a pious, although perhaps more or less apocryphal, bond. Yet the highest praise that it seems right to bestow upon Thomas Heywood is that which was happily expressed by Tieck when he described him as the "model of a light and rapid talent." Carried, it may be, by fortune or by choice from the tranquil court of Peterhouse to a very different scene of intellectual effort, he worked during a long and laborious life with an energy in itself deserving of respect, and manifestly also with a facility attesting no ordinary natural endowment. His creative power was, however, of that secondary order which is content with accommodating itself to conditions imposed by the prevailing tastes of the day. It may be merely his prenticed hand that he tried on a dramatic reproduction of chronicles and popular storybooks; but though even here the simplicity of his workmanship was due to a natural directness of touch by no means to be confounded with rudeness of hand, he cannot be said to have done much to revive a species that though still locally popular was already doomed to decay. . . . Of humor, he had his

share—or he would have been no master of pathos; but he cannot be said to have excelled in humorous characterization; there is as a rule little individuality in his comic figures at large; and his clowns, although good examples of their kind, are made to order. Indeed, the inferior sort of wit—which of all writers, dramatists most readily acquire as a literary accomplishment his practiced inventiveness displays with the utmost abundance; of all the Elizabethan playwrights, he is one of the most unwearied, and to my mind one of the most intolerable punsters. In outward form he is nearly as Protean as in choice of subject and of treatment; his earlier plays more especially abound with rimes; in general, fluent verse and easy prose are freely intermixed. But—apart from the pathetic force of particular passages and scenes, and a straightforward naturalness that lends an irresistible charm to a writer as it does to a friend in real life—his strength lies in a dramatic insight that goes far toward the making of a master of the playwright's art, while it has undoubtedly been possessed by some not entitled to rank as dramatic poets.

109. It can be inferred that the author of the article thinks that Thomas Heywood was

    A. a great poet.
    B. a very poor playwright.
    C. a very insightful playwright.
    D. an average poet.

110. The period of time in which Thomas Heywood wrote was the

    A. present.
    B. Elizabethan.
    C. nineteenth century.
    D. eighteenth century.

111. The author's attitude toward Thomas Heywood is one of

    A. admiration.
    B. ridicule.
    C. criticism.
    D. dislike.

112. According to the author of the article, Thomas Heywood's greatest strength as a writer was his

    A. humor.
    B. pathos.
    C. dramatic insight.
    D. comic figures.

113. The main theme of the article is Heywood's

    A. emotional lifestyle.
    B. sense of humor.
    C. creative powers.
    D. reputation as an intolerable punster.

114. It can be inferred from the article that the author believes that a truly great writer must be able to

    I. develop universal themes that will live through the ages.
    II. develop characters with which the audience can identify.
    III. rise above the taste of the times rather than cater to them.

    A. I only
    B. III only
    C. I and II only
    D. II and III only

Passage VI (Questions 115–122)

During the past four decades, the fishery scientists of the West have studied the dynamics of fish populations with the objective of determining the relationship between the amount of fishing and the sustainable catch. They have developed a substantial body of theory that has been applied successfully to a large number of animal populations and has led to significant improvement in the management of some of the major marine fisheries.

The theory has been developed for single-species populations with man as a predator. Much of it is based on the Darwinian concept of a constant overpopulation of young that is reduced by density-dependent mortality resulting from intraspecific competition. The unfished population tends toward a maximum equilibrium size and proportions of large, old individuals. As fishing increases, both population size and proportions of large, old individuals are reduced. Fishing mortality eventually takes the place of most natural mortality. If the amount of fishing is increased too much, the individuals will tend to be taken before realizing their potential growth, and total yield will be reduced. The maximum sustainable yields can be taken at an intermediate population size that in some populations is about one-third to one-half the unfished population size.

G. V. Nikolskii, of Moscow State University, develops his theory from a different approach. He is a non-Darwinian and is (he says) a nonmathematician; rather he considers himself an ecologist and a morphologist. He argues that Darwin's concept of constant overpopulation has led to the neglect of the problem of protecting spawners and young fish. He argues also that Darwin's concept of a variety as an incipient species has led to extensive mathematical analysis of racial characteristics without an understanding of the adaptive significance of the characters. Nikolskii considers the main laws of population dynamics to be concerned with the succession of generations: their birth, growth, and death. The details are governed by the relative states of adaption and environmental change. The mass and age structure of a population are the result of adaptation to the food supply. The rate of growth of individuals, the time of sexual maturity, and the accumulation of reserves vary according to the food supply. These factors, in turn, influence the success of reproduction in ways that tend to bring the size of the population into balance with its food supply.

GO ON TO THE NEXT PAGE

115. Fishing experts have been studying the dynamics of fish populations with the goal of discovering

    A. the conditions under which fish survive best.
    B. how environmental change affects fish populations.
    C. how different species of fish interact.
    D. the maximum sustainable level of fishing that will keep the fish population constant.

116. According to Nikolskii, the rate of growth of individuals and the time of sexual maturity is based on

    I. food supply.
    II. how many males are in the population.
    III. number of predators.

    A. I only
    B. I and II only
    C. III only
    D. II and III only

117. The research done by western scientists is based on

    A. mathematical concepts.
    B. concepts of space and density.
    C. Darwinian concepts of constant overpopulation of the young.
    D. non-Darwinian concepts of ecology.

118. G. V. Nikolskii believes that the Darwinians have failed to take into account

    A. the size of the body of water the fish live in.
    B. whether the fish are freshwater or saltwater fish.
    C. the impact of other predators besides man.
    D. how to protect spawners and young fish.

119. The article states that this kind of marine research has been done by western scientists over the last

    A. decade.
    B. four decades.
    C. two decades.
    D. five decades.

120. Nikolskii considers the main laws of population dynamics to be concerned with

    A. size, age, and genetic traits.
    B. the succession of generations, number of predators, and rate of habitat destruction.
    C. the succession of generations: their birth, growth, and death.
    D. ecology, evolution, and death.

121. It can be inferred from the article that one main difference between the Darwinians and Nikolskii is the

    A. influence that the food supply will have on the success of a fish population's maintaining its level.
    B. role of the environment on a fish population's ability to sustain itself.
    C. role that predators other than man play.
    D. mass of the body of water that the fish inhabit.

122. According to Nikolskii, mass and age structure of populations are the result of

    A. the number of predators in the environment.
    B. whether the fish is environmentally well adapted.
    C. adaptation to the food supply.
    D. size of the species of fish.

Passage VII (Questions 123–128)

The cultural life of modern democratic societies is a pluralistic enterprise. Fortunately, no central direction is imposed on the creation of art and ideas. Instead, we see an apparently limitless number of forces competing in a dynamic struggle of creation and consumption.

Precisely because modern democratic society is so diverse, a peculiar component of our cultural situation—criticism—has emerged. So powerful, indeed, is this force in today's society that we are undoubtedly justified in asking, "Who will criticize the critic?" Before we can criticize the critic, however, we must try to understand what he does.

The first task of the critic is to see the work of art and describe its qualities and attributes as clearly as possible. This is the task of elucidation, and it is fundamental to all criticism worthy of the name. Yet the task of elucidation is not easily separable from another important function of criticism, evaluation. Even the most objectively conceived critical elucidation is bound to contain signs of a judgment. Therefore, so as not to conceal this admixture of description and judgment, critical evaluation is best performed as honestly as possible with reasoned arguments and detailed examples.

In our own time, when all of the institutions of society—the museums, the media, the universities, the galleries, the collectors, and all government agencies concerned with the arts—are prejudiced in favor of whatever is deemed on any grounds new and innovative in the arts, the challenge to criticism is monumental.

The question in a democratic society is not whether criticism has a role to play; that is taken for granted. The real question concerns, rather, the responsibility of criticism to defend the integrity of art against all encroachments—especially, in our day, the ideological encroachments. By concentrating in the most disinterested way on its traditional tasks of elucidation and evaluation, criticism will make its necessary contribution to the life of art and the freedom of the spirit.

123. It can be inferred that the author's major point in the article is that

   A. critics stifle creativity.
   B. criticism of art tends to keep art traditional.
   C. the most important role of critics is to define art.
   D. the critic's role is to defend art's integrity against all encroachments.

124. The author believes that critics

   I. have a difficult but important task in a democratic society.
   II. need to be controlled by the government so that their evaluation of art will be fair.
   III. should play a part in our societies whether the societies are democratic or dictatorial.

   A. I only
   B. II only
   C. I and II only
   D. II and III only

125. According to the author, because of the great power critics have, their criticism should be performed

   A. in a totally objective manner.
   B. with reasoned arguments and detailed examples.
   C. with comparisons to other criticism of the same work.
   D. in a manner that is balanced and fair to all concerned.

126. It would be reasonable to infer from the article that the writer believes that critics are likely to look more positively at art that is

   A. traditional.
   B. in a museum's exhibit.
   C. new and innovative.
   D. able to appeal to a wide audience.

GO ON TO THE NEXT PAGE

127. According to the article, the first task of the critic is

    A. objectivism.
    B. evaluation.
    C. elucidation.
    D. criticism.

128. According to the article, in which type of society can criticism flourish?

    A. Oligarchy
    B. Totalitarian
    C. Dictatorial
    D. Democratic

Passage VIII (Questions 129–135)

After a century, the message first enunciated by John Muir is sinking in: "When you dip your hand into nature, you find that everything is connected to everything else." But until recently, few comprehended the implications of the naturalist's words.

The message first found institutional expression on a global scale in the 1972 United Nations Conference on the Human Environment at Stockholm. There, 130 nations solemnly acknowledged a mutual obligation in maintaining a livable global environment. They promulgated a host of recommendations for steps that should be taken. But they created no comprehensive mechanism or procedure for realizing the measures recommended. Some important measures have been implemented. But meanwhile, new environmental problems with global ramifications have surfaced faster than problems have been resolved.

It has taken an ominously accelerating succession of calamities, accidents, and incipient crises—the diminishing stratospheric ozone layer and the greenhouse effect, Chernobyl and Bhopal, desertification and deforestation, famines and oil spills—to remind us forcefully that the implications of Muir's words and the good intentions of Stockholm have not been effectively heeded.

Although Americans tend to bask in the notion that we are environmentally progressive, in truth the United States is in many ways a mirror of global environmental problems—a story of too little and too late, of disarray and confusion, of human welfare treated as a shuttlecock or left to the problematical mercies of "the marketplace."

The United States did move quickly, as the Environmental Revolution dawned in the late 1960s, to enact constructive measures: the epochal National Environmental Policy Act; laws to abate air and water pollution and even noise; laws to deal with solid waste, to protect wildlife, to save coasts from degradation; and more. But the ensuing years have painfully demonstrated that environmental quality is much easier sought than achieved. Although we have been spending roughly $85 billion a year—$340 per capita—on pollution controls, we are far short of our goals of clean air and water. Disposal of everyday solid waste has become a nightmare. Raw sewage and worse despoil our shores.

The United States exemplifies the worldwide conflict of interests standing in the way of environmental reforms: the conflict between professed desires for environmental quality versus an addiction to lifestyles that are environmentally destructive in every aspect, from industrial activity to forest destruction and the reckless use of chemicals. Lack of a coherent national energy policy has contributed to problems extending from the Alaska oil spill to Detroit auto manufacturing, and from acid rain in the Adirondacks to a stymied nuclear power industry from coast to coast.

In the last decade, a wave of environmental populism has swept across Western Europe. Under the loose generic appellation "the Greens," the movement has become an important political force in a score of nations, drawing support from both the left and the right. Greens have been elected to legislative bodies in West Germany, France, Italy, Austria, Luxembourg, Switzerland, Belgium, Finland, and Portugal. Some 3,000 Greens have been counted in the federal, state, and local legislative bodies in West Germany alone. "Environmentalists have become Europe's most formidable and best-organized pressure group," a correspondent wrote in June.

Despite the long prevalence in America of old-line organizations like the Sierra Club and the Audubon Society, the Green movement is getting a portentous foothold in the United States. Its original spawning ground in New England is reported to have expanded to 200 chapters throughout the country.

In recent public opinion surveys, two Americans out of three said they believed that "protecting the environment is so important that requirements and standards cannot be too high, and the continued environmental improvements must be made regardless of cost."

With such environmental populism gathering such momentum, it seems only a matter of time, and not too long a time, until it brings significant changes in national lifestyles that are *conspicuously* inimical to environmental quality. Such conspicuous habits include demands for gas-guzzling cars, a voracious pattern of energy consumption, throw-away consumerism, recreational vehicles designed to ravage deserts, the equation of growth with good, and all the rest.

The Green Wave that is changing the face of politics in Europe has the potential to do the same thing in other parts of the world—knitting the political muscle and consolidating the all-important consensus.

129. John Muir said, "When you dip your hand into nature, you find that everything is connected to everything else." The reader could assume the author uses this quote to emphasize

    A.   the beauty of nature.

    B.   the interrelationship of different components of the environment.

    C.   a commitment to clean air.

    D.   the need for international action to save the environment.

130. Although the United States likes to bask in the notion that we are environmentally progressive, the author suggests that

    A.   we have, in fact, been environmentally reactionary.

    B.   we have failed to appropriate funds for pollution control.

    C.   while we were progressive in the late 1960s and early 1970s, we reversed our stand in the late 1970s and 1980s.

    D.   while we have been progressive, we have not done enough.

131. It would be reasonable to infer from the article that the author believes which of the following?

    I.   The United States has played a very positive role in the environmental movement.

    II.   The United States must follow the example of Europe in passing more aggressive environmental legislation.

    III.   While the rest of the world has done a lot about the environment, the United States has lagged behind.

    A.   I only

    B.   III only

    C.   I and II only

    D.   II and III only

132. On the basis of this article, it would be reasonable to say that

    A.   our lifestyles are developing in a way appropriate to helping the environment.

    B.   based on the money the United States is spending on the environment, we can expect that rapid improvement in the environmental quality of life will occur in the near future.

    C.   the United States does not have environmental problems similar to those of the rest of the world.

    D.   though most Americans claim a strong commitment to improving the environment, our lifestyles are often harmful to it.

GO ON TO THE NEXT PAGE

133. Greens have been elected to the legislatures of all of the following countries except

    A. Germany.
    B. the United States.
    C. Belgium.
    D. France.

134. The author attributes the relatively slow growth of the Green movement in the United States to which of the following causes?

    A. Americans are always reluctant to follow European trends.
    B. Americans tend to pursue a lifestyle that abuses rather than preserves the environment.
    C. The movement provides insufficient political power.
    D. The movement appeals only to nature lovers.

135. According to the article, the United States spends

    A. 65 billion dollars a year protecting the environment.
    B. $340 per person a year protecting the environment.
    C. $330 per capita protecting the environment.
    D. 75 billion dollars a year to protect the environment.

Passage IX (Questions 136–142)

The way we live is profoundly affected by our climate. When and where we farm, how much we heat and cool our homes, and how we obtain our water all depend on the climate we experience. Climate determines whether we have a bumper crop or a shortage. It affects the severity of our pollution problems. It determines where the sea meets the shore and the makeup of our forests and our wetlands.

Everyone contributes to greenhouse gas concentrations. The activities leading to rising concentrations of greenhouse gases occur in every country in the world. In some, it may be the burning of wood for heating and cooking. In others, it may be automobile use. But both the source of the problem and its impacts are global in scope. No one country dominates in the emission of greenhouse gases, and any country that takes action to control emissions will achieve only limited success if other countries do not follow suit. It is thus necessary that, if action needs to be taken, it should be taken on a global scale with the participation of as many countries as possible for a sustained period of time.

While we know that much is at stake if the climate changes, there is uncertainty concerning the rate and magnitude of climate change. This poses a major dilemma since the longer we wait before taking action, the larger the amount of warming we will have to live in. Already, we have seen an increase in greenhouse gas concentrations which means that some climate change may be inevitable. Since there is a great deal of year-to-year variation in climate from purely natural causes, it will also be difficult to detect the early signs of a global warming. If we wait until we can actually measure warming before we take action, then we may have to live with warmings for many generations, since it takes many years before emission reductions could have an impact on atmospheric concentrations and the climate system.

In short, global climate change is an issue with potentially profound consequences for mankind and nature. Limiting climate change would require sustained concerted action by many nations for a long period of time.

Given these facts, a number of actions must urgently be undertaken. We must continue to build our scientific research capabilities and to develop an international scientific consensus on the nature of the climate change problem—the kind of consensus that can endure changes in governments and incorporate a wide number of nations. This international understanding of the problem is necessary before effective policy responses can be developed.

Yet, we do not have the luxury of sitting on our hands while a scientific consensus emerges. Rather, the United States and other countries should begin to think of ways to reduce greenhouse gas emissions, in the event that it ultimately proves necessary to do so. The source of these reductions would be different for every country. For one, it may be changing land-use patterns to reduce tropical deforestation. For another, it may be improving energy efficiency. In many cases, actions that may be found to be effective in reducing greenhouse gas concentrations may make sense on their own, for totally independent reasons. For example, reducing production of chlorofluoro-carbons (CFCs) will slow the depletion of the stratospheric ozone layer and have the ancillary benefit of potentially limiting global warming.

Finally, we must improve our understand-ing of the effects of warming in case we find that we need to adapt to climate changes. Since greenhouse gas emissions have already in-creased, some amount of adaptation may be necessary even if we limited emissions today. Moreover, if concerted action on an interna-tional level is to be undertaken, then a consen-sus must emerge on the seriousness of the climate change problem. Only through interna-tionally coordinated research on the impacts of climate change can this be accomplished.

136. The author argues that if action is to be taken on the greenhouse effect, it must be taken

   A.   by those countries that contribute most to the greenhouse effect.
   B.   by those countries that use high concentrations of fossil fuels.
   C.   by those countries that can best afford to take action.
   D.   on a global scale.

137. The article suggests various approaches to achieving global control of increased greenhouse gas emissions. Which of the following is not a suggested approach?

   A.   Change the source of reduction of greenhouse gas emissions in cooper-ating countries.
   B.   Allow individual nations to have the option of initiating any approaches to solving climate change problems.
   C.   Utilize varied methods of adaptation even if limited emissions are re-duced.
   D.   Reach a consensus on the serious-ness of the problem and undertake concerted action on an international level.

138. According to the author, the major dilemma as to what action to take concerning global warming is that

   A.   if we wait until we are sure how much warming will take place, we may have to live with the effects of global warming for generations.
   B.   we do not really have any clear idea of what action we should take.
   C.   any action taken will hamper developing countries.
   D.   too much global warming has already taken place for action to be of significant value.

139. The author discusses the effect of climate on all of the following aspects of our lives except

   A.   how much food we can grow.
   B.   how much we heat and cool our houses.
   C.   the kind of clothing we buy.
   D.   how we obtain water.

GO ON TO THE NEXT PAGE

140. The author believes that if we wait for the final results of scientific research before acting to control greenhouse gas emissions

    A. we will not have the consensus required to enact the necessary changes.

    B. it may be too late to reverse the greenhouse effect.

    C. the level of chlorofluorocarbons will be too high.

    D. the rain forest will be gone and we will not be able to replace it.

141. The tone of the article stresses the urgent need to address global climate change

    A. through international cooperative efforts at decreasing greenhouse gas emissions.

    B. by limiting greenhouse gas emissions through an international scientific consensus.

    C. through United States leadership working with international governments.

    D. through coordinated research leading to understanding of the problem and some degree of adaptation on an international level.

142. According to the article, which of the following actions should be taken in order to effect a global reduction of greenhouse gas emissions?

    I. A global cooperative organization should be formed to provide appropriate measures.

    II. The United States should assume the responsibility of providing leadership.

    III. The United Nations should sponsor a global cooperative action.

    A. I only

    B. III only

    C. I and II only

    D. II and III only

END OF TEST 2.

IF YOU FINISH BEFORE THE TIME IS UP, YOU MAY CHECK YOUR WORK ON THIS TEST ONLY.

WRITING SAMPLE

TIME: 60 MINUTES   2 ESSAYS

Directions: This test consists of two parts. You will have 30 minutes to complete each part. During the first 30 minutes, you may work on Part 1 only. During the second 30 minutes, you may work on Part 2 only. You will have three pages for each essay answer, but you do not have to fill all three pages. Be sure to write legibly; illegible essays will not be scored.

Part 1

Consider this statement:

Know the truth and it shall set you free.

Write a unified essay in which you perform the following tasks. Explain what you think the above statement means. Describe a specific situation in which knowing the truth does *not* set you free. Discuss what you think determines whether knowledge of the truth allows one to be free.

DO NOT START THE NEXT TOPIC UNTIL THE TIME IS UP.

Part 2

Consider this statement:

He has not learned the first lesson of life who does not every day surmount a fear.

Write a unified essay in which you perform the following tasks. Explain what you think the above statement means. Describe a specific situation in which the first lesson of life does *not* involve conquering a fear. Discuss what you think determines whether life is or is not governed by a daily conquest of fear.

END OF TEST 3.
DO NOT RETURN TO PART 1.

BIOLOGICAL SCIENCES

> **Directions:** This test contains 77 questions. Most of the questions consist of a descriptive passage followed by a group of questions related to the passage. For these questions, study the passage carefully and then choose the best answer to each question in the group. Some questions in this test stand alone. These questions are independent of any passage and independent of each other. For these questions, too, you must select the one best answer. Indicate all your answers by blackening the corresponding circles on your answer sheet.
>
> A Periodic Table is provided at the beginning of this unit (page 564). You may consult it whenever you wish.

Passage I (Questions 143–149)

Enzymes act as biological catalysts that help speed up reactions by lowering the activation energy needed to bring reactants to their "transition state." In this unstable condition, bonds can break and the reaction proceeds. The reaction itself is often described in the following way:

$$E + S \rightarrow ES \rightarrow P + E$$

E = Enzyme   ES = Enzyme-Substrate Complex
S = Substrate(s)   P = Product(s)

Enzymes can carry out their catalytic functions only with particular substrates, and only under particular environmental (pH, temperature, etc.) conditions. This characteristic of enzymes is referred to as enzyme specificity. The enzyme specificity in four different enzymes is shown in the figure here.

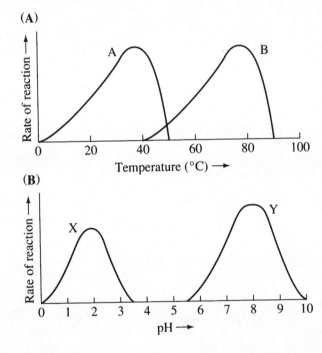

143. Enzymes *X* and *Y* in the figure are both protein-digesting enzymes found in humans. Where would they most likely be at work?

A. *X* in the mouth; *Y* in the small intestine

B. *X* in the small intestine; *Y* in the mouth

C. *X* in the stomach; *Y* in the small intestine

D. *X* in the small intestine; *Y* in the stomach

144. Which statement is true concerning enzymes *X* and *Y*?

A. They could not possibly be at work in the same part of the body at the same time.

B. They have different temperature ranges at which they work best.

C. At a pH of 4.5, enzyme *X* works slower than enzyme *Y*.

D. At their appropriate pH ranges, both enzymes work equally fast.

145. What conclusion may be drawn concerning enzymes *A* and *B*?

A. Neither enzyme is likely to be a human enzyme.

B. Enzyme *A* is more likely to be a human enzyme.

C. Enzyme *B* is more likely to be a human enzyme.

D. Both enzymes are likely to be human enzymes.

146. At which temperatures might enzymes *A* and *B* both work?

A. Above 40°C

B. Below 50°C

C. Above 50°C and below 40°C

D. Between 40°C and 50°C

147. An enzyme-substrate complex can form when the substrate(s) bind(s) to the active site of the enzyme. Which environmental condition might alter the conformation of an enzyme in the figure to the extent that its substrate is unable to bind?

A. Enzyme *A* at 40°C

B. Enzyme *B* at pH 2

C. Enzyme *X* at pH 4

D. Enzyme *Y* at 37°C

148. At 35°C, the rate of the reaction catalyzed by enzyme *A* begins and levels off. Which hypothesis best explains this observation?

A. The temperature is too far below optimum.

B. The enzyme has become saturated with substrate.

C. Both A and B

D. Neither A nor B

149. In which of the following environmental conditions would digestive enzyme *Y* be unable to bring its substrate(s) to the transition state?

A. At any temperature below optimum

B. At any pH where the rate of reaction is not maximum

C. At any pH lower than 5.5

D. At any temperature higher than 37°C

Passage II (Questions 150–156)

A set of experiments was performed to examine the effects of ultraviolet radiation (UV) on the bacterium *E. coli*. It is known that purines and pyrimidines absorb UV radiation at 260 nanometers (nm). Fewer colonies suggest that cells have died, while smaller colonies suggest that growth has been inhibited.

Experiment 1

The undersides of two glass petri dishes (*A* and *B*) were divided in half (each dish divided into sides 1 and 2) using a marking pencil. Melted agar and nutrients were poured into the dishes and allowed to harden. A sample of bacterial culture was streaked across the entire surface of each dish before covering with the glass lid. Treatment was as follows: With the lid removed, dish *A* was radiated with UV (260 nm) on side 1 only, while dish *B* was radiated with green light (550 nm) on side 1 only. Both dishes were then covered and incubated in a dark container.

Experiment 2

The procedures used in Experiment 1 were repeated except that the dishes were exposed to regular incandescent light for 20 minutes before being incubated in a dark container. The results of both experiments are summarized in the table below.

Number and Characteristics of Bacterial Colonies

	Dish A		Dish B	
	Side 1	Side 2	Side 1	Side 2
Experiment 1	5 large 5 small	30 large	31 large	29 large
Experiment 2	10 large 10 small	29 large	30 large	30 large

150. The results of Experiment 1 demonstrate that UV light (260 nm)

    A. can inhibit growth in *E. coli*.
    B. can kill *E. coli*.
    C. Both A and B.
    D. Neither A nor B.

151. A total of 40 colonies on dish *A* can be observed in Experiment 1. Which statement is true concerning these colonies?

    A. Of the colonies exposed to UV light, 25 percent show the effects of radiation.
    B. Exposure to UV light results in one-third the number of colonies that result in bacteria not exposed to UV light.
    C. Two-thirds of the colonies on the plate were not affected by exposure to UV light.
    D. Exposure to UV light results in one-eighth of all cells dying.

152. Based on the results of both experiments, what conclusions can be drawn about the effects of green light on bacterial colony formation?

    A. It has no effects when bacteria are incubated in the dark.
    B. It has no effects when bacteria are incubated in the light.
    C. Both A and B.
    D. Neither A nor B.

153. Identify the control(s) in this set of experiments.

    A. Side 1 of dish *A*
    B. Side 2 of dish *B*
    C. Side 1 of both dish *A* and dish *B*
    D. Side 2 of both dish *A* and dish *B*

154. Which hypothesis is a reasonable interpretation of results observed when comparing dish *A* in both experiments?

A. Exposure to incandescent light helps magnify the effects of UV damage.

B. Exposure to incandescent light helps repair the effects of UV damage.

C. Exposure to UV light does twice as much damage as exposure to incandescent light.

D. Exposure to UV light does one-half the damage of exposure to incandescent light.

155. UV light probably affects what part(s) of the bacterium?

A. Most covalent molecules in the cell wall

B. Proteins in the membrane

C. DNA in the chromosome

D. All of the above

156. Experiment 1 was repeated without removing the glass lid prior to UV radiation. The results in dish *A* were as follows: After incubation, side 1 had 29 large colonies and side 2 had 30 large colonies. What do these results suggest when compared to data from the earlier experiments?

A. UV radiation has no effect on bacterial colony formation.

B. UV radiation can inhibit growth, but it does not kill.

C. Glass has no effect on bacterial colony formation.

D. Glass blocks the effects of UV radiation.

Passage III (Questions 157–162)

The small intestine is one of many organs that has endocrine functions in addition to its more familiar roles in the body. By producing such hormones as intestinal gastrin, gastric inhibitory peptide (GIP), secretin, and cholecystokinin, the small intestine regulates the activities of neighboring digestive organs and their secretions.

The thymus gland secretes thymosin, a protein hormone that stimulates the maturation and differentiation of T-lymphocytes. These cells of the immune system provide cell-mediated immunity, which not only includes attacks on infectious agents, but on infected cells as well.

Other endocrine-producing structures include the pineal gland, the kidney, and the heart. In response to light stimuli entering the eye, the pineal gland (located in the brain) releases melatonin, which is believed to play a role in regulating daily circadian rhythms. The kidney regulates red blood cell production through the secretion of erythropoietin. The heart, by secreting atrial natriuretic factor (ANF), helps regulate blood pressure, salt, and water balance.

157. The factor(s) that these structures have in common is that they

A. are all glands.

B. release chemicals into the blood.

C. have a secretory function regulated by the hypothalamus.

D. All of the above.

158. An indirect effect of erythropoietin is the increase in blood volume that accompanies increased red blood cell production. This, in turn, helps raise blood pressure. In contrast, ANF helps lower blood pressure by increasing the kidneys'

A. reabsorption of sodium and excretion of water.

B. reabsorption of water and excretion of sodium.

C. reabsorption of sodium and water.

D. excretion of sodium and water.

GO ON TO THE NEXT PAGE

159. Secretin acts as a signal to the pancreas to release bicarbonate ions through the pancreatic duct. The release of secretin is itself stimulated because

    A.   acidic chyme arrives in the small intestine.

    B.   digestive pancreatic enzymes require a slightly alkaline environment.

    C.   Both A and B.

    D.   Neither A nor B.

160. When cells from the pineal gland of various vertebrates are cultured in a dish under conditions of darkness, they release melatonin in a cyclic pattern. This suggests that

    A.   the pineal cells themselves have an intrinsic rhythmic property.

    B.   melatonin production varies proportionately with light and dark cycles.

    C.   melatonin production is not cyclic during daylight.

    D.   pineal tissue probably has neural connections with the hypothalamus.

161. Thymosin can directly

    A.   respond to specific foreign antigens and bind to receptors on invading organisms.

    B.   destroy infected host cells.

    C.   produce chemical (humoral) antibodies.

    D.   None of the above.

162. Cholecystokinin stimulates the gallbladder to release bile when fats arrive in the small intestine. While in the gallbladder, bile can become overly concentrated and gallstones may form. If this necessitates removal of the gallbladder, which of the following statements is true?

    A.   Fats can no longer be emulsified before digestion in the small intestine.

    B.   Bile can still reach the small intestine from the liver.

    C.   Fats can no longer be digested.

    D.   None of the above.

Passage IV (Questions 163–169)

The immune response is part of the body's "specific defense system." Two aspects of this defense mechanism are the primary and secondary immune responses. When the body is first exposed to a foreign antigen (primary immune response), B-lymphocytes or B-cells, as well as macrophages, come in contact with the antigen. When the macrophages digest the antigen-bearing agent and display the antigen on their surface, T-helper cells (one kind of T-cell) become activated. The T-helper cells assist other types of T-cells in responding to the agent and interact with B-cells, causing some of them to differentiate into antibody-secreting plasma cells. Such humoral antibodies (immunoglobulins) can be produced and released by plasma cells for many weeks as other effector components of the immune system help destroy the invading organisms. During this time, the host suffers through various symptoms (depending on the invader), but in addition, sensitized memory cells are produced that can remain dormant for decades. Upon second exposure to the same antigen, the memory cells (various T-cells and B-cells) can give rise to clones of appropriate effector cells much more rapidly than the first time; this is a secondary immune response.

The figure below characterizes both primary and secondary responses.

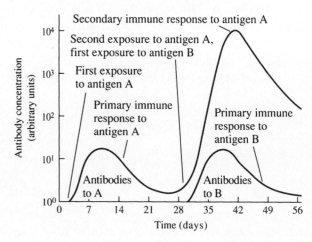

163. On approximately which day would the peak of the secondary immune response to antigen B occur?

    A. 40
    B. 56
    C. 63
    D. 70

164. According to the figure, which answer most closely approximates the number of days between the initial exposure to a foreign antigen and the peak primary immune response?

    A. Less than 5 days
    B. Less than 12 days
    C. Less than 19 days
    D. Less than 28 days

165. Which answer most closely approximates how many more antibodies the peak secondary immune response produces in comparison to the peak primary response?

    A. More than 10 times as many
    B. More than 100 times as many
    C. More than 1,000 times as many
    D. More than 10,000 times as many

166. Referring to the passage, what types of cells are the macrophages, and by what process do they help fight off invading organisms?

    A. Red blood cells/hemolysis
    B. White blood cells/phagocytosis
    C. Platelets/coagulation (clotting)
    D. White blood cells/agglutination

167. The ability of our immune system to carry out a "secondary immune response" provides a direct theoretical basis for

    A. how cells differentiate.
    B. regeneration technology.
    C. vaccine technology.
    D. most recessive lethal genes.

168. The AIDS virus (HIV) can infect T-helper cells, preventing them from functioning properly and often killing them. Which aspect(s) of the body's defenses will be affected by the virus?

    A. Primary immune response
    B. Secondary immune response
    C. Both A and B
    D. Neither A nor B

169. Which conclusion can be drawn concerning the danger at hand if a serious allergy to a drug such as penicillin is discovered during initial treatment?

    A. When the drug is administered a second time, the patient's allergic response can be even more severe.
    B. When the drug is administered a second time, the patient should be able to receive the benefits even faster.
    C. Both A and B.
    D. Neither A nor B.

Passage V (Questions 170–175)

Loss of muscular movement may be caused by numerous agents including microorganisms, poisons, and both environmental and genetic factors that manifest themselves by interfering with normal function. Changes in function can occur at various locations that contribute to muscular activity, such as the motor neurons, neuromuscular junctions, and within the muscle cells themselves.

170. *Clostridium botulinum* is the bacterium associated with botulism, a disease that leads to flaccid paralysis. The organism prevents the release of acetylcholine by motor neurons at the neuromuscular junction. The physiological effect of this action is to

    A. prevent repolarization of the sarcolemma.
    B. prevent depolarization of the sarcolemma.
    C. inhibit the active transport needed to return calcium to the sarcoplasmic reticulum.
    D. inhibit neurons of the sympathetic autonomic nervous system.

GO ON TO THE NEXT PAGE

171. The polio virus can infect and destroy cell bodies located in the anterior horn of the spinal cord. These motor neurons are vital because they stimulate

    A. the part of the brain that controls voluntary movement.
    B. receptors found in freely movable joints.
    C. skeletal muscles.
    D. interneurons along circuits leading to the cerebrum.

172. When athletes overexert themselves on hot days, they often suffer immobility from painful muscle cramping. Which of the following is a reasonable hypothesis to explain such cramps?

    A. Muscle cells do not have enough ATP for normal muscle relaxation.
    B. Excessive sweating has affected the salt balance within the muscles.
    C. Prolonged contractions have temporarily interrupted blood flow to parts of the muscle.
    D. All of the above.

173. Myasthenia gravis is a heritable disorder in which autoantibodies (antibodies to one's own tissues) bind to receptors at the motor end plate. This disease *directly* affects

    A. motor neurons.
    B. brain cells.
    C. muscle insertions.
    D. neuromuscular junctions.

174. Multiple sclerosis is another disease associated with an autoimmune response. Antibodies cause the destruction of myelin sheaths in the central nervous system. This affects

    A. axons in the brain and spinal cord.
    B. axons and dendrites in the brain only.
    C. axons and dendrites in the brain and spinal cord.
    D. axons in the brain, spinal cord, and spinal nerves.

175. Duchenne muscular dystrophy is a sex-linked recessive disorder associated with severe deterioration of muscle tissue. The gene for the disease

    A. is inherited by males from their mothers.
    B. should be more common in females than in males.
    C. Both A and B.
    D. Neither A nor B.

Passage VI (Questions 176–181)

The role of chlorophyll, a light-absorbing pigment, in photosynthesis was investigated in a pair of experiments. Pigment was extracted from a leaf preparation and examined using paper chromatography and spectrophotometric techniques.

Experiment 1

In order to analyze the composition of leaf extract, a sample of the pigment was applied near the bottom of a strip of chromatographic filter paper and allowed to dry. This was repeated a number of times to ensure that an adequate amount of pigment was present. The strip was suspended in a test tube containing the solvent acetone. As the experiment proceeded, the acetone soaked into the filter paper and slowly moved up across the pigment sample, eventually reaching the top of the paper. This technique is designed to separate substances in a mixture based on differences in their tendency to adhere to the material over which they are passed (adsorption), as well as on their solubility in the solvent used. Substances with color can easily be detected on the paper. The experiment revealed three separate bands of color on the filter paper: a green band, a yellow-green band, and an orange band.

Experiment 2

Samples of each band were examined using a spectrophotometer. This instrument can send light of various wavelengths (375 nm to 750 nm) through a sample. For each wavelength, the amount of light passing through (percentage of transmittance) can be monitored and then converted to absorbance. Absorbance is a measure of the amount of light absorbed as it passes through a sample. Unless light is absorbed, the energy in the light cannot be utilized. A sample's absorption spectrum indicates the range of its ability to absorb different wavelengths of light. The absorption spectra of all three samples are shown in the figure below.

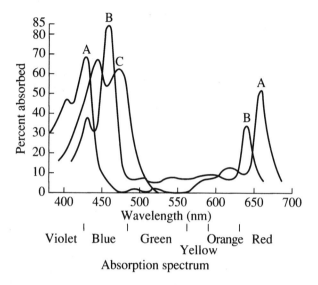

Absorption spectrum

176. Which statement is true concerning the paper chromatography technique used in Experiment 1?

A. All other factors being equal, the most soluble substance travels fastest and will likely be highest on the paper.

B. All other factors being equal, the substance with the greatest adsorptive tendency will likely be highest on the paper.

C. Both A and B.

D. Neither A nor B.

177. The most reasonable hypothesis that addresses the results of Experiment I is which of the following?

A. The chlorophyll extract may contain three different pigments.

B. Chlorophyll has three different solubility/adsorption patterns.

C. The chlorophyll applied to the filter paper was not allowed to dry properly.

D. Chlorophyll can have three different conformations.

178. As seen in the figure, the three samples from Experiment 1 have different absorption spectra. Which of the following statements is correct?

A. Each substance shows at least two different absorbance peaks of 40 percent or higher.

B. Substance A shows a low level of transmittance across a broad range of wavelengths.

C. Each pigment shows an absorbance peak at both ends of the spectrum.

D. Substance B shows its greatest absorption in the blue range of wavelengths.

179. Which colors of light are most likely utilized in photosynthesis by substance A?

A. Blue-green

B. Blue-green and red

C. Violet-blue and red

D. Violet-blue and orange

180. What do the results of Experiment 2 suggest about the question "Why are green plants green"?

A. The light wavelengths utilized by each pigment mix to form green.

B. The pigments absorb green.

C. The pigments do not absorb green.

D. Green light is the most utilized light in photosynthesis.

GO ON TO THE NEXT PAGE

181. Which hypothesis best interprets the presence of more than one pigment in green leaves?

   A. The ability of different pigments to use the same wavelengths equally well makes photosynthesis more efficient.
   B. Making small amounts of more than one pigment is energetically less expensive than making a large amount of the same pigment.
   C. When light is absorbed by more than one pigment, heat can be dissipated in the plant more easily.
   D. The ability of different pigments to use different wavelengths makes photosynthesis more efficient.

Passage VII (Questions 182–187)

Phenylalanine is an amino acid that is necessary in small amounts for proper human nutrition. The normal metabolism of this substance requires the enzyme phenylalanine hydroxylase. The ability to produce the enzyme is controlled by an autosomal dominant trait. Approximately one in 15,000 whites in the United States is born without the capacity to produce the enzyme due to a homozygous recessive condition called phenylketonuria (PKU). In people with PKU, phenylalanine accumulates in the blood, and phenylpyruvic acid accumulates in the urine—giving it a distinctive odor. High levels of phenylalanine in the brain and spinal fluid during the first weeks after birth causes mental retardation in PKU individuals. Since PKU can be identified by a blood test at birth, dietary treatment can be administered to prevent this damage. If placed on a low-phenylalanine diet for the first few years of life, symptoms can be avoided.

182. If a couple, both heterozygous for PKU, have a child, what is the probability that the child will have *at least one normal allele*?

   A. 100 percent
   B. 75 percent
   C. 50 percent
   D. 0 percent

183. If the same couple were to have two children, what is the probability that *both children* will be carriers (heterozygotes) of the disease?

   A. 100 percent
   B. 75 percent
   C. 50 percent
   D. 25 percent

184. A woman, homozygous for PKU, was successfully treated after birth to avoid symptoms of the disorder. If she becomes pregnant, why must similar precautions be taken to control her diet again?

   A. The fetus must have the genotype for the disorder.
   B. High levels of phenylalanine in her blood can cause brain damage in the fetus, regardless of its genotype.
   C. High levels of phenylalanine in her blood can stimulate her body to overproduce phenylalanine hydroxylase, which causes damage in the fetus.
   D. Phenylpyruvic acid in her urine can cause damage to the fetus.

185. Polydactyly (extra toes or fingers) is an autosomal dominant trait. Identify the correct statement concerning this trait.

   A. All children of homozygotes must have the trait.

   B. Affected children must have at least one affected parent.

   C. Seventy-five percent of the children of two heterozygote parents must have the trait.

   D. All of the above

186. Holandric traits are Y-linked. Which of the following statements is correct concerning such traits?

   A. Holandric traits will only appear in males.

   B. Every holandric gene that is present will be expressed.

   C. Both A and B.

   D. Neither A nor B.

187. Amyotrophic lateral sclerosis (Lou Gehrig's Disease) is caused by an autosomal recessive gene. Which of the following statements is correct concerning family members of individuals with this disorder?

   A. If not affected themselves, both parents of an affected individual have to be carriers.

   B. If not affected themselves, all siblings of an affected individual must be carriers.

   C. Both A and B.

   D. Neither A nor B.

Passage VIII (Questions 188–193)

Tautomers are compounds that differ in their arrangement of atoms and undergo rapid equilibrium reactions. An example is enol–keto tautomerism:

$$-\overset{|}{C}=\overset{|}{C}-OH \rightleftharpoons -\overset{|}{C}-\underset{\underset{H}{|}}{\overset{|}{C}}=O$$

enol tautomer   keto tautomer

Because the equilibrium lies to the right, usually the reactions that produce the enol tautomer end up mostly with the keto form. The rearrangement takes place because of the polarity of the O-H bond, which enables H^+ to separate readily from oxygen:

$$-\overset{|}{C}=\overset{|}{C}-OH \rightleftharpoons -\overset{|}{C}=\overset{|}{C}-O^{\ominus}$$

$$\updownarrow$$

$$-\underset{\underset{H}{|}}{\overset{|}{C}}-\overset{|}{C}=O \rightleftharpoons -\overset{|}{C}-\underset{\underset{\ominus}{..}}{\overset{|}{C}}=O + H^+$$

When the H^+ returns, it can join with the negatively charged carbon in the anion or go back to the oxygen. However, when H^+ attaches to carbon, it tends to stay on much longer, favoring the keto tautomer.

188. Adding one mole of water to one mole of acetylene produces mostly

   A. vinyl alcohol.

   B. a diol.

   C. acetaldehyde.

   D. acetone.

GO ON TO THE NEXT PAGE

189. Which of the following statements best explains why the above equilibrium favors the keto form?

    A. Ketones are, in general, more stable than alcohols.

    B. Ketones are stronger acids.

    C. Equilibrium favors the weaker acid.

    D. Equilibrium favors the stronger acid.

190. Phenol is favored over its keto form:

$$\text{}\bigcirc\!\!\!-OH \rightleftharpoons \bigcirc\!\!\!=O$$

Which of the following statements best explains this exception?

    A. Weaker acids tend to form from stronger acids.

    B. Extra stability associated with the aromatic phenyl ring makes phenol more stable.

    C. Oxygen does not have an octet in the keto form.

    D. Enols tend to be favored over their keto tautomers.

191. Another example of tautomerism is the enamine-imine equilibrium system:

$$
\begin{array}{c}
\overset{\displaystyle H}{\overset{\displaystyle |}{}} \quad \overset{\displaystyle H}{\overset{\displaystyle |}{}} \\
-C\!=\!C\!-\!N\!-\!R' \rightleftharpoons -C\!-\!C\!=\!N\!-\!R' \\
2\quad 1\quad | \qquad\qquad | \\
\quad\quad H \qquad\qquad H \\
\text{enamine} \qquad\quad \text{imine}
\end{array}
$$

The acidic proton on the enamine form is attached to

    A. R'.

    B. C—2.

    C. N.

    D. C—1.

192. Carbonyl compounds react with 1° and 2° amines by nucleophilic addition. The addition product then undergoes dehydration. Which pair of reactions best describes these reactions?

A.

$$-\overset{|}{C}-\overset{|}{C}\!=\!O + RNH_2 \rightarrow -\overset{|}{C}-\overset{|}{C}-\overset{|}{N}-R$$

$$-\overset{|}{C}-\overset{|}{C}-\overset{|}{N}-R \rightarrow -C\!=\!C-\overset{|}{N}-R + H_2O$$

B.

$$-C\!=\!O + RNH_2 \rightarrow -\overset{|}{C}-\overset{|}{N}-H$$

$$-\overset{|}{C}-\overset{|}{N}-H \rightarrow -C\!=\!NH + ROH$$

C.

$$-\overset{|}{C}-\overset{|}{C}\!=\!O + RNH_2 \rightarrow -\overset{|}{C}-\overset{|}{C}-\overset{|}{N}-R$$

$$-\overset{|}{C}-\overset{|}{C}-\overset{|}{N}-R \rightarrow -\overset{|}{C}-C\!=\!NR + H_2O$$

D.

$$-\overset{|}{C}-\overset{|}{C}\!=\!O + RNH_2 \rightarrow -\overset{|}{C}-\overset{|}{C}-R$$

$$-\overset{|}{C}-\overset{|}{C}-R \rightarrow -C\!=\!C-R + H_2O$$

193. Which of the following enamines does not form an imine tautomer?

A. 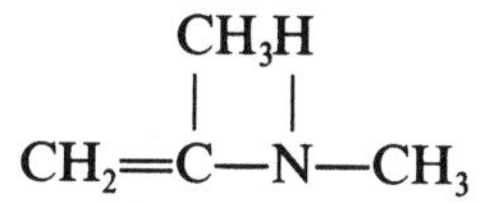
$$CH_2=C-N-CH_3$$
with CH_3H above

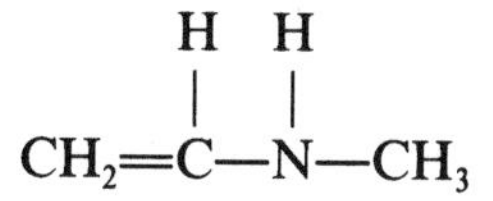

B.
$$CH_2=C-N-CH_3$$
with H H above

C.
$$H-C=C-N-CH_3$$
with CH_3CH_3H above

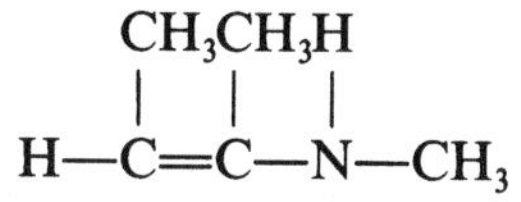

D. 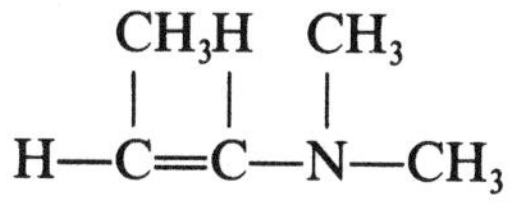
$$H-C=C-N-CH_3$$
with CH_3H CH_3 above

Passage IX (Questions 194–199)

A student titrates one liter of a 1.0 M amino acid solution, which is acidified with HCl with a NaOH solution. He plots pH versus moles of NaOH added to give the following graph:

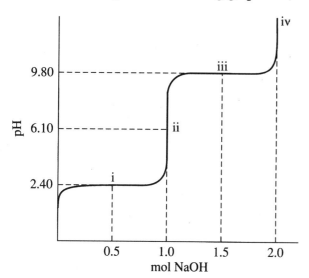

194. The titration curve indicates that the amino acid is

A. triprotic.
B. diprotic.
C. a base.
D. monoprotic.

195. The amino acid can be identified by comparing

A. the first full neutralization point with pK_{a_1}.
B. the second full neutralization point with pK_{a_2}.
C. the isoelectric point (pI) with pK_{a_1}.
D. the pK_{a_1}, and pK_{a_2} of the amino acid with the pH after addition of 0.5 mol and 1.5 mol of NaOH.

196. At which isoelectric point (pH) does the amino acid have a dipolar or zwitterioric form?

A. 6.10
B. 2.40
C. 7.00
D. 9.80

197. Which of the following is the predominant form of the amino acid after 0.60 mol of NaOH is added?

A. 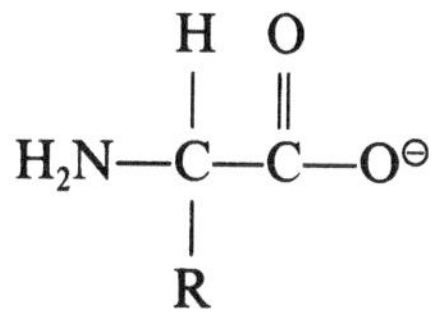
$$H_2N-C-C-O^{\ominus}$$
with H O (double bond) above and R below

B.
$$H_3N^{\oplus}-C-C-OH$$
with H O (double bond) above and R below

C.
$$H_3N^{\oplus}-C-C-O^{\ominus}$$
with H O (double bond) above and R below

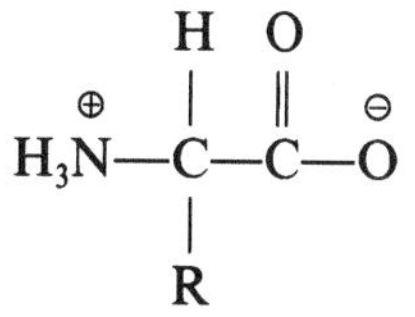

D. 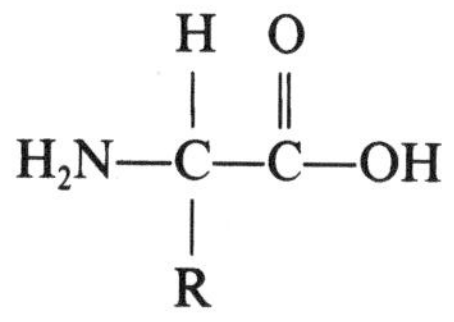
$$H_2N-C-C-OH$$
with H O (double bond) above and R below

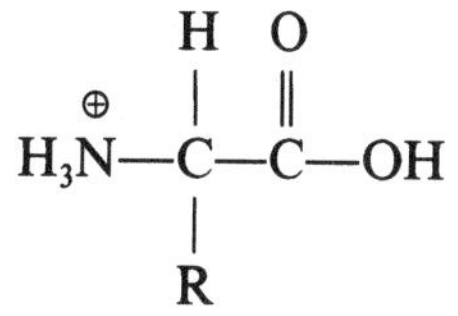

GO ON TO THE NEXT PAGE

198. After 2.0 mol of NaOH is added, the pH of the solution is

- A. higher than pI.
- B. lower than I but lower than pK_{a2}.
- C. higher than pK_{a2}.
- D. lower than pK_{a1}.

199. A buffer solution is produced after the addition of how much NaOH?

- A. 1.0 mol
- B. 1.5 mol
- C. 2.0 mol
- D. 2.5 mol

Passage X (Questions 200–204)

An organic chemistry student conducts a free-radical reaction by exposing a mixture of 2-methylpropane and Br_2 to light. She separates the products and obtains the NMR spectrum of a dibromo substituted propane. The spectrum contains two singlets with a peak ratio of 3:1.

200. The NMR spectrum is of

- A. 1,1-dibromo-2-methylpropane.
- B. 1,3-dibromo-2-methylpropane.
- C. 1,2-dibromo-2-methylpropane.
- D. 2-bromo-2-methylpropane.

201. A dehydrohalogenation reaction produces 2-methyl-3-bromo-1-propane. How many signals will its NMR spectrum contain?

- A. 4
- B. 3
- C. 2
- D. 1

202. The NMR spectrum of 1,1-dideutero-2-methyl-3-bromo-1-propane contains

- A. a quartet and a triplet.
- B. two singlet peaks.
- C. three singlet peaks.
- D. a singlet, a quartet, and a triplet.

203. The effect of bromine on the chemical shift of a proton bonded to the same carbon is to

- A. move the absorption downfield.
- B. move the absorption upfield.
- C. cause a singlet peak to split into a doublet peak.
- D. increase the intensity of the peak.

204. Which of the following statements is false?

- A. The area under an NMR signal depends on the number of protons causing the signal.
- B. Splitting of NMR signals is caused by nearby protons.
- C. Equivalent protons have the same chemical shift.
- D. Only protons give rise to NMR spectra.

Questions 205–219 are independent of any passage and independent of each other.

205. Microfilaments and microtubules form a complex network of fibers within the eukaryotic cell that can be disassembled and reassembled. If this were to occur, what is likely to be the immediate result?

- A. Depolarization
- B. Protein synthesis
- C. Absorption
- D. Change in cell shape

206. The semiconservative hypothesis of replication refers to

- A. the process of transcription.
- B. the formation of chromatids.
- C. one aspect of protein formation.
- D. the activity of lysogenic viruses.

207. In general, each cell synthesizes its own macromolecules and does not receive them previously formed from other cells. For example, muscle cells make their own glycogen, rather than receiving it intact from the

A. pancreas.
B. kidney.
C. liver.
D. small intestine.

208. Which statement is true concerning the sites at which muscles attach to bones?

A. The origin of a muscle is never on a bone that forms part of a movable joint.
B. The insertion of a muscle is usually on the same bone as the body of the muscle.
C. The same bone can serve as the origin for one muscle and the insertion for a different muscle.
D. No muscles are attached to bones forming immovable joints.

209. In certain insects, juvenile hormone suppresses metamorphosis from larva to adult. Instead, this hormone allows the young organism to grow in size while remaining in the immature larval stage. Eventually, the juvenile hormone decreases, causing metamorphosis to take place. If the corpora allata, the site of juvenile hormone production and release, is surgically removed at an early larval stage, what is expected to happen?

A. A tiny adult will form.
B. The larva will continue to grow, and metamorphosis will occur at the normal age.
C. The larva will no longer grow or undergo metamorphosis.
D. The larva will continue to grow until it looks like a giant, adult-sized larva.

210. Which statement is most likely to be true concerning obligate anaerobes?

A. These organisms can use oxygen if it is present in their environment.
B. These organisms cannot use oxygen as their final electron acceptor.
C. These organisms carry out fermentation for at least 50 percent of their ATP production.
D. Most of these organisms are vegetative fungi.

211. A countercurrent mechanism in the kidney helps maintain a high concentration of salt in the interstitial fluid of the medulla, the site adjacent to where the hypotonic tiltrate passes before its elimination out of the body. This permits efficient

A. secretion of excess salts.
B. adjustment of filtrate pH.
C. filtration of venous blood returning to the heart.
D. reabsorption of water.

212. Point mutations are changes in a single DNA nucleotide base pair. An addition results in an extra base pair, while a deletion results in an omitted base pair along the DNA molecule. In contrast, a substitution results in an incorrect base pair replacing the correct one. Which point mutations have the highest probability of causing drastic results?

A. Substitutions
B. Deletions
C. Additions and deletions
D. All three have equal chances of causing drastic results

GO ON TO THE NEXT PAGE

213. Foods rich in fiber are basically plant materials high in cellulose, a cell wall polysaccharide that we cannot digest. The nutritional benefit(s) provided by such foods result from

A. other macromolecules present that can be digested and absorbed.

B. macromolecules (like cellulose) that are absorbed without digestion and then catabolized inside the cells.

C. microbes that are the normal symbionts of plant tissues.

D. All of the above.

214. Water and small proteins leak out of capillaries at their arterial ends because hydrostatic pressure (exerted mainly by blood pressure pushing outward against the capillary walls) is greater than colloid osmotic pressure (a fluid-retaining force caused by large solutes in the blood). Most of the fluid returns at the venule end because blood pressure

A. increases and large solutes decrease.

B. decreases and large solutes decrease.

C. increases and large solutes stay the same.

D. decreases and large solutes stay the same.

215. The most stable isomer of 1,3-dimethylcyclo-hexane is

A.

B.

C.

D.

216. The dehydration of

$$CH_3{-}CH_2{-}\overset{\overset{\displaystyle CH_3}{|}}{\underset{\underset{\displaystyle OH}{|}}{C}}{-}CH_3$$

yields mostly which of the following?

A.

$$CH_2{=}CH{-}\overset{\overset{\displaystyle CH_3}{|}}{\underset{\underset{\displaystyle OH}{|}}{C}}{-}CH_3$$

B.

$$CH_3{-}CH{=}\overset{\overset{\displaystyle CH_3}{|}}{C}{-}CH_3$$

C.

$$CH_3{-}CH_2{-}\overset{\overset{\displaystyle CH_3}{|}}{C}{=}CH_2$$

D.

$$CH_3{-}CH_2{-}\overset{\overset{\displaystyle CH_2}{\|}}{C}{-}CH_3$$

217. The aldohexoses shown below are examples of which of the following?

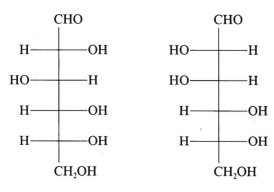

A. Enantiomers
B. Optically inactive isomers
C. Anomers
D. Epimers

218. Which of the following is the oxidation product of CH_3—CH—CH_2—CH_2OH?
    |
    OH

A.

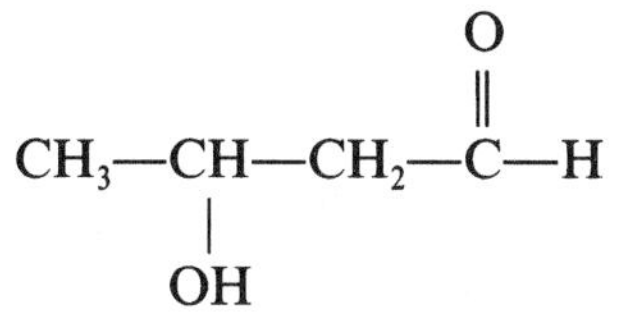

CH_3—CH—CH_2—C—H
    | ||
    OH   O

B.

CH_3—C—CH_2—C—OH
    || ||
    O   O

C.

CH_3—CH—CH_2—C—OH
    | ||
    OH   O

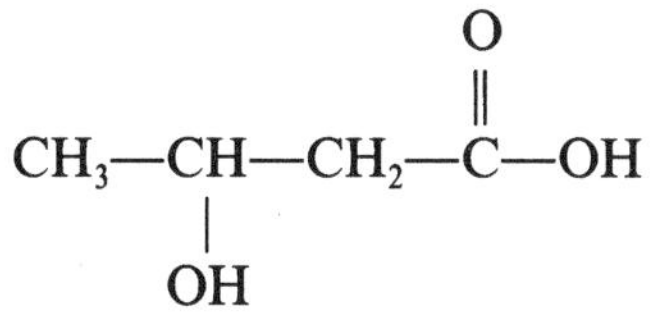

D. CH_3—CH—CH_2—CH_2OH
        |
        OH

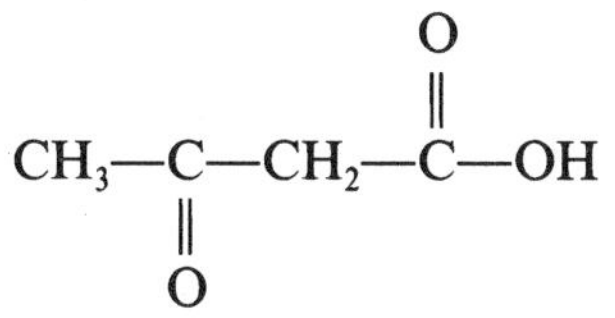

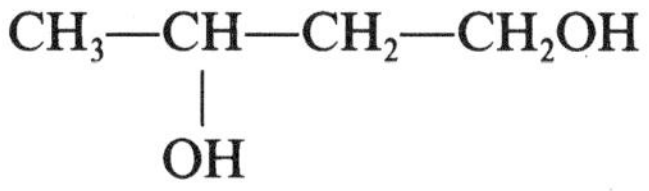

219. The following two reactions were carried out.

Reaction I

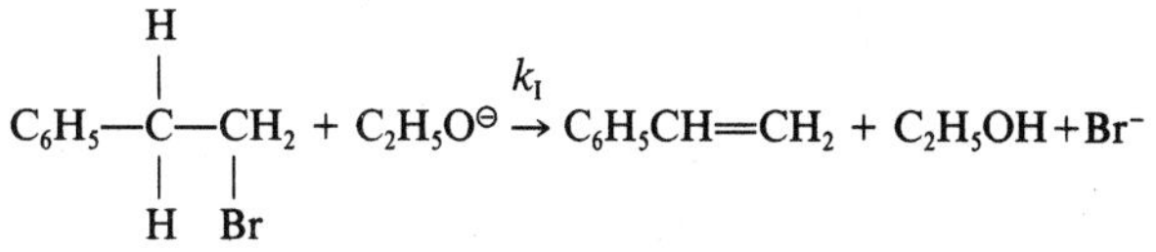

        H
        | k_I
C_6H_5—C—CH_2 + $C_2H_5O^{\ominus}$ → C_6H_5CH=CH_2 + C_2H_5OH + Br^-
        | |
        H   Br

Reaction II

        D
        | k_{II}
C_6H_5—C—CH_2 + $C_2H_5O^{\ominus}$ → C_6H_5CD=CH_2 + C_2H_5OD + Br^-
        | |
        D   Br

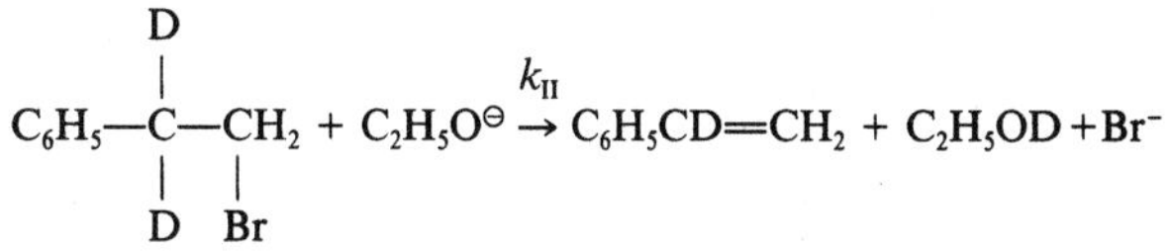

The rate constant k_I was seven times greater than the rate constant k_{II}. Therefore

A. the rate-determining step involves the breaking of a β-carbon-hydrogen bond.
B. the rate-determining step involves the breaking of the carbon-bromine bond.
C. the rate of the reaction does not depend on the breaking of a carbon-hydrogen bond.
D. the rate of the reaction does not depend on the breaking of the carbon-bromine bond.

END OF TEST 4.
IF YOU FINISH BEFORE THE TIME IS UP,
YOU MAY CHECK YOUR WORK ON THIS TEST ONLY.

ANSWER KEY

Physical Sciences		Verbal Reasoning		Biological Sciences	
1. D	40. D	78. B	111. A	143. C	182. B
2. C	41. C	79. B	112. C	144. A	183. D
3. B	42. A	80. B	113. C	145. B	184. B
4. B	43. C	81. B	114. B	146. D	185. D
5. A	44. B	82. C	115. D	147. C	186. C
6. D	45. C	83. B	116. A	148. B	187. A
7. A	46. A	84. B	117. C	149. C	188. C
8. A	47. B	85. A	118. D	150. C	189. C
9. B	48. D	86. B	119. B	151. B	190. B
10. B	49. A	87. C	120. C	152. A	191. C
11. C	50. C	88. B	121. A	153. D	192. C
12. B	51. B	89. D	122. C	154. B	193. D
12. A	52. A	90. D	123. D	155. C	194. B
14. B	53. A	91. B	124. A	156. D	195. D
15. A	54. A	92. D	125. B	157. B	196. A
16. A	55. D	93. A	126. C	158. D	197. C
17. C	56. A	94. D	127. C	159. C	198. C
18. C	57. C	95. A	128. D	160. A	199. B
19. D	58. C	96. C	129. B	161. D	200. D
20. B	59. A	97. B	130. D	162. B	201. A
21. B	60. B	98. D	131. A	163. D	202. B
22. C	61. A	99. B	132. D	164. B	203. A
23. A	62. D	100. C	133. B	165. B	204. D
24. B	63. B	101. D	134. B	166. B	205. D
25. D	64. D	102. C	135. B	167. C	206. B
26. B	65. C	103. D	136. D	168. C	207. C
27. B	66. B	104. A	137. B	169. A	208. C
28. B	67. A	105. D	138. A	170. B	209. A
29. C	68. C	106. A	139. C	171. C	210. B
30. D	69. D	107. A	140. B	172. D	211. D
31. A	70. D	108. B	141. D	173. D	212. C
32. B	71. B	109. C	142. A	174. A	213. A
33. A	72. A	110. B		175. A	214. D
34. B	73. B			176. A	215. B
35. C	74. A			177. A	216. B
36. B	75. B			178. D	217. D
37. B	76. C			179. C	218. B
38. C	77. C			180. C	219. A
39. A				181. D	

ANSWERS AND EXPLANATIONS

PHYSICAL SCIENCES

1. **The correct answer is (D).** $6.6 \times 10^{-7}/3.89 \times 10^{-7} = 1.7$

2. **The correct answer is (C).** $389 \times 10^{-9} m = 3.89 \times 10^{-7}$ m

3. **The correct answer is (B).** Higher energy differences correspond to higher frequencies and thus shorter wavelengths.

4. **The correct answer is (B).** $E = hv = hc/\lambda$

5. **The correct answer is (A).** No spectral line occurs at 610 nm; to Scientist 1, this fact means no corresponding transition exists.

6. **The correct answer is (D).** Scientist 2 believes hydrogen to have a broad range of emissions, only a few of which pass through the glass in the measuring instrument.

7. **The correct answer is (A).** If other atoms showed the same spectra in the same spectrometer, there would be proof that the device, not the atoms, was the source of the spectral lines.

8. **The correct answer is (A).** Evidently, the spectrometer *will* pass a broad spectrum of wavelengths. Thus, Scientist 2's objection to Scientist 1's position is refuted.

9. **The correct answer is (B).** PbS has the smaller K_{sp}, so the tendency for its separate ions to combine is greater.

10. **The correct answer is (B).** The sulfide concentration is maintained at 0.1 so A is incorrect, and the powers of 2 are not needed as in C and D.

11. **The correct answer is (C).** $(1 \times 10^{-20}$ M/L$)(6 \times 10^{23}$ ions/mol$)$ $(10^{-3}$ L/cc$) = 6$ ions

12. **The correct answer is (B).** If pH is low, $[H^+]$ is high, and $[S^{2-}]$ is low.

13. **The correct answer is (A).** $[S^{2-}] = (1 \times 10^{-23})/(10^{-2})^2 = 1 \times 10^{-19}$M

14. **The correct answer is (B).** $[H^+] = (10^{-23})/(10^{-20})^{\frac{1}{2}} = 0.032$ M

15. **The correct answer is (A).** The solubility in this case is equal to the number of moles per liter of magnesium ion liberated by a dissociation. Note that K_{sp} is not wanted.

16. **The correct answer is (A).** Since hydroxide is a product in the equilibrium, adding more of it will drive the equilibrium to the left, with the result that less of the salt will dissociate.

17. **The correct answer is (C).** The student needs to insert "0.1" as the concentration of hydroxide, then square it, since there are 2 OH⁻'s in the solubility equation. It is not correct to double the concentration of hydroxide before squaring, as in D.

18. **The correct answer is (C).** The strong acid will remove hydroxide ions from solution, pulling the equilibrium to the right.

19. **The correct answer is (D).** Here $[OH^-] = K_w/[H^+]$.

20. **The correct answer is (B).** Solubility is surely pH-dependent, but K_{sp} is not. Since other magnesium salts would not necessarily have hydroxides in their formulas, these concerns need not apply to them.

21. **The correct answer is (B).** $n = PV/RT$, so n decreases as T increases.

22. **The correct answer is (C).** Note pressure, temperature.

23. **The correct answer is (A).** $MW = g/mol$

24. **The correct answer is (B).** Use $MW = g/n = gRT/PV$. All answers except B give an error in the wrong direction.

25. **The correct answer is (D).** There would be fewer of the aggregated molecules than there would be if the molecules did not bind to each other. Since the aggregates would be more massive, they would move more slowly.

26. **The correct answer is (B).** Since the measured MW is about three times the correct MW, on average three molecules must bind together.

27. **The correct answer is (B).** Concentrations of reactants, not products, determine rate in both theories, according to the text.

28. **The correct answer is (B).** Here you must have understood the relation of numbers of reactants in the overall equation to exponents in the rate law.

29. **The correct answer is (C).** The theories differ in that the first calls for the use of the coefficients in the *overall* reaction as exponents in the rate law, while the second asks that the coefficients from the *slow step* be employed. In a single-step reaction, the theories predict the same thing.

30. **The correct answer is (D).** Theory 1 requires that the coefficients in the overall equation be used as exponents in the rate law.

31. **The correct answer is (A).** The slow stage controls the overall rate, according to Theory 2.

32. **The correct answer is (B).** Be sure to use column 3, not column 4. The value for PbS is clearly the lowest in the column; it takes more examination to see that the value for BaF_2 is the highest.

33. **The correct answer is (A).** You need to find the ratio of the column 3 value to the column 1 value; this ratio is 10, not $\frac{1}{10}$.

34. **The correct answer is (B).** This considerable difference in solubility is found for all rows of the table.

35. **The correct answer is (C).** Each value in column 4 is 10 times greater than the corresponding value in column 2; choice C reflects this fact.

36. **The correct answer is (B).** Use column 2, and divide K_{sp} for PbS by K_{sp} for $CaSO_4$.

37. **The correct answer is (B).** Here you can look for the greatest pure-water solubility, i.e., the greatest value in column 3 among the three lead salts.

38. **The correct answer is (C).** The chart shows the pure-water solubility of BaF_2 to be greater than that when .1 M Ba^{2+} is present. Therefore, as $Ba(NO_3)_2$ is added, solid BaF_2 precipitates.

39. **The correct answer is (A).** Since K_{sp} is smaller for $BaSO_4$ than for $CaSO_4$, $BaSO_4$ will precipitate. Only if the Ba^{2+} in solution is effectively used up will Ca^{2+} precipitate. As an alternative solution, examine the solubilities in column 4.

40. **The correct answer is (D).** Weight is the product of mass and the acceleration of gravity.

$$F_{gravity} = Wgt = mg = (100 \text{ kg}) (9.8 \text{ m/s}^2)$$
$$Wgt = 980 \text{ kg m s}^{-2} = 980 \text{ N}$$

41. **The correct answer is (C).** The entire 200-N force was used to overcome the frictional force. The applied force of 200 N is parallel to the direction of motion of the block. Therefore, none of the applied force was used to overcome gravity. Since the velocity is constant, none of the force was used to accelerate the block.

42. **The correct answer is (A).** Work is force times distance in the same direction of force. The applied force and the direction of motion are both horizontal, so the work performed is

$$W = Fd = (200 \text{ N})(8 \text{ m}) = 1600 \text{ N-m} = 1600 \text{ J}$$

43. **The correct answer is (C).** $v^2 = v_0^2 + 2ax = 0 + 2 (9.8 \text{ m/s}^2) (8\text{m})$ $v = 12.5$ m/s

44. **The correct answer is (B).** $E = \frac{1}{2}mv^2 = \frac{1}{2} (100 \text{ kg}) (12.5 \text{ m/s})^2$ $E = 7840$ J

45. **The correct answer is (C).** $P_2 = I_2^2 R_2 = (2 \text{ A})^2 (60 \text{ }\Omega) = 240$ W

46. **The correct answer is (A).** Energy is the product of power and time:

$$E = Pt = I^2Rt = 240 \text{ W } (3 \text{ s}) = 720 \text{ W}-\text{s} = 720 \text{ J}$$

47. **The correct answer is (B).** Since R_1 and R_2 are connected in parallel, the voltage drop across each must be identical: $V_1 = V_2 = I_2R_2 = (2 \text{ A}) (60 \text{ }\Omega) = 120$ V

48. **The correct answer is (D).** The parallel resistors R_1 and R_2 can be replaced by a single resistance, R_{eq}, which will be in series with R_3. The current in R_{eq} must equal the sum of the currents in R_1 and R_2. Once this current is found, the voltage of R_{eq} can be computed. The voltage of the source is the sum of the voltages for R_3 and R_{eq}.

$V_1 = V_2 = I_1R_1 = I_2R_2$, therefore

$$I_1 = \frac{I_2R_2}{R_1} = \frac{(2 \text{ A})(60 \text{ }\Omega)}{30 \text{ }\Omega} = 4\text{A}$$

$$I_{eq} = I_1 + I_2 = 4\text{A} + 2\text{A} = 6\text{A}$$

Since R_3 and R_{eq} are in series, the same current must flow through both resistors, so that $I_{tot} = 6$A. The total resistance of the circuit is given by

$$R_{tot} = R_3 + R_{eq}$$

We can either stop and calculate R_{eq} so we can get R_{tot}, or we can use the value of I_3 and R_3 to find V_3, then find

$$V_{tot} = V_3 + V_{eq}$$
$$V_3 = I_3R_3 = (6\text{A}) (40 \text{ }\Omega) = 240 \text{ V}$$
$$V_{tot} = V_3 + V_{eq} = 240 \text{ V} + 120 \text{ V} = 360 \text{ V}$$

49. **The correct answer is (A).** The terminal voltage is the voltage when the source is connected in a closed circuit. The terminal voltage equals the emf minus Ir, produced by current flowing through the source. For the circuit shown, I_{tot} was 6A so Ir = (6A) (4Ω) = 24 V. And the emf is found from

terminal voltage = emf − Ir

so emf = term. volt. + Ir = 360 V + 24 V = 384 V

50. **The correct answer is (C).** Since all of the walls of the apparatus through which the ray passes are parallel, and since the ray exits into the same medium it originally entered from (air), the path of the ray as it exits must be parallel to its path when it entered from the air into chamber 1. This angle is given as 45° to the normal of the first wall. Therefore, the ray should exit into the air with an angle of 45° to the normal of the outside wall. Trace F looks closest to 45°.

51. **The correct answer is (B).** By definition, the refractive index, n, is the ratio of the speed of light in a vacuum, c, to its speed in the medium of interest, water, v. Therefore,

    $v = c/n$

    $v = (3.00 \times 10^8 \text{ m/s})/1.33 = 2.26 \times 10^8 \text{ m/s}$

    Choices C and D are easily eliminated because they are too large. We don't expect light to travel as fast in a physical medium as it does in a vacuum, so that eliminates C. And, nothing travels faster than the speed of light in a vacuum, so that eliminates choice D. The product of n and v equals c. This eliminates choice A as too small. Since $n \sim 1$, we expect v to be fairly close to c.

52. **The correct answer is (A).** The greater the refractive index, n, the greater the optical density of the medium and the greater the extent to which the medium will slow down light. As light slows, its refraction angle at an interface decreases. D is the only choice that can be immediately eliminated since n_x is greater than n_{H_2O}, sin x must be less than the refractive angle in water, sin 45°.

    Using Snell's law we get

    sin x/sin 45° $= n_{H_2O}/n_x$ where x represents medium 2

    sin $x = (1/2)(.707) = 0.353 < .500 = $ sin 30°

53. **The correct answer is (A).** The sine of the critical angle is the reciprocal of the refractive index: sin $0_{crit} = 1/2.00 = 0.500$

54. **The correct answer is (A).** Stress $= F/A$ where F is the tension on the wire and A is the cross-section al area of the wire:

    $A = \pi^2 = \pi(2.00 \times 10^{-3} \text{ m}/2)^2$

    $= 3.14 \times 10^{-6} \text{ m}^2$ stress $= F/A$

    $= 628 \text{ N}/3.14 \times 10^{-6} \text{ m}^2 = 2.00 \times 10^8 \text{ N/m}^2$

    Choice D can be eliminated because it has no units, which fits the property of strain. Similarly, choice B can also be eliminated because it has the wrong units for stress.

55. **The correct answer is (D).** Strain is the fractional change in length to the original length

    strain $= \Delta\ell/\ell = 0.24 \text{ m}/240 \text{ m} = 1.0 \times 10^{-3}$

    Choices A and B can be eliminated because strain has no units.

56. **The correct answer is (A).** Any modulus is the ratio of stress to strain $= 2.0 \times 10^{11} \text{ N/m}^2$.

57. **The correct answer is (C).** The elastic modulus being described is for a change in length, which is given by Young's modulus. By definition, Young's modulus is the ratio of the tensile stress to the tensile strain

    $Y = (F/A)/(\Delta\ell/\ell)$

58. **The correct answer is (C).** The ability of a substance to return to its original shape once a deforming force is removed is called elasticity.

59. **The correct answer is (A).** The shortest pipe length will be associated with the wavelength for the fundamental tone. For a closed-end pipe, this is: $\lambda = 4\ell$. The wavelength is the ratio of the speed to the frequency: $\lambda = v/\nu$. Therefore, the shortest length is:

$$\ell = v/4\nu = \frac{360 \text{ m/s}}{4 \, (450 \text{ s}^{-1})} = 0.20 \text{ m} = 20 \text{ cm}$$

60. **The correct answer is (B).** Acceleration is the change in velocity; therefore,

$$a = \frac{\Delta v}{\Delta t} = \frac{100 \text{ m/s} - 80 \text{ m/s}}{2s} = 10 \text{ m/s}^2$$

Choice C can be eliminated immediately because the unit meter per second is for velocity, not acceleration.

61. **The correct answer is (A).** $v = v_0 + at$. Estimate the acceleration due to gravity using $a = -g = -9.8 \text{ m/s}^2 \sim -10 \text{ m/s}^2$. The velocity is approximately

$$v = 40.0 \text{ m/s} - 10 \text{ m/s}^2 \, (2 \text{ s})$$
$$= 40\text{m/s} - 20\text{m/s} = 20\text{m/s}$$

The closest choice to 20 m/s is A.

$$v = 40.0 \text{ m/s} - 9.80 \text{ m/s}^2 \, (2.00 \text{ s}) = 20.4 \text{ m/s}$$

62. **The correct answer is (D).** From Newton's second law, $F = ma$, so the acceleration is

$$a = F/m = \frac{10 \text{ N}}{2.0 \text{ kg}} = \frac{10 \text{ kg m s}^{-2}}{2.0 \text{ kg}} = 5.0 \text{ m/s}^2$$

The velocity is $v = v_0 + at$ where $v_0 = 0$ so that

$$v = at \frac{(5.0 \text{ m})}{s^2} 5.0 \text{ s} = 25 \text{ m/s}$$

63. **The correct answer is (B).** This expression gives the number of moles of $NiCl_2$ (and therefore of Ni). It must equal the number of moles of product, which has 1 Ni per molecule. There is no need to work with the MW of the product, since its weight is not requested.

64. **The correct answer is (D).** Only choice D shows each of the oxygens surrounded by an octet as well as showing the required 14 electrons.

65. **The correct answer is (C).** This solution is a buffer, for which
$$[H^+] = K_a \, [\text{HFor}]/[\text{For}^-] = K_a$$
$$pH = -\log \, (1.8 \times 10^{-4}) = 3.7$$

66. **The correct answer is (B).** Heat lost by graphite = heat gained by water

(1.0 mol) (heat cap. for graphite) (temperature drop for graphite) =
(1.0 mol) (heat cap. for water) (temp gain for water)

67. **The correct answer is (A).** A 0th-order reaction proceeds with a constant rate, so the time to go from one-half to one-quarter of the original amount will be only half the time needed to go from all of the reactants to one-half of them. (Had the reaction been first-order, the answer would have been 5 minutes.)

68. **The correct answer is (C).** Since the egg is cooked in water, it can't be heated above the boiling temperature of the liquid. The boiling temperature is lower at high altitudes, where the external pressure is lower and molecules can more easily escape from the liquid phase into the vapor.

69. **The correct answer is (D).** The "m" quantum number is used as the beginning of the orbital's name: "4." The value of "ℓ" is translated into the second designation; when "ℓ" = 2, the orbital is called "d." Hence, "$4d$."

70. **The correct answer is (D).** The first two choices will decrease the solubility owing to the common ion effect. The third will have no effect, since as long as some solid is present at equilibrium, any more will not change the concentrations of ions.

71. **The correct answer is (B).** The force of interaction between two charges is:

$F = \dfrac{kq_1 q_2}{r^2}$. Since the charges are alike, the force is repulsive (positive sign). This eliminates choice D immediately.

$$F = \left(9 \times 10^9 \, \frac{Nm^2}{C^2}\right)$$

$$= \frac{(10 \times 10^{-6}C)(10 \times 10^{-6}C)}{(10 \times 10^{-2}m)^2}$$

$$= \frac{(9 \times 10^9)(10^{-10})}{10^{-2}}N$$

$$= 9 \times 10^9 \times 10^{-10} \times 10^2 N$$

$$= 9 \times 10^1 N = 90 \, N$$

72. **The correct answer is (A).** Power can be expressed as $P = V^2/R$. Solving for R gives

$$R = \frac{V^2}{P} = \frac{120 \, V}{1200 \, W} = \frac{(120 \, V)(120 \, V)}{1200 \, W} = \frac{120 \, V^2}{10 \, W} = 12 \, \Omega$$

73. **The correct answer is (B).** Intensity, power, and radial distance between source and observer are related by

$$I = \frac{P}{4\pi r^2}$$

Since the source doesn't change, the power is constant; therefore, the ratio of the two intensities becomes

$$\frac{I_{6 \, feet}}{I_{3 \, feet}} = \frac{P/(4\pi(6 \, ft)^2)}{P/(4\pi(3 \, ft)^2)} = \frac{(6 \, ft)^2}{(3 \, ft)^2} = \frac{36 \, ft^2}{9 \, ft^2} = 4$$

Choices C and D can be eliminated immediately because the brightness must increase, not decrease, as the source is brought closer to the observer.

74. **The correct answer is (A).** Conservation of mass means you get $\frac{4}{2}x$, which corresponds to an alpha particle being emitted.

75. **The correct answer is (B).** Because the resistors are in series, the same current must flow through both resistors. Apply Ohm's law to find the voltage across the 40 Ω resistor.

$V = IR = (2.0 \, A)(40 \, \Omega) = 80 \, V$

76. **The correct answer is (C).** Conservation of mass and charge means that the sum of mass numbers on the reactant side must add up to $235 + 1 = 236$. Since $144 + 89 + x = 236$, x must equal 3. There are 3 neutrons emitted.

77. **The correct answer is (C).** Choices A and D are immediately eliminated because they represent the difference and the sum of the two vectors and only occur if they are both collinear. The resultant is equivalent to the hypotenuse of a right triangle with the adjacent legs of 6 N and 8 N. This is an example of a 3-4-5 right triangle where each side is multiplied by the constant 2. The result is $2 \times 5 = 10$ N.

VERBAL REASONING

78. **The correct answer is (B).** The answer to this question is based on the following statements made in paragraphs 2 and 3 and on the overall tone of the article. "It is only with respect to those laws that offend the fundamental values of human life that moral defense of civil disobedience can be rationally supported." (paragraph 2) "The assumption that a law is a valid target of civil disobedience is filled with moral and legal responsibility that cannot be taken lightly. To be morally justified in such a stance one must be prepared to submit to legal prosecution for violation of the law and accept the punishment if his attack is unsuccessful." (paragraph 3)

79. **The correct answer is (B).** The answer to this question is based on the following statement in paragraph 2: "However, disobedience of laws not the subject of dissent, but merely used to dramatize dissent, is regarded as morally as well as legally unacceptable."

80. **The correct answer is (B).** The answer to this question is based on the following statement in paragraph 2: "It is only with respect to those laws that offend the fundamental values of human life that moral defense of civil disobedience can be rationally supported."

81. **The correct answer is (B).** The answer to this question is based on the following statement in paragraph 3: "To be morally justified in such a stance, one must be prepared to submit to legal prosecution for violation of the law."

82. **The correct answer is (C).** The answer to this question is based on the following statement in paragraph 4: "For a just society to exist, the principle of tolerance must be accepted, both by the government in regard to properly expressed individual dissent and by the individual toward legally established majority verdicts."

83. **The correct answer is (B).** The answer to this question is based on the same statement from paragraph 2 that answers Question 3 (refer to the answer for Question 80).

84. **The correct answer is (B).** The answer to this question can be inferred from the statement from paragraph 4 that answers Question 5 (refer to the answer for Question 82).

85. **The correct answer is (A).** The answer to this question is based on the following statement in paragraph 3: "One should even demand that the law be enforced and then be willing to acquiesce in the ultimate judgment of the courts."

86. **The correct answer is (B).** The answer to this question is supported by this statement in the first paragraph: "Sooner or later on the basis of observation and analysis, what astronomers detect finds its way into theory . . ."

87. **The correct answer is (C).** The answer to this question is based on the following statement in paragraph 5: "Even such indirect observations need elaborate and highly sensitive equipment that wasn't in place until about five years ago."

88. **The correct answer is (B).** The answer to this question can be inferred from this statement in the last paragraph: "Certain quantities that physicists insist should be the same after an interaction as before—momentum, energy, and angular momentum—could be conserved only if another particle of zero charge and negligible mass were emitted."

89. **The correct answer is (D).** The answer to this question is based on the following statement in paragraph 4: "Having no charge, it does not interact with the fields around which most particle detection experiments are built; it can be detected only inferentially, by identifying the debris from its rare interaction with matter."

90. **The correct answer is (D).** The answer to this question is based on the following statement in paragraph 2: "Despite the construction, finally, of a string of elaborate observatories, some buried in the earth from southern India to Utah to South America, the last five years as well have produced not a single, validated observation of an extraterrestrial neutrino."

91. **The correct answer is (B).** The answer to this question is based on the following statement in paragraph 5: "The goal is worth the effort; however, once detected, extraterrestrial neutrinos will provide solid, firsthand information on the sources and conditions that spawned them."

92. **The correct answer is (D).** The answer to this question is based on the statement found in paragraph 7 that is given also as the answer to Question 11 (refer to the statement given in Question 88).

93. **The correct answer is (A).** The answer to this question is based on the statement in paragraph 7 that is given in the answer to Question 88.

94. **The correct answer is (D).** The answer to this question is based on the following statement in paragraph 1: ". . . cannot overlook the absence of common sense and impartiality. . . ."

95. **The correct answer is (A).** The answer to this question is based on the following statement in paragraph 1: "Many persons who appreciate and admire Mr. Swinburne's genius cannot help regretting that he should ever have descended from the serene heights of poetry into the arena of criticism."

96. **The correct answer is (C).** The answer to this question is based on the following statement in paragraph 3: "A careful comparison of *Essays and Studies* with another volume published about eleven years later, under the title of *Miscellanies*, shows that their author has either deliberately or unconsciously contradicted many of the opinions he had previously expressed . . . ."

97. **The correct answer is (B).** The answer to this question is based on the following two statements in paragraphs 2 and 5: "Mr. Swinburne's criticism is characterized by an utter want of proportion and aggressive dogmatism that finds vent in offensive and vituperative language quite unsuited to the dignity of literature. . . ." (paragraph 2) ". . . he is too one-sided, too extravagant, too unrestrained." (paragraph 5)

98. **The correct answer is (D).** The answer to this question is based on the statement in paragraph 1, which is quoted in the answer to Question 94.

99. **The correct answer is (B).** This inference is based on the following statement made in paragraph 4: "Indeed, nearly all that he has written about this rather overrated representative of the French romanticist school is little better than hysterical declamation."

100. **The correct answer is (C).** This assumption can be made based on the following statement in paragraph 5: "This fact, however, remains; his judgments upon books and their authors are the reverse of impartial, and it is manifest that Nature never intended him for a critic."

101. **The correct answer is (D).** The last two paragraphs of the article clearly state that Mr. Swinburne was not an impartial, astute, nor perceptive critic.

102. **The correct answer is (C).** The answer to this question is based on the following statements in paragraph 2: "A prolific photographer, he also took thousands of photographs documenting the daily lives and customs of the peoples he saw. After his death, James's unique pictorial history of the region was donated to the Southwest Museum in Los Angeles . . . founded to preserve and interpret the art, artifacts, and documentary material of the prehistoric and historic cultures of the Americas."

103. **The correct answer is (D).** The answer to this question is based on the following statement in paragraph 8: "The more than eleven thousand nitrate-based negatives in the museum's collection 'are still in good condition . . .' but experts have already detected . . . signals of deterioration."

104. **The correct answer is (A).** The answer to this question is based on the following statements in paragraph 5: ". . . James and many other photographers of the early 1900s often used a nitrate-based film. . . . Within decades, however, the nitrate-based film begins to deteriorate . . . the early photographers . . . 'just didn't realize it would deteriorate so quickly.' "

105. **The correct answer is (D).** The answer to this question is based on the following statement in paragraph 1: "A proper, English-born minister, George Wharton James seemed out of his element when he arrived in the still-wild West in 1881."

106. **The correct answer is (A).** The answer to this question is based on the following statements in paragraph 8: ". . . experts have already detected early warning signals of deterioration. 'The negatives could turn to powder before we know it,' she [Moneta] notes, adding the museum's anxiety over the film has increased greatly in the past five years."

107. **The correct answer is (A).** The answer to this question is based on the following statement in paragraph 2: "After his death, James's unique pictorial history of the region was donated to the Southwestern Museum in Los Angeles . . . founded . . . to preserve . . . the art, artifacts, and documentary material of the prehistoric and historic cultures of the Americas."

108. **The correct answer is (B).** The answer to this question can be inferred from the following statements in paragraphs 4 and 6: "There is very little documentation of that period remaining. . . ." (paragraph 4) "The photo library is a treasure house for researchers—particularly those living in the West—since it contains vintage prints that show . . . the daily life of the Native Americans." (paragraph 6)

109. **The correct answer is (C).** The answer to this question is based on the following statement in the passage: "But . . . his strength lies in a dramatic insight that goes far toward the making of a master of the playwright's art . . . ."

110. **The correct answer is (B).** The answer to this question is based on the following statement in the passage: ". . . of all the Elizabethan playwrights he is one of the most unwearied . . . ."

111. **The correct answer is (A).** The answer to this question can be inferred from the following statements in the passage: "It would grieve me to seem unjust toward a writer to whom I have long felt very specially attracted . . . ." and " . . . his strength lies in a dramatic insight that goes far toward the making of a master of the playwright's art . . ."

112. **The correct answer is (C).** The answer to this question is based on the following statement in the passage: ". . . his strength lies in a dramatic insight that goes far toward the making of a master playwright's art. . . ."

113. **The correct answer is (C).** The answer to this question is found in the article as a whole as it discusses almost nothing else but Heywood's creative ability. The following two statements are an example of this focus. The first statement says, "His creative power was, however, of that secondary order which is content with accommodating itself to conditions imposed by the prevailing tastes of the day." The second states ". . . his practiced inventiveness displays with the utmost abundance; of all the Elizabethan playwrights he is one of the most unwearied . . . ."

114. **The correct answer is (B).** This inference could be based on many statements in the article, but the following two statements give the best basis for the inference: "Yet the highest praise that it seems right to bestow upon Thomas Heywood is that which was happily expressed by Tieck when he described him as the 'model of the light and rapid talent' " and "His creative power was, however, of that secondary order which is content with accommodating itself to conditions imposed by the prevailing tastes of the day."

115. **The correct answer is (D).** The answer to this question is based on the following statement in paragraph 1: "During the past four decades the fishery scientists of the West have studied the dynamics of fish populations with the objective of determining the relationship between the amount of fishing and the sustainable catch."

116. **The correct answer is (A).** The answer to this question is based on the following statement in paragraph 3: "The rate of growth of individuals, the time of sexual maturity, and the accumulation of reserves vary according to the food supply."

117. **The correct answer is (C).** The answer to this question is based on the following statement in paragraph 2: "Much of it (theory) is based on the Darwinian concept of a constant overpopulation of young that is reduced by density-dependent mortality resulting from intraspecific competition."

118. **The correct answer is (D).** The answer to this question is based on the following statement in paragraph 3: "He argues that Darwin's concept of constant overpopulation has led to the neglect of the problem of protecting spawners and young fish."

119. **The correct answer is (B).** The answer to this question is based on the following statement in paragraph 1: "During the past four decades the fishery scientists of the West have studied the dynamics of fish populations with the objective of determining the relationship between the amount of fishing and the sustainable catch."

120. **The correct answer is (C).** The answer to this question is based on the following statement in paragraph 3: "Nikolskii considers the main laws of population dynamics to be concerned with the succession of generations: their birth, growth, and death."

121. **The correct answer is (A).** This inference is based on the following statements in paragraphs 2 and 3. In paragraph 2, the Darwinian point of view and food supply are not mentioned. "Much of it [the theory] is based on the Darwinian concept of a constant overpopulation of young that is reduced by density-dependent mortality resulting from intraspecific competition." In paragraph 3, part of the explanation of the non-Darwinian point of view of G. V. Nikolskii is stated: "The mass and age structure of a population are the result of adaptation to the food supply. The rate of growth of individuals, the time of sexual maturity, and the accumulation of reserves vary according to the food supply."

122. **The correct answer is (C).** The answer to this question is based on the following statement in paragraph 3: "The mass and age structure of a population are the result of adaptation to the food supply." The answer is also listed above as part of the answer to Question 121.

123. **The correct answer is (D).** The answer to this question is based on the following statement in paragraph 5: "The real question concerns, rather, the responsibility of criticism to defend the integrity of art against all encroachments. . . ."

124. **The correct answer is (A).** The answer to this question is based on the following statement in paragraph 5: "By concentrating in the most disinterested way on its traditional tasks of elucidation and evaluation, criticism will make its necessary contribution to the life of art and the freedom of the spirit."

125. **The correct answer is (B).** The answer to this question is based on the following statement in paragraph 3: "Therefore, so as not to conceal this admixture of description and judgment, critical evaluation is best performed as honestly as possible with reasoned arguments and detailed examples."

126. **The correct answer is (C).** The answer is based on the following statement: ". . . when all the institutions of society—the museums, the media, the universities, the galleries, the collectors, and all government agencies . . .—are prejudiced in favor of whatever is deemed on any grounds new and innovative in the arts, the challenge to criticism is monumental."

127. **The correct answer is (C).** The answer to this question is based on the following statement in paragraph 3: "The first task of the critic is to see the work of art and describe its qualities . . . This is the task of elucidation, and it is fundamental to all criticism worthy of the name."

128. **The correct answer is (D).** The answer to this question is based on a number of statements, but the following statement in paragraph 5 best sums up the answer: "The question in a democratic society is not whether criticism has a role to play; that is taken for granted."

129. **The correct answer is (B).** The answer to this question can be inferred from the following statements in paragraph 2: The "message" in Muir's quote "first found institutional expression on a global scale in the 1972 United Nations Conference on the Human Environment . . ." "There, 130 nations . . . acknowledged a mutual obligation in maintaining a livable global environment."

130. **The correct answer is (D).** The answer to this question is found in the following statement in paragraph 4: "Although Americans tend to bask in the notion that we are environmentally progressive, in truth the United States is in many ways a mirror of global environmental problems—a story of too little and too late . . ."

131. **The correct answer is (A).** The answer to this question can be inferred in the following statement in paragraph 5: "The United States did move quickly, as the Environmental Revolution dawned in the late 1960s, to enact constructive measures: the epochal National Environmental Policy Act; laws to abate air and water pollution and even noise; laws to deal with solid waste, to protect wildlife, to save coasts from degradation; and more."

132. **The correct answer is (D).** The answer is based on the following statement: "The United States exemplifies the worldwide conflict . . . between professed desires for environmental quality versus addiction to lifestyles that are environmentally destructive in every aspect. . . ."

133. **The correct answer is (B).** The answer to this question can be inferred from the following statement in paragraph 7: "Greens have been elected to legislative bodies in West Germany, France, Italy, Austria, Luxembourg, Switzerland, Belgium, Finland, and Portugal."

134. **The correct answer is (B).** This answer is based on the following statements in paragraph 10: ". . . it seems only a matter of time . . . until it brings significant changes in national lifestyles that are conspicuously inimical to environmental quality. Such conspicuous habits include demands for gas-guzzling cars, a voracious pattern of energy consumption, throwaway consumerism, recreational vehicles designed to ravage deserts, the equation of growth with good, and all the rest."

135. **The correct answer is (B).** The answer to this question is based on the following statement in paragraph 5: "Although we have been spending roughly $85 billion a year—$340 per capita—on pollution controls, we are still far short of our goals of clean air and water."

136. **The correct answer is (D).** The answer to this question is based on the following statement in paragraph 2: "It is thus necessary that, if action needs to be taken, it should be taken on a global scale with the participation of as many countries as possible for a sustained period of time."

137. **The correct answer is (B).** The answer is based on the process of eliminating choices A, C, and D, which are supported by statements in the article. Choice B is the remaining possible answer, as it is not supported by any statement in the article. Choice A is supported by the following statements in paragraph 6: ". . . the United States and other countries should begin to think of ways to reduce greenhouse gas emissions . . . The source of these reductions would be different for every country." Choice C is inferred by several statements in paragraph 6 and supported directly by a statement in paragraph 7: "The source of these reductions would be different for every country. For one, it may be changing land-use patterns to reduce tropical deforestation. For another, it may be improving energy efficiency" (paragraph 6). "Since greenhouse gas emissions have already increased, some amount of adaptation may be necessary even if we limited emissions today." (paragraph 7) Choice D is supported by the following statements in paragraph 7: "Moreover, if concerted action on an international level is to be undertaken, then a consensus must emerge on the seriousness of the climate change problem. Only through internationally coordinated research on the impacts of climate change can this be accomplished."

138. **The correct answer is (A).** The answer to this question is based on the following statement in paragraph 3: "If we wait until we can actually measure warming before we take action, then we may have to live with warmings for many generations, since it takes many years before emission reductions could have an impact on atmospheric concentrations and the climate system."

139. **The correct answer is (C).** The answer to this question is based on a number of statements in paragraph 1: "The way we live is profoundly affected by our climate. When and where we farm, how much we heat and cool our homes, how we obtain our water—all depend on the climate we experience. Climate determines whether we have a bumper crop or a shortage." There is no mention of climate and clothing.

140. **The correct answer is (B).** The answer to this question is found in several statements in paragraph 6: "Yet, we do not have the luxury of sitting on our hands while a scientific consensus emerges. Rather, the United States and other countries should begin to think of ways to reduce greenhouse gas emissions, in the event that it ultimately proves necessary to do so."

141. **The correct answer is (D).** The correct answer is based on summarization of paragraphs 5 and 7.

142. **The correct answer is (A).** The answer to this question can be found in several statements in paragraph 2: "No one country dominates in the emission of greenhouse gases, and any country that takes action to control emissions will achieve only limited success if other countries do not follow suit. It is thus necessary that, if action needs to be taken, it should be taken on a global scale with the participation of as many countries as possible for a sustained period of time."

BIOLOGICAL SCIENCES

143. **The correct answer is (C).** A basic knowledge of digestive processes is required, i.e., the stomach is a highly acidic environment, whereas the small intestine is slightly alkaline. The lower part of the graph shows that enzyme X works best at a pH close to 2, while enzyme Y works best at a pH closer to 8.

144. **The correct answer is (A).** Because the two enzymes have two different, non-overlapping pH ranges, they could not be at work in the same place at the same time. In addition, the graph does not refer to the temperature ranges of X and Y (only A and B). Although enzyme X generally works more slowly than enzyme Y, neither enzyme works at all at a pH of 4.5.

145. **The correct answer is (B).** The key to this question is the temperature range at which the two enzymes work. Only enzyme A has a temperature range encompassing human body temperature (37°C). An enzyme whose peak activity is close to 75°C–80°C (enzyme B) is unlikely to be found in the human body.

146. **The correct answer is (D).** Both enzymes overlap between 40°C and 50°C. Choices A and B are too broad, and each includes a range of temperatures beyond which one of the enzymes cannot work.

147. **The correct answer is (C).** When an enzyme is not active in a particular environment, it may be because that environment affects its conformation. The only possible answer, therefore, is C. For choices B and D, no information is provided in the graph.

148. **The correct answer is (B).** Some knowledge about factors that affect enzyme activity is needed here. Within an enzyme's normal range of activity, a clear indication that all enzyme molecules are saturated with substrate is a leveling off of the rate of reaction curve (an increase in enzyme concentration would help increase activity again).

149. **The correct answer is (C).** When enzymes are at work, they help bring their substrate(s) to the "transition state," at which time bonds can break and the reaction can proceed. To be able to do this, the enzyme must be in an environment compatible with its range of activity. A pH below 5.5 is not within the activity range of enzyme Y. Therefore, it would be unable to bring its substrate(s) to the transition state.

150. **The correct answer is (C).** The understanding that each single bacterial cell can give rise to an entire colony is helpful. The passage states that the presence of fewer colonies is indicative of cells dying, while smaller colonies suggests that growth has been inhibited. Side 1 (the UV radiated side) has *fewer and smaller colonies* compared to the unradiated side, as well as compared to the dish irradiated with green light.

151. **The correct answer is (B).** Only side 1 was exposed to UV light. Therefore, ten colonies grew compared to 30 on the unexposed side (1/3).

152. **The correct answer is (A).** The observation that the number and size of colonies exposed to green light (dish B/ side 1) is about the same as the number and size of colonies not exposed to anything (dish A/side 2; dish B/side 2) demonstrates that green light has no effects. What should also be clear is that in both experiments, cultures were only incubated in the dark (exposure to light in Experiment 2 took place *before* incubation).

153. **The correct answer is (D).** In both experiments, side 2 was always treated identically to side 1 *except* for the variable being tested—the type of radiation.

154. **The correct answer is (B).** In *both* experiments, dish A/side 1 was exposed to *UV radiation*. In Experiment 2, exposure to incandescent light took place *after* UV. Therefore, any change (in this case, a restorative effect) was due to the incandescent light. This effect is referred to as photoreactivation. (Neither experiment compared exposure to UV light versus exposure to incandescent light.)

155. **The correct answer is (C).** The passage states that UV radiation is absorbed by purines and pyrimidines. Since these bases are part of nucleotide structure in the DNA, choice C is correct.

156. **The correct answer is (D).** The only difference in procedure between the new experiment and Experiment 1 is the presence of the glass lid prior to UV radiation. Since the number and size of colonies on the UV-exposed side (in the new experiment) were equivalent to those on the unexposed side, one must conclude that the glass lid protected the bacterial cells (glass does absorb UV—that's why we can't get a sunburn through a window!).

157. **The correct answer is (B).** If each of these structures has endocrine functions, the secretions must enter the blood. The hypothalamus only regulates the activity of the pituitary gland.

158. **The correct answer is (D).** The question states that an increase in blood volume will increase blood pressure. When reabsorption of sodium occurs, reabsorption of water usually follows (increasing blood volume). Therefore, without knowing anything about ANF, you know choice D is the only possible answer.

159. **The correct answer is (C).** Knowledge about the role of bicarbonate ion (here, in the form of sodium bicarbonate) as an alkaline secretion that helps neutralize acidity is helpful. The arrival of acidic chyme signals the small intestine to release secretin ("proximate" reason). The fact that pancreatic enzymes are most active in the slightly alkaline pH of the small intestine (they require a slightly alkaline environment to function properly) is the "ultimate" reason.

160. **The correct answer is (A).** When cells in a noncyclic environment (darkness) display a cyclic pattern of response, an "internal" cyclic rhythm is suggested. Choices B and C do not apply to the conditions described in the question. There is no relevant basis for selecting choice D.

161. **The correct answer is (D).** The passage states that thymosin only influences the differentiation of T-lymphocytes. Choices A, B, and C are each specific roles of lymphocytes (either T- or B-lymphocytes).

162. **The correct answer is (B).** Knowledge of the source and function of bile is important. The liver produces bile, while the gallbladder stores and concentrates bile. The role of bile is to emulsify fats so that they can be efficiently digested by pancreatic lipase. Without the gallbladder, bile can still be sent to the small intestine via the liver directly.

163. **The correct answer is (D).** According to the figure, the peak secondary response to antigen A (day 40) came approximately 30 days after the peak primary response (days 9–10). The peak primary response to antigen B appears to occur on day 40. Therefore, day 70 is the appropriate answer for this question.

164. **The correct answer is (B).** Initial exposure to antigen A occurs prior to day 2, while peak primary response is approximately at day 9–10. Similarly, the initial exposure to antigen B occurs at day 28, while peak primary response is approximately at days 37–38. Thus, choice B is the correct answer.

165. **The correct answer is (B).** The peak primary response is approximately 20 units. The peak secondary response is somewhat less than 10,000 units. Therefore, it is between 100 and 1000 times as great.

166. **The correct answer is (B).** Since macrophages ". . . digest the antigen-bearing agent . . . ," it should immediately be recognized that they carry out phagocytosis. Neither red blood cells nor platelets take part in this process. The macrophages are most likely neutrophils or monocytes (granular and nongranular white blood cells, respectively).

167. **The correct answer is (C).** Initial contact with a dead or weakened form of the antigen in the form of a vaccine provides effective immunity when the "real" organism makes contact the second time.

168. **The correct answer is (C).** Careful referral to the passage reveals that T-cells play important roles during both stages of the immune response.

169. **The correct answer is (A).** The ability to draw inferences from previous information is important here. If the primary immune response (response to initial treatment) to penicillin causes an allergic response, the secondary immune response (response to the drug the next time it is administered) may be much more severe and extremely dangerous (as shown earlier, the secondary response can produce between 100 and 1000 times as many antibodies).

170. **The correct answer is (B).** When acetylcholine is released by motor neurons, it initiates depolarization of the sarcolemma. Calcium returns to the sarcoplasmic reticulum only *after* depolarization has occurred. Additionally, neurons of the sympathetic nervous system would never be on the "receiving" side of a neuromuscular junction.

171. **The correct answer is (C).** Basic knowledge of the organization of the nervous system is needed. Motor neurons, by definition, carry impulses *from* the CNS *to* the effectors. Only choice C is a plausible answer.

172. **The correct answer is (D).** Each answer is a reasonable option. ATP is needed for a variety of processes involved in muscle relaxation (repolarization of the sarcolemma, return of calcium to the SR, events at the neuromuscular junction, etc.). Interrupted blood flow can prevent efficient delivery of oxygen needed for ATP production during cellular respiration. Salt imbalances (sodium, potassium, calcium) can also prevent normal muscle function.

173. **The correct answer is (D).** Knowledge about neuromuscular junctions is required. The motor end plate is the site directly under the axon terminals of the motor neuron (where the motor neuron and muscle cell membrane meet).

174. **The correct answer is (A).** To answer this question correctly, knowledge that the CNS consists of the brain and spinal cord, and that myelin sheaths are found on axons, is necessary.

175. **The correct answer is (A).** Understanding the inheritance pattern of sex-linked traits is essential. Males always inherit sex-linked traits (on the X-chromosome) from their mothers. In addition, sex-linked traits are much more commonly expressed in males since they only have one X chromosome.

176. **The correct answer is (A).** The more soluble a substance is, the further it will be carried in solution. Additionally, the passage states that adsorption is the tendency of substances in a mixture to adhere to the material over which they are passed. Thus, the greater the adsorptive tendency, the sooner they will leave the mixture (and the *lower* they will be on the paper).

177. **The correct answer is (A).** Since chromatography is designed to separate substances from a mixture, the three colored bands most likely represent three separate pigments ("Substances with color can easily be detected on the paper.") found in leaves.

178. **The correct answer is (D).** A careful reading of the graph reveals that this is the only correct answer. Choice B is incorrect because substance A has a broad range of low absorbance (high transmittance). Although the three substances each have two major absorbance peaks, the second peak of substance B (in the red range) does not reach 40-percent absorbance.

179. **The correct answer is (C).** The passage states that unless light is absorbed, its energy cannot be put to use. Substance A has absorbance peaks in the red and violet-blue range. These are the wavelengths used by this pigment (chlorophyll a) to run the light reactions of photosynthesis.

180. **The correct answer is (C).** Green wavelengths are among the *least* absorbed by the plant pigments, especially substances A and B (chlorophylls a and b, respectively). The appearance of the leaves is due to those wavelengths of light that are *reflected* and thus, visible to the eye. Substance C (a carotenoid pigment) mostly reflects the yellows, oranges, and reds, thereby contributing to the color changes seen in autumn when the chlorophylls are no longer present.

181. **The correct answer is (D).** If different pigments absorb different wavelengths, more of the light energy reaching the plant can be harnessed at the same time. The light absorbed for photosynthesis has nothing to do with heat dissipation. Similarly, making different pigments would probably be energetically more expensive since a different synthetic pathway would also require the anabolism of different enzymes and different "machinery" for dealing with new metabolites, etc.

182. **The correct answer is (B).** This question is about a typical Mendelian cross. Having "at least one normal allele" is simply another way of referring to the probability of a child having the normal phenotype (3:1 ratio).

183. **The correct answer is (D).** The probability of one child being a carrier is 1/2 or 50% (the child has a two-in-four chance of receiving the Pp genotype). Each subsequent child will have the same chances. However, it should be understood that the probability of two children being carriers (considering the two events together) is the product of the two events happening separately ($1/2 \times 1/2 = 1/4$).

184. **The correct answer is (B).** Amino acids do cross the placenta into the embryo's circulation (that is how the baby gets the building blocks for synthesizing its own proteins!). However, since the mother cannot make the enzyme to metabolize phenylalanine (remember, she has PKU), she must be careful with her diet. Otherwise, the high levels of the amino acid again in her blood can pass to the baby's blood (regardless of the baby's genotype) and cause the same situation that confronts PKU children.

185. **The correct answer is (D).** It must be understood that any individual with one allele (it is a dominant trait) for polydactyly will express the trait.

186. **The correct answer is (C).** A basic knowledge of human sex-determination and the general characteristics of the sex chromosomes is required. Only males have a Y chromosome. Therefore, only males can express holandric traits. Similarly, since the Y chromosome is not homologous to the X chromosome, every trait will be expressed (as are all X-linked traits carried by a male).

187. **The correct answer is (A).** An affected individual must be homozygous recessive. If the parents are heterozygotes, one in four offspring can be homozygous dominant (all offspring do not have to be heterozygous).

188. **The correct answer is (C).**

$$H-C\equiv C-H + HOH \rightarrow H_2C=C-H \rightleftarrows H_3C-C=O$$
$$\underset{\text{enol form}}{\overset{|}{OH}} \qquad \underset{\text{keto form}}{\overset{|}{H}}$$

189. **The correct answer is (C).** The weaker acid holds on more tightly to its proton than the stronger acid does, which will release its proton more readily. As a result, the concentration of the weaker acid will increase over the stronger acid.

190. **The correct answer is (B).** The aromatic structure is lost in the keto form so that the enol structure is favored.

191. **The correct answer is (C).**

192. **The correct answer is (C).** The imine is the chief product.

193. **The correct answer is (D).** There is no hydrogen joined to N.

194. **The correct answer is (B).** There are two equivalence points (or full neutralization points), ii and iv, indicating two acidic protons.

195. **The correct answer is (D).** When the amino acid is acidified, its structure is

$$\overset{\oplus}{H_3N}-CH-COOH$$
$$|$$
$$R$$

It therefore behaves like a diprotic acid with two acid dissociation constants, K_{a1}, and K_{a_2}. The pK_a values are

$$pK_{a_1} = -\log K_{a_1}$$
$$pK_{a_2} = -\log K_{a_2}$$

Each amino acid has its characteristic pK_a values. At each 1/2 neutralization or equivalence point (after adding 0.50 mol and 1.50 mol of NaOH) pH = pK_a. Therefore, by measuring the pH after addition of 0.50 mol of NaOH, you have the value of pK_{a_1}. After the addition of 1.50 mol of NaOH, pH = pK_{a_2}.

196. **The correct answer is (A).** $pI = \dfrac{pK_{a_1} + pK_{a_2}}{2}$ At this pH the amino acid is a zwitterion

$$\overset{\oplus}{H_3N}-CH-COO^{\ominus}$$
$$|$$
$$R$$

$$pI = \frac{2.40 + 9.80}{2} = 6.10$$

197. **The correct answer is (C).** At this point in the titration, the first 1/2 equivalence point has been passed. At the first 1/2 equivalence point, one-half of the diprotic acid

$$\overset{\oplus}{H_3N}-CH-COOH$$
$$|$$
$$R$$

has been converted into its conjugate base.

$$\overset{\oplus}{H_3N}-CH-COO^{\ominus} \text{ by OH}^-:$$
$$|$$
$$R$$

$$\overset{\oplus}{H_3N}-CH-COOH + OH^{\ominus} \rightarrow \overset{\oplus}{H_3N}-CH-COO^{\ominus}$$
$$| \qquad\qquad\qquad\qquad\qquad |$$
$$R \qquad\qquad\qquad\qquad\qquad R$$

Therefore, at the first 1/2 equivalence point

$$[\overset{\oplus}{H_3N}-CH-COOH]=[\overset{\oplus}{H_3N}-CH-COO^{\ominus}]$$
$$| \qquad\qquad\qquad\qquad |$$
$$R \qquad\qquad\qquad\qquad R$$

As you add more NaOH, you increase

$$[\overset{\oplus}{H_3N}-CH-COO^{\ominus}]$$
$$|$$
$$R$$

so that it exceeds the concentration of the diprotic form.

198. **The correct answer is (C).**

199. **The correct answer is (B).** After the addition of 1.5 mol of NaOH,

$$[H_3\overset{\oplus}{N}-CH-COO^{\ominus}] \rightleftharpoons [H_2N-CH-COO^{\ominus}]$$

$$\begin{array}{cc} \quad\quad | & \quad\quad | \\ \quad\quad R & \quad\quad R \\ \text{acid} & \text{conjugate base} \end{array}$$

A buffer solution contains similar concentrations of an acid and its conjugate base (or a base and conjugate acid).

200. **The correct answer is (D).**

$$\begin{array}{c} \quad\quad CH_3 \\ \quad\quad | \\ CH_3-C-CH_2Br \\ \quad\quad | \\ \quad\quad Br \end{array}$$

There are two kinds of protons in this molecule: the six methyl protons and the two —CH_2— protons. Splitting is not observed because these nonequivalent protons are not on adjacent carbons. Hence, two NMR signals are observed in a 3:1 ratio.

201. **The correct answer is (A).** There are four nonequivalent protons: methyl protons, —CH_2— protons, and the two vinyl protons. The vinyl protons are nonequivalent because of their different chemical environments.

$$\begin{array}{ccc} (a)\text{H} & & \overset{(c)}{CH_3} \\ \diagdown & & \diagup \\ & C=C & \\ \diagup & & \diagdown \\ (b)\text{H} & & CH_2BR \\ & & (d) \end{array}$$

Consequently, 4 NMR signals will be observed.

202. **The correct answer is (B).** A deuteron gives no signal in a proton NMR spectrum because it absorbs at a much higher field. Consequently, by replacing H with D, signals are removed from the spectrum so that only two NMR signals will appear in a 3:2 peak ratio. No splitting will occur because the nonequivalent hydrogens are not attached to adjacent carbon atoms.

$$\begin{array}{ccc} \text{D} & & \overset{(a)}{CH_3} \\ \diagdown & & \diagup \\ & C=C & \\ \diagup & & \diagdown \\ \text{D} & & CH_2BR \\ & & (b) \end{array}$$

203. **The correct answer is (A).** The Br atom withdraws negative charge via an inductive effect, deshielding the proton and causing a downfield shift.

204. **The correct answer is (D).** Nuclei of some elements generate a magnetic moment. When such nuclei are exposed to a magnetic field, their magnetic moment can be aligned with *or* against the field. The magnetic moment of the nucleus is aligned with the field in the more stable state. Energy can be absorbed to excite the nucleus into a higher energy state in which the magnetic moment of the nucleus is aligned against the field. An NMR spectrum records these absorptions. Some examples of nuclei that generate a magnetic field include protons, ^{13}C, and ^{19}F.

205. **The correct answer is (D).** Familiarity with the parts of a eukaryotic cell is required. The microtubules and microfilaments make up part of the cell's cytoskeleton. A change in their arrangement can lead to cell movement or a change in cell shape.

206. **The correct answer is (B).** It should be known that the semiconservative hypothesis refers to the accepted model of how DNA replication occurs. This takes place at the onset of mitosis or meiosis—when chromatids are synthesized.

207. **The correct answer is (C).** Knowledge about the roles of the liver is required. In addition, it should be understood that the liver first catabolizes its stored glycogen back to glucose. The monosaccharides, not the entire insoluble polysaccharide, enter the bloodstream.

208. **The correct answer is (C).** Basic knowledge about muscle and joint anatomy is required. The origin of a muscle is the end that attaches to a site (bone) that does not move when the muscle contracts. In contrast, the insertion is the end that does move when the muscle contracts. The same bone can serve as the origin (site) for one muscle while serving as the insertion (site) for a different muscle.

209. **The correct answer is (A).** No previous knowledge about insects, hormones, or metamorphosis is necessary. The ability to logically apply the given information is required. If juvenile hormone inhibits metamorphosis, removal of the hormone (and its source) should cause metamorphosis to occur.

210. **The correct answer is (B).** An understanding of the role of oxygen in cellular respiration is needed, as is familiarity with microbiology terminology. Obligate anaerobes can survive only in the absence of oxygen.

211. **The correct answer is (D).** A basic understanding of kidney function and osmotic interactions is required. If a hypotonic filtrate (less solute, more water) passes a hypertonic tissue (more solute, less water), water will move from filtrate to surrounding tissue.

212. **The correct answer is (C).** Substitutions affect only one codon, and as a result, only one amino acid. Both additions and deletions affect the codons in which they occur, and every codon thereafter (frameshift mutations).

213. **The correct answer is (A).** An understanding of the relationship between digestion and absorption is helpful. Except for the associated beneficial effects of maintaining normal digestive function and regularity, fiber itself provides little or no nutrition. The foods containing fiber, however, have other nutritional substances that we are able to digest and absorb.

214. **The correct answer is (D).** A basic knowledge about the major osmotic components of blood plasma is important, as is an understanding of the relationship between blood pressure and blood vessel distance from the heart. The major osmotic blood proteins (such as albumin) are too large to leave the capillaries. Thus, colloid osmotic pressure (COP) normally remains the same at both ends of the capillary. However, blood pressure decreases in vessels as distance from the heart increases, resulting in hydrostatic pressure being lower than COP at the venule end.

215. **The correct answer is (B).** In this isomer, the bulky methyl groups are in equatorial positions where they have more room.

216. **The correct answer is (B).** The most substituted alkene is favored in elimination reactions.

217. **The correct answer is (D).** Epimers are diastereomeric aldoses that differ only in their configuration about carbon-2.

218. **The correct answer is (B).**

219. **The correct answer is (A).** A bond to deuterium is broken more slowly than a bond to protium (H). Observation of such a primary hydrogen isotope effect elucidates the rate-determining step in a reaction.

Practice Exam II

TEST	QUESTIONS	MINUTES
Physical Sciences	1–77	100 minutes
Verbal Reasoning	78–142	85 minutes
Writing Sample	2 Essays	60 minutes
Biological Sciences	143–219	100 minutes

ANSWER SHEET

PRACTICE EXAM II

Physical Sciences	Verbal Reasoning	Biological Sciences

Physical Sciences

1. Ⓐ Ⓑ Ⓒ Ⓓ   40. Ⓐ Ⓑ Ⓒ Ⓓ
2. Ⓐ Ⓑ Ⓒ Ⓓ   41. Ⓐ Ⓑ Ⓒ Ⓓ
3. Ⓐ Ⓑ Ⓒ Ⓓ   42. Ⓐ Ⓑ Ⓒ Ⓓ
4. Ⓐ Ⓑ Ⓒ Ⓓ   43. Ⓐ Ⓑ Ⓒ Ⓓ
5. Ⓐ Ⓑ Ⓒ Ⓓ   44. Ⓐ Ⓑ Ⓒ Ⓓ
6. Ⓐ Ⓑ Ⓒ Ⓓ   45. Ⓐ Ⓑ Ⓒ Ⓓ
7. Ⓐ Ⓑ Ⓒ Ⓓ   46. Ⓐ Ⓑ Ⓒ Ⓓ
8. Ⓐ Ⓑ Ⓒ Ⓓ   47. Ⓐ Ⓑ Ⓒ Ⓓ
9. Ⓐ Ⓑ Ⓒ Ⓓ   48. Ⓐ Ⓑ Ⓒ Ⓓ
10. Ⓐ Ⓑ Ⓒ Ⓓ   49. Ⓐ Ⓑ Ⓒ Ⓓ
11. Ⓐ Ⓑ Ⓒ Ⓓ   50. Ⓐ Ⓑ Ⓒ Ⓓ
12. Ⓐ Ⓑ Ⓒ Ⓓ   51. Ⓐ Ⓑ Ⓒ Ⓓ
13. Ⓐ Ⓑ Ⓒ Ⓓ   52. Ⓐ Ⓑ Ⓒ Ⓓ
14. Ⓐ Ⓑ Ⓒ Ⓓ   53. Ⓐ Ⓑ Ⓒ Ⓓ
15. Ⓐ Ⓑ Ⓒ Ⓓ   54. Ⓐ Ⓑ Ⓒ Ⓓ
16. Ⓐ Ⓑ Ⓒ Ⓓ   55. Ⓐ Ⓑ Ⓒ Ⓓ
17. Ⓐ Ⓑ Ⓒ Ⓓ   56. Ⓐ Ⓑ Ⓒ Ⓓ
18. Ⓐ Ⓑ Ⓒ Ⓓ   57. Ⓐ Ⓑ Ⓒ Ⓓ
19. Ⓐ Ⓑ Ⓒ Ⓓ   58. Ⓐ Ⓑ Ⓒ Ⓓ
20. Ⓐ Ⓑ Ⓒ Ⓓ   59. Ⓐ Ⓑ Ⓒ Ⓓ
21. Ⓐ Ⓑ Ⓒ Ⓓ   60. Ⓐ Ⓑ Ⓒ Ⓓ
22. Ⓐ Ⓑ Ⓒ Ⓓ   61. Ⓐ Ⓑ Ⓒ Ⓓ
23. Ⓐ Ⓑ Ⓒ Ⓓ   62. Ⓐ Ⓑ Ⓒ Ⓓ
24. Ⓐ Ⓑ Ⓒ Ⓓ   63. Ⓐ Ⓑ Ⓒ Ⓓ
25. Ⓐ Ⓑ Ⓒ Ⓓ   64. Ⓐ Ⓑ Ⓒ Ⓓ
26. Ⓐ Ⓑ Ⓒ Ⓓ   65. Ⓐ Ⓑ Ⓒ Ⓓ
27. Ⓐ Ⓑ Ⓒ Ⓓ   66. Ⓐ Ⓑ Ⓒ Ⓓ
28. Ⓐ Ⓑ Ⓒ Ⓓ   67. Ⓐ Ⓑ Ⓒ Ⓓ
29. Ⓐ Ⓑ Ⓒ Ⓓ   68. Ⓐ Ⓑ Ⓒ Ⓓ
30. Ⓐ Ⓑ Ⓒ Ⓓ   69. Ⓐ Ⓑ Ⓒ Ⓓ
31. Ⓐ Ⓑ Ⓒ Ⓓ   70. Ⓐ Ⓑ Ⓒ Ⓓ
32. Ⓐ Ⓑ Ⓒ Ⓓ   71. Ⓐ Ⓑ Ⓒ Ⓓ
33. Ⓐ Ⓑ Ⓒ Ⓓ   72. Ⓐ Ⓑ Ⓒ Ⓓ
34. Ⓐ Ⓑ Ⓒ Ⓓ   73. Ⓐ Ⓑ Ⓒ Ⓓ
35. Ⓐ Ⓑ Ⓒ Ⓓ   74. Ⓐ Ⓑ Ⓒ Ⓓ
36. Ⓐ Ⓑ Ⓒ Ⓓ   75. Ⓐ Ⓑ Ⓒ Ⓓ
37. Ⓐ Ⓑ Ⓒ Ⓓ   76. Ⓐ Ⓑ Ⓒ Ⓓ
38. Ⓐ Ⓑ Ⓒ Ⓓ   77. Ⓐ Ⓑ Ⓒ Ⓓ
39. Ⓐ Ⓑ Ⓒ Ⓓ

Verbal Reasoning

78. Ⓐ Ⓑ Ⓒ Ⓓ   111. Ⓐ Ⓑ Ⓒ Ⓓ
79. Ⓐ Ⓑ Ⓒ Ⓓ   112. Ⓐ Ⓑ Ⓒ Ⓓ
80. Ⓐ Ⓑ Ⓒ Ⓓ   113. Ⓐ Ⓑ Ⓒ Ⓓ
81. Ⓐ Ⓑ Ⓒ Ⓓ   114. Ⓐ Ⓑ Ⓒ Ⓓ
82. Ⓐ Ⓑ Ⓒ Ⓓ   115. Ⓐ Ⓑ Ⓒ Ⓓ
83. Ⓐ Ⓑ Ⓒ Ⓓ   116. Ⓐ Ⓑ Ⓒ Ⓓ
84. Ⓐ Ⓑ Ⓒ Ⓓ   117. Ⓐ Ⓑ Ⓒ Ⓓ
85. Ⓐ Ⓑ Ⓒ Ⓓ   118. Ⓐ Ⓑ Ⓒ Ⓓ
86. Ⓐ Ⓑ Ⓒ Ⓓ   119. Ⓐ Ⓑ Ⓒ Ⓓ
87. Ⓐ Ⓑ Ⓒ Ⓓ   120. Ⓐ Ⓑ Ⓒ Ⓓ
88. Ⓐ Ⓑ Ⓒ Ⓓ   121. Ⓐ Ⓑ Ⓒ Ⓓ
89. Ⓐ Ⓑ Ⓒ Ⓓ   122. Ⓐ Ⓑ Ⓒ Ⓓ
90. Ⓐ Ⓑ Ⓒ Ⓓ   123. Ⓐ Ⓑ Ⓒ Ⓓ
91. Ⓐ Ⓑ Ⓒ Ⓓ   124. Ⓐ Ⓑ Ⓒ Ⓓ
92. Ⓐ Ⓑ Ⓒ Ⓓ   125. Ⓐ Ⓑ Ⓒ Ⓓ
93. Ⓐ Ⓑ Ⓒ Ⓓ   126. Ⓐ Ⓑ Ⓒ Ⓓ
94. Ⓐ Ⓑ Ⓒ Ⓓ   127. Ⓐ Ⓑ Ⓒ Ⓓ
95. Ⓐ Ⓑ Ⓒ Ⓓ   128. Ⓐ Ⓑ Ⓒ Ⓓ
96. Ⓐ Ⓑ Ⓒ Ⓓ   129. Ⓐ Ⓑ Ⓒ Ⓓ
97. Ⓐ Ⓑ Ⓒ Ⓓ   130. Ⓐ Ⓑ Ⓒ Ⓓ
98. Ⓐ Ⓑ Ⓒ Ⓓ   131. Ⓐ Ⓑ Ⓒ Ⓓ
99. Ⓐ Ⓑ Ⓒ Ⓓ   132. Ⓐ Ⓑ Ⓒ Ⓓ
100. Ⓐ Ⓑ Ⓒ Ⓓ   133. Ⓐ Ⓑ Ⓒ Ⓓ
101. Ⓐ Ⓑ Ⓒ Ⓓ   134. Ⓐ Ⓑ Ⓒ Ⓓ
102. Ⓐ Ⓑ Ⓒ Ⓓ   135. Ⓐ Ⓑ Ⓒ Ⓓ
103. Ⓐ Ⓑ Ⓒ Ⓓ   136. Ⓐ Ⓑ Ⓒ Ⓓ
104. Ⓐ Ⓑ Ⓒ Ⓓ   137. Ⓐ Ⓑ Ⓒ Ⓓ
105. Ⓐ Ⓑ Ⓒ Ⓓ   138. Ⓐ Ⓑ Ⓒ Ⓓ
106. Ⓐ Ⓑ Ⓒ Ⓓ   139. Ⓐ Ⓑ Ⓒ Ⓓ
107. Ⓐ Ⓑ Ⓒ Ⓓ   140. Ⓐ Ⓑ Ⓒ Ⓓ
108. Ⓐ Ⓑ Ⓒ Ⓓ   141. Ⓐ Ⓑ Ⓒ Ⓓ
109. Ⓐ Ⓑ Ⓒ Ⓓ   142. Ⓐ Ⓑ Ⓒ Ⓓ
110. Ⓐ Ⓑ Ⓒ Ⓓ

Biological Sciences

143. Ⓐ Ⓑ Ⓒ Ⓓ   182. Ⓐ Ⓑ Ⓒ Ⓓ
144. Ⓐ Ⓑ Ⓒ Ⓓ   183. Ⓐ Ⓑ Ⓒ Ⓓ
145. Ⓐ Ⓑ Ⓒ Ⓓ   184. Ⓐ Ⓑ Ⓒ Ⓓ
146. Ⓐ Ⓑ Ⓒ Ⓓ   185. Ⓐ Ⓑ Ⓒ Ⓓ
147. Ⓐ Ⓑ Ⓒ Ⓓ   186. Ⓐ Ⓑ Ⓒ Ⓓ
148. Ⓐ Ⓑ Ⓒ Ⓓ   187. Ⓐ Ⓑ Ⓒ Ⓓ
149. Ⓐ Ⓑ Ⓒ Ⓓ   188. Ⓐ Ⓑ Ⓒ Ⓓ
150. Ⓐ Ⓑ Ⓒ Ⓓ   189. Ⓐ Ⓑ Ⓒ Ⓓ
151. Ⓐ Ⓑ Ⓒ Ⓓ   190. Ⓐ Ⓑ Ⓒ Ⓓ
152. Ⓐ Ⓑ Ⓒ Ⓓ   191. Ⓐ Ⓑ Ⓒ Ⓓ
153. Ⓐ Ⓑ Ⓒ Ⓓ   192. Ⓐ Ⓑ Ⓒ Ⓓ
154. Ⓐ Ⓑ Ⓒ Ⓓ   193. Ⓐ Ⓑ Ⓒ Ⓓ
155. Ⓐ Ⓑ Ⓒ Ⓓ   194. Ⓐ Ⓑ Ⓒ Ⓓ
156. Ⓐ Ⓑ Ⓒ Ⓓ   195. Ⓐ Ⓑ Ⓒ Ⓓ
157. Ⓐ Ⓑ Ⓒ Ⓓ   196. Ⓐ Ⓑ Ⓒ Ⓓ
158. Ⓐ Ⓑ Ⓒ Ⓓ   197. Ⓐ Ⓑ Ⓒ Ⓓ
159. Ⓐ Ⓑ Ⓒ Ⓓ   198. Ⓐ Ⓑ Ⓒ Ⓓ
160. Ⓐ Ⓑ Ⓒ Ⓓ   199. Ⓐ Ⓑ Ⓒ Ⓓ
161. Ⓐ Ⓑ Ⓒ Ⓓ   200. Ⓐ Ⓑ Ⓒ Ⓓ
162. Ⓐ Ⓑ Ⓒ Ⓓ   201. Ⓐ Ⓑ Ⓒ Ⓓ
163. Ⓐ Ⓑ Ⓒ Ⓓ   202. Ⓐ Ⓑ Ⓒ Ⓓ
164. Ⓐ Ⓑ Ⓒ Ⓓ   203. Ⓐ Ⓑ Ⓒ Ⓓ
165. Ⓐ Ⓑ Ⓒ Ⓓ   204. Ⓐ Ⓑ Ⓒ Ⓓ
166. Ⓐ Ⓑ Ⓒ Ⓓ   205. Ⓐ Ⓑ Ⓒ Ⓓ
167. Ⓐ Ⓑ Ⓒ Ⓓ   206. Ⓐ Ⓑ Ⓒ Ⓓ
168. Ⓐ Ⓑ Ⓒ Ⓓ   207. Ⓐ Ⓑ Ⓒ Ⓓ
169. Ⓐ Ⓑ Ⓒ Ⓓ   208. Ⓐ Ⓑ Ⓒ Ⓓ
170. Ⓐ Ⓑ Ⓒ Ⓓ   209. Ⓐ Ⓑ Ⓒ Ⓓ
171. Ⓐ Ⓑ Ⓒ Ⓓ   210. Ⓐ Ⓑ Ⓒ Ⓓ
172. Ⓐ Ⓑ Ⓒ Ⓓ   211. Ⓐ Ⓑ Ⓒ Ⓓ
173. Ⓐ Ⓑ Ⓒ Ⓓ   212. Ⓐ Ⓑ Ⓒ Ⓓ
174. Ⓐ Ⓑ Ⓒ Ⓓ   213. Ⓐ Ⓑ Ⓒ Ⓓ
175. Ⓐ Ⓑ Ⓒ Ⓓ   214. Ⓐ Ⓑ Ⓒ Ⓓ
176. Ⓐ Ⓑ Ⓒ Ⓓ   215. Ⓐ Ⓑ Ⓒ Ⓓ
177. Ⓐ Ⓑ Ⓒ Ⓓ   216. Ⓐ Ⓑ Ⓒ Ⓓ
178. Ⓐ Ⓑ Ⓒ Ⓓ   217. Ⓐ Ⓑ Ⓒ Ⓓ
179. Ⓐ Ⓑ Ⓒ Ⓓ   218. Ⓐ Ⓑ Ⓒ Ⓓ
180. Ⓐ Ⓑ Ⓒ Ⓓ   219. Ⓐ Ⓑ Ⓒ Ⓓ
181. Ⓐ Ⓑ Ⓒ Ⓓ

WRITING SAMPLE

Part 1

_____

_____

_____

_____

_____

_____

_____

_____

_____

_____

_____

_____

_____

_____

_____

_____

_____

_____

_____

TURN PAGE FOR ADDITIONAL SPACE →

648

END OF PART 1

WRITING SAMPLE

Part 2

_____
_____
_____
_____
_____
_____
_____
_____
_____
_____
_____
_____
_____
_____
_____
_____
_____
_____
_____
_____
_____
_____
_____
_____
_____
_____
_____

TURN PAGE FOR ADDITIONAL SPACE

_____

_____

_____

_____

_____

_____

_____

_____

_____

_____

_____

_____

_____

_____

_____

_____

_____

_____

_____

_____

_____

_____

_____

_____

END OF PART 2

PHYSICAL SCIENCES

Directions: This test contains 77 questions. Most of the questions consist of a descriptive passage followed by a group of questions related to the passage. For these questions, study the passage carefully and then choose the best answer to each question in the group. Some questions in this test stand alone. These questions are independent of any passage and independent of each other. For these questions, too, you must select the one best answer. Indicate all your answers by blackening the corresponding circles on your answer sheet.

A Periodic Table is provided at the beginning of this unit (page 564). You may consult it whenever you wish.

Passage I (Questions 1–10)

By tabulating standard thermodynamic functions, we gain the ability to calculate thermodynamic properties for a broad range of reactions. We can calculate not only the basic state functions, but also related quantities, such as the equilibrium constant.

The table below lists various thermodynamic properties—standard enthalpies and free energies of formation, absolute entropies, and standard heat capacities—for a range of hydrocarbons and oxygen-containing compounds. All compounds are in the gaseous state unless otherwise noted.

Compound	$\Delta H_f°$ (kJ/mol)	$\Delta G_f°$ (kJ/mol)	$S°$ (J/mol K)	$C_p°$ (kJ/mol K)
C (gas)	715	67.1	158	20.9
C (graphite)	0	0	57.3	8.4
CO	−110	−137	197	29.2
CO_2	−394	−395	214	37.2
CH_4	−749	−50.6	186	35.1
C_2H_6	−84.5	−32.9	229	52.7
C_2H_4	51.9	68.1	220	43.5
C_3H_8	−103.8	−23	270	73.6
C_6H_6	82.9	130	269	81.6
CH_3OH	−201	162	240	43.9
CH_3Cl	−808	−57.3	234	40.6
CH_2Cl_2	−92.5	−66.1	270	51.0
$CHCl_3$	−103	−70.2	295	65.6
HCHO	−116	−113	219	35.6
H_2	0	0	131	28.9
H_2O	−242	−228	189	33.5
O_2	0	0	205	29.3
O_3	143	163	239	39.3

GO ON TO THE NEXT PAGE

1. Under standard conditions, how many of the substances listed in the table can be formed spontaneously from their constituent elements?

   A. 6
   B. 9
   C. 10
   D. 11

2. Using the values in the table, what is $\Delta S°$ (in J/mol K) for the following reaction?

   $$2H_2(g) + O_2(g) \rightarrow 2H_2O(g)$$

   A. -89
   B. -147
   C. -484
   D. -456

3. According to the table, the amount of heat needed, at constant pressure, to raise the temperature of 10 g of gaseous carbon 10K would raise the temperature of the same mass of graphite by how many degrees?

   A. 2K
   B. 4K
   C. 10K
   D. 25K

4. For the data shown in the table, the molar heat capacities of saturated hydrocarbons

   A. decrease with increasing chain length.
   B. increase with increasing chain length.
   C. do not show a consistent trend.
   D. remain constant with increasing chain length.

5. The value of $\Delta H_f°$ for C_2H_2 is considerably higher than that for C_2H_4. The heat capacities for the two compounds are very similar. Therefore, which of the following is (are) likely to be true?

   I. The energy of a double bond differs substantially from that of a triple bond.
   II. When heat is added to each of these compounds at 298K, more of the heat will be absorbed by the triple bond than by the double bond.
   III. When each compound is decomposed into its elements at their standard states, more energy is released by C_2H_2.

   A. I only
   B. II only
   C. III only
   D. I and III only

6. Among the halogenated hydrocarbons shown in the table, which of the following increases as the number of chlorines increases?

   A. $\Delta H°$ only
   B. $\Delta H°$ and $\Delta G°$ only
   C. $S°$ and $C_p°$ only
   D. All four thermodynamic functions shown

7. The free energy change (in kJ) when 2 moles of C_2H_6 are oxidized to CO_2 and H_2O is approximately which of the following?

   A. -1375
   B. -1442
   C. 2750
   D. -2880

8. The difference in the values of the thermodynamic functions between gas-phase carbon and graphite can be explained by which of the following?

   I. Covalent bonding in the graphite lattice stabilizes the solid relative to the gas phase.

   II. The free motion and greater molar volume of the gaseous atoms are reflected in a greater value of the entropy for the gas.

   III. The greater molar volume of the gas leads to a lower absolute entropy.

   A. I only
   B. II only
   C. III only
   D. I and II only

9. Which of the following graphs best illustrates the formation of CH_4 from its elements?

A.
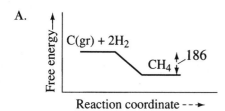

B.
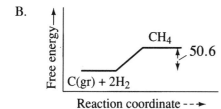

C.
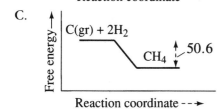

D.
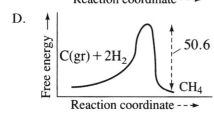

10. Which of the following expressions can be used to calculate the equilibrium constant for the following reaction?

$$CO(g) + \frac{1}{2} O_2(g) \rightarrow CO_2(g)$$

   A. $10^{-258/RT}$
   B. $10^{258/2.3RT}$
   C. $10^{532/RT}$
   D. $258/RT$

Passage II (Questions 11–17)

The kinetic theory predicts that gas molecules will move in all directions at a range of speeds. The average kinetic energy of the molecules is $3/2RT$ per mole, where R (the gas constant) = 8.31 J/mol K. Since the kinetic energy is related to speed, we can show that for an ideal gas, the root-mean-square speed (a quantity that is usually very close to the average speed) is given by

$$(3RT/M)^{\frac{1}{2}}$$

where M is the molar mass in g/mol.

In the following graph, the curves show the fraction of molecules having a given speed, for the temperatures of 300K and 600K.

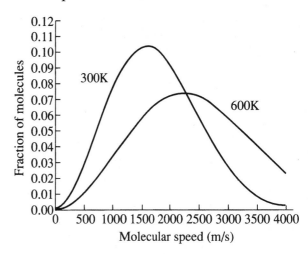

GO ON TO THE NEXT PAGE

11. Which of the following expresses the ratio of average speeds of a molecule of O_2 to a molecule of H_2 when both are at the same temperature?

    A. $\dfrac{1}{16}$
    B. 16
    C. $\dfrac{1}{4}$
    D. 4

12. If the temperature of a mole of gaseous O_2 is raised from 100°C to 200°C, the average speed of the molecules is

    A. lowered by the factor 100/200.
    B. raised by the factor 200/100.
    C. raised by the factor 473/373.
    D. raised by the factor $(473/373)^{\frac{1}{2}}$.

13. Based on the graph, the most probable speed at 600K is closest to which of the following?

    A. 0 m/s
    B. 0.075 m/s
    C. 1,600 m/s
    D. 2,300 m/s

14. Based on the graph, for 600K, what is the approximate fraction of molecules having speeds greater than 1,600 m/s?

    A. 0.10
    B. 0.25
    C. 0.50
    D. 0.75

15. Based on the graph, the curve for 1,200K is most likely to peak at which of the following?

    A. 165 m/s
    B. 1,000 m/s
    C. 1,600 m/s
    D. 3,200 m/s

16. The fact that there are no negative speeds on the graph reflects the

    A. experimenter's failure to measure negative speeds.
    B. fact that speed is the magnitude of velocity.
    C. fact that all molecules in a diatomic gas travel in a positive direction.
    D. fact that kinetic energy must always be positive or zero.

17. Which of the following may be inferred from the speed distributions shown on the graph?

    I. At higher temperatures, the average speed is higher.
    II. At lower temperatures, the speed distribution is more widely distributed.
    III. The average speed is proportional to the absolute temperature.

    A. I only
    B. II only
    C. III only
    D. I and II only

Passage III (Questions 18–26)

The following graph shows a titration of 100 mL of an unknown weak acid of undetermined concentration with 0.20 M NaOH.

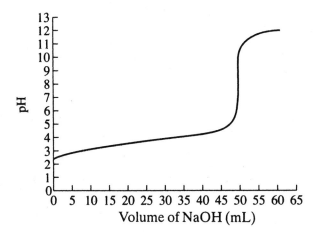

A student is told that the unknown acid is one of those listed in the following table.

Acid	K_a	pK_a
hydrogen sulfate	1.2×10^{-2}	1.92
formic	1.8×10^{-4}	3.74
acetic	1.8×10^{-5}	4.74
dihydrogen phosphate	6.2×10^{-8}	7.21

18. Which of the following is the number of moles of NaOH added at the endpoint of the titration shown in the graph?

    A. 0.0050
    B. 0.010
    C. 0.10
    D. 1.0

19. The data in the graph indicates that the concentration of the unknown acid is which of the following?

    A. 0.010
    B. 0.050
    C. 0.10
    D. 0.20

20. In the titration shown in the graph, as the volume of NaOH added is changed from 8 to 30 mL, the change in $[H^+]$ is

    A. an increase of about 30 percent.
    B. a decrease of about 30 percent.
    C. an increase of about a factor of 10.
    D. a decrease of about a factor of 10.

21. Based on the graph, the ratio $\Delta V_{OH^-}/\Delta pH$ is smallest when V_{OH^-} equals

    A. 0 mL
    B. 5 mL
    C. 25 mL
    D. 50 mL

22. Based on the information given, what is the pH when $V_{OH^-} = 100$ mL?

    A. 12
    B. 13
    C. 14
    D. Cannot be determined.

23. Based on the data in the table and the titration curve shown in the graph, which of the following is the unknown acid?

    A. Hydrogen sulfate
    B. Formic acid
    C. Acetic acid
    D. Dihydrogen phosphate

24. A second sample of the unknown acid is titrated with NaOH of the same concentration, and the endpoint is found to occur at 60 mL. The solution is then titrated with 30 mL of 0.20 M HCl. The resulting pH is closest to which of the following?

    A. 3
    B. 4
    C. 5
    D. 7

GO ON TO THE NEXT PAGE

25. At the 40-mL point on the graph, the solution most closely resembles which of the following mixtures (where "conjugate acid/base" refers to the unknown acid)?

A. 4 parts strong base to 1 part strong acid

B. 4 parts conjugate base to 1 part conjugate acid

C. 1 part conjugate base to 4 parts conjugate acid

D. 1 part conjugate base to 5 parts conjugate acid

26. The student wishes to choose an indicator to signal the equivalence point of the titration. Indicators that change color at pH 7.5 or 8.5 are available. Which should she choose?

A. 7.5 only

B. 8.5 only

C. Either 7.5 or 8.5

D. Neither would be accurate.

Passage IV (Questions 27–31)

An investigator studies several properties related to silver and chlorine and to their salt, AgCl.

Experiment 1
The investigator determines the first ionization energy, ΔH_{IE}, of gas-phase Ag.

$$Ag(g) \rightarrow Ag^+ + e^- \quad \Delta H_{IE} = 728 \text{ kJ/mol}$$

Experiment 2
The investigator determines the heat of sublimation of solid silver:

$$Ag(s) \rightarrow Ag(g) \quad \Delta H_{subl} = 286 \text{ kJ/mol}$$

Experiment 3YXYF
Next, the investigator determines the dissociation energy of diatomic chlorine, Cl:

$$Cl_2(g) \rightarrow 2Cl(g) \quad \Delta H_{diss} = 239 \text{ kJ/mol}$$

Experiment 4
The investigator finds the solubility product of solid AgCl in water:

$$AgCl(s) = Ag^+ (aq) + Cl^- (aq) \quad K_{sp}$$
$$= 1.8 \times 10^{-10}$$

Experiment 5
Finally, the investigator measures the value of the heat of formation of AgCl:

$$Ag(s) + \frac{1}{2} Cl_2 \rightarrow AgCl(s) \quad \Delta H_f = -128 \text{ kJ}$$

27. Of the reactions for which ΔH is given, how many can be said with certainty to proceed spontaneously?

A. 1

B. 2

C. 3

D. Cannot say without further information.

28. Find the energy taken in or given off when 20 moles of gaseous chlorine atoms are converted to gaseous Cl_2 molecules.

A. 2390 kJ given off

B. 2390 kJ taken in

C. 4780 kJ given off

D. 4730 kJ taken in

29. Use the data given to calculate the concentration of silver ion, $[Ag^- (aq)]$, expected in pure water.

A. 1.8×10^{-10} M

B. 1.3×10^{-10} M

C. 1.3×10^{-5} M

D. 728 kJ

30. Using the results of the experiments, what energy would be necessary to produce 0.10 mol of gas-phase silver ion (Ag^+) from metallic silver?

A. 28.6 kJ

B. 72.8 kJ

C. 101.4 kJ

D. 1014 kJ

31. Find the heat added or given off when 0.5 mol AgCl(s) is converted to gaseous Ag atoms and gaseous Cl atoms.

A. 139 kJ

B. 267 kJ

C. 278 kJ

D. 534 kJ

Passage V (Questions 32–36)

A "phase diagram" is used by chemists to display graphically the different solid, liquid, and gas phases—as well as mixtures of these—that exist in a pure compound or combination of compounds. Depending on the situation, the diagram may show the variation of phases with temperature, pressure, percentage of one component of a mixture, or other variables.

Figure 1 shows a temperature-pressure phase diagram for Substance 1, a pure compound. Figure 2 is a similar diagram for Substance 2. Figure 3 shows the temperature behavior of the phases in a mixture of aluminum, which contains a small, variable amount of silicon. Note that this diagram refers to two different solids, labeled "solid 1" and "solid 2." Each of these solids contains a mixture of aluminum and silicon, but they differ in percent composition and in crystal structure.

Figure 1

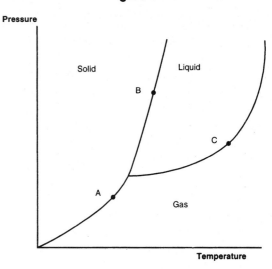

Figure 2

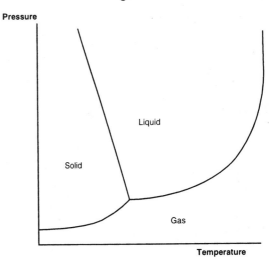

32. In Figure 1, which point corresponds to a pressure and temperature at which sublimation is taking place?

   A. Point A
   B. Point B
   C. Point C
   D. Point D

33. Consider Figures 1 and 2, Which would best describe water, given that water has the unusual property of expanding as it freezes?

   A. Figure 1, owing to the slope of boundary between solid and liquid
   B. Figure 1, owing to the slope of boundary between gas and liquid
   C. Figure 2, owing to the slope of boundary between solid and liquid
   D. Figure 2, owing to the slope of boundary between solid and gas

34. Figure 3 displays the phases that result when small amounts of silicon are added to aluminum at different temperatures. One property of these substances that helps to determine the shape of the diagram is the atomic radius. Which of

Figure 3

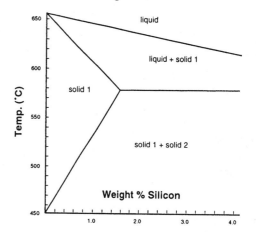

GO ON TO THE NEXT PAGE

the following best predicts the relationship of the radii of aluminum and silicon?

A. The radius of aluminum is larger, since as one moves to the right on the Periodic Table, there is an increase in nuclear charge that tends to pull the outer electrons more closely toward the nucleus.

B. The radius of silicon is larger, since as one moves to the right on the Periodic Table, there is a decrease in nuclear charge that tends to pull the outer electrons more closely toward the nucleus.

C. The radius of aluminum is larger, since as one moves to the right on the Periodic Table, electrons are added to a new shell, one that puts them farther from the nucleus.

D. The radius of silicon is larger, since as one moves to the right on the Periodic Table, electrons are added to a new shell, one that puts them farther from the nucleus.

35. Referring to Figure 3, determine the phase that will exist in a mixture of aluminum and 1.00% silicon at 550°C.

A. Liquid only
B. Liquid plus solid 1
C. Liquid plus solid 2
D. Solid 1 only

36. Which of the following statements may be inferred from the diagram?

According to the diagram, as the percentage of silicon increases:

I. The minimum temperature needed for the existence of any solid decreases.
II. The maximum temperature at which solid 2 appears increases sharply, then levels out.
III. The minimum temperature at which liquid is found decreases at a roughly constant rate.

A. I only
B. II only
C. III only
D. I and II only

Passage VI (Questions 37–43)

The state function entropy measures the increase (or decrease) in "disorder" of a system when it undergoes a change, such as a chemical reaction. Generally, reactions such as gas-phase dissociations proceed with a positive entropy change, since several fragments are created from an initial molecule. (Dissociations in a solvent are not easy to predict, however, as you will see as you work some examples.)

Is a positive entropy change enough to ensure that a reaction will proceed? No. Entropy enters into one of the terms in the expression for the free energy, which determines spontaneity.

The table below shows the entropy changes associated with a number of reactions.

Reaction	ΔS°_{298} (J/mol K)
1. $Cu(s) \rightarrow Cu(g)$	133
2. $H_2(g) \rightarrow 2H(g)$	98.6
3. $NaCl(s) \rightarrow Na^+ + Cl^-$	43
4. $H_2O(g) \rightarrow H_2O(l)$	−119
5. $HCl(g) \rightarrow HCl(aq)$	−131
6. $C(diamond) \rightarrow C(graphite)$	3.25
7. $MgCl_2 \rightarrow Mg^2 + 2Cl^-$	−97.1
8. $LiCl \rightarrow Li^+ + Cl^- 14$	

37. How many of the reactions in the table are spontaneous?

A. 0
B. 5
C. 8
D. Cannot be determined.

38. An investigator who wishes to test the hypothesis that the entropy change is positive for a reaction that results in more product molecules or ions than reactants would find what pattern in the data?

A. Confirming instances: reactions 1,2,3
   Disconfirming instances: reactions 7,8
B. Confirming instances: reactions 2,3,7,8
   Disconfirming instances: none
C. Confirming instances: reactions 2,3,8
   Disconfirming instances: reaction 7
D. Confirming instances: reactions 2,3
   Disconfirming instances: reactions 7,8

39. An investigator wishing to predict the direction of entropy change as dry ice (solid CO_2) sublimes to its vapor would get the best prediction from which of the following reactions?

A. 1
B. 3
C. 4
D. 6

40. Given the value of ΔS° for reaction 3 and the high solubility of NaCl in water, it can be said that the enthalpy change of NaCl solution

A. must be negative.
B. must be positive.
C. must be zero.
D. could be negative, zero, or positive.

GO ON TO THE NEXT PAGE

41. The ΔS for a phase change equals the enthalpy change for the phase change divided by the temperature at the phase change. In order to predict the melting point of ice, an investigator would need to know

A. only data given in the table.
B. the data given, plus the enthalpy of fusion of ice at its boiling point.
C. the data given, plus the enthalpy of fusion of ice at its melting point.
D. both the enthalpy and entropy of fusion of ice at its melting point.

42. In order to explain the difference between the S° values given for the two forms of carbon, an investigator might reasonably suggest which of the following?

I. A mole of diamond consists of fewer particles than a mole of graphite.
II. Diamond is a more stable structure than graphite.
III. The structure of diamond is more ordered than that of graphite.

A. I only
B. II only
C. III only
D. I and III only

43. An investigator wishes to account for the difference in $\Delta S°$ between NaCl and $MgCl_2$. Which of the following would not help to explain the difference?

I. Entropy changes increase as the number of product molecules increase.
II. When Mg^{2+} is dissolved, its large positive charge causes a more orderly arrangement of water molecules around it than in the case of Na^+.
III. The heat of solution is greater for $MgCl_2$ than for NaCl.

A. I only
B. II only
C. III only
D. I and III only

44. What is the half-life of $^{30}_{15}P$?

A. 7.5 rain
B. 5.0 rain
C. 2.5 rain
D. 2.0 rain

45. A second particle, $^{0}_{1}X$, is emitted along with silicon in the decay process. What is the most likely identity of this second particle?

A. Electron
B. Positron
C. Neutron
D. α-particle

46. What is the mass number for the silicon isotopes?

A. 30
B. 15
C. 14
D. 16

47. How many neutrons are present in the silicon isotope produced?

    A. 29
    B. 16
    C. 15
    D. 14

48. What is the atomic number of the silicon?

    A. 30
    B. 16
    C. 15
    D. 14

49. The silicon isotope given above falls

    A. above the belt of stability.
    B. below the belt of stability.
    C. on the belt of stability.
    D. None of the above.

50. What is the atomic number of a stable phosphorus nucleus?

    A. 30
    B. 14
    C. 15
    D. 29

Passage VII (Questions 51–55)

Miguel is taking a high school physics class. His teacher has told him to design and carry out any simple experiment that will allow him to observe an aspect of physics. Miguel goes home feeling quite perplexed because he can't think of an experiment. While sitting in the kitchen, he notices his baby sister trying first to pull and then to push a box across the highly polished kitchen floor. The little girl is trying to give a ride to her stuffed bear that is sitting in the box. Miguel suddenly "sees" his experiment. He decides to follow his sister's progress across the kitchen floor by plotting the estimated velocity of the box versus time.

In his report, Miguel notes that he is assuming that the kitchen floor is perfectly horizontal and frictionless. When his sister is through playing, Miguel measures the combined mass of the box and stuffed bear and finds that the total is 4.0 kg. The graph of his observed velocity vs. time is shown below.

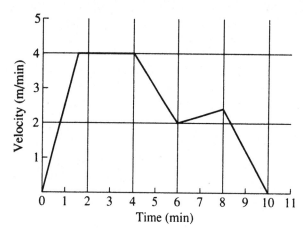

51. What is the best estimate of the distance the box moved during the last two recorded minutes?

    A. 1.0 m
    B. 2.0 m
    C. 3.0 m
    D. 4.0 m

52. Over which of the following time intervals was the kinetic energy of the box greatest?

    A. Minutes 0 to 1
    B. Minutes 2 to 3
    C. Minutes 5 to 6
    D. Minutes 7 to 8

53. What was the net force acting on the box over the interval of 1.5 minutes to 4 minutes?

    A. 0 N
    B. 0.5 N
    C. 2 N
    D. 8 N

GO ON TO THE NEXT PAGE

54. What was the momentum of the box over the interval of 1.5 minutes to 4 minutes?

    A.   0 kg m/min

    B.   4 kg m/min

    C.   8 kg m/min

    D.   16 kg m/min

55. During which of the following intervals was no work being done on the box?

    A.   Minutes 1 to 2

    B.   Minutes 2 to 3

    C.   Minutes 4 to 5

    D.   Minutes 7 to 8

Passage VIII (Questions 56–62)

An instructor in an introductory physics course makes up a set of five simple graphs with unlabeled axes to represent various functions. The graphs are shown below. She then asks her students to answer the following questions.

A.
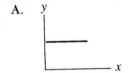

B.
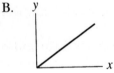

C.
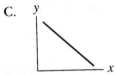

D.
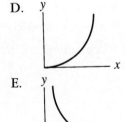

E.

56. If the x and y axes are volts and amperes, respectively, which graph best represents Ohm's law?

    A.   A

    B.   B

    C.   C

    D.   D

57. Which graph gives the closest approximation of the relationship between the force of gravity and the radial distance from the center of the Earth?

    A.   B

    B.   C

    C.   D

    D.   E

58. If the x and y axes are time and velocity, respectively, which graph describes the behavior of a ball thrown vertically upward?

    A.   B

    B.   C

    C.   D

    D.   E

59. For Einstein's mass-energy equation $E = mc^2$, which graph provides the best representation of the relationship between energy and mass?

    A.   A

    B.   B

    C.   C

    D.   D

60. For a body in dynamic equilibrium, which graph gives the expected relationship between velocity and time?

    A.   A

    B.   B

    C.   C

    D.   D

61. Which graph shows the relationship between pressure and volume of a gas at constant temperature?

A. B
B. E
C. D
D. C

62. Which graph shows the increase in pressure as increasing force pushes water through a hose?

A. A
B. B
C. C
D. E

Questions 63–77 are independent of any passage and independent of each other.

63. What is the maximum number of electrons in an atom that can have quantum numbers of $n = 5$ and $l = 2$?

A. 5
B. 8
C. 10
D. 15

64. Which of the following are arranged in decreasing order of expected dipole moment?

A. F_2, Cl_2, Br_2
B. H_2, HBr, HF
C. HF, HBr, H_2
D. K, Na, Li

65. The solubility product for $BaSO_4$ is 1.5×10^{-9}. Which of the following is correct?

I. The solubility of $BaSO_4$ in pure water is greater than the solubility in 0.1 M $Ba(NO_3)_2$.
II. The solubility product of $BaSO_4$ in pure water is greater than the solubility product in 0.1 M $Ba(NO_3)_2$.
III. The reaction of Ba^{2+} with SO_4^{2-} has an equilibrium constant greater than 1.0.

A. I only
B. II only
C. III only
D. I and III only

66. A student finds that $MgCO_3$ is more soluble in HNO_3 than in plain water. Which of the following is a likely explanation for this effect?

A. The NO_3^- ion attaches preferentially to the Mg^{2+}.
B. Mg^{2+} is a strong base and reacts completely with the H^+ from the nitric acid, causing the magnesium salt to dissociate.
C. Carbonate is a weak base and reacts with the H^+ from the strong acid, causing the barium salt to dissociate.
D. The HNO_3 reduces the Mg^{2+} to magnesium metal.

67. For the reaction $E + 2F \rightarrow G$, it is found that doubling the concentration of E quadruples the rate, while doubling the concentration of F has no effect. The rate law is which of the following?

A. rate $= k[E]$
B. rate $= k[E]^2$
C. rate $= k[E]^2[F]$
D. rate $= k[E][F]^2$

GO ON TO THE NEXT PAGE

68. An electron in a p_z orbital is least likely to be found in the

A. positive lobe.
B. xy plane.
C. negative lobe.
D. same side of the xy plane as another electron.

69. The pH of a solution of 0.1 M HNO_3 is closest to which of the following?

A. 0.1
B. 1
C. 7
D. 13

70. A gas mixture containing 1 mole of H_2 and 3 moles of N_2 has a total pressure of P atm. Which of the following are the partial pressures of each gas?

A. N_2: 3 atm; H_2: 1 atm
B. N_2: $(2P/3)$ atm; H_2: $(P/3)$ atm
C. N_2: $(P/3)$ atm; H_2: $(2P/3)$ atm
D. N_2: $(3P/4)$ atm; H_2: $(P/4)$ atm

71. Four media are separated from each other by horizontal surfaces. The path of a ray of light passing through the media system is illustrated below. In which medium is the speed of light greatest?

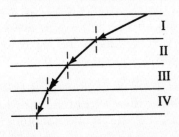

A. I
B. II
C. III
D. IV

72. Ball A is thrown horizontally from the roof of a building. At the same time, ball B, which weighs half as much as ball A, is dropped from the roof. Air resistance is negligible. Since both balls start at the same height and time, which statement is most accurate?

A. A and B will hit the ground simultaneously.
B. Ball A will hit the ground first.
C. Ball B will hit the ground first.
D. There is not enough information to determine which ball will hit the ground first.

73. Which of the following units cannot be used to represent energy?

A. Joule
B. kilowatt-hour
C. kilogram meter per second squared
D. Newton-meter

74. How far can light travel in a vacuum during the same time it takes sound to travel 660 meters in air?

A. 1.0×10^8 m
B. 1.5×10^8 m
C. 3.0×10^8 m
D. 6.0×10^8 m

75. What is the average power output of a 70-kg woman who runs up an incline to a height of 2 meters in 2 seconds?

A. 343 W
B. 686 W
C. 1372 W
D. 1715 W

76. Assume that a pole vaulter can convert all of his kinetic energy into potential energy. If a 70.0-kg pole vaulter approaches the vault with a velocity of 9.80 m/s, about how high can he vault?

A. 2.45 m
B. 4.90 m
C. 9.80 m
D. 19.6 m

77. A car drives around a circular track at a constant speed of 20 m/s. If the track is flat and has a radius of 200 m, what is the acceleration of the car?

A. 2.0 m/s^2
B. 10 m/s^2
C. 1.0 m/s^2
D. 0.10 m/s^2

END OF TEST 1.

IF YOU FINISH BEFORE THE TIME IS UP,
YOU MAY CHECK YOUR WORK ON THIS TEST ONLY.

VERBAL REASONING

Time: 85 minutes   **Questions 78–142**

> **Directions:** There are nine passages in this test. Each passage is followed by questions based on its content. After reading a passage, choose the one best answer to each question and indicate your selection by blackening the corresponding circle on your answer sheet.

Passage I (Questions 78–83)

If the world experiences significant temperature increases due to the greenhouse effect, both people and nature will have to adapt. One way people will need to adapt is in the way they use energy.

For example, everyone uses energy in ways that are affected directly by weather conditions. Heating, cooking, refrigerating, and water heating are important uses of energy that are affected directly by temperature, humidity, and other weather conditions. One consequence of higher temperatures caused by global warming would be lowered demand for energy used for heating in the winter and increased demand for energy used for cooling in the summer. Under the greenhouse effect, the changing seasonal patterns in energy use—less energy needed in winter and more consumed in summer—and the overall impact on total energy demand could have important implications for energy planning and ultimately on the cost of energy for individuals and businesses.

While climate change could affect a wide range of energy sources and uses, the implications for the demand for electricity are particularly significant. This is because the primary weather-sensitive energy uses—space heating and cooling, water heating, and refrigerating—make up a significant portion of total electricity sales for public utilities. These "end-uses" can account for as much as one-third of a power company's total sales and even more during daily and seasonal peak-usage periods.

Also, because of the large investments by utilities in long-lived capital-intensive power plants, the industry must focus on long-term planning. In other words, utilities must begin planning their investments now to meet their power generation needs into the new century.

To address these issues, the Environmental Protection Agency (EPA) and ICF Incorporated, an environmental and energy consulting firm, have assessed the potential impacts of the greenhouse effect on the demand for electricity and the consequences of these impacts for utility planning. Based on this study, preliminary regional and natural estimates were developed for a period from the present to the middle of the century (2055).

By the year 2055, the greenhouse effect could measurably change regional demands for electricity in the United States. A principal factor in generating capacity requirements is the peak (highest hourly) demand the utility must meet. For most utilities in the United States, this occurs on a day during a summer hot spell. Peak electricity demands are driven largely by peak use of air conditioning. Because the greenhouse effect is expected to have a significant influence on air conditioning and other summertime uses of electricity, higher temperatures in the future could lead to significant increases in the capacity needed to satisfy those uses.

Capacity requirements would not increase in all states, however. Because of greater demands for heating than cooling in colder regions, some utilities experience peak demands in the winter. In these cases, warmer winter

PRACTICE EXAM II: VERBAL REASONING

temperatures caused by the greenhouse effect could reduce the amount of generating capacity required. Such reductions in new capacity requirements induced by the greenhouse effect are restricted to a few states in the Northeast (Maine, New Hampshire, and Vermont) and in the Northwest (Washington, Oregon, Montana, and Wyoming).

The EPA-ICF study estimated that the investment in new power plants necessitated by the greenhouse effect could total several hundred billion dollars (not including any increase in costs due to inflation) over the next fifty years. In addition, increased fuel and operating and maintenance costs to generate electricity with these plants could reach several billion dollars per year by 2055. Much of these costs would undoubtedly be reflected in higher electric bills for consumers.

Of course, it is difficult, if not impossible, to predict the future. The extent and rate of climate change that will occur are very uncertain. Nonetheless, the picture painted by the study results is a very real possibility. The findings suggest that a substantial amount of our resources could be devoted to planning for and adapting to the greenhouse effect in this one sector alone. There are a number of other ways the greenhouse effect could make an impact on electric utilities (for example, reductions in the availability of water in rivers used to generate hydropower), and there are many other sectors of the world economy and environment that will feel the effects of climate change.

Designing and implementing strategies that will help to mitigate the greenhouse effect and to adapt to climate changes that do occur are the challenges facing policy makers and planners today.

78. The passage states that in some parts of the country, peak demand for electricity might decrease under the greenhouse effect because:

   A. these regions use more electricity for heating than for cooling and the need to heat would be reduced.
   B. conservation efforts might eliminate the need for more electricity.
   C. increases in rainfall might increase the number of cloudy days and reduce temperatures.
   D. we might switch from electric power to solar power.

79. The passage indicates that electricity demands caused by the greenhouse effect:

   A. will not be felt for fifty years.
   B. may result in greater dependence on hydropower.
   C. are most likely to increase in the Northeast and Northwest.
   D. could be significantly changed by the year 2055.

80. It would be reasonable to take the writer's argument further and assume that the writer

   A. would advocate planning for the greenhouse effect in other areas of our society.
   B. believes that the only aspect of our society that will be affected by the greenhouse effect is the use of electricity.
   C. does not believe the greenhouse effect is going to occur.
   D. believes adjustment to the greenhouse effect will not cause major disruption in our society.

GO ON TO THE NEXT PAGE

81. If the greenhouse effect takes place, the author believes that peak demand for electricity will decrease in the Northeast United States during the

   I. winter.
   II. summer.
   III. spring.

   A. I only
   B. II only
   C. I and II only
   D. II and III only

82. It can be assumed from the article that the author

   A. thinks the greenhouse effect is a near certainty.
   B. believes we should stop the greenhouse effect before it is too late.
   C. believes utilities have not planned enough in the past and need to do a better job in the future.
   D. believes that nonelectrical sources of energy need to be found to reduce the demand for electricity.

83. According to the article, long-range planning is important to utilities because

   A. without it, they would run out of electricity.
   B. huge capital investments will be needed to build new generating facilities.
   C. the government needs to know well in advance if there are going to be any shortfalls in power generation.
   D. of the time it takes to build generating facilities.

Passage II (Questions 84–92)

As a child of the frontier, it was natural for George Caleb Bingham (1811–79), the "Missouri painter," to paint the fur trappers, flatboatmen, country politicians, and squatters he knew so well. He portrayed them as rugged and self-reliant Americans, emblems of the frontier spirit.

Bingham came of age in the Golden Age of American painting (1830–60), when the work of American artists was, for the first time, appreciated and purchased not only by the wealthy—whose taste tended toward European works and artists—but also by an emerging and increasingly affluent middle class with an appetite for art that reflected the American spirit.

Today, Bingham ranks among the best of the nineteenth-century American narrative painters. "He was a powerful figure who broke new ground in illustrating the simple joys of American life and who prepared the way for the giants—Winslow Homer and Thomas Eakins—to follow," says E. Maurice Bloch, emeritus professor of art history at the University of California at Los Angeles. Bloch is author of *The Paintings of George Caleb Bingham: A Catalogue Raisonné*, published by the University of Missouri Press.

Bloch's catalogue raisonné places Bingham's life and work in the context of the social, artistic, and political climate of nineteenth-century America. The catalogue also reflects on Bingham's philosophy of art and examines the issue of patronage and national support for artists.

To his foes, Bingham was volatile, irascible, and pugnacious—with a colorful vocabulary to match. "He never attempted to mitigate the combative part of his personality," says Bloch. To his close friends, though, he was fiercely loyal and often charming, witty, and even affectionate.

Like many American artists, Bingham was largely self-taught and "he was proud of it," according to Bloch. Inspired by an itinerant painter, Bingham started out as a journeyman portraitist, traveling from town to town through Missouri and Mississippi. The stiffness of his early work began to soften after he studied for several months at the Philadelphia Academy of Art. He was also exposed to other artists while he worked as a portraitist for several years in Washington, D.C.

Bingham gained a national reputation through the American Art Union, an important corporate patron that encouraged artists to paint works appealing to patriotic feeling. The Art Union bought such works and distributed them by lottery to its members. The Art Union bought nineteen of Bingham's paintings between 1845 and 1851, exhibited them for long periods, promoted his work in its magazine, and engraved *The Jolly Flatboatman* in an edition of 10,000.

Despite national recognition, Bingham never achieved federal patronage. He sought, but did not win, a commission "to paint a western subject by a western artist" for a new extension to the Capitol in Washington, D.C. Although he has always been well known in Missouri, his national reputation began to fade even before his death in 1879. Not until 1935, after an exhibition of American realists at the Museum of Modern Art, did contemporary scholars become interested in Bingham's work.

Having studied Bingham's life and work for more than forty years, Bloch notes, "It would have been possible to write an excellent book on Bingham by noting only a narrow circle of authentic works. But the much greater mass of questionable works and copies acted as a magnet and a challenge." The catalogue raisonné, which supersedes an earlier version written by Bloch, includes one hundred works discovered in recent years. In addition, the attribution of twenty works previously thought to be by Bingham has been changed.

Because most of Bingham's paintings are held in private collections, this catalogue raisonné with its 370 black-and-white and 34 color illustrations may become indispensable to students and scholars.

84. According to the passage, the golden age of American painting

    A. lasted for most of the nineteenth century.

    B. was the period from 1830 to 1860.

    C. was over before George Caleb Bingham came of age.

    D. benefited from the patronage of the Philadelphia Academy of Art.

85. Based on reading the article, it would be reasonable to say that Bloch believes Bingham was

    I. an artist whose works varied enormously in quality.

    II. a very important early American artist.

    III. worth remembering as a historic figure in the art movement but not as an artist.

    A. I only

    B. II only

    C. I and II only

    D. I and III only

86. Bloch describes Bingham as

    A. nice, social, dedicated, and kind.

    B. calm, diligent, sensitive, and distant.

    C. aggressive, talented, cultured, and caustic.

    D. loyal, charming, witty, and affectionate.

87. Bingham's training as an artist was reflective of most American artists of the time in that he was

    A. largely self-taught.

    B. trained by itinerant artists.

    C. molded by the art schools dominant in the East.

    D. commissioned by wealthy patrons.

GO ON TO THE NEXT PAGE

88. The article states that Bingham gained his national reputation

 A. through the American Art Union.
 B. by getting a commission from the federal government to paint western scenes.
 C. by studying at the Philadelphia Academy of Art.
 D. by traveling and painting scenes all over the United States.

89. It can be inferred from the article that Bingham did much of his painting in

 A. Texas and New Mexico.
 B. Missouri and Kansas.
 C. Missouri and Mississippi.
 D. Mississippi and Texas.

90. According to the article, E. Maurice Bloch

 A. dubbed Bingham the "Missouri painter."
 B. studied the work of Winslow Homer and Thomas Eakins.
 C. taught art history at the University of Missouri.
 D. studied Bingham's life and work for over forty years.

91. The recognition of Bingham's reputation as one of the U.S.'s leading 19th-century narrative painters is a testament to Bingham's

 A. ability to depict in his art the spirit of American individualism and self-reliance.
 B. ability to incorporate patriotic themes in his art, thereby promoting a sense of vibrant nationalism.
 C. ability to create an appreciation of American artistic talent.
 D. creative artistic drive that coincided with the American public's gradual preference for American over European art.

92. According to the article, Bingham's paintings were highly reflective of the

 A. nineteenth-century American middle class.
 B. early nineteenth-century American city dweller.
 C. frontier-American pioneer spirit.
 D. mid-nineteenth-century mercantile class.

Passage III (Questions 93–98)

Throughout the nation, the current focus in education is on excellence. Recommendations from four independent national panels call for increased emphasis on: the five new basics (English, mathematics, science, social studies, and computer science); increased graduation requirements; a longer school day and school year; performance-based pay; incentives for outstanding teacher achievement; and alternate career ladders.

A master teacher plan is one of several procedures recommended to improve the quality of teachers and instruction in the classroom and to raise the achievement of students. A master teacher plan would provide a reward system for excellent teaching and make the profession more attractive to bright, talented college students seeking a professional career. It would also aid in retaining outstanding tenured teachers.

In response to the recommendations of the President's Commission on Excellence in Education, the Department of Defense Dependents School has implemented several educational reforms, one of which is a Master Teacher Pilot Program. In the development of the pilot program in the Department of Defense Dependents School's Panama Region, 374 classroom teachers and special area teachers responded to a 25-item questionnaire on issues related to the Master Teacher Pilot Program. The survey revealed:

 • The professional community is uncertain about its readiness for a master teacher program.

- Elementary teachers are more receptive to the concept of a master teacher plan than are secondary teachers.

- Almost 75 percent of the teachers believe an alternate career path is needed in the teaching profession.

- The ultimate professional goal for 50 percent of the teachers is to remain classroom teachers.

- Fewer than 10 percent of all teachers aspire to be administrators.

- Fifty percent of the teachers believe that a master teacher program could provide for professional growth.

- The majority of teachers believe that a master teacher program is likely to create tension, jealousy, favoritism, competition, and low morale.

- About two-thirds of the teachers believe the major problem in the development of a master teacher program is the construction of accurate, impartial, and fair evaluation instruments.

- Measurement and selection issues were the biggest concerns reported by the teachers.

- About one-third of the teachers would like to be considered for a master teacher position.

- Approximately 70 percent of the teachers prefer to have their building principal perform the observation and evaluation for the selection of master teachers.

- The majority of teachers believe that at least half the master teacher's time should be spent in the classroom.

Teachers in the Panama Region then responded to a second survey about the criteria to be used in selecting master teachers.

What is to be the profile of a master teacher? First and foremost, the master teacher would have comprehensive knowledge about his or her subject. The master teacher would be highly skilled in managing and instructing a class of students. Management of the total class as well as individual student behavior was deemed important. The master teacher would also excel in organizational planning, use of class time, and knowledge and use of instructional materials.

The most significant instructional skill of a master teacher would be the application and adaptation of major educational concepts and theories to provide for individual student differences, when designing lessons and in using instructional strategies to implement lessons. Students of master teachers would learn content as measured by teacher-developed tests. The master teacher would demonstrate clarity in both verbal and written expression. The master teacher would work well with students, would show consideration for others, and would have a commitment to professional growth and to the school program. The master teacher would frequently initiate and complete educational tasks and would show support for other group members. He or she would be well informed of recent developments in education.

The Department of Defense Dependents School has accepted the challenge for educational reform; the Master Teacher Program is one small step in an overall plan for excellence. In this endeavor, active teacher participation is vital to the success of a master teacher program.

GO ON TO THE NEXT PAGE

93. Recommendations from four independent national panels call for increased emphasis on all of the following subjects except

   A. science.
   B. computer science.
   C. mathematics.
   D. foreign language study.

94. According to the author, a master teacher plan would provide

   I. a reward for excellence.
   II. professional development for new teachers.
   III. specialized teachers for the elementary schools.

   A. I only
   B. I and II only
   C. II only
   D. II and III only

95. Based on the article, it would be reasonable to assume that the author

   A. is strongly opposed to the concept of a master teacher.
   B. is mildly critical of the master teacher concept.
   C. believes that the master teacher idea is good, but disagrees with the way it is being used by the armed forces.
   D. believes that the master teacher concept is a positive step toward improving education.

96. According to the author, which one of the following is the most important attribute of the master teacher?

   A. The ability to train other teachers
   B. Skill in classroom management
   C. The ability to communicate well with students
   D. Comprehensive knowledge of the subject areas taught

97. Which of the following was not one of the findings of the Panama Region survey?

   A. High school teachers were not as receptive to the master teacher concept as were elementary school teachers.
   B. Development of fair and impartial evaluation instruments is a major problem in implementing a master teacher program.
   C. The majority of teachers aspire to be administrators.
   D. More than 50 percent of all the teachers surveyed believe a master teacher program will result in low morale.

98. According to the article, the ideal master teacher would be highly skilled in

   I. managing and instructing a class of students.
   II. providing for individual students' needs.
   III. verbal and written expression.
   IV. administrative techniques.

   A. I and II only
   B. I, II, and III only
   C. I, II, and IV only
   D. III only

Passage IV (Questions 99–106)

Consider for a moment these chemicals: safrole, hydrazine, tannin, and ethyl carbamate. We ingest them every day when we consume pepper, mushrooms, tea, and bread. Now consider this: Each of these chemicals is a naturally occurring carcinogen. Do they jeopardize human health? Should this information lead to a movement to eliminate tea, outlaw mushrooms, condemn pepper, and banish bread from our tables?

Of course not. Yet that's where a manipulation of the numbers, and a misinterpretation of the facts, can take us. The numbers can be made to show that a substance is killing us—even when there isn't the remotest possibility. How, then, can a mother be sure that her food purchases will nourish her family and not contribute to its morbidity?

If you listen to every restrictive environmental report that has received media attention, you know that in addition to apples, you shouldn't eat most other fruits, not to mention meats, fish, fowl, vegetables, eggs, or milk products. You shouldn't even drink the water. This brings up the question, how can we make intelligent choices about risk?

Determining levels of safety in the environment, which is broadly defined to include lifestyle, must start with some basic premises. The first is that public health means preventing premature disease and death. The second is that public health policy should ensure safety, not harass industry or needlessly terrify the public.

What Americans suffer from is not a lack of data. It's something else entirely. The malady that needs immediate attention is called nosophobia. It's akin to hypochondria, but different.

Hypochondriacs think they are sick. Nosophobics think they will be sick in the future because of lurking factors in their diet and general environment. They fixate on an array of allegedly health-threatening gremlins. Due to this phobia, they believe that living—and eating and drinking—in America is inherently hazardous to their health. They are sure there is a death-dealing carcinogen on every plate, a life-sapping toxin under every pillow. They see salvation only in ever-increasing federal regulations and bans.

The nosophobics' fears of alar and other agricultural chemicals used in the United States are obviously purely emotional. These are fears of "invisible hazards," which have always played a special role in the mass psychology of paranoia, according to Park Elliott Dietz, Professor of Law and Psychiatry at the University of Virginia. Yesterday's invisible hazards give rise to monster legends, claims of witchcraft, and vampire myths. Today, notes Dr. Dietz, we see the same phenomenon among those who exaggerate the hazards of radiation, chemicals, toxic waste, and food additives.

The most deadly public health issues that threaten our lives have been obscured in the face of trumped-up charges against the food we eat, the water we drink, and the air we breathe. They fall under the category of hazardous lifestyles. And the data detailing the toll they take on human lives—not the lives of laboratory rats and mice—are compelling and truly frightening.

Cigarette smoking claims 1200 lives a day. In just one year, over 400,000 will perish because they'd rather die than switch. Another obvious example of a hazardous lifestyle habit is excessive or abusive alcohol consumption, which claims 100,000 lives annually. Add to this the use of addictive substances, such as heroin, cocaine, and crack, which claim some 50,000 lives each year.

These numbers are in. They aren't hypothetical. They aren't based on probability theories that require one to suspend disbelief. These data detail a real loss of life. Clearly, our focus should be on environmental lifestyle issues that, left unchecked, are systematically and prematurely killing our population. As a society, however, we seem more willing to assume the enormous and deadly risks of smoking or not wearing seatbelts—risks that are within our power to avoid taking. Ironically, what we appear to be unwilling to tolerate are the minute, infinitesimal risks we perceive to be outside our control. Today's prime example is the risk the public perceives when chemicals are married to food.

What most don't understand is that food is 100-percent chemicals. Even the foods on our holiday dinner tables—from mushroom soup to roasted turkey to apple pie—contain naturally occurring chemicals that are toxic when taken in high doses. Undoubtedly, there are some who may think we should start worrying about levels of allyl isothiocyanate in broccoli, because this naturally produced chemical is, in high doses, an animal carcinogen. Where does it end? Worrying about more numbers to focus more attention on non-issues accomplishes absolutely nothing.

GO ON TO THE NEXT PAGE

99. According to the article, public health policy should not

   A. needlessly harass industry or terrify the public.

   B. avoid controversial issues just to protect industry.

   C. hide dangers in eating certain foods from the public simply to keep the public from becoming fearful.

   D. try to change people's lifestyles.

100. According to the author, which of the following foods naturally contain toxic chemicals?

   I. Grains and dairy products
   II. Mushrooms and bread
   III. Salmon and trout

   A. I only

   B. II only

   C. III only

   D. II and III only

101. The article defines nosophobics as those who are

   A. environmentally conscious.

   B. committed to improving the quality of life.

   C. overly concerned about their lifestyle.

   D. fearful of future illness due to current hazards in their food or environment.

102. It would be reasonable to infer from this article that the author thinks we should

   A. spend more time regulating carcinogens that occur naturally in food.

   B. spend more time worrying about the quality of our air than worrying about additives in food.

   C. not worry so much about the potential effects of what we add to food.

   D. more closely regulate what we allow to be added to food.

103. The author implies that our current fear of chemicals in the food and the environment is similar to which of the following?

   A. The fear of technology exhibited in the seventeenth and eighteenth centuries

   B. The fear of the study of science throughout the European Renaissance period

   C. The fear of witchcraft and vampires in past centuries

   D. The fear of the unknown

104. The author believes that one of the most important steps we can take to lengthen our lives is to

   A. eat only organic produce.

   B. change our lifestyles by avoiding smoking, drinking, and other drug-taking.

   C. pay more attention to the fat content of the food we eat.

   D. pay more attention to exercise.

105. One possible explanation of the fear of chemicals in food and the environment can be interpreted as a

   A. legitimate public concern.

   B. symptom of a paranoia among an isolated segment of the population.

   C. public-oriented fear substantiated by reliable studies performed by consumer food organizations.

   D. hoax perpetuated by a disgruntled few.

106. According to the author, cigarette smoking kills

   A. 1200 people a year.

   B. 50,000 people a year.

   C. 100,000 people a year.

   D. 400,000 people a year.

Passage V (Questions 107–113)

How can a society's economic system produce the greatest good for the largest number of its members? Can the Aristotelian idea of the "good life" be conceived independently of the ability to acquire wealth? What is the happiness that Americans believe they have the right to pursue? The people of Seattle are confronting questions like these in an adult education program created by the Metrocenter YMCA in conjunction with the continuing education program at the University of Washington.

In 1981, during a City Fair program sponsored by the YMCA, some of the citizens of Seattle examined the hard economic questions facing their city. "People felt that decisions about economic growth involved more than statistics," says Richard Conlin, a project director for Metrocenter YMCA. They discovered that economic questions are not only technical and political, but ethical and religious as well. "People wanted to talk about the economy in terms of values," Conlin says. "Yet when they began to discuss the economy, they felt they lacked the ability to understand and articulate the philosophical issues that lie at the heart of the social contract."

To make the readings more accessible, the scholars included commentaries that place them in social and historical contexts. "When Plato and Aristotle examined the question, 'What is the good life?' they were living in an age of anxiety. The city-state of Athens was in decline. Their best hopes were a society that could ensure a reasonable quality of life for individuals despite a political environment threatening chaos," says Heyne. "When Aristotle asserted that 'man is by nature a political animal,' he meant that man, who is neither beast nor god, does not live in isolation," says Heyne, "but in a community." Thus, according to Aristotle, the pursuit of material wealth should be a means to strengthen the community, the *polis*. People who pursue material wealth for its own sake, Aristotle wrote, "are intent upon living only and not living well."

"Adam Smith, on the other hand, did not believe that the desire for wealth was in any way unnatural or a threat to the well-being of the society," says Heyne. Increasing wealth was a universal urge, Smith wrote in his classic treatise of 1776, *The Wealth of Nations*. People want to "better their condition . . . a desire that comes with us from the womb and never leaves us till we fall into the grave." "But Smith knew something that Aristotle couldn't consider," says Heyne. "Smith had observed the process of economic growth visible in Europe in the sixteenth and seventeenth centuries. He had seen how a society could increase the production power over time, expanding the supply of 'necessities and conveniences of life.' This was not unnatural or a threat to the well being of future generations. 'Capital has been silently and gradually accumulated by the private frugality . . . of individuals to better their own condition . . . This effort, protected by law and allowed by liberty . . . has maintained the progress of England toward opulence and improvement . . . ,' Smith wrote."

"We won't find simple answers for our age in the writing of these philosophers," says Heyne. "Their worlds differed so much from ours. But those differences can be instructive. If we can understand why Aristotle opposed economic growth and why Adam Smith extolled it, it will prompt us to think about how decisions are actually made in modern democracies."

Arlis Steward, director of Metrocenter YMCA's community development programs, says that "the challenge of this project was to select an anthology that people would not only read, but would also reflect upon before coming to get things done. Our economic system, as Adam Smith noted, depends basically upon self-interested behavior. Could a system based on nobler obligations be as effective in coordinating the everyday details of a highly specialized economic system?"

GO ON TO THE NEXT PAGE

107. The article implies that a basic reason for setting up the program was to

   A. develop an adult education program that discussed philosophy.

   B. develop a program that would help the public to be better informed on social questions.

   C. help adults better understand economic questions particularly as they concerned the city of Seattle.

   D. allow the University of Washington to effectively reach out to the adult community.

108. The inclusion by the YMCA's community adult education programs of the works of philosophers of diverse thinking and historical periods, such as Aristotle and Adam Smith, was a reflection of

   A. an effort to instruct the public's general understanding of contemporary economic issues through analysis of different philosophical approaches.

   B. a realization that philosophers offered solutions to economic problems that apply today.

   C. a commitment to reintroducing classical writers no longer read by the general public.

   D. an effort to help the general public accept the growing policy of harsh economic reforms occurring in Seattle.

109. According to Richard Conlin, people in Seattle found that economic questions were not only technical and political but also

   A. cultural and social.

   B. philosophical and historical.

   C. were based on knowledge of the past, present, and future.

   D. ethical and religious.

110. According to the article, which of the following correctly reflects the views of Adam Smith and Aristotle toward economic growth?

   A. Adam Smith opposed economic growth and Aristotle extolled it.

   B. Both Aristotle and Adam Smith extolled economic growth, but for different reasons.

   C. Both Aristotle and Adam Smith opposed economic growth, but for different reasons.

   D. Aristotle opposed economic growth while Adam Smith extolled it.

111. One can infer from the article that we can better understand our modern-day society by exploring the works of philosophers of the past because these works offer

   I. viable solutions to contemporary problems.

   II. ways of viewing variable approaches to contemporary decision-making.

   III. idealized answers applicable to today's realistic situations.

   A. I only

   B. II only

   C. I and II only

   D. II and III only

112. Based on the article, it would be reasonable to assume that the author

   A. supports the program that the YMCA created.

   B. opposes the kind of program the YMCA created.

   C. supports the concept of the program, but is not satisfied with the program as implemented.

   D. believes that programs such as the one that the YMCA developed should be developed by universities instead of YMCAs.

113. Which of the following expresses one of the basic differences between the philosophies of Adam Smith and Aristotle?

    A. Adam Smith felt that wealth should be accumulated for the good of society if it was to have any real value, and Aristotle believed that the accumulation of wealth was of value in itself.

    B. Aristotle thought that wealth had value only when it was accumulated for the good of society, and Adam Smith felt the accumulation of wealth was of value in its own right.

    C. Aristotle was more philosophical and Adam Smith was more pragmatic.

    D. Adam Smith was more interested in money than Aristotle.

Passage VI (Questions 114–121)

One hallmark of the Southern literary tradition has been the varied ways that writers have drawn upon Southerners' almost instinctive relationship to their surroundings. Working within a land-oriented cultural ethos, Southern writers have evoked a familiar, often haunting sense of place that gives the South a distinctive regional identity. Writers as well as artists have variously envisioned the land as a nostalgic emblem of the past, a source of goodness or a reflection of the divine, a product of decay, an exemplar of the bizarre, and a symbol of the human condition. Their portrayals range from the mythic and romantic to the factual and realistic.

"What is distinctive about the South," says Robert C. Stewart, executive director of the Alabama Humanities Foundation, "and about the Southerners' response to it, is that it remained primarily agricultural well into the twentieth century, long after the rest of the nation had become urbanized. This has kept much of the South poor economically, though not poor in spirit. Memories of defeat in the Civil War and of poverty during the Reconstruction and Depression eras have sometimes figured predominantly in the Southern consciousness. Consequently, Southerners have had mixed feelings about the land rather than purely idealized reactions, with pastoral myths often giving way to hard reality."

To help Alabamians examine their traditional relation to the land, Stewart directed the development of "In View of Home: Twentieth-Century Visions of the Alabama Landscape," a public program that combines a traveling photography exhibition with a seven-week series of reading and discussion programs, continuing through May at eight public libraries across the state . . . The program introduces participants to some of the major works of twentieth-century Southern literature and to a renewed sense of their roots in the land and its continuing vitality.

In selected readings, Stewart worked with Kieran Quinlan, an assistant professor of English at the University of Alabama at Birmingham. Southern literature, Quinlan says, is a particularly effective tool for grappling with a sense of regional identity: "Southern literature came into its own after the First World War, when Southern writers stopped blaming the Northeast for the South's problems and instead turned a critical eye on themselves."

What these writers found in the South, however, makes today's Southerner uncomfortable. "There is a tendency to deny what Faulkner or Agee found to be quintessentially Southern," Quinlan says. "The progressive South is uncomfortable with its rural heritage. Our program is an attempt to look squarely at its complicated past."

Participants are learning that Southern writers do not present a uniform view of "home." Among the works being read is William Faulkner's *The Bear* (1942), which depicts a mythic landscape and treats the theme of humanity's withdrawal from civilization. Jean Toomer's *Cane* (1923) portrays the spiritual landscape and the folk rhythms of black life in rural Georgia. And the Agrarians, represented by John Crowe Ransom's essay "Reconstructed but Unregenerate" (1930) and Andrew Lytle's short story "Jericho, Jericho, Jericho" (1984), who present the rural South as the philosophic preserve of the Jeffersonian values that first formed this nation.

GO ON TO THE NEXT PAGE

"With Walker Percy's *The Last Gentleman* (1966) and Mary Ward Brown's *Tongues of Flame* (1986), Southern literature reaches the point at which it ceases to be distinctively Southern and becomes broadly American," says Quinlan.

As chronicled in the works of these and other contemporary Southern writers, the South is moving inexorably into the urban, industrial mainstream. With fewer people living close to the land, the experiences that in many ways made Southerners "Southern" are becoming alien. "This program enables participants to think about some crucial cultural issues now that the great majority of Alabamians are living in urban areas," says Stewart. "As we move farther from the land of our parents and grandparents, we need to reflect on their special relationships with the land, whether we will have it today, and what will become of it as we move into the 1990s."

"In View of Home" is part of Alabama Reunion, a year-long, state-wide celebration.

114. According to the article, which of the following is true?

A. The South became industrial before the North.

B. The South has never become industrialized.

C. The South remained agricultural long after the North had become largely urban.

D. The South is still predominately agricultural while the rest of the country is predominately urban.

115. The article states that Southern writing has slowly evolved since World War I from a tendency to criticize the North for the South's problems to a self-assessment of the South's virtues and faults. The implication is that contemporary Southern writers

A. are no longer concerned with the South's regional identity and urge moving away from Southern literary tradition.

B. acknowledge the South's rural literary past as their writings become more mainstream.

C. have disavowed their regional heritage in a gradual effort to become more "American."

D. have become prolific in writings that renew their literary ties to a nostalgic and romantic view of the past.

116. According to the author, which two books mark the point at which Southern literature stops being regional and becomes broadly national?

A. *Cane* and *The Bear*

B. *Their Eyes Were Watching God* and *Mules and Men*

C. *Tobacco Road* and *God's Little Acre*

D. *The Last Gentleman* and *Tongues of Flame*

117. The author suggests that today's progressive South

A. is uncomfortable with the process of urbanization that has taken place during this century.

B. is uncomfortable with its rural past.

C. would prefer to forget its history of slavery and segregation.

D. feels that remembering past literary history is important to understanding the present.

118. Based on the article, it would be reasonable to assume that the author believes that what made Southerners quintessentially Southerners was

   I. the segregation of black and white society.
  II. the South's antagonism to the North.
 III. the predominately rural culture that dominated through the early part of the twentieth century.

A. I only
B. III only
C. I and II only
D. II and III only

119. As shown through "In View of Home," Southern writers offered a

A. romantic view of an antebellum aristocratic society that dominated the region.
B. picture of a homespun, frolicking, spirited rural society.
C. variety of images of the South that reflected its wide diversity.
D. view of a society still tormented by its historical support of slavery.

120. According to the article, the work of contemporary Southern writers is a reflection of the South's

A. moving into the urban, industrial mainstream.
B. moving further into the nationalistic mainstream of literature.
C. reevaluating its rural beginnings.
D. losing its vital, regional character.

121. Based on what the author stated, which of the following is most likely to occur?

A. Southern literature will remain distinctive from Northern literature.
B. In the future there will be no distinctive Southern literature and Southern writers will be largely indistinguishable from Northern writers.
C. In the future, the basic difference in writing styles will be between rural and urban writers rather than between Southern and Northern writers.
D. While there has been much talk about the historic difference between Southern writers and Northern writers, realistically there has been very little difference.

Passage VII (Questions 122–128)

Since 1977, Richard D. Brown, a professor of history at the University of Connecticut, has been reading through diaries from the various social strata. Most of these diaries have been used by historians only to gauge reactions to a specific event—how the scholar-clergyman William Bentley felt about Shays' Rebellion, for example—and few have been studied closely. Brown's perspective is much wider. Among the eleven chapters from his work, *The Diffusion of Information in Early America, 1700–1865*, there are discussions of declining isolation among Yankee farmers, the development of the legal profession as seen through the careers of John Adams and Robert Treat Paine, and the flow of information among merchants and mariners in port cities.

Diaries are the best sources of this type of inquiry, according to Brown, because they enable one "to see a person whole, to see how print and oral communication fit together in a person's life, to determine which is more important and exactly how both are used." Up to this point, scholars of journalism have written the history of communications, and they have tended to focus on particular forms, such as

GO ON TO THE NEXT PAGE

how newspapers developed from a primitive state to the present.

Brown finds long diaries like that kept by Boston judge Samuel Sewall from 1685 until 1729 especially valuable because they provide a constant against which changing mores can be examined over time. "For the first part of Sewall's diary," Brown says, "there are no newspapers in America. When the first newspaper is published, he gets one. So you can trace the effect of newspapers in Sewall's life over the next twenty-five years, and you see that they didn't make a whole lot of difference for him. People in Sewall's time did not read newspapers for news. Word of mouth was much faster. What newspapers did provide was the text of official documents, such as laws or treaties, and the speeches of high officials."

Because keeping a diary was a good deal more common during the eighteenth and nineteenth centuries than at present, Brown had to choose from the multitude available in university libraries and historical societies. The vast majority, being of the line-a-day or weather-report variety, were clearly of little interest. He also avoided the atypical experiences found in battle or travel diaries and screened out the many diaries concerned chiefly with the writer's spiritual health, concentrating instead on those that offer a reasonably full record of the author's experiences over at least a year. In particular, Brown sought out generic types—ordinary folks, such as farmers, merchants, women, artisans—rather than notables. There were, however, a few major figures—Sewall, Bentley, John Adams, William Byrd II—whose diaries, while frequently studied, were so revealing about patterns of social intercourse that they could not be ignored.

Based on a full reading of these diaries, about eighty altogether, Brown has revised some of his preconceptions about the movement of information. "Initially, I thought I would see successive stages in an information revolution over the period," he recalls. "During much of the eighteenth century, information was a scarce commodity, and its dispersal was hierarchical: A community's leaders controlled important communications and diffused them by word of mouth to other people. Then, with the Revolution and the explosion of printing in the 1780s and 1790s, came a much more egalitarian flow of information.

"Instead of this rather simple model of one system being supplanted by another, however, I found a picture of overlap and layering. Things were different in the 1800s not because the old face-to-face ways had been erased but because new developments had multiplied ways of diffusing information. The radical difference between the America of 1700 and 1850 was the extraordinary abundance of information. People gradually became selectors of information according to their individual temperament, their occupation, their social class. For example, a New England farmer thought that it was far more important to be informed about the land in his area than about the Constitution. In these farmers' diaries, one can see a tremendous information network that had little to do with print. Every time they left the farm they spoke with all sorts of people about local matters—the marriage market for their daughters, births and deaths, the availability of land. In short, people acquire the information pertinent to their lives.

"By the nineteenth century a dramatic change had occurred," Brown says. "The ideology of the Revolution required that the people—that is, all sorts of people, who run the nation in a democracy—be well-informed. It was the beginning of the idea that we should worry if a high percentage of people don't know who their senator is. This notion had many implications: It led to the public-school movement, the founding of academies, the rise of the lecture circuit, all aimed at upgrading the knowledge of the average citizen."

122. Diaries are a good source for gaining a better understanding of how people lived in the early eighteenth century because

- A. they are the only written record that remains from that period.
- B. diaries were widely written during this period of time and often captured the day-to-day experiences of the average person.
- C. diaries were written by those who were on the bottom of society and books and newspapers were written by those who were on the top.
- D. all the decision makers of the period kept diaries, and by reading these diaries we can learn how the important decisions were made.

123. On the basis of the fact that the number of newspapers in America increased dramatically between 1700 and the middle of the eighteenth century, we can reasonably assume all of the following except

- A. more people in America could read in 1850 than in 1700.
- B. newspapers became an increasingly important source of information during this period.
- C. the quality of writing in newspapers improved during the period in discussion.
- D. one of the results of the American Revolution was to encourage people to be better informed; one way to be better informed was to read the newspaper.

124. All but which one of the following are mentioned as means by which Americans selected their own information by the mid-nineteenth century?

- A. Individual temperament
- B. Occupation
- C. Social class
- D. Geographical location

125. Although Richard Brown usually read diaries of little-known people, he did study the diaries of a few major figures, including

- A. Alexander Hamilton and Benjamin Franklin.
- B. John Adams and Samuel Sewall.
- C. Patrick Henry and Thomas Jefferson.
- D. George Washington and Henry Clay.

126. In the early 1700s, in what is today the United States, people read newspapers to

- A. better understand the views of others.
- B. get the official text of treaties and speeches.
- C. read the political satire of the time.
- D. follow literary events.

127. The idea that the people need to be well informed developed during the

- A. eighteenth century as newspapers became more widely available.
- B. eighteenth century because new technologies made information more available.
- C. early nineteenth century because of an expanded need for leadership in the United States.
- D. early nineteenth century as a product of the American Revolution.

128. According to the article, the primary method of obtaining information in the eighteenth century was

- I. word of mouth.
- II. newspapers.
- III. town meetings.

- A. I only
- B. II only
- C. I and II only
- D. II and III only

GO ON TO THE NEXT PAGE

Passage VIII (Questions 129–135)

In order to understand and deal with the acid rain problem, programs that examine possible control measures and increase scientific knowledge have been developed and are being carried out cooperatively by the United States and Canada.

Initially, sulphur and sulphuric compounds were selected for study because they were known to be capable of causing damage over large areas of eastern North America and because of the prospect for substantial increases in the atmospheric sulphur load in connection with the United States's plans to increase the use of coal. Scientists in both the United States and Canada are also examining other major pollutants, such as the oxides of nitrogen, heavy metals, hydrocarbons, and fine particles. Similar studies are being made in Scandinavia.

Results of these early studies enabled the two countries to recognize and clarify the time-sensitive nature and the ultimate irreversibility of the impact of acid rain. A national program was recently modified to meet two clearly stated objectives; one aimed at short-term efforts and the other at long-term efforts. Elements of this program include emission inventories, the systematic study of precipitation, and the study of the progressive deterioration of the watersheds and fish population.

Long-range transport of air pollution represents a serious environmental problem for Canada. While much scientific work still needs to be carried out, some action must be taken as soon as possible. Such action not only should prevent further increases in emissions but also should reduce emissions from their current levels. Action by Canada alone will be insufficient in view of the continental dimension of the problem and the climatic behavior that favors transport of United States's pollutants over Canada.

In recognition of the importance of the task at hand, Canada looks forward to close cooperation with the United States, particularly through the development of a bilateral agreement.

129. According to the article, a planned United States increase in its burning of coal will increase the atmospheric load of

A. hydrocarbons.
B. sulphuric compounds.
C. fine particles.
D. sulphur.

130. The article emphasizes the ability of the United States and Canada to work cooperatively on the acid-rain program. Which of the following offers the best assessment of the advantage of such cooperation?

A. Neighboring countries can develop and implement mutually beneficial programs that increase understanding and control of environmental problems.
B. Neighboring countries can reinforce close working relations based on governmental research.
C. Neighboring countries working together increase and strengthen their nationalistic programs on environmental issues.
D. Neighboring countries have no choice but to work together to confront mutual environmental concerns.

131. The first compounds that were selected for study were

A. sulphur and sulphuric compounds.
B. ozone and hydrocarbons.
C. sulphur and hydrochloric acid.
D. sulphuric compounds and oxides of nitrogen.

132. The article points out that climatic conditions result in transport of pollutants from

A. Canada to the United States.
B. the United States to Canada.
C. the United States to Sweden.
D. east to west across the United States.

133. The article states that the damage done by acid rain to ponds and forests is

    A.   irreversible.
    B.   reversible over a short period of time.
    C.   reversible with bilateral action.
    D.   reversible over a long period of time.

134. The article implies that a forceful, aggressive program to resolve problems with acid rain must be undertaken

    I.   with close cooperation between the United States and Canada.
    II.   with the United States always taking the initiative.
    III.   among governments of the world despite its great cost.

    A.   I only
    B.   II only
    C.   I and II only
    D.   I and III only

135. The writer of the article suggests that while more research must be done, the two actions that must be taken are a

    A.   ban on the burning of coal and an increase in the budget for research.
    B.   bilateral action by the United States and Canada to freeze emissions at their current level and to work to reduce those emissions in the future.
    C.   multinational agreement between Sweden, the United States, and Canada to freeze emissions at their current level and then to reduce them.
    D.   unilateral commitment to studying water sheds and fish population.

Passage IX (Questions 136–142)

In 1855, when the population of the United States was about one-ninth what it is today, and when nineteen states had yet to join the Union, Thomas Bulfinch's *The Age of Fable; or, Stories of Gods and Heroes* began its long and influential life. Americans may confuse the author with his architect father, Charles Bulfinch; nevertheless, in the American mind, the name of Bulfinch is indelibly associated with classical mythology.

Without a doubt, *The Age of Fable* formed the image that millions of Americans had of the classical gods and heroes . . . . The mythology learned by Americans was Bulfinch's mythology . . . Bulfinch did not . . . simply adapt the myths for contemporary readers, . . . he wrote to instruct by making the material entertaining. "Thus we hope to teach mythology," he explains in his preface, "not as a study, but as a relaxation from study; to give our work the charm of a story-book, yet by means of it to impart a knowledge of an important branch of education." Bulfinch recreated dozens of myths, discussed their use in modern poetry, and wrote for both adults and young people.

The Age of Fable consists of prose narratives of classical myths, chiefly from Ovid (as well as some stories from Norse, Oriental, and Egyptian mythologies); information about ancient classical writers and artists; and lists for reference. Intertwined with Bulfinch's narrative are myth-related quotations from poetry, chiefly British. The subject of the book, he emphasizes in his preface, is not just mythology, but "mythology as connected with literature."

Bulfinch's strong background in classical literature, especially Roman, accounts for his success in adapting Ovid for American readers. Although he included material from other ancient authors, notably Homer and Virgil, the majority of the myths in *The Age of Fable* are his own translations from the *Metamorphoses*, the chief source for classical myth in Western literature and art. Bulfinch abridged, bowdlerized, and rearranged Ovid, and at times he added a tidbit or two from other sources. Yet, his translations of the ancient author's power-

GO ON TO THE NEXT PAGE

fully wrought details of physical description and human behavior convey Ovidian sprightliness and charm.

Having retold Ovid's story, Bulfinch notes in passing that it is an allegory for the seasons, and he then shifts into "poetical citations," as he calls them in his preface, which illustrate the use of the myth of Proserpine by modern poets. Annotating as he quotes, he cites short passages from Milton (whom he quotes forty times in *The Age of Fable*); Thomas Hood; Coleridge; and, in two separate passages, one of his favorites, the Irish poet Thomas Moore.

Bulfinch drew his 188 "citations" from the work of forty poets. All were British except for three—Longfellow, Lowell, and Stephen Greenleaf Bulfinch, brother of the author. The shining lights of English literature—Milton, Coleridge, Spenser, Shakespeare, Dryden, Pope, Swift, Wordsworth, Keats, Shelley, and Tennyson—dominate. Also included, however, are some of the minor poets popular in Bulfinch's time, for example, Erasmus Darwin, Charles Darwin's uncle.

In using poetry as a counterpoint in *The Age of Fable*, Bulfinch was tapping into an interest of the general educated public. His criterion for choosing selections, he explains in his preface, was popularity; these are passages that "are most frequently quoted or alluded to in reading or conversation." Many of the poets who appear in *The Age of Fable* are represented in William Holmes McGuffey's *Eclectic Readers* and also in the "gift books." A phenomenon of Bulfinch's era, those literary annuals containing poetry, stories, and moral maxims were great favorites with middle-class Americans and helped create, in that level of society, a demand for literature and art.

What led Bulfinch . . . to put together the combination of ancient myth and modern poetry that is *The Age of Fable*? . . . Unquestionably, he was following the altruistic example of his architect father and hoping to serve an American public confronted by enormous societal change. He was responding, in particular, to the rise of science and technology, a decline in classical learning and increasing educational opportunities . . . For the purpose of educating his fellow citizens, Bulfinch directed his book to . . . out-of-school audiences. He imagined *The Age of Fable* not in a classroom, but in the "parlor." His audience was not to be schoolchildren, but "the reader of English literature, of either sex," others "more advanced" who may require mythological knowledge when they visit museums or "mingle in cultivated society," and also, readers "in advanced life."

The presence of *The Age of Fable* . . . across America for well over a hundred years has assured for Bulfinch a place as progenitor of the strong American fascination with classical mythology in art and literature . . . What Bulfinch proves is that in America the poetry and story of our common classical past are not for the few, but for the many.

136. The popularity of *The Age of Fable* during the latter part of the nineteenth century can be interpreted as being due to all of the following reasons except

- A. the public's acceptance of the combination of classical mythology and modern poetry as devised by Bulfinch.
- B. the growth of an educated public and its interest in and use of references from the book in everyday speech and reading material.
- C. the appeal of the book to an increasingly sophisticated adult audience.
- D. a reflection of the waning influence of classical learning due to the Industrial Revolution.

137. Which of the following was not one of Bulfinch's intents in writing *The Age of Fable*?

- A. To provide didactic entertainment
- B. To generate interest in translations of a classical work
- C. To reach an audience of adults and young people
- D. To educate schoolchildren in particular

138. One can infer from the article that the predominance of the poets cited by Bulfinch indicates a

    I. strongly American influence.
    II. heavily British influence.
    III. distinctly European influence.

    A. I only
    B. II only
    C. III only
    D. II and III only

139. The widespread appeal of Bulfinch's rewriting of ancient mythology during the nineteenth century does not reflect which one of the following?

    A. A fairly well-read and well-educated middle class of Americans
    B. A demand for writings reflecting a tradition in classical works
    C. A strong feeling among Americans of the necessity to revamp the educational system
    D. A trend among most Americans to quote or read passages for conversation

140. Using classical literature as his basis, Bulfinch was demonstrating the nineteenth-century's educational tendency to

    A. borrow from the past to explain the present.
    B. look upon a foundation in the classics as a reflection of a proper education.
    C. inculcate a teaching method accessible to the affluent.
    D. generate learning through memorization of ancient works.

141. The author suggests that the enduring popularity of *The Age of Fable* cannot be attributed to which one of the following?

    A. American interest in and attraction to classical literature
    B. An interplay of interesting narrative stories and poetry
    C. Bulfinch's ability to interpret and translate classical work with skill and intelligence
    D. The inclusion of well-known British writers

142. One can infer from the article that the author believes Bulfinch's legacy to the American public is a work that

    A. successfully introduced classical mythology interspersed with literature.
    B. was dedicated to preserving a segment of classical mythology in order to educate the American people.
    C. reflected the importance of both classical mythology and mid-nineteenth-century British writers.
    D. successfully preserved classical mythology while instructing the educated.

END OF TEST 2.

IF YOU FINISH BEFORE THE TIME IS UP,
YOU MAY CHECK YOUR WORK ON THIS TEST ONLY.

WRITING SAMPLE

TIME: 60 MINUTES   **2 ESSAYS**

Directions: This test consists of two parts. You will have 30 minutes to complete each part. During the first 30 minutes, you may work on Part 1 only. During the second 30 minutes, you may work on Part 2 only. You will have three pages for each essay answer, but you do not have to fill all three pages. Be sure to write legibly; illegible essays will not be scored.

Part 1

Consider this statement:

> Most bad habits are tools to help us through life.

Write a unified essay in which you perform the following tasks. Explain what you think the above statement means. Describe a specific situation in which most bad habits are *not* tools that help individuals through life. Discuss what you think determines whether such habits become useful in assisting individuals through life.

DO NOT START THE NEXT TOPIC UNTIL THE TIME IS UP.

Part 2

Consider this statement:

> If you don't learn, you will always find someone else to do it for you.

Write a unified essay in which you perform the following tasks. Explain what you think the above statement means. Describe a specific situation in which one learns on his or her own without relying on another individual to do it. Discuss what you think determines whether learning on one's own enables someone to avoid relying on others.

END OF TEST 3.
DO NOT RETURN TO PART 1.

BIOLOGICAL SCIENCES

Directions: This test contains 77 questions. Most of the questions consist of a descriptive passage followed by a group of questions related to the passage. For these questions, study the passage carefully and then choose the best answer to each question in the group. Some questions in this test stand alone. These questions are independent of any passage and independent of each other. For these questions, too, you must select the one best answer. Indicate all your answers by blackening the corresponding circles on your answer sheet.

A Periodic Table is provided at the beginning of this unit (page 564). You may consult it whenever you wish.

Passage I (Questions 143–148)

Carbohydrates, fats, and proteins can all be utilized as sources of material for making ATP in cellular respiration. The figure below shows how each of these food molecules can enter the respiratory pathway.

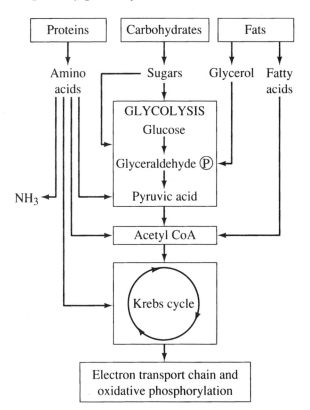

143. Beta oxidation is the process in which fatty acids are converted to a substance that feeds into the respiratory pathway. What is the name of this substance?

   A.   Glycerol
   B.   Glyceraldehyde phosphate (PGAL)
   C.   Acetyl CoA
   D.   Glucose

144. One reason fatty acids are excellent sources of fuel is that, gram for gram, they are richer in hydrogens than in glucose. Which of the following is the best estimate of how many ATP molecules a 6-carbon fatty acid would yield if it were completely metabolized in cellular respiration?

   A.   Between 2 and 18
   B.   Between 18 and 24
   C.   Between 24 and 36
   D.   More than 36

GO ON TO THE NEXT PAGE

145. When utilized in cellular respiration, amino acids are deaminated before being metabolized further. After deamination, alanine becomes pyruvic acid, glutamate is converted to alpha-ketoglutarate, and aspartate yields oxaloacetate. Based on information in the figure, alpha-ketoglutarate and oxaloacetate are probably

- A. acetyl CoA.
- B. hydrogen acceptors in the electron transport chain.
- C. Krebs cycle intermediates.
- D. None of the above.

146. In the human body, what happens to the ammonia (NH_3) that results from the deamination of amino acids?

- A. Most is converted to uric acid before being eliminated in the urine.
- B. Most is converted to urea before being eliminated in the urine.
- C. Most is converted to creatinine before being eliminated in the urine.
- D. Most is eliminated in the urine without further conversion.

147. According to information in the figure, where in the cell does glycerol enter the respiratory pathway?

- A. In the cytoplasm
- B. Inside the mitochondrial matrix
- C. Along the inner mitochondrial membranes (cristae)
- D. In the intermembranous space of the mitochondria

148. If the same molecule forms as an intermediate in more than one catabolic pathway, it can often be used in the conversion of one type of substance to another. Therefore, acetyl CoA should enable the body to convert

- A. amino acids to fat.
- B. glucose to fat.
- C. starch to fat.
- D. All of the above.

Passage II (Questions 149–154)

A number of historic experiments were designed to identify characteristics of the genetic material. In 1928, Frederick Griffith showed that genetic information could be transferred from dead bacteria (heat-killed) to living bacteria of a different strain. It was not until years later that this genetic material was finally confirmed to be DNA.

Experiments 1 and 2

In 1952, Hershey and Chase examined how the bacteriophage T2 infects the intestinal bacterium *E. coli*. They knew that viruses were composed of proteins and DNA, and they used radioactive isotopes of phosphorus and sulfur to label the viral components. After previously labeled phage was mixed in a test tube with bacterial cells long enough to ensure infection, the mixture was agitated in a blender in order to dislodge all viral components that had not entered the bacterial cell. The mixture was then centrifuged at high speed, separating the dislodged viral fraction and bacterial fraction from each other. Two similar experiments were carried out separately. In Experiment 1, only radioactive sulfur was used. In Experiment 2, only radioactive phosphorus was used.

149. After centrifugation, which of the organisms would be expected in each of the two separated fractions (sedimentary pellet at the bottom vs. suspended supernatant at the top)?

- A. Heavier bacterial cells in the supernatant; lighter dislodged viral particles in the pellet
- B. Heavier dislodged viral particles in the supernatant; lighter bacterial cells in the pellet
- C. Lighter bacterial cells in the supernatant; heavier dislodged viral particles in the pellet
- D. Lighter dislodged viral particles in the supernatant; heavier bacterial cells in the pellet

150. Based on how viruses infect bacteria, which fraction would be expected to contain radioactively labeled material in Experiment 1?

A. The fraction containing dislodged viral particles of protein
B. The fraction containing infected *E. coli* cells made of bacterial proteins and DNA
C. Both A and B
D. Neither A nor B

151. In Experiment 2, only the fraction containing infected bacterial cells should be labeled. Which of the following best explains this expectation?

A. Viral DNA and proteins were labeled and both are inside the bacteria.
B. Vital and bacterial DNA were labeled and both are inside the bacteria.
C. Only vital DNA was labeled and it is now inside the bacteria.
D. Viral and bacterial proteins were labeled and are both being synthesized by the bacteria.

152. If the infected *E. coli* were returned to a normal, unlabeled culture medium so that the infection had additional time to run its course, the bacterial cells (after growing for many generations) would lyse and many new phages would be released. Which hypothesis is most reasonable?

A. All released phages would contain labeled DNA.
B. No released phages would contain labeled DNA.
C. Most released phages would contain labeled DNA.
D. Most released phages would contain unlabeled DNA.

153. In the 1940s, Beadle and Tatum, working with the red bread mold *Neurospora*, used irradiation to cause mutations in various biosynthetic pathways. When one of the mutant strains could grow on *complete medium* (all essential nutritional ingredients included), but not on *minimal medium* (various nutrients missing that the organism can normally synthesize on its own), a mutation in such a synthetic pathway was suggested. To identify the specific nutrient no longer being synthesized by the organism, an experimenter might try to grow samples of

A. different strains (each with a different biosynthetic mutation) together on the same minimal medium.
B. one strain on different minimal media (each medium having one different nutrient added).
C. different strains (each with a different biosynthetic mutation) together on the same complete medium.
D. one strain on different media with different combinations of nutrients.

154. In their experiments, Beadle and Tatum occasionally observed *different* mutant strains that could not synthesize the exact same nutrient. Since such biosynthetic pathways were known to involve many steps, these observations provided evidence suggesting that

A. different mutations affect different synthetic pathways.
B. different mutations affect different enzymes involved in the same pathway.
C. different nutrients are synthesized in different pathways.
D. All of the above.

GO ON TO THE NEXT PAGE

Passage III (Questions 155–161)

Imagine a species of plant with two varieties: dark flowers (due to the dominant allele A) and light flowers (due to the recessive allele a). If the two purebred varieties were pollinated in a typical monohybrid cross, dark flowers would be expected to outnumber light flowers 3:1 in the F_2 generation. It would seem reasonable, therefore, that after a number of generations, the dominant allele would become increasingly prevalent at the expense of the recessive allele. According to the Hardy-Weinberg Equilibrium, however, unless "evolutionary" factors are at work, the two allele frequencies in the breeding population should not change from generation to generation.

Since A and a are the only alleles present in the population for flower shade (algebraically represented by p and q, respectively), the sum of these two allele frequencies, regardless of the genotypes in which they are found, must be 100% ($p + q = 1$). All individuals in this population must have one of these genotypes: AA, Aa, or aa. A homozygous dominant (AA) individual can only come about at fertilization if both gametes carry the A allele. The probability of this occurring is $p \times p = p^2$. Similarly, the probability of an individual being homozygous recessive is $q \times q = q^2$. A heterozygote (Aa) can result from both an $A \times a$ cross or an $a \times A$ cross. Thus, the probability of either of these combinations occurring is $(q \times p) + (p \times q) = 2pq$. The sum of all genotypes in the population is:

$$p^2 + 2pq + q^2 = 1$$

155. In a population of 1000 plants in which 910 have dark flowers, there can only be 90 with light flowers. What are the frequencies of each allele?

A. $p = .7$; $q = .3$
B. $p = .3$; $q = .7$
C. $p = .9$; $q = .1$
D. $p = .1$; $q = .9$

156. Referring to the plant population described in Question 155, how many plants are homozygous dominant?

A. .49
B. .81
C. 490
D. 810

157. In the plant population described in Question 155, what proportion of individuals will be heterozygotes?

A. .18
B. .09
C. .50
D. .42

158. Which of the following would have no effect on the allele frequencies observed in the next generation of the plant population described in Question 155?

A. Predatory caterpillars that preferred the dark- flowered variety
B. Insect pollinators that could see the light flowers more easily
C. The dark-flowered variety's pollen grains, which are dispersed more easily by winds
D. None of the above.

159. If approximately one in every 2500 white individuals in the United States is affected by the autosomal recessive disease cystic fibrosis, what are the frequencies of both the dominant and recessive alleles in the population?

A. $p = 2499$; $q = 1$
B. $p = .9996$; $q = .0004$
C. $p = .98$; $q = .02$
D. $p = .96$; $q = .04$

160. Based on the information in Question 159, how many white Americans (out of 2500) are carriers for cystic fibrosis?

A. Approximately 1
B. Approximately 4
C. Approximately 10
D. Approximately 100

161. The cystic fibrosis allele originated as a result of

A. genetic drift.
B. mutation.
C. nonrandom mating.
D. gene migration.

Passage IV (Questions 162–167)

The evolutionary origin of viruses remains a mystery.

Hypothesis A

One hypothesis is that the ancestors of modern viruses were free-living heterotrophs that evolved in the early seas and fed on the organic molecules around them. By the time these nutrients became depleted, other heterotrophic and autotrophic forms may have begun to appear, and viruses adapted to a parasitic lifestyle.

Hypothesis B

A second hypothesis favors the idea that viruses evolved from a cellular form and subsequently became highly specialized parasites. So specialized were they, that they "lost" almost all of their cellular components except the nuclear (genetic) material.

Hypothesis C

A third hypothesis is that viruses arose from bits of nucleic acid that escaped from cellular organisms. They may have survived at first without any form of outer covering before evolving their specialized coats. Various viruses may have arisen this way from different kinds of organisms.

162. Which hypothesis views viruses as having evolved independently from prokaryotes and eukaryotes?

A. Hypothesis A
B. Hypothesis B
C. Hypothesis C
D. None of the above

163. Which of the following questions would be especially difficult to answer for a proponent of the view that viruses predate cells?

A. Why are viruses so much smaller than cellular forms?
B. How could viruses reproduce before cells evolved?
C. From what precursor molecules could viral DNA and viral proteins have formed?
D. From what source could viruses have obtained nourishment?

164. Which piece of evidence would strongly support only hypothesis C?

A. Viral genetic material is usually made of the same type of nucleic acid as that of the viruses' hosts.
B. Sometimes, viral genes are virtually identical to host-cell genes.
C. Viruses are well adapted as parasites to their host cells.
D. Viruses are all very similar in their genetic makeup.

GO ON TO THE NEXT PAGE

165. Which hypothesis views cells as having evolved *before* viruses?

   A. Hypothesis A
   B. Hypothesis B
   C. Hypothesis C
   D. Hypotheses B and C

166. Which hypothesis appears strongest in view of the frequent observation today that there is greater genetic similarity between viruses and their hosts than between types of viruses?

   A. Hypothesis A
   B. Hypothesis B
   C. Hypothesis C
   D. Hypotheses B and C

167. Which of the following is not implied by hypothesis A?

   A. Photosynthetic organisms evolved after viruses.
   B. Viral ancestors could absorb.
   C. Viral ancestors required host cells to reproduce.
   D. Viral ancestors could metabolize food on their own.

Passage V (Questions 168–174)

A survivorship curve is a representation of the age structure of a population. It shows the number of individuals still alive at each age. The pattern exhibited by a survivorship curve can provide valuable information about an organism's life history characteristics. By examining these curves, we can deduce information concerning a population's average life expectancy, mortality rate, proportion surviving at each age, number dying at each age, potential for growth, and vulnerable periods within the life cycle. The following figure shows three generalized types of survivorship curves, each representing organisms with different combinations of life history characteristics. Each type of organism successfully mates, reproduces, and leaves adequate numbers of offspring to maintain species continuity in its environment.

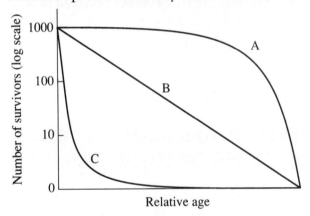

168. Which curve represents a species in which most individuals die before reaching reproductive age?

   A. Curve A
   B. Curve B
   C. Curve C
   D. Curves B and C

169. Which of the following life history characteristics would assure the survival of a species in which most individuals die before reaching reproductive age?

   A. Individuals mate and produce few offspring at a late age.
   B. Individuals produce high numbers of offspring with each mating episode.
   C. Individuals have long courtship periods before carefully choosing mates.
   D. Breeding pairs have few mating episodes but pairs are well distributed across the breeding grounds.

170. Which survivorship curve suggests that mortality occurs as a result of relatively random events with little age bias?

   A. Curve A
   B. Curve B
   C. Curve C
   D. None of the above

171. According to the figure, the highest mortality rate appears to be associated with

   A. curve A—late in life.
   B. curve B—from midlife to late in life.
   C. curve C—early in life.
   D. Both A and C.

172. Which of the following combinations of environmental and life history characteristics is likely to be associated with survivorship curve A?

   A. Late reproductive age, severe predation of young
   B. Few offspring, extensive parental care
   C. Many offspring, limited resources
   D. Limited parental care, severe predation of young

173. "Individuals alive halfway through the average maximum life span can expect little or no increase in their probability of dying." For which survivorship curves is this statement correct?

   A. Curves A and B
   B. Curves A and C
   C. Curves B and C
   D. Curves A, B, and C

174. Which of the survivorship curves represents the longest maximum life span?

   A. Curve A
   B. Curve B
   C. Curve C
   D. Maximum life spans are the same

Passage VI (Questions 175–181)

A number of experiments have been performed to examine possible mechanisms of development.

Experiment 1

In amphibians, the first cleavage division produces two blastomeres that equally divide the gray crescent, a region near the equator of the egg. When the two blastomeres are separated, each can develop into a normal tadpole. If the zygote is manipulated so that the first cleavage division does not pass through the gray crescent, and these two blastomeres are separated as before, only the one containing the gray crescent develops normally.

Experiment 2

Skin cells from a spotted frog were grown in tissue culture. The nuclei from the cells were transplanted into unfertilized eggs of an unspotted frog whose nuclei had been removed. When grown in the proper environment, a small percentage of these eggs subsequently formed blastulas and eventually developed into tadpoles and adults.

GO ON TO THE NEXT PAGE

Experiment 3

In the 1920s, it was found that the dorsal lip of the blastopore acts as an organizer of early amphibian development in such a way that surrounding cells eventually form the notocord, neural plate, and neural tube. Later in development, the neural tube gives rise to the brain and spinal cord. When dorsal lip cells from one embryo were transplanted to another embryo (into a region where these cells are not usually found), a second brain and spinal cord often developed. In some cases, a second head could be seen growing out of the belly!

175. Which of the following is one conclusion that can be drawn from Experiment 1?

    A. Under normal circumstances, the fate of embryonic cells is determined by the first division of the zygote.
    B. Materials outside cells can have a profound effect on the fate of cells.
    C. After the first division, cells normally retain the potential to form all parts of the organism (totipotency).
    D. The directional plane of the first cleavage division plays no role in determining the developmental fate of cells.

176. Experiment 1 also clearly demonstrates that

    A. cytoplasmic contents are not important at this stage of development.
    B. totipotency can be transferred from one cell to another.
    C. the absence of nuclear material does not limit the developmental potential of a blastomere.
    D. cytoplasmic contents affect the developmental fate of cells at this stage.

177. In Experiment 2, what is the expected appearance of frogs that successfully completed development?

    A. All should be unspotted.
    B. 50% should be spotted, 50% should be unspotted (1:1 ratio).
    C. 75% should be spotted, 25% should be unspotted (3:1 ratio).
    D. All should be spotted.

178. Were any findings from Experiment 1 also demonstrated by Experiment 2?

    A. Yes, cells can retain their totipotency (even after development has been completed).
    B. Yes, different cytoplasmic ingredients in the enucleated cells clearly affected the fates of the developing cells.
    C. No, too many of the enucleated eggs did not successfully develop.
    D. No, nuclei from spotted frogs were no longer affected by their own normal cellular environment.

179. Results from Experiment 3 demonstrate that

    A. cytoplasmic factors are of major importance in determining the developmental fate of cells.
    B. nuclear material is secondary to environmental cues in development.
    C. tissue induction takes place in development.
    D. totipotency can be nullified by environmental factors.

180. The organizing effects of the dorsal lip cells can normally be observed

   A. during cleavage.
   B. in the early blastula.
   C. during early gastrulation.
   D. during early organogenesis.

181. Experiments 1-3 indicate that although cells can retain the genetic potential to form all parts of the organism during development

   A. environmental factors inside and outside the cell influence the expression of that potential.
   B. interaction between genes and cytoplasmic factors occurs.
   C. interaction between genes and other tissues occurs.
   D. All of the above.

Passage VII (Questions 182–187)

Animals move in a variety of ways. Each method of movement results in an energy cost to the organism that is dependent, in part, on the size of the organism. Some organisms are specialized for aquatic movement, others for terrestrial movement, still others for flight. The following figure shows the energy costs of different methods of locomotion for animals of different size.

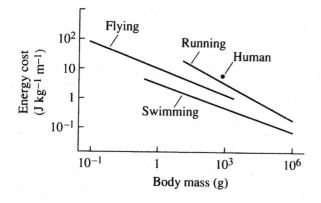

182. Based on the figure, what seems to be the most efficient mode of locomotion, pound for pound?

   A. Running
   B. Flying
   C. Swimming
   D. Flying and swimming (both activities have similar slopes)

183. In J/kg/m (log scale), what is the energy cost of flying for a 1-g (log scale) beast?

   A. 10^2
   B. 10
   C. 1
   D. Less than 1

184. According to the figure, which is the more efficient mode of locomotion for a human?

   A. Running
   B. Swimming
   C. Both are equally efficient
   D. Cannot be determined

185. Based on the figure, which statement is correct?

   A. If two individuals use the same method of movement, the smaller individual is usually more efficient.
   B. If two individuals use the same method of movement, the larger individual is always more efficient.
   C. Body mass is inversely proportional to energy cost.
   D. Neither A, B, nor C is correct for all methods of movement.

GO ON TO THE NEXT PAGE

186. Which of the following would be expected to move with the greatest energy cost (J/kg/m)?

    A. A running human
    B. A 1-g flyer
    C. A 10^3-g swimmer
    D. A 10^6-g runner

187. Which of the following would be expected to move with the least energy cost (J/kg/m)?

    A. A mosquito
    B. A horse
    C. A blue whale
    D. A cheetah

Passage VIII (Questions 188–193)

A heterocyclic compound contains a ring with more than one kind of atom. The ring of heterocyclic amines contains carbon and nitrogen. They are a very important kind of amino compound; for example, the bases of DNA are heterocyclic amines. The most important property of heterocyclic amines is their basicity due to the presence of nitrogen. Some examples are shown below.

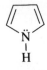 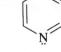 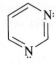

   Pyrrole   Pyridine   Pyrimidine

188. Pyrrole, pyridine, and pyrimidine all have abnormally low heats of combustion and tend to undergo reactions in which their ring is retained, i.e., substitution reactions. These properties are consistent with

    A. conjugated dienes.
    B. aromatic compounds.
    C. bases.
    D. alkenes.

189. Which of the following statements is true about the extra pair of electrons in pyrrole and pyridine?

    A. In pyrrole, an sp^2 orbital contains the pair of electrons, while in pyridine, they are involved in the π cloud.
    B. In both pyrrole and pyridine, an sp^2 orbital contains the pair of electrons.
    C. In both pyrrole and pyridine, they are involved in the π cloud.
    D. In pyrrole, they are involved in the π cloud, while in pyridine, an $sp^2$2 orbital contains the pair of electrons.

190. Pyridine is a much stronger base than pyrrole because

    A. pyrrole will lose its aromatic character if nitrogen accepts H^+.
    B. pyridine has a pair of electrons in an sp^2 orbital that is available for sharing.
    C. the extra pair of electrons on nitrogen in pyrrole is involved in the π cloud and therefore less available for sharing.
    D. All of the above.

191. Pyrrole undergoes electrophilic substitution at position 2 because

    A. the carbocation intermediate has more resonance structures than the intermediate formed when the electrophile attacks position 3.
    B. the inductive effect of N is greater.
    C. the aromatic ring is maintained in the carbocation.
    D. resonance structures cannot be drawn for the carbocation intermediate formed by the attack at position 3.

192. Pyridine undergoes nucleophilic substitution more readily than electrophilic substitution. Which of the following is a reasonable explanation?

    A. The N atom can better stabilize the carbanion intermediate than the carbocation intermediate.

    B. No resonance structures can be drawn for the intermediate formed by the attack of an electrophile.

    C. Nitrogen cannot expand its octet.

    D. The nitrogen atom repels electrophiles.

193. Piperidine $\overset{\frown}{N}$ is formed by the catalytic
             |
             H
reduction of pyridine. It is found in some alkaloids, such as nicotine and cocaine. One would expect the basicity of piperidine to be similar to that of

    A. pyridine.
    B. pyrrole.
    C. dimethylamine.
    D. aniline.

Passage IX (Questions 194–199)

These experiments were performed to study esterification reactions.

Experiment 1

Labeled $CH_3{}^{18}OH$ reacted with acetic acid to form methyl acetate enriched in ^{18}O

$$CH_3-\overset{O}{\overset{\|}{C}}-OH + CH_3{}^{18}OH \rightleftarrows CH_3-\overset{O}{\overset{\|}{C}}-{}^{18}OCH_3 + H_2O$$

Experiment 2

Acetic acid was reacted with several alcohols. The rate of esterification increased according to

$$CH_3-\underset{\underset{OH}{|}}{\overset{\overset{CH_3}{|}}{C}}-CH_3 < CH_3-\overset{\overset{CH_3}{|}}{CH}-OH < CH_3CH_2OH < CH_3OH$$

Experiment 3

Ethanol was reacted with several carboxylic acids. The rate of esterification increased according to

$$(CH_3)_3CCOOH < (CH_3)_2CHCOOH < CH_3CH_2COOH < CH_3COOH$$

194. The results of Experiment 1 indicate that in esterification, the bond that is cleaved
                           O
                           ‖
in the carboxylic acid, $R-\overset{O}{\overset{\|}{C}}-OH$, is which of the following?

    A. C$\nmid$OH
    B. R$\nmid$C
    C. CO$\nmid$H
    D. O
        $\overset{\text{⫪}}{C}$

195. The mechanism for the acid-catalyzed
                           O
                           ‖
hydrolysis of ester, $R-\overset{O}{\overset{\|}{C}}-OR'$, involves the breaking of which of the following bonds?

    A. R$\nmid$C
    B. C$\nmid$OR'
    C. CO$\nmid$R'
    D. O
        $\overset{\text{⫪}}{C}$

GO ON TO THE NEXT PAGE

196. Strong acids catalyze both esterification and hydrolysis because

    A.   they add to the carbonyl carbon.

    B.   they protonate the alcoholic oxygen.

    C.   the carbonyl carbon is made more susceptible to attack by a nucleophile when the carbonyl oxygen is protonated.

    D.   they remove OH^- ions.

197. The results of Experiments 2 and 3 support which of the following statements?

    A.   The presence of bulky groups near the site of the reaction slows both esterification and hydrolysis reactions.

    B.   The presence of bulky groups on only the alcohol slows both esterification and hydrolysis reactions.

    C.   The presence of bulky groups near the site of the reaction slows esterification with no effect on hydrolysis.

    D.   The presence of bulky groups near the site of the reaction slows hydrolysis with no effect on esterification.

198. Basic hydrolysis of esters involves attack of OH^- and is essentially irreversible.

$$R-\overset{\overset{\textstyle O}{\|}}{C}-OR' + OH^- \rightarrow R-\overset{\overset{\textstyle O}{\|}}{C}-O^{\ominus} + R'OH$$

A basic hydrolysis reaction is carried out using a labeled ester:

$$CH_3-\overset{\overset{\textstyle O}{\|}}{C}-{}^{18}OC_2H_5 + OH^- \rightarrow CH_3-\overset{\overset{\textstyle O}{\|}}{C}-O^{\ominus} + C_2H_5\,{}^{18}OH$$

Therefore, in basic hydrolysis of an ester, cleavage occurs between

    A.   oxygen and the alkyl group of the alcohol.

    B.   the carbonyl carbon and the alkyl group of the acid.

    C.   the carbonyl carbon and the carbonyl oxygen.

    D.   oxygen and the acyl group.

199. Esterification and both acidic and basic hydrolysis reactions can be described as attack of

    A.   a nucleophile on the carbonyl carbon.

    B.   a nucleophile on an alkyl carbon.

    C.   an electrophile on the carbonyl carbon.

    D.   an electrophile on an alkyl carbon.

Infrared Absorption by Some Oxygen-Containing Compounds

Compound	O—H	C—O	C═O
Alcohols	3200-3600cm^{-1}	1000-1200cm^{-1}	—
Phenols	3200-3600	1140-1230	—
Ethers, aliphatic	—	1060-1150	—
Ethers, aromatic	—	1200-1275 1020-1075	—
Aldehydes, ketones	—	—	1675-1725cm^{-1}
Carboxylic acids	2500-3000	1250	1680-1725
Esters	—	1050-1300 (two bands)	1715-1740
Acid chlorides	—	—	1750-1810
Amides (RCONH$_2$)	(N—H 3050-3550)	—	1650-1690

Passage X (Questions 200–204)

The infrared spectrum of an organic compound composed of carbon, oxygen, and hydrogen shows strong absorptions at about 3350 cm^{-1}; 1000 cm^{-1}; and 675-870 cm^{-1}. The absorption at 3350 cm^{-1} is both strong and broad. The compound also exhibits strong absorption bonds in the ultraviolet region.

200. Based on the table, the infrared spectrum indicates which of the following oxygen-containing functional groups is (are) present?

A. Carbonyl and hydroxyl
B. Hydroxyl and ether
C. Carboxyl group
D. Hydroxyl group

201. Absorption in the ultraviolet region indicates the presence of

A. a conjugated structure or aromatic group.
B. an alkyl group.
C. one double bond.
D. an ether group.

202. The NMR spectrum contains several signals, one of which exhibits splitting only when a dry, pure sample is used. The splitting disappears on the addition of a trace acid or base. This same signal is absent in the NMR spectrum of the product formed by reaction with a carboxylic acid. The functional group that can account for this behavior is which of the following?

A.
$$\begin{array}{c} O \\ \parallel \\ H-C- \end{array}$$

B.
$$\begin{array}{c} O \\ \parallel \\ -C-OH \end{array}$$

C.
$$\begin{array}{c} | \\ -C-OH \\ | \end{array}$$

D.
$$\begin{array}{c} \quad\quad H \\ | \quad\quad | \\ -C-O-C- \\ | \quad\quad | \end{array}$$

GO ON TO THE NEXT PAGE

203. The infrared spectrum of the compound also contains moderate and weak bands associated with a mono-substituted benzene. Which of the following is the most likely structure of the compound?

A. ⬡—COOH

B. ⬡—CH₂OH

C. ⬡—O—CH₃

D. ⬡—CH₃

204. Which of the following spectroscopic techniques should be used to establish the presence of a carbonyl group in an organic molecule?

A. NMR
B. Ultraviolet spectroscopy
C. Infrared spectroscopy
D. Mass spectrometry

Questions 205–219 are independent of any passage and independent of each other.

205. Eukaryotic chromosomes consist of DNA in association with histone proteins. This association enables the genetic material to remain either tightly coiled, condensed, and visible as distinct chromosomes (only during mitosis), or loose and unwound as chromatin (during the rest of the cell cycle). DNA remains *uncoiled* during most of a cell's life so that

A. exposed nucleotides can efficiently provide phosphate groups for ATP production.
B. the larger surface area covered by the chromatin acts as a more efficient osmotic attractant.
C. transcription can take place when necessary.
D. ER channels cannot penetrate the nucleus.

206. During respiratory ventilation, impulses along the phrenic nerves stimulate the diaphragm, causing it to contract and move downward. When this occurs, which of the following takes place in the thoracic cavity and lungs?

A. Volume increases, pressure increases, and air moves out.
B. Volume decreases, pressure decreases, and air moves out.
C. Volume increases, pressure decreases, and air moves in.
D. Volume decreases, pressure increases, and air moves in.

207. Blood pressure is a function of cardiac output (heart rate × stroke volume), as well as peripheral resistance (a measure of friction between the blood and the blood vessel walls). Factors that can increase peripheral resistance include

A. vasoconstriction and low blood viscosity.
B. vasoconstriction and high blood viscosity.
C. vasodilation and low blood viscosity.
D. vasodilation and high blood viscosity.

208. Cerebrospinal fluid (CSF) is produced by special capillary networks in the brain called *choroid plexuses*. CSF circulates through the hollow regions of the brain and spinal cord and around the central nervous system, within its protective coverings. Areas that are part of the CSF pathway include the

A. ventricles, spinal canal, and cranial nerves.
B. ventricles, spinal canal, and meninges.
C. ventricles, spinal canal, and spinal nerves.
D. meninges, spinal canal, and cranial nerves.

209. The pedigree in the following diagram represents the inheritance of deaf-mutism over three generations within a family. (An arrow on a circle is a male, and a cross below a circle is a female; affected individuals have blackened circles). What kind of trait is deaf-mutism?

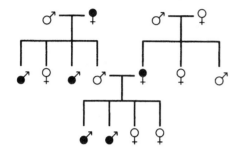

- A. Autosomal dominant
- B. Autosomal recessive
- C. Sex-linked dominant
- D. Sex-linked recessive

210. The human body has various ways to protect itself against pathogens, including specific and nonspecific defense mechanisms. The nonspecific defenses do not distinguish one pathogen from another. Which of the following would not be considered a component of the nonspecific defenses?

- A. Macrophages
- B. Inflammation
- C. Antibodies
- D. Interferon

211. The following diagram represents a major role played by enzymes in living systems. Which statement best describes this role?

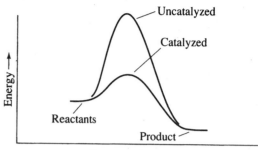

- A. Enzymes lower the barrier of activation energy.
- B. Enzymes allow metabolic reactions to be exergonic.
- C. Enzymes act as energy producers.
- D. Enzymes act as catalysts to slow down reactions.

212. Parkinsonism is a degeneration of the cerebrum's basal ganglia, which help regulate contractions of skeletal muscles through the release of the neurotransmitter dopamine. Symptoms can include tremor and/or rigidity, wide-eyed staring, and drooling. Intelligence, vision, and hearing remain unaffected by this disorder, which suggests that Parkinsonism does not attack

- A. the medulla oblongata.
- B. the diencephalon (thalamus and hypothalamus).
- C. the dorsal root ganglia.
- D. the cerebral cortex.

GO ON TO THE NEXT PAGE

213. Individuals with Turner's syndrome have 45 chromosomes (one sex chromosome is missing in the cells of these "XO" individuals). This usually is caused by meiotic nondisjunction during gametogenesis. Which statement is not correct concerning people with this disorder?

A. They are genetic females.
B. They are subject to sex-linked disorders at frequencies similar to those predicted for normal females.
C. The nondisjunction event could have occurred during meiosis in either the male or female parent.
D. If meiosis occurs in Turner's syndrome individuals, one daughter cell resulting from the first meiotic division will have no sex chromosome.

214. Rigor mortis, a condition in which skeletal muscles temporarily remain in a rigid state of partial contraction due to the absence of ATP, occurs a few hours after death. Which of the following steps is not necessary for muscle relaxation?

A. Repolarization of the sarcolemma
B. The return of calcium to the sarcoplasmic reticulum
C. The detachment of the troponin-tropomyosin complex from actin
D. The decomposition of acetylcholine by cholinesterase

215. In the presence of a base, two molecules of an aldehyde or a ketone can combine to form a β-hydroxyaldehyde or β-hydroxyketone in an aldol condensation. Which of the following compounds will not react in an aldol condensation?

A.
$$CH_3-\overset{\overset{\displaystyle O}{\|}}{C}-CH_3$$

B.
$$CH_3-\overset{\overset{\displaystyle O}{\|}}{C}-CH_2-\overset{\overset{\displaystyle O}{\|}}{C}-H$$

C.
$$CH_3-\overset{\overset{\displaystyle CH_3}{|}}{\underset{\underset{\displaystyle CH_3}{|}}{C}}-\overset{\overset{\displaystyle O}{\|}}{C}-H$$

D.
$$CH_3-\overset{\overset{\displaystyle CH_3}{|}}{\underset{\underset{\displaystyle H}{|}}{C}}-\overset{\overset{\displaystyle O}{\|}}{C}-H$$

216. How many amide linkages are in Ala-Gly-Phe?

A. 1
B. 3
C. 0
D. 2

217. The alcohol produced upon basic or acidic hydrolysis of a fat is which of the following?

A.
$$\underset{\underset{\displaystyle OH}{|}}{CH_2}-\underset{\underset{\displaystyle OH}{|}}{CH_2}$$

B. $CH_3-CH_2CH_2OH$

C.
$$CH_3-\underset{\underset{\displaystyle OH}{|}}{CH}-\underset{\underset{\displaystyle OH}{|}}{CH_2}$$

D.
$$\underset{\underset{\displaystyle OH}{|}}{CH_2}-\underset{\underset{\displaystyle OH}{|}}{CH}-\underset{\underset{\displaystyle OH}{|}}{CH_2}$$

218. Ortho-nitrophenol has a low boiling point and aqueous solubility due to

    A.   intermolecular H-bonding.
    B.   intramolecular H-bonding.
    C.   van der Waals forces.
    D.   London dispersion forces.

219. In the rod cells of the retina of a mammal, the conjugated protein rhodopsin is present. The prosthetic group of rhodopsin is 11-*cis*-retinal:

When light impinges on the retina, 11-*cis*-retinal is transformed into 11-*trans*-retinal:

Energy is then required to convert the *trans* isomer back into the less stable *cis* isomer. The difference in stability of the two isomers is due to

    A.   an inductive effect.
    B.   a resonance effect.
    C.   an isotope effect.
    D.   steric hindrance.

END OF TEST 4.

IF YOU FINISH BEFORE THE TIME IS UP, YOU MAY CHECK YOUR WORK ON THIS TEST ONLY.

ANSWER KEY

Physical Sciences		Verbal Reasoning		Biological Sciences	
1. C	40. D	78. A	111. B	143. C	182. C
2. A	41. D	79. D	112. A	144. D	183. B
3. D	42. C	80. A	113. B	145. C	184. B
4. B	43. D	81. A	114. C	146. B	185. B
5. D	44. C	82. A	115. B	147. A	186. B
6. C	45. B	83. B	116. D	148. D	187. C
7. D	46. A	84. B	117. B	149. D	188. B
8. D	47. B	85. B	118. B	150. A	189. D
9. C	48. D	86. D	119. C	151. C	190. D
10. B	49. B	87. A	120. A	152. D	191. A
11. C	50. C	88. A	121. B	153. B	192. A
12. D	51. B	89. C	122. B	154. B	193. C
13. D	52. B	90. D	123. C	155. A	194. A
14. D	53. A	91. A	124. D	156. C	195. B
15. D	54. D	92. C	125. B	157. D	196. C
16. B	55. B	93. D	126. B	158. D	197. A
17. A	56. B	94. A	127. D	159. C	198. D
18. B	57. D	95. D	128. A	160. D	199. A
19. C	58. B	96. D	129. D	161. B	200. D
20. D	59. B	97. C	130. D	162. A	201. A
21. D	60. A	98. B	131. A	163. B	202. C
22. B	61. B	99. A	132. B	164. B	203. B
23. B	62. B	100. B	133. A	165. D	204. C
24. B	63. C	101. D	134. A	166. C	205. C
25. B	64. C	102. C	135. B	167. C	206. C
26. C	65. D	103. C	136. D	168. C	207. B
27. D	66. C	104. B	137. D	169. B	208. B
28. A	67. B	105. B	138. B	170. B	209. B
29. C	68. B	106. D	139. C	171. D	210. C
30. C	69. B	107. C	140. B	172. B	211. A
31. B	70. D	108. A	141. D	173. C	212. D
32. A	71. A	109. D	142. D	174. D	213. B
33. C	72. A	110. D		175. C	214. C
34. A	73. C			176. D	215. C
45. D	74. D			177. D	216. D
36. D	75. B			178. A	217. D
37. D	76. B			179. C	218. B
38. C	77. A			180. D	219. D
39. A				181. D	

ANSWERS AND EXPLANATIONS

PHYSICAL SCIENCES

1. **The correct answer is (C).** Look for negative values of the standard free energy.

2. **The correct answer is (A).** Remember to use the fourth column and to use the factors of 2 in the equation.

3. **The correct answer is (D).** Use $[\left(\frac{10}{12}\right) C_p \Delta T]_{graphite} = [\left(\frac{10}{12}\right) C_p \Delta T]_{gaseous}$ C.

4. **The correct answer is (B).** Be careful to select only the three "saturated" hydrocarbons, i.e., those having the maximum hydrogens for a given number of carbons: CH_4, C_2H_6, and C_3H_8.

5. **The correct answer is (D).** Note that II is ruled out since double- and triple-bonded compounds in the examples have similar C_p's.

6. **The correct answer is (C).** $\Delta G°$ decreases as the number of Cl's increases: $\Delta H°$ follows an irregular trend.

7. **The correct answer is (D).** The balanced equation is $C_2H_6 + \frac{7}{2} O_2 \rightarrow$ $.3H_2O + 2CO_2$. Be certain to use $\Delta G°$ values from column 3, paying attention to coefficients.

8. **The correct answer is (D).** I is reflected in the lower values of $\Delta G°$ for the solid. II (but not III) is reflected in the higher $S°$ for the gas.

9. **The correct answer is (C).** The standard free energy of formation is 0 for both C and H_2, while for methane the value is -50.6. Thus, the free energy of the system decreases by 50.6 kJ/mol when methane is formed, as indicated in choice C.

10. **The correct answer is (B).** Use $K = \exp(-\Delta G°/RT) = 10^{-\Delta G°/2.3RT}$, where $\Delta G° = -258$. Note that choice C uses $\Delta H°$ (an error) and also ignores the factor of 2.3.

11. **The correct answer is (C).** The speed is lower for a heavier molecule:
$$\frac{v_{O_2}}{v_{H_2}} = \sqrt{\frac{mH_2}{m_{O_2}}} = \sqrt{\frac{2}{32}}$$

12. **The correct answer is (D).** Speed is proportional to $T^{\frac{1}{2}}$, where T is in K. So $v_2/v_1 = (T_2/T_1)^{\frac{1}{2}}$.

13. **The correct answer is (D).** Choose the point on the horizontal axis that corresponds to the peak of the "600K" curve.

14. **The correct answer is (D).** Estimate the fraction of the area under the curve that lies to the right of 1600 m/s.

15. **The correct answer is (D).** Refer to the answer to 12; if the temperature goes up by a factor of 4, from 300K to 1200K, the average speed will roughly double.

16. **The correct answer is (B).** Speed is the absolute value of velocity, so it is always zero or positive.

17. **The correct answer is (A).** The spread is greater for higher temperatures, not lower, and the most probable speed is proportional to the square root of the absolute temperature.

18. **The correct answer is (B).** 0.05 liter $\times$ 0.20 mol/liter = 0.010 mol NaOH added at endpoint.

19. **The correct answer is (C).** $V_aC_a = V_bC_b$ at endpoint, since moles of hydroxide added must equal moles of monoprotic weak acid initially present.

20. **The correct answer is (D).** The pH increases by about 1 unit, corresponding to a decrease in $[H^+]$ of a factor of 10.

21. **The correct answer is (D).** The ratio requested is the reciprocal slope of the curve.

22. **The correct answer is (B).** We will have added 50 mL of NaOH past the endpoint, so $[OH^-]$ will be the original concentration of NaOH diluted by a factor of 2, or 0.10. Then pOH = 1 and pH = 13.

23. **The correct answer is (B).** Halfway through the titration, at the 25-mL mark, pH closely approximates pK_a. Look for a pK_a close to 3.7 and you find formic acid.

24. **The correct answer is (B).** This route to the halfway point in the titration involves going all the way to the endpoint of a second sample, and then going halfway back: pH = pK_a.

25. **The correct answer is (B).** All but 20 percent of the original weak acid has been converted to weak base at 40 mL, since 40 mL is 80 percent of the way to the endpoint.

26. **The correct answer is (C).** Since the curve is so steep, either indicator should signal the value of V_{OH-} at the endpoint with equal accuracy.

27. **The correct answer is (D).** Although one of the four values of ΔH is negative, indicating that heat is released and that the reaction is *likely* to be spontaneous, we cannot answer the question with certainty unless we learn the value of the *entropy* for each reaction. A reaction is spontaneous if $\Delta G < 0$, where = $\Delta H - T\Delta S$.

28. **The correct answer is (A).** The question refers to Experiment 3, but in this case the products of the reaction as written are being converted to the reactants; thus, heat will be given off. There are 20 moles of Cl atoms compared with the 2 moles in the original equation, so ΔH_{diss} must be multiplied by 10 to determine the heat released.

29. **The correct answer is (C).** In pure water, $[Ag^+] = [Cl^-] = x$

$$x^2 = K_{sp} = 1.8 \times 10^{-10}$$
$$x = 1.3 \times 10^{-5} \text{ M}$$

30. **The correct answer is (C).** To answer this question, we need to add the equations referring to the sublimation of Ag(s) and the ionization of Ag(g):

$$\frac{\begin{aligned}Ag(s) \rightarrow Ag(g) \qquad & 286 \text{ kJ/mol}\\ Ag(g) \rightarrow Ag^+ + e^- \qquad & 728 \text{ kJ/mol/}\end{aligned}}{Ag(s) \rightarrow Ag^+ + e^- \qquad 1014 \text{ kJ/mol}}$$

Since only 0.10 mol of silver ion is produced, the energy required is (0.10)(1014) = 101.4 kJ/mol

31. **The correct answer is (B).** We need to add the following reactions to obtain the reaction desired:

$$AgCl(s) \rightarrow Ag(s) + \frac{1}{2}Cl_2(g) \rightarrow \qquad -\Delta H_f = 128 \text{ kJ/mol}$$

$$Ag(s) \rightarrow Ag(g) \qquad\qquad \Delta H_{subl} = 286 \text{ kJ/mol}$$

$$\frac{1}{2}Cl_2(g) \rightarrow Cl(g) \qquad (0.5)\, \Delta H_{diss} = 120 \text{ kJ/mol}$$

$$\overline{AgCl(s) \rightarrow Ag(g) + Cl(g) \qquad\qquad \Delta H = 534 \text{ kJ/mol}}$$

Since 0.5 mol AgCl(s) reacts, the result is $(0.5)(534) = 267$ kJ/mol.

32. **The correct answer is (A).** Since sublimation is the process by which a solid is changed directly to a gas, without passing through the liquid phase, we look for a point on the boundary between solid and gas.

33. **The correct answer is (C).** To see why the negatively-sloping solid-liquid boundary explains the fact that water expands when it freezes (i.e., is denser as a liquid than as a solid), consider liquid water in equilibrium with its solid form at 1.00 atm and 0°K:

$$H_2O(s) = H_2O(l)$$

Suppose we increase the pressure—as when the blade of an ice skate presses on ice. Then the equilibrium will shift in a direction that will best relieve the pressure, which in this case will be the state having the smaller volume per mole or, put another way, the greater density. Thus, an increase in pressure causes solid water to melt to form the liquid. This effect is illustrated by the solid-liquid boundary of Figure 1.

34. **The correct answer is (A).** As nuclear charge increases from 13 (aluminum) to 14 (silicon), it pulls the outer electrons more closely toward the nucleus. (The extra electron added to the outer shell of the atom does not completely shield this additional nuclear charge.)

35. **The correct answer is (D).** The coordinates of temperature and percent silicon that are given place the point in the left-hand region of solid 1.

36. **The correct answer is (D).** To see that I is true, examine the downward-sloping line at the top of the diagram. To verify II, examine the line that begins at the lower left corner and continues up and to the right. To rule out III, examine the line that starts at the upper left, slants down and to the right, then changes its slope to become approximately flat as it moves to the right. Note that the uppermost downward sloping line is not the one specified here.

37. **The correct answer is (D).** Spontaneity is determined by $\Delta G = \Delta H - T\Delta S$. We know nothing about the enthalpy changes, and so we cannot determine the spontaneity of these reactions.

38. **The correct answer is (C).** For confirming instances, look for reactions that (a) have $\Delta S° > 0$ and (b) have more product species than reactant species in their balanced reactions.

39. **The correct answer is (A).** Reaction 1 shows solid copper changing directly to copper vapor, without passing through the liquid phase. This is analogous to the carbon dioxide sublimation described.

40. **The correct answer is (D).** Since the entropy change for the (evidently spontaneous) process is favorable, the enthalpy change is not well determined.

41. **The correct answer is (D).** From the discussion, we need to know both the entropy and enthalpy of fusion of ice at its melting point.

42. **The correct answer is (C).** Entropy measures disorder, not stability.

43. **The correct answer is (D).** II could be an explanation for the difference since it predicts a lower $\Delta S°$ for $MgCl_2$ than NaCl. I predicts the reverse effect, and III is a statement about enthalpy, not entropy.

44. **The correct answer is (C).** The relation between the initial and final masses of an isotope with a half-life is

$$m_{final} = \left(\frac{1}{2^n}\right) m_{initial}$$

where n is the number of half-lives. Using this calculation we get

$$\frac{2\text{ g}}{32\text{ g}} = \frac{1}{16} = \frac{1}{2^4}$$

There were four half-lives in the ten-minute period; therefore, each half-life is 2.5 minutes. In this problem it is just as easy to count up the half-lives. That is, it takes one half-life to get from 32 g to 16 g; a second to get from 16 g to 8 g; a third to get from 8 g to 4 g; and finally, a fourth to get from 4 g to 2 g.

45. **The correct answer is (B).** The second particle has a mass of 0 amu (atomic mass units) and a positive charge. This fits the description of the antielectron, or positron.

46. **The correct answer is (A).** The mass number is given by the superscript A. The law of conservation of mass requires that the sum of mass numbers before the decay equal the number after the decay. Therefore

$$30 = A + 0 \text{ so that } A = 30$$

47. **The correct answer is (B).** The number of neutrons in the nucleus must be the mass number, A, minus the atomic number, Z, where $Z = 15 - 1 = 14$. This gives $30 - 14 = 16$.

48. **The correct answer is (D).** The atomic number is the number of protons in the nucleus, Z. Conservation of mass requires that $15 = Z + 1$, so that $Z = 14$.

49. **The correct answer is (B).** The emitted particle decreases the number of protons by 1, while keeping the number of neutrons constant. Therefore, n/p increases so that the radioactive isotope $^{30}_{15}P$ lies below the belt of stability.

50. **The correct answer is (C).** All nuclei of phosphorus have the same atomic number. A different atomic number means a different element.

51. **The correct answer is (B).** Distance traveled is the product of the average speed and the time traveled. $D = v_{average}t$ The average speed in turn is found by taking the average of the velocity at the beginning and at the end of the interval:

$$v_{aver} = (2.3\text{ m/min} + 0\text{ m/min})/2 = 1.15\text{ m/min}$$
$$d = (1.15\text{ m/min})\, 2\text{ min} = 2.3\text{ m} \sim 2\text{ m}$$

52. **The correct answer is (B).** Kinetic energy is directly proportional to the square of the velocity. The maximum velocity for any of the intervals listed is 4 m/min, which occurs during the interval 2 min to 3 min.

53. **The correct answer is (A).** During this interval, the velocity is constant. Therefore, the acceleration is zero, so that the net force acting on the box must be zero over this interval of time.

54. **The correct answer is (D).** Momentum is the product of mass and velocity = (4.0 kg)(4 m/min) = 16 kg m/min.

55. **The correct answer is (B).** Since the velocity is constant over this interval, the acceleration is zero, which means the force acting on the box must be zero. Since work is force times distance, the work over this interval must also be zero.

56. **The correct answer is (B).** Ohm's law states that the voltage is equal to the product of the current and the resistance. Since the axes given are for voltage and current, this rearranges to $R = V/I$. V and I are both linear, so the graph will be a straight line. They are also directly proportional so that the slope will be positive.

57. **The correct answer is (D).** The force of gravity is given by

$$F_{grav} = GM_{earth}m/r^2$$

The force is inversely related to the square of the radial distance. Since the term for r is NOT linear, the graph will be a curve. Since the relation between F and r^2 is inversely proportional, the slope of the curve will be negative.

58. **The correct answer is (B).** For any body thrown vertically upward near the surface of the Earth, due to gravity the initial velocity is working in opposition to the acceleration. This means the upward velocity will decrease as the height above the ground increases. At the maximum height, the velocity is zero and the body will then start to fall back toward the ground. Velocity and time are linearly related, so the graph will be a straight line. They are also inversely related, so that the slope will be negative.

59. **The correct answer is (B).** Be careful. The variables are mass and energy, which are linear and directly proportional, so the graph is a straight line with a positive slope, c^2 is the constant value of the slope.

60. **The correct answer is (A).** Since equilibrium requires that no net force act on the body, a body in dynamic equilibrium must be moving with a constant velocity.

61. **The correct answer is (B).** Boyle's law $PV = k$ is shown by this graph for a particular temperature.

62. **The correct answer is (B).** Because $P = F/A$ for a given area, P and F are directly proportional.

63. **The correct answer is (C).** These quantum numbers refer to the $5d$ electrons. The value of n is not used directly to answer the question. From $+2$ through -2, m can have 5 values. Each m value can have 2 values of m^s associated with it, for a total of 10 states.

64. **The correct answer is (C).** In choice C the electronegativity between the bonded atoms decreases from HF through H_2. Note that the answers in D are atoms, not molecules, so no dipole moment is defined for them. Note also that the dipole moment is zero for each of the homonuclear diatomic molecules in A.

65. **The correct answer is (D).** II is ruled out because the solubility product, unlike the solubility, does not depend on concentration.

66. **The correct answer is (C).** CO_3^{2-} from the $BaCO_3$ reacts with H^+ to form HCO_3^- (and, if enough strong acid is available, H_2CO^3), causing the $MgCO_3$ to dissociate more than it would in neutral water.

67. **The correct answer is (B).** If doubling of a concentration leads to quadrupling of the rate, then the reaction is 2nd-order in that concentration. If changing another concentration has no effect, then the rate must be 0th-order in that concentration.

68. **The correct answer is (B).** The p_z orbital has a nodal plane in the xy-plane. Choice D is unfavorable but not impossible.

69. **The correct answer is (B).** HNO_3 is a strong acid, so $[H^+] = .1$ Therefore, $pH = -\log(.1) = 1$

70. **The correct answer is (D).** Use $P_i = X_i PT$ where $X(N_2) = 3/(3 + 1)$ and $X(H_2) = 1/(3 + 1)$.

71. **The correct answer is (A).** The angle between the light ray and the normal to the medium's surface decreases as the speed of the light decreases. The ray is traveling fastest in medium I (largest angle with respect to the normal) and slowest in medium IV (smallest angle to normal).

72. **The correct answer is (A).** Vertical motion is independent of horizontal motion, and for both balls the vertical acceleration is due to gravity. The balls hit the ground at the same time.

73. **The correct answer is (C).** This is the definition of the Newton, N, which is a unit of force, not work or energy.

74. **The correct answer is (D).** The speed of sound in air at 0°C is 330 meters/s, so it takes 2 seconds for sound to travel 660 meters. Light has a speed of 3.00×10^8 m/s, so in 2.0 seconds it would cover 6.0×10^8 meters.

75. **The correct answer is (B).** $P_{av} = \dfrac{\Delta w}{t}$, but the work done ($\Delta w$) is mgh; therefore,

$$P_{av} = \frac{(70 \text{ kg})(9.8 \text{ m/s}^2)(2 \text{ m})}{2s} = 686 \frac{\text{kg m}^2}{s^3}$$

$$P_{av} = 686 \text{ J/s} = 686 \text{ W}$$

This problem can be more readily answered by estimating the value

$$P_{av} \sim \frac{(70 \text{ kg})(10 \text{ m/s}^2)(2 \text{ m})}{2s} = 700 \text{ W}$$

which is closest to choice (B).

76. **The correct answer is (B).** Conservation of energy means the sum of the kinetic and potential energies must be the same at the start of the jump and at its maximum height

$$\frac{1}{2}mv_0^2 + mgh_0 = \frac{1}{2}mv^2 + mgh$$

where subscript 0 stands for the initial state. This becomes $\frac{1}{2}mv_0^2 + 0 = 0 + mgh$. Thus,

$$h = \frac{v_0^2}{2g} = \frac{(9.8 \text{ m/s})^2}{2(9.8 \text{ m/s}^2)} = 4.9 \text{ m}$$

The mass of the vaulter cancels out.

77. **The correct answer is (A).** The speed is constant but the direction of the car is constantly changing; thus, the velocity is constantly changing, which in turn means the car undergoes acceleration. Since only the direction, but not the magnitude of the velocity, is changing, only the radial acceleration component is nonzero. The tangential acceleration component is zero.

$$a_r = \frac{v^2}{r} = \frac{(20 \text{ m/s})^2}{200 \text{ m}} = 2.0 \text{ m/s}^2$$

VERBAL REASONING

78. **The correct answer is (A).** The answer to this question is found in the following statement in paragraph 7: "Because of greater demands for heating rather than cooling in colder regions, some utilities experience peak demands in the winter. In these cases, warmer winter temperatures caused by the greenhouse effect could reduce the amount of generating capacity required."

79. **The correct answer is (D).** The answer to this question is found in the following statement in paragraph 6: "By the year 2055, the greenhouse effect could measurably change regional demands for electricity in the United States."

80. **The correct answer is (A).** It is unreasonable to assume that someone so aware of one consequence of the greenhouse effect would be completely unaware of its other effects. The writer specifically mentions possible reduction of the flow of rivers.

81. **The correct answer is (A).** The answer to this question is found in the following statement in paragraph 7: "Such reductions in new capacity requirements induced by the greenhouse effect are restricted to a few states in the Northeast . . . and in the Northwest . . . ."

82. **The correct answer is (A).** The answer to this question is based on the fact that the author does not question the assumption anywhere in the article and on the following statement in paragraph 6: "Because the greenhouse effect is expected to have a significant influence on air conditioning and other summertime uses of electricity, higher temperatures in the future could lead to significant increases in the capacity needed to satisfy those uses." Notice that this statement assumes higher temperatures in the future and only questions how much electricity will be needed to supply the needs of the population in the warmer environment.

83. **The correct answer is (B).** The answer to this question is based on the following statement in paragraph 4: "Also, because of the large investments by utilities in long-lived capital-intensive power plants, the industry must focus on long-term planning."

84. **The correct answer is (B).** The answer to this question is based on the following statement in paragraph 2: "Bingham came of age in the Golden Age of American painting (1830–60), when the work of American artists was, for the first time, appreciated. . . ."

85. **The correct answer is (B).** The answer to this question is based on several statements in paragraph 3: "Today, Bingham ranks among the best of the nineteenth-century American narrative painters. 'He was a powerful figure who broke new ground in illustrating the simple joys of American life and who prepared the way for the giants—Winslow Homer and Thomas Eakins—to follow,' says E. Maurice Bloch. . . ."

86. **The correct answer is (D).** The answer to this question is based on the following statement in paragraph 5: "To his close friends, though, he was fiercely loyal and often charming, witty, and even affectionate."

87. **The correct answer is (A).** The answer to this question is in paragraph 6: "Like many American artists, Bingham was largely self-taught and 'he was proud of it,' according to Bloch."

88. **The correct answer is (A).** The answer to this question is based on the following statement in paragraph 7: "Bingham gained a national reputation through the American Art Union, an important corporate patron that encouraged artists to paint works appealing to patriotic feeling."

89. **The correct answer is (C).** The answer to this question is based on a number of statements. In paragraph 1, Bingham is called the "Missouri painter," and in paragraph 8 ". . . he has always been well known in Missouri. . . ." But the statement that best answers this question is in paragraph 6: ". . . Bingham started out as a journeyman portraitist, traveling from town to town through Missouri and Mississippi."

90. **The correct answer is (D).** The answer to this question is based on the following statement in paragraph 9: "Having studied Bingham's life and work for more than forty years, Bloch notes, 'It would have been possible to write an excellent book on Bingham by noting only a narrow circle of authentic works.' "

91. **The correct answer is (A).** Paragraph 1 supplies the answer: "He portrayed them as rugged and self-reliant Americans, emblems of the frontier spirit."

92. **The correct answer is (C).** The answer to this question is implied in several statements in paragraph 1: "As a child of the frontier, it was natural for George Caleb Bingham . . . to paint the fur trappers, flatboatmen, country politicians, and squatters he knew so well. He portrayed them as rugged and self-reliant Americans, emblems of the frontier spirit."

93. **The correct answer is (D).** The answer to this question is based on the following statement in paragraph 1: "Recommendations from four independent national panels call for increased emphasis on: the five new basics (English, mathematics, science, social studies, and computer science). . . ."

94. **The correct answer is (A).** The answer to this question is based on the following statement in paragraph 2: "A master teacher plan would provide a reward system for excellent teaching and make the profession more attractive to bright, talented college students seeking a professional career."

95. **The correct answer is (D).** The answer to this question is implied by the following statements in paragraphs 2 and 7: "A master teacher plan would provide a reward system for excellent teaching and make the profession more attractive to bright, talented college students seeking a professional career." (paragraph 2) "The Department of Defense Dependents School has accepted the challenge for educational reform; the Master Teacher Program is one small step in an overall plan for excellence. In this endeavor, active teacher participation is vital to the success of a master teacher program." (paragraph 7)

96. **The correct answer is (D).** The answer to this question is in the following statement in paragraph 5: "First and foremost, the master teacher would have comprehensive knowledge about his or her subject."

97. **The correct answer is (C).** The answer to this question is based on the following statement in paragraph 3: "Fewer than 10 percent of all teachers aspire to be administrators."

98. **The correct answer is (B).** The answer to this question is found in the profile of a master teacher in paragraphs 5 and 6. All of the attributes are mentioned except administrative skill.

99. **The correct answer is (A).** The answer to this question is based on the following statement in paragraph 4: ". . . public health policy should ensure safety, not harass industry or needlessly terrify the public."

100. **The correct answer is (B).** The answer to this question is found in the following statement in paragraph 1: "Consider, for a moment, these chemicals: safrole, hydrazine, tannin, and ethyl carbamate. We ingest them every day when we consume pepper, mushrooms, tea, and bread."

101. **The correct answer is (D).** The answer to this question is based on the following statement in paragraph 6: "Nosophobics think they will be sick in the future because of lurking factors in their diet and general environment."

102. **The correct answer is (C).** This inference is based on the following statements in paragraphs 2 and 3, plus the overall tone of the article: "The numbers can be made to show that a substance is killing us—even when there isn't the remotest possibility." (paragraph 2) "If you listen to every restrictive environmental report that has received media attention, you know that in addition to apples, you shouldn't eat most other fruits, not to mention meats, fish, fowl, vegetables, eggs, or milk products." (paragraph 3)

103. **The correct answer is (C).** The answer to this question is based on the following statement in paragraph 7: "Yesterday's invisible hazards give rise to monster legends, claims of witchcraft, and vampire myths."

104. **The correct answer is (B).** The answer to this question can be inferred from two statements in paragraph 8 and several statements in paragraph 9. From paragraph 8 are the following statements: "The most deadly public health issues that threaten our lives have been obscured in the face of trumped-up charges against the food we eat, the water we drink, and the air we breathe. They fall under the category of hazardous lifestyles." From paragraph 9 are these statements: "Cigarette smoking claims 1,200 lives a day. . . . Another obvious example of a hazardous lifestyle habit is excessive or abusive alcohol consumption, which claims 100,000 lives annually. Add to this the use of addictive substances, such as heroin, cocaine, and crack, which claim some 50,000 lives each year."

105. **The correct answer is (B).** The answer to this question can be inferred from the following statements found in paragraph 6: "Nosophobics think they will be sick in the future because of lurking factors in their diet and general environment. They fixate on an array of allegedly health-threatening gremlins. Due to this phobia, they believe that living—and eating and drinking—in America is inherently hazardous to their health. They are sure there is a death-dealing carcinogen on every plate, a life-sapping toxin under every pillow."

106. **The correct answer is (D).** The answer to this question can be found from a statement in paragraph 9: "Cigarette smoking claims 1,200 lives a day. In just one year, over 400,000 will perish. . . ."

107. **The correct answer is (C).** The answer to this question is based on the following statements in paragraph 2: "In 1981, . . . some of the citizens of Seattle examined the hard economic questions facing their city. . . . They discovered that economic questions are not only technical and political, but ethical and religious as well. . . . When they began to discuss the economy, they felt they lacked the ability to understand and articulate the philosophical issues that lie at the heart of the social contract." In addition to these statements, the tenor of the article implies this answer.

108. **The correct answer is (A).** The answer in paragraph 5 states: "Their worlds differed so much from ours. But those differences can be instructive. If we can understand why Aristotle opposed economic growth and why Adam Smith extolled it, it will prompt us to think about how decisions are actually made in modern democracies."

109. **The correct answer is (D).** The answer to this question is based on the following statement in paragraph 2: "They discovered that economic growth questions are not only technical and political, but ethical and religious as well."

110. **The correct answer is (D).** The answer to this question is based on several statements in paragraphs 3 and 4. In paragraph 3 are the statements that ". . . according to Aristotle, the pursuit of material wealth should be a means to strengthen the community, the polis. People who pursue material wealth for its own sake, Aristotle wrote, 'are intent upon living only and not living well.' " In paragraph 4 are these statements: " 'Adam Smith . . . did not believe that the desire for wealth was in any way unnatural or a threat to the well-being of the society. . . .' " "Increasing wealth was a universal urge. . . ." " 'Smith had observed the process of economic growth visible in Europe in the sixteenth and seventeenth centuries . . . (and) how a society could increase the production power over time. . . .' "

111. **The correct answer is (B).** The answer to this question is based on the following statements in paragraph 5: " 'We won't find simple answers for our age in the writing of these philosophers. . . . Their worlds differed so much from ours. . . . If we can understand why Aristotle opposed economic growth and why Adam Smith extolled it, it will prompt us to think about how decisions are actually made in modern democracies.' "

112. **The correct answer is (A).** The answer to this question is based on the positive tone of the article. The article gives no criticism of the program.

113. **The correct answer is (B).** The answer to this question is supported by several statements in paragraphs 4 and 5: "Thus, according to Aristotle, the pursuit of material wealth should be a means to strengthen the community, the polis. People who pursue material wealth for its own sake . . . are intent upon living only and not living well." (paragraph 4) "Adam Smith . . . did not believe that the desire for wealth was in any way unnatural or a threat to the well-being of the society. . . . Smith had observed the process of economic growth . . . in Europe in the sixteenth and seventeenth centuries. He had seen how a society could increase the production power over time, expanding the supply of necessities and conveniences of life." (paragraph 5)

114. **The correct answer is (C).** The answer to this question is based on the following statement in paragraph 2: " 'What is distinctive about the South,' says Robert C. Stewart, executive director of the Alabama Humanities Foundation, 'and about the Southerners' response to it, is that it remained primarily agricultural well into the twentieth century, long after the rest of the nation had become urbanized.' "

115. **The correct answer is (B).** In paragraph 7: "With Walker Percy's *The Last Gentleman* (1966) and Mary Ward Brown's *Tongues of Flame* (1986), Southern literature reaches the point at which it ceases to be distinctively Southern and becomes broadly American. . . ."

116. **The correct answer is (D).** The answer to this question is supported by the following statement from paragraph 7: " 'With Walker Percy's *The Last Gentleman* (1966) and Mary Ward Brown's *Tongues of Flame* (1986), Southern literature reaches the point at which it ceases to be distinctly Southern and becomes broadly American,' says Quinlan."

117. **The correct answer is (B).** The answer to this question is based on the following statement in paragraph 5: " 'The progressive South is uncomfortable with its rural heritage.' "

118. **The correct answer is (B).** The answer to this question can be inferred from statements made throughout the article. In paragraph 1 are the following statements: ". . . writers have drawn upon Southerners' almost instinctive relationship to their surroundings. Working within a land-oriented cultural ethos, Southern writers have evoked a familiar, often haunting sense of place that gives the South a distinctive regional identity." In paragraph 2 are these statements: " 'What is distinctive about the South . . . and about the Southerners' response to it, is that it remained primarily agricultural . . .' " and ". . . Southerners have had mixed feelings about the land rather than purely idealized reactions, with pastoral myths often giving way to hard reality.' " In paragraph 3 there is reference to the Alabama Humanities Foundation helping ". . . Alabamians examine their traditional relation to the land . . ." and a statement that the Foundation ". . . introduces participants to some of the major works of twentieth-century Southern literature and to a renewed sense of their roots in the land and its continuing vitality."

119. **The correct answer is (C).** The answer to this question is based on paragraph 6: "Participants are learning that Southern writers do not present a uniform view of 'home.' Among the works being read is William Faulkner's *The Bear* (1942), which depicts a mythic landscape. . . . Jean Toomer's *Cane* (1923) portrays the spiritual landscape and folk rhythms of black life in rural Georgia. . . . John Crowe Ransom's essay 'Reconstructed but Unregenerate' (1930) and Andrew Lytle's short story 'Jericho, Jericho, Jericho' (1984), who present the rural South. . . ."

120. **The correct answer is (A).** The answer to this question is supported by the following statement in paragraph 8: "As chronicled in the works of these and other contemporary Southern writers, the South is moving inexorably into the urban, industrial mainstream."

121. **The correct answer is (B).** The answer to this question can be inferred from the following statements from paragraph 8: ". . . the South is moving inexorably into the urban, industrial mainstream. With fewer people living close to the land, the experiences that in many ways made Southerners 'Southern' are becoming alien. . . . 'As we move farther from the land of our parents and grandparents, we need to reflect on their special relationship with the land, whether we will have it today, and what will become of it as we move into the 1990s.'"

122. **The correct answer is (B).** The answer to this question is based on the following statements in paragraphs 2 and 4: "Diaries are the best sources of this type of inquiry, according to Brown, because they enable one 'to see a person whole, to see how print and oral communication fit together in a person's life to determine which is more important and exactly how both are used.'" (paragraph 2) "Because keeping a diary was a good deal more common during the eighteenth and nineteenth centuries than at present. . . ." (paragraph 4)

123. **The correct answer is (C).** Though it may be true that newspapers were better written in 1850 than in 1700, there is nothing in the article to indicate this. On the other hand, the article states that more people read the newspaper in 1850, implying that more people could read. The writer states that there was an explosion of newspapers in the 1780s and '90s, implying that more people used newspapers as a source of information. In the final paragraph, the writer mentions that the American Revolution encouraged the concept that the people should be well informed.

124. **The correct answer is (D).** The answer to this question is based on the following statements in paragraph 6: " 'The radical difference between the America of 1700 and 1850 was the extraordinary abundance of information. People gradually became selectors of information according to their individual temperament, their occupation, their social class.'"

125. **The correct answer is (B).** The answer to this question is based on the following statements from paragraph 4: "In particular, Brown sought out generic types . . . rather than notables. There were, however, a few major figures—Sewall, Bentley, John Adams, William Byrd II—whose diaries . . . could not be ignored."

126. **The correct answer is (B).** The answer to this question is based on the following statements in paragraph 3: " 'People in Sewall's time did not read newspapers for news. Word of mouth was much faster. What newspapers did provide was the text of official documents, such as laws or treaties, and the speeches of high officials.'"

127. **The correct answer is (D).** The answer to this question is supported by statements in paragraph 7: " 'By the nineteenth century a dramatic change had occurred,' Brown says. 'The ideology of the Revolution required that the people—that is, all sorts of people, who run the nation in a democracy—be well-informed.'"

128. **The correct answer is (A).** The answer to this question is supported by the following statement in paragraph 5: " 'During much of the eighteenth century, information was a scarce commodity . . . a community's leaders controlled important communications and diffused them by word of mouth to other people.' "

129. **The correct answer is (D).** The answer to this question is based on the following statement in paragraph 2: "Initially, sulphur and sulphuric compounds were selected for study because they were known to be capable of causing damage over large areas of eastern North America and because of the prospect for substantial increases in the atmospheric sulphur load in connection with the United States's plans to increase the use of coal."

130. **The correct answer is (D).** The answer is based on inferences from the first and last paragraphs: ". . . programs that examine possible control measures and increase scientific knowledge have been developed and are being carried out cooperatively by the United States and Canada." And ". . . Canada looks forward to close cooperation with the United States. . . ."

131. **The correct answer is (A).** The answer to this question is based on the following statement in paragraph 2: "Initially, sulphur and sulphuric compounds were selected for study because they were known to be capable of causing damage over large areas of eastern North America. . . ."

132. **The correct answer is (B).** The answer to this question is based on the following statement in paragraph 4: "Long-range transport of air pollution represents a serious environmental problem for Canada."

133. **The correct answer is (A).** The answer to this question can be inferred by the following statement in paragraph 3: "Results of these early studies enabled the two countries to recognize and clarify the time-sensitive nature and the ultimate irreversibility of the impact of acid rain."

134. **The correct answer is (A).** The answer to this question is based on the following statement in paragraph 4: "Action by Canada alone will be insufficient in view of the continental dimension of the problem and the climatic behavior that favors transport of United States's pollutants over Canada."

135. **The correct answer is (B).** The answer to this question is supported by the following statement in paragraph 4: "Such action not only should prevent further increases in emissions but also should reduce emissions from their current levels."

136. **The correct answer is (D).** The passage makes no reference at all to the Industrial Revolution nor its effect on classical learning.

137. **The correct answer is (D).** The answer to this question is based on the following statements in paragraph 9: "He imagined *The Age of Fable* not in a classroom, but in the 'parlor.' His audience was not to be schoolchildren, but 'the reader of English literature, of either sex,' others 'more advanced' who may require mythological knowledge when they visit museums or 'mingle in cultivated society,' and also readers 'in advanced life.' "

138. **The correct answer is (B).** The answer to this question is based on the following statements in paragraph 6: "Bulfinch drew his 188 'citations' from the work of forty poets. All were British except for three."

139. **The correct answer is (C).** The answer to this question is inferred because all of the other reasons listed as possible answers are stated in the reading. This answer is not stated but, in addition, the author of the reading specifically states that this book was not written for the classroom (see the answer to Question 137 and paragraph 8).

140. **The correct answer is (B).** The answer can be inferred from several statements throughout the reading and by one particular statement in paragraph 8. The reading's general implication is that during Bulfinch's time, an educated individual was expected to be knowledgeable about classical literature, as shown in the following statements: ". . . in the American mind, the name of Bulfinch is indelibly associated with classical mythology." (paragraph 1) "Without a doubt, *The Age of Fable* formed the image that millions of Americans had of the classical gods and heroes. . . . The mythology learned by Americans was Bulfinch's mythology. . . . Bulfinch recreated dozens of myths. . . ." (paragraph 2) "*The Age of Fable* consists of prose narratives of classical myths." (paragraph 3) "Bulfinch's strong background in classical literature, especially Roman, accounts for his success in adapting Ovid for American readers." (paragraph 4) The answer is best inferred from the following statement in paragraph 8: "He [Bulfinch] was responding, in particular, to the rise of science and technology, a decline in classical learning and increasing educational opportunities. . . ."

141. **The correct answer is (D).** The answer to this question is based on statements made by the author listing all of the other reasons given as answers. While the author mentions the high number of British writers used, the author does not give this as a reason for the popularity of the book.

142. **The correct answer is (D).** The answer to this question is based on the following statements made in paragraphs 2 and 7: " 'Thus we hope to teach mythology,' he explains in his preface, 'not as a study, but as a relaxation from study; to give our work the charm of a story-book, yet by means of it to impart a knowledge of an important branch of education.' " (paragraph 2) "In using poetry as a counterpoint in *The Age of Fable*, Bulfinch was tapping into an interest of the general educated public." (paragraph 7)

BIOLOGICAL SCIENCES

143. **The correct answer is (C).** Following the arrow in the flow chart immediately reveals that fatty acids can be converted to acetyl CoA.

144. **The correct answer is (D).** You must know that the net gain in ATP molecules by the complete metabolism of glucose during cellular respiration is 36. Because fatty acids are richer in hydrogens (it is the treatment of hydrogens during the electron transport chain that provides most of the ATP), the best estimate would be *higher than 36.*

145. **The correct answer is (C).** Recognizing the names of some amino acids is helpful, but not essential. The flow chart shows that after deamination (when NH_3 is formed), amino acids can be converted to pyruvic acid or acetyl CoA, or they can feed into the Krebs cycle. They do not feed into the transport chain.

146. **The correct answer is (B).** Basic knowledge of metabolic processes and/or urine content is required. Ammonia is too toxic to be transported directly. Urea is the nitrogenous waste resulting from the metabolism of amino acids. Uric acid is produced during metabolism of nucleic acids, and creatinine results from the metabolism of creatine (creatine phosphate can be used as a source of energy in muscle cells).

147. **The correct answer is (A).** General understanding of the location of each stage of cellular respiration is needed. Glycolysis occurs in the cytoplasm (cytosol), the Krebs cycle takes place within the mitochondrial matrix, and the transport chain is found along the mitochondrial cristae. Since the flow chart shows glycerol entering the pathway at glycolysis, it must be in the cytoplasm.

148. **The correct answer is (D).** You should understand that catabolic intermediates can often be used as building blocks during anabolic processes (synthesis). Acetyl CoA is found on the flow chart at the juncture where protein, carbohydrate, and fat metabolism can all intersect. Since starch is a polysaccharide carbohydrate that is eventually broken down to glucose, all routes mentioned in the question can lead to each other.

149. **The correct answer is (D).** The supernatant at the top will contain the lighter viral protein coats that did not enter the host cell, while the much larger and heavier bacterial cells (now also containing the injected viral DNA) will be in the pellet on the bottom.

150. **The correct answer is (A).** The radioactive sulfur used in Experiment 1 will be found in protein material (sulfur is not found in nucleic acids). Since the radioactive labeling involved the virus and not the bacteria, only viral proteins (which remained outside the host cell and were dislodged by agitation) will be labeled.

151. **The correct answer is (C).** Experiment 2 used radioactive phosphorus, a component of nucleic acids like DNA. As stated in the passage (and in Question 150), only the virus was labeled. Upon infection, the vital DNA is injected into the host cell. Therefore, choice C is the only possible answer.

152. **The correct answer is (D).** Two general points must be understood to answer this question properly: (1) Bacterial growth for many generations involves many cycles of cell division, and (2) DNA replication occurs with each cycle of division in a semiconservative manner. The infected bacterial cells have a limited amount of viral DNA inside them as they begin to be cultured. *No new strands of DNA* can be labeled since the bacterial medium contains only normal nutrients. As division continues for generations, a higher and higher percentage of cells will have their DNA synthesized only from ingredients in the fresh medium (and lower and lower percentages will contain labeled DNA that was present in the first generation of cells placed in the medium).

153. **The correct answer is (B).** The abilities to formulate hypotheses and to see which variable is being examined in an experimental design are important here. If the ability to produce a specific substance is lost, and that inability prevents growth on minimal medium, then adding that particular substance should enable the cells to grow again. Choice B is the only procedure that will identify the "lost" ability. Growing different strains together will always confound which strain needs what! Similarly, growing one strain on different media (when they are not minimal media) can be unfruitful and endless.

154. **The correct answer is (B).** The question states that different strains lack the ability to synthesize the same substance. By definition, different strains have mutations at different points in the genetic material. Therefore, since it is known that the synthesis of this "lost" substance requires many steps, it is not unreasonable to hypothesize that each mutation may have affected a different gene coding for a different enzyme involved with a different step in the synthetic pathway! Choices A and C are irrelevant to the information addressed in the question.

155. **The correct answer is (A).** The 90 plants with light flowers are those with the double recessive genotype (*aa*). The frequency of this genotype in the population can be represented by q_2. Therefore, $90/1000 = q^2 = .09$. If $q^2 = .09$, then $q = .3$. It is known that if the frequency of the q allele is .3, then the frequency of the p allele must be .7 ($p + q = 1$).

156. **The correct answer is (C).** From the response to Question 155, it was learned that the frequency of $p = .7$. Homozygous dominant individuals have a frequency of $p^2 = (.7)(.7) = .49$. This question asks for the number of individuals with this genotype. Thus, $.49 \times 1000$ individuals $= 490$.

157. **The correct answer is (D).** The proportion of heterozygous individuals will be $2pq = 2(.7)(.3) = .42$.

158. **The correct answer is (D).** All of the factors *would* have an effect on the number of each plant type (more dark flowers being preyed upon by caterpillars; more light flowers being pollinated by insects; more dark plant pollen being dispersed). Therefore, *none* of the choices will have *no effect*!

159. **The correct answer is (C).** One individual out of 2500 (.0004) has the double recessive genotype. Thus, $q^2 = .0004$ and $q = .02$. If $q = .02$, then $p = .98$. These are the allele frequencies in the population.

160. **The correct answer is (D).** It should be understood that "carriers" are heterozygotes. If $q = .02$ and $p = .98$, then $2pq = 2(.98)(.02) = .0392$. The number of individuals of this genotype will be $.0392 \times 2500 = 98$.

161. **The correct answer is (B).** New alleles *originate* by mutation. A new allele represents a change in the DNA sequence of the former allele. Any change in the DNA sequence is considered a mutation.

162. **The correct answer is (A).** Hypothesis A proposes that viruses (and their ancestors) were present *before* other heterotrophs and autotrophs. It is implied that these other forms were cellular, since the hypothesis goes on to state that viruses then adapted to a parasitic lifestyle (the heterotrophs and autotrophs became the hosts).

163. **The correct answer is (B).** It is known today that viruses can reproduce only after infecting a host cell. A proposal that places viruses earlier in evolutionary time than cellular forms would also have to suggest a different method of reproduction.

164. **The correct answer is (B).** Hypothesis C suggests that different viruses may have originated in different hosts. If some genes were identical to the hosts, this would be strong supportive evidence. Simply having the same type of nucleic acid is too broad a similarity (DNA? RNA?). Hypothesis B says nothing about differing origins for different viruses (". . . viruses evolved from a cellular form. . . .").

165. **The correct answer is (D).** Hypothesis B proposes that viruses evolved *from* a cellular form, as does hypothesis C (nucleic acid that escaped from the host cell). As discussed in the explanation of Question 162, hypothesis A suggests that viruses predated cellular forms.

166. **The correct answer is (C).** Again, *genetic* similarity with the host cell is strong evidence for hypothesis C. If other kinds of similarities were at issue (environmental, temperature, pH, etc.), the highly specialized host-parasite relationships emphasized by hypothesis B would gain support as well.

167. **The correct answer is (C).** Hypothesis A refers to viruses preceding photosynthetic organisms (autotrophs), feeding on nutrients in the surrounding seas (absorption), and surviving this way (taking care of business on their own). What is *implied* is that they did not need a host cell for anything!

168. **The correct answer is (C).** Curve C shows that most individuals die (no longer survive) very early in life. The straight line in curve B suggests that survival, as well as the rate of death (mortality rate), is the same at all ages.

169. **The correct answer is (B).** Logical thinking will definitely help here. If most individuals die at a young age, mating at a late age will not do the trick! Similarly, long courtships would probably result in unconsummated love! However, by producing large numbers of offspring, *some* of them will survive to reproductive age (fish eggs, frog eggs, insects, etc.). Choice D seems irrelevant.

170. **The correct answer is (B).** The rate of mortality is equivalent at all ages *only* for curve B. This suggests that random events play a role in the death of individuals. If these events were not random, some ages would have greater survival (and some, higher mortality) than others.

171. **The correct answer is (D).** Severe drops in survival (increases in mortality) are clearly shown early in curve C and late in curve A.

172. **The correct answer is (B).** Species (or life-history patterns) represented by curve A show high survival (and low mortality) in early life. All choices *except* B include some variable that will contribute to low survival of young (predation of young, many offspring with limited resources, limited care, and high predation). Only choice B fits the survival data represented by curve A.

173. **The correct answer is (C).** Species represented by curve B have the same probability of dying (or living) regardless of age. Living 50% through the average maximum life span has no effect. In species represented by curve C, if an individual makes it to the halfway mark, there is little subsequent change in the chances of dying (the curve is basically a horizontal line after that point). In curve A species, however, once the halfway mark is reached, the chances of dying start to *increase*.

174. **The correct answer is (D).** Each curve ends (maximum life span) in the same place on the graph.

175. **The correct answer is (C).** After separation, both cells were able to develop into complete organisms. Thus, their fate was not yet determined. Additionally, materials outside the cells were not even considered in Experiment 1 (the gray crescent was part of the cytoplasm *inside* the cells). Clearly, the direction of the cleavage plane *did* have a powerful influence.

176. **The correct answer is (D).** As stated in the explanation of Question 175, the gray crescent was an extremely important region in the cytoplasm. Choices B and C are irrelevant.

177. **The correct answer is (D).** The only piece of information relevant to this question is that the genes determining skin pattern are all located in the implanted nucleus donated by the spotted frog. All frogs will be spotted.

178. **The correct answer is (A).** Experiment 2 showed that even the nuclei from *adult* skin cells had the potential to produce complete organisms when implanted into an egg. Experiment 2 did not address the question of cytoplasmic factors, so choice B is incorrect. As long as one adult cell nucleus produced an entire organism, totipotency is demonstrated, and choice C is eliminated as well. Choice D only addresses the cytoplasmic issue. The question asks about any findings from Experiment 2 (cytoplasmic influences—*no,* totipotency—*yes!*).

179. **The correct answer is (C).** Induction refers to the phenomenon of one group of cells influencing the development of other cells. This was clearly demonstrated in Experiment 3 (cytoplasmic factors inside the cell were not examined). Choices B and D imply that genetic factors have been affected by environmental conditions. However, the experiment provided no evidence that either statement is correct. The importance of environmental factors does not negate the effects of genetic factors. There clearly must be an interaction between the inducing factors and the genes in the developing cells. Similarly, a loss of totipotency would only be demonstrated if the induced cells were removed and then used unsuccessfully to grow a complete organism.

180. **The correct answer is (D).** The effects described in the passage (formation of notochord, neural plate, neural tube, etc.) mark the process of neurulation. This development of the nervous system begins after gastrulation, early in organogenesis.

181. **The correct answer is (D).** Cytoplasmic factors inside the cell (Experiment 1) and induction processes due to surrounding tissues outside the cell (Experiment 3) were shown to have significant effects on the genetic potential underlying development.

182. **The correct answer is (C).** Efficiency, in terms of modes of locomotion, is solely based on the energy costs of each mode at a particular size (body mass). At all sizes, swimming "costs" less than running and flying. The slopes of the lines suggest the rate of change in energy costs related to size.

183. **The correct answer is (B).** All that is needed to answer this question is the ability to read the graph. First, find 1 g on the *x*-axis (body mass), then look to see where the "flying line" intersects the *y*-axis (energy cost).

184. **The correct answer is (B).** On the graph, humans have a body mass just under 1000 g. At this body mass, the swimming line reflects the lowest energy cost (less than 1 J/kg/m).

185. **The correct answer is (B).** An examination of the graph reveals that for any single mode of locomotion, the energy costs decrease as body mass increases. This holds true for all three modes of locomotion.

186. **The correct answer is (B).** If each potential answer is identified on its appropriate line graph, the 1-g flyer has the greatest energy cost. This should in no way imply that the smaller animal spends more total energy. Efficiency refers to energy cost/body mass (J/kg/m).

187. **The correct answer is (C).** A large swimmer clearly is the most efficient "mover" among the possible choices. Again, in terms of J/kg/m, the blue whale wins it "flippers down."

188. **The correct answer is (B).** Pyrrole, pyridine, and pyrimidine contain the aromatic sextet. In pyrrole, the sigma bonds around N are formed by sp^2 hydrid orbitals. An N electron participates in each of the sigma bonds. The remaining N electrons are in an N $2p$ orbital that overlaps with the carbon $2p$ orbitals in the ring to form π bonds and the aromatic sextet. In pyridine, the nitrogen atom donates one electron to each of the two sigma bonds by use of sp_2 orbitals. The third sp_2 orbital contains two electrons, which are available for acids. One electron of N is present in a p orbital, which interacts with the carbon p orbitals to form the π structure and give rise to the aromatic sextet. The bonding of the N atoms in pyrimidine is equivalent to that in pyridine.

189. **The correct answer is (D).** See the explanation of Question 188.

190. **The correct answer is (D).** See the explanation of Question 188.

191. **The correct answer is (A).** Attack at position 2 gives three resonance structures.

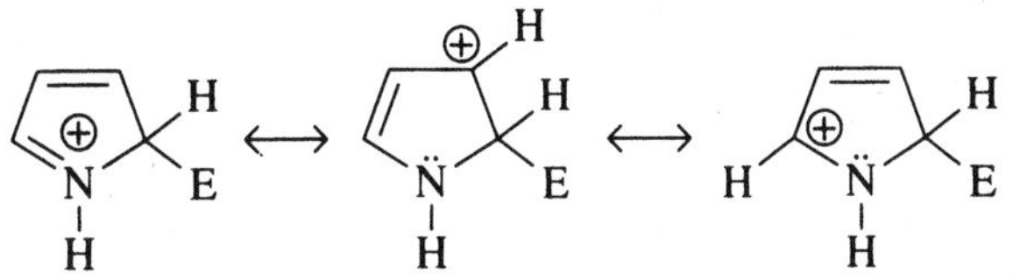

Attack at position 3 gives only two.

192. **The correct answer is (A).** The pyridine ring behaves much like a benzene ring that is joined to strongly electron-withdrawing groups. Nucleophilic substitution occurs most readily at the 2— and 4— positions. Attack at the 4— position gives the following resonance stabilized carbanion:

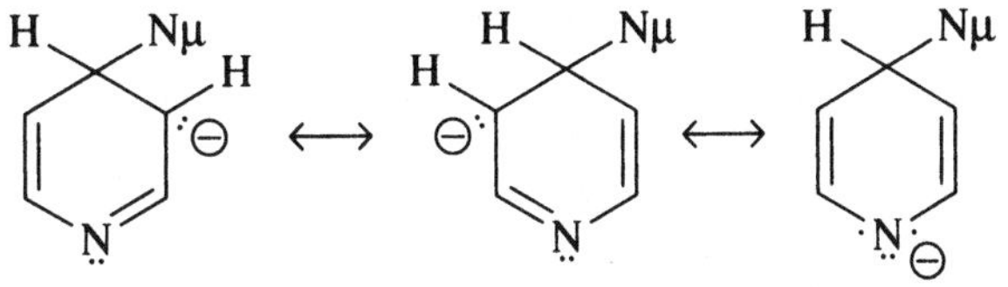

The structure in which N carries the negative charge is particularly stable. A similar structure can be drawn for attack of the nucleophile at the 2 position.

193. **The correct answer is (C).** Piperidine is a secondary amine like dimethylamine. Pyridine is a stronger base than pyrrole but is much weaker than aliphatic amines.

194. **The correct answer is (A).** This bond must be broken in order to account for the labeled alcohol oxygen appearing in the ester.

195. **The correct answer is (B).** The mechanism of acidic hydrolysis must be the exact reverse of the mechanism of esterification catalyzed by acid. If a labeled oxygen of an alcohol appears in the ester, hydrolysis of the ester will form the labeled alcohol back again.

196. The correct answer is (C). Protonation of an ester yields:

$$
\begin{array}{cc}
\text{H}^+ & \\
\searrow & \\
\text{O} & \text{OH}^{\oplus} \\
\parallel & \parallel \\
\text{R—C—OR}' \rightleftharpoons \text{R—C—OR}'
\end{array}
$$

The carbon is then rendered more susceptible to attack by a nucleophile because the oxygen will not need to carry a negative charge. The nucleophile in acidic hydrolysis is H_2O, while in esterification the alcohol is the nucleophile.

197. The correct answer is (A). Special methods are often needed to prepare esters of tertiary alcohols or esters of acids containing bulky groups.

198. The correct answer is (D).

$$
\begin{array}{c}
\text{O} \\
\parallel \\
\text{R—C}\!\!+\!\!{}^{18}\text{OC}_2\text{H}_5 \\
\text{acyl} \\
\text{group}
\end{array}
$$

199. The correct answer is (A).

200. The correct answer is (D).

$$3350 \text{ cm}^{-1} \qquad \text{—OH stretch (H—bonded)}$$
$$1000 \text{ cm}^{-1}\text{C} \qquad \text{—O stretch}$$

According to the table provided, the above two bonds are associated with alcohols.

201. The correct answer is (A). The ultraviolet spectrum of an unknown compound is used chiefly to identify conjugation or the presence of an aromatic group.

202. The correct answer is (C). Proton exchange occurs very rapidly in the presence of an acid or base. Consequently, the hydroxyl proton sees only an averaged chemical environment and thus gives rise to a singlet. If proton exchange is slowed, the hydroxyl proton signal will be split by nearby protons. The hydroxyl proton will also cause splitting in the signals of these nearby protons.

203. The correct answer is (B).

204. The correct answer is (C). IR is the best method to detect a —C$=$O group. The strong band due to C$=$O stretching is generally seen at about 1700 cm^{-1} where it seldom is hidden by other absorptions.

205. The correct answer is (C). A fundamental understanding of the relationship between genes and cell function is required. The uncoiled DNA exposes the nucleotide sequence of the gene so that it can be transcribed and translated into the gene product: a protein (or protein subunit). Since different parts of the genome are constantly being activated (depending on the needs of the cell and the needs of the organism), the chromosomes must constantly have their active genes exposed (uncoiled).

206. The correct answer is (C). Basic knowledge of respiratory anatomy and the gas laws are required. When the diaphragm contracts (moves downward), the volume in the thoracic cavity (and lungs) increases, causing the pressure to decrease. As a result, the air outside the body is under higher pressure than the air in the lungs, and air rushes in (inspiration).

207. **The correct answer is (B).** A general understanding of blood pressure concepts, and the factors that influence blood pressure, is required. If peripheral resistance reflects friction between the blood and the walls of the blood vessels, both narrower blood vessels (vasoconstriction) and a thicker, more viscous blood will increase peripheral resistance.

208. **The correct answer is (B).** Basic knowledge of central nervous system (CNS) anatomy and the protective coverings of the CNS are required. The organs of the CNS (brain and spinal cord) have hollow regions (ventricles and spinal canal, respectively). The CNS also has three layers of protective covering (the meninges). The question states that cerebrospinal fluid circulates in these areas. Thus, choice B is the correct answer. The spinal nerves and cranial nerves are not considered part of the CNS.

209. **The correct answer is (B).** The question requires a solid foundation in Mendelian genetics and a familiarity with the interpretation of pedigrees. By process of elimination, the trait must be an autosomal recessive trait. The affected female in the second generation (third from the fight on the second line) could not have an autosomal dominant trait if neither parent has the allele (both parents are unaffected). Similarly, the same affected female could not result from such a cross if the trait is either sex-linked dominant or sex-linked recessive (the father would also have to be affected in either case). Only an autosomal recessive trait successfully works its way through the pedigree in the pattern presented.

210. **The correct answer is (C).** A basic knowledge of the immune system is required. Although specific defense vs. nonspecific defense is defined in the question, one still must have some understanding of the roles of the various choices. Phagocytosis by macrophages, inflammation, and interferon are all general, nonspecific responses by the immune system. Each type of antibody, on the other hand, is normally produced in response to a specific antigen (usually associated with a specific invading organism).

211. **The correct answer is (A).** This question calls for a general understanding of the function of enzymes, as well as the characteristics of chemical reactions. Enzymes catalyze reactions by lowering the activation energy required to initiate them. They speed reactions rather than slow them. Enzymes do not produce energy, nor can they make an endergonic reaction exergonic.

212. **The correct answer is (D).** Familiarity with brain structure and function is required. Although most information in the question relates to the effects of Parkinsonism, the question really asks which part of the brain is associated with "intelligence, vision, and hearing . . . unaffected by this disorder. . . ."

213. **The correct answer is (B).** A familiarity with the events of meiosis and the factors that influence sex determination are helpful, but a clear understanding about the pattern of inheritance for sex-linked traits is essential. Since normal females have two X chromosomes, Turner's syndrome females (XO) *do not* have the same probabilities of inheriting sex-linked disorders (they actually have the same chances as males).

214. **The correct answer is (C).** A basic understanding of the events involved with muscle contraction is required. Choices A, B, and D are all necessary for a muscle cell to return to its resting state. The troponin–tropomyosin complex must return to its original position on the actin (the position it occupied before calcium was released from the sarcoplasmic reticulum). When the complex *detaches*, muscle *contraction* occurs.

215. **The correct answer is (C).** If only $(CH_3)_3CCHO$ and a strong base are present, no reaction can occur. For an aldol condensation to occur, the aldehyde or ketone must contain an α-hydrogen. The α-hydrogen is acidic and will combine with the base to form a carbanion. The carbanion is the nucleophile in the reaction that attacks the carbonyl carbon of another aldehyde or ketone molecule. The generally accepted mechanism follows, using acetone as an example.

$$CH_3-\overset{\overset{\displaystyle O}{\|}}{C}-CH_3 + OH^- \rightleftarrows CH_3-\overset{\overset{\displaystyle O}{\|}}{C}-\underset{\underset{\displaystyle \ominus}{\cdot\cdot}}{CH_2} + H_2O$$

$$CH_3-\overset{\overset{\displaystyle O}{\|}}{C}-\underset{\underset{\displaystyle \ominus}{\cdot\cdot}}{CH_2} + CH_3-\overset{\overset{\displaystyle O}{\|}}{C}-CH_3 \rightleftarrows CH_3-\overset{\overset{\displaystyle O^{\ominus}}{|}}{\underset{\underset{\displaystyle CH_3}{|}}{C}}-CH_2-\overset{\overset{\displaystyle O}{\|}}{C}-CH_3$$

$$CH_3-\overset{\overset{\displaystyle O^{\ominus}}{|}}{\underset{\underset{\displaystyle CH_3}{|}}{C}}-CH_2-\overset{\overset{\displaystyle O}{\|}}{C}-CH_3 + H_2O \rightleftarrows CH_3-\overset{\overset{\displaystyle OH}{|}}{\underset{\underset{\displaystyle CH_3}{|}}{C}}-CH_2-\overset{\overset{\displaystyle O}{\|}}{C}-CH_3$$

216. **The correct answer is (D).** The amino acid residues are joined by amide linkages.

$$-NH-\overset{\overset{\displaystyle O}{\|}}{C}-$$

217. **The correct answer is (D).** Glycerol: a fat is a triglyceride.

$$\begin{array}{l} H_2C-O-\overset{\overset{\displaystyle O}{\|}}{C}-R \\ | \\ HC-O-\overset{\overset{\displaystyle O}{\|}}{C}-R' \\ | \\ H_2C-O-\overset{\overset{\displaystyle O}{\|}}{C}-R'' \end{array}$$

218. **The correct answer is (B).**

219. **The correct answer is (D).**

Practice Exam III

TEST	QUESTIONS	MINUTES
Physical Sciences	1–77	100 minutes
Verbal Reasoning	78–142	85 minutes
Writing Sample	2 Essays	60 minutes
Biological Sciences	143–219	100 minutes

ANSWER SHEET

PRACTICE EXAM III

Physical Sciences	Verbal Reasoning	Biological Sciences

Physical Sciences

1. Ⓐ Ⓑ Ⓒ Ⓓ
2. Ⓐ Ⓑ Ⓒ Ⓓ
3. Ⓐ Ⓑ Ⓒ Ⓓ
4. Ⓐ Ⓑ Ⓒ Ⓓ
5. Ⓐ Ⓑ Ⓒ Ⓓ
6. Ⓐ Ⓑ Ⓒ Ⓓ
7. Ⓐ Ⓑ Ⓒ Ⓓ
8. Ⓐ Ⓑ Ⓒ Ⓓ
9. Ⓐ Ⓑ Ⓒ Ⓓ
10. Ⓐ Ⓑ Ⓒ Ⓓ
11. Ⓐ Ⓑ Ⓒ Ⓓ
12. Ⓐ Ⓑ Ⓒ Ⓓ
13. Ⓐ Ⓑ Ⓒ Ⓓ
14. Ⓐ Ⓑ Ⓒ Ⓓ
15. Ⓐ Ⓑ Ⓒ Ⓓ
16. Ⓐ Ⓑ Ⓒ Ⓓ
17. Ⓐ Ⓑ Ⓒ Ⓓ
18. Ⓐ Ⓑ Ⓒ Ⓓ
19. Ⓐ Ⓑ Ⓒ Ⓓ
20. Ⓐ Ⓑ Ⓒ Ⓓ
21. Ⓐ Ⓑ Ⓒ Ⓓ
22. Ⓐ Ⓑ Ⓒ Ⓓ
23. Ⓐ Ⓑ Ⓒ Ⓓ
24. Ⓐ Ⓑ Ⓒ Ⓓ
25. Ⓐ Ⓑ Ⓒ Ⓓ
26. Ⓐ Ⓑ Ⓒ Ⓓ
27. Ⓐ Ⓑ Ⓒ Ⓓ
28. Ⓐ Ⓑ Ⓒ Ⓓ
29. Ⓐ Ⓑ Ⓒ Ⓓ
30. Ⓐ Ⓑ Ⓒ Ⓓ
31. Ⓐ Ⓑ Ⓒ Ⓓ
32. Ⓐ Ⓑ Ⓒ Ⓓ
33. Ⓐ Ⓑ Ⓒ Ⓓ
34. Ⓐ Ⓑ Ⓒ Ⓓ
35. Ⓐ Ⓑ Ⓒ Ⓓ
36. Ⓐ Ⓑ Ⓒ Ⓓ
37. Ⓐ Ⓑ Ⓒ Ⓓ
38. Ⓐ Ⓑ Ⓒ Ⓓ
39. Ⓐ Ⓑ Ⓒ Ⓓ
40. Ⓐ Ⓑ Ⓒ Ⓓ
41. Ⓐ Ⓑ Ⓒ Ⓓ
42. Ⓐ Ⓑ Ⓒ Ⓓ
43. Ⓐ Ⓑ Ⓒ Ⓓ
44. Ⓐ Ⓑ Ⓒ Ⓓ
45. Ⓐ Ⓑ Ⓒ Ⓓ
46. Ⓐ Ⓑ Ⓒ Ⓓ
47. Ⓐ Ⓑ Ⓒ Ⓓ
48. Ⓐ Ⓑ Ⓒ Ⓓ
49. Ⓐ Ⓑ Ⓒ Ⓓ
50. Ⓐ Ⓑ Ⓒ Ⓓ
51. Ⓐ Ⓑ Ⓒ Ⓓ
52. Ⓐ Ⓑ Ⓒ Ⓓ
53. Ⓐ Ⓑ Ⓒ Ⓓ
54. Ⓐ Ⓑ Ⓒ Ⓓ
55. Ⓐ Ⓑ Ⓒ Ⓓ
56. Ⓐ Ⓑ Ⓒ Ⓓ
57. Ⓐ Ⓑ Ⓒ Ⓓ
58. Ⓐ Ⓑ Ⓒ Ⓓ
59. Ⓐ Ⓑ Ⓒ Ⓓ
60. Ⓐ Ⓑ Ⓒ Ⓓ
61. Ⓐ Ⓑ Ⓒ Ⓓ
62. Ⓐ Ⓑ Ⓒ Ⓓ
63. Ⓐ Ⓑ Ⓒ Ⓓ
64. Ⓐ Ⓑ Ⓒ Ⓓ
65. Ⓐ Ⓑ Ⓒ Ⓓ
66. Ⓐ Ⓑ Ⓒ Ⓓ
67. Ⓐ Ⓑ Ⓒ Ⓓ
68. Ⓐ Ⓑ Ⓒ Ⓓ
69. Ⓐ Ⓑ Ⓒ Ⓓ
70. Ⓐ Ⓑ Ⓒ Ⓓ
71. Ⓐ Ⓑ Ⓒ Ⓓ
72. Ⓐ Ⓑ Ⓒ Ⓓ
73. Ⓐ Ⓑ Ⓒ Ⓓ
74. Ⓐ Ⓑ Ⓒ Ⓓ
75. Ⓐ Ⓑ Ⓒ Ⓓ
76. Ⓐ Ⓑ Ⓒ Ⓓ
77. Ⓐ Ⓑ Ⓒ Ⓓ

Verbal Reasoning

78. Ⓐ Ⓑ Ⓒ Ⓓ
79. Ⓐ Ⓑ Ⓒ Ⓓ
80. Ⓐ Ⓑ Ⓒ Ⓓ
81. Ⓐ Ⓑ Ⓒ Ⓓ
82. Ⓐ Ⓑ Ⓒ Ⓓ
83. Ⓐ Ⓑ Ⓒ Ⓓ
84. Ⓐ Ⓑ Ⓒ Ⓓ
85. Ⓐ Ⓑ Ⓒ Ⓓ
86. Ⓐ Ⓑ Ⓒ Ⓓ
87. Ⓐ Ⓑ Ⓒ Ⓓ
88. Ⓐ Ⓑ Ⓒ Ⓓ
89. Ⓐ Ⓑ Ⓒ Ⓓ
90. Ⓐ Ⓑ Ⓒ Ⓓ
91. Ⓐ Ⓑ Ⓒ Ⓓ
92. Ⓐ Ⓑ Ⓒ Ⓓ
93. Ⓐ Ⓑ Ⓒ Ⓓ
94. Ⓐ Ⓑ Ⓒ Ⓓ
95. Ⓐ Ⓑ Ⓒ Ⓓ
96. Ⓐ Ⓑ Ⓒ Ⓓ
97. Ⓐ Ⓑ Ⓒ Ⓓ
98. Ⓐ Ⓑ Ⓒ Ⓓ
99. Ⓐ Ⓑ Ⓒ Ⓓ
100. Ⓐ Ⓑ Ⓒ Ⓓ
101. Ⓐ Ⓑ Ⓒ Ⓓ
102. Ⓐ Ⓑ Ⓒ Ⓓ
103. Ⓐ Ⓑ Ⓒ Ⓓ
104. Ⓐ Ⓑ Ⓒ Ⓓ
105. Ⓐ Ⓑ Ⓒ Ⓓ
106. Ⓐ Ⓑ Ⓒ Ⓓ
107. Ⓐ Ⓑ Ⓒ Ⓓ
108. Ⓐ Ⓑ Ⓒ Ⓓ
109. Ⓐ Ⓑ Ⓒ Ⓓ
110. Ⓐ Ⓑ Ⓒ Ⓓ
111. Ⓐ Ⓑ Ⓒ Ⓓ
112. Ⓐ Ⓑ Ⓒ Ⓓ
113. Ⓐ Ⓑ Ⓒ Ⓓ
114. Ⓐ Ⓑ Ⓒ Ⓓ
115. Ⓐ Ⓑ Ⓒ Ⓓ
116. Ⓐ Ⓑ Ⓒ Ⓓ
117. Ⓐ Ⓑ Ⓒ Ⓓ
118. Ⓐ Ⓑ Ⓒ Ⓓ
119. Ⓐ Ⓑ Ⓒ Ⓓ
120. Ⓐ Ⓑ Ⓒ Ⓓ
121. Ⓐ Ⓑ Ⓒ Ⓓ
122. Ⓐ Ⓑ Ⓒ Ⓓ
123. Ⓐ Ⓑ Ⓒ Ⓓ
124. Ⓐ Ⓑ Ⓒ Ⓓ
125. Ⓐ Ⓑ Ⓒ Ⓓ
126. Ⓐ Ⓑ Ⓒ Ⓓ
127. Ⓐ Ⓑ Ⓒ Ⓓ
128. Ⓐ Ⓑ Ⓒ Ⓓ
129. Ⓐ Ⓑ Ⓒ Ⓓ
130. Ⓐ Ⓑ Ⓒ Ⓓ
131. Ⓐ Ⓑ Ⓒ Ⓓ
132. Ⓐ Ⓑ Ⓒ Ⓓ
133. Ⓐ Ⓑ Ⓒ Ⓓ
134. Ⓐ Ⓑ Ⓒ Ⓓ
135. Ⓐ Ⓑ Ⓒ Ⓓ
136. Ⓐ Ⓑ Ⓒ Ⓓ
137. Ⓐ Ⓑ Ⓒ Ⓓ
138. Ⓐ Ⓑ Ⓒ Ⓓ
139. Ⓐ Ⓑ Ⓒ Ⓓ
140. Ⓐ Ⓑ Ⓒ Ⓓ
141. Ⓐ Ⓑ Ⓒ Ⓓ
142. Ⓐ Ⓑ Ⓒ Ⓓ

Biological Sciences

143. Ⓐ Ⓑ Ⓒ Ⓓ
144. Ⓐ Ⓑ Ⓒ Ⓓ
145. Ⓐ Ⓑ Ⓒ Ⓓ
146. Ⓐ Ⓑ Ⓒ Ⓓ
147. Ⓐ Ⓑ Ⓒ Ⓓ
148. Ⓐ Ⓑ Ⓒ Ⓓ
149. Ⓐ Ⓑ Ⓒ Ⓓ
150. Ⓐ Ⓑ Ⓒ Ⓓ
151. Ⓐ Ⓑ Ⓒ Ⓓ
152. Ⓐ Ⓑ Ⓒ Ⓓ
153. Ⓐ Ⓑ Ⓒ Ⓓ
154. Ⓐ Ⓑ Ⓒ Ⓓ
155. Ⓐ Ⓑ Ⓒ Ⓓ
156. Ⓐ Ⓑ Ⓒ Ⓓ
157. Ⓐ Ⓑ Ⓒ Ⓓ
158. Ⓐ Ⓑ Ⓒ Ⓓ
159. Ⓐ Ⓑ Ⓒ Ⓓ
160. Ⓐ Ⓑ Ⓒ Ⓓ
161. Ⓐ Ⓑ Ⓒ Ⓓ
162. Ⓐ Ⓑ Ⓒ Ⓓ
163. Ⓐ Ⓑ Ⓒ Ⓓ
164. Ⓐ Ⓑ Ⓒ Ⓓ
165. Ⓐ Ⓑ Ⓒ Ⓓ
166. Ⓐ Ⓑ Ⓒ Ⓓ
167. Ⓐ Ⓑ Ⓒ Ⓓ
168. Ⓐ Ⓑ Ⓒ Ⓓ
169. Ⓐ Ⓑ Ⓒ Ⓓ
170. Ⓐ Ⓑ Ⓒ Ⓓ
171. Ⓐ Ⓑ Ⓒ Ⓓ
172. Ⓐ Ⓑ Ⓒ Ⓓ
173. Ⓐ Ⓑ Ⓒ Ⓓ
174. Ⓐ Ⓑ Ⓒ Ⓓ
175. Ⓐ Ⓑ Ⓒ Ⓓ
176. Ⓐ Ⓑ Ⓒ Ⓓ
177. Ⓐ Ⓑ Ⓒ Ⓓ
178. Ⓐ Ⓑ Ⓒ Ⓓ
179. Ⓐ Ⓑ Ⓒ Ⓓ
180. Ⓐ Ⓑ Ⓒ Ⓓ
181. Ⓐ Ⓑ Ⓒ Ⓓ
182. Ⓐ Ⓑ Ⓒ Ⓓ
183. Ⓐ Ⓑ Ⓒ Ⓓ
184. Ⓐ Ⓑ Ⓒ Ⓓ
185. Ⓐ Ⓑ Ⓒ Ⓓ
186. Ⓐ Ⓑ Ⓒ Ⓓ
187. Ⓐ Ⓑ Ⓒ Ⓓ
188. Ⓐ Ⓑ Ⓒ Ⓓ
189. Ⓐ Ⓑ Ⓒ Ⓓ
190. Ⓐ Ⓑ Ⓒ Ⓓ
191. Ⓐ Ⓑ Ⓒ Ⓓ
192. Ⓐ Ⓑ Ⓒ Ⓓ
193. Ⓐ Ⓑ Ⓒ Ⓓ
194. Ⓐ Ⓑ Ⓒ Ⓓ
195. Ⓐ Ⓑ Ⓒ Ⓓ
196. Ⓐ Ⓑ Ⓒ Ⓓ
197. Ⓐ Ⓑ Ⓒ Ⓓ
198. Ⓐ Ⓑ Ⓒ Ⓓ
199. Ⓐ Ⓑ Ⓒ Ⓓ
200. Ⓐ Ⓑ Ⓒ Ⓓ
201. Ⓐ Ⓑ Ⓒ Ⓓ
202. Ⓐ Ⓑ Ⓒ Ⓓ
203. Ⓐ Ⓑ Ⓒ Ⓓ
204. Ⓐ Ⓑ Ⓒ Ⓓ
205. Ⓐ Ⓑ Ⓒ Ⓓ
206. Ⓐ Ⓑ Ⓒ Ⓓ
207. Ⓐ Ⓑ Ⓒ Ⓓ
208. Ⓐ Ⓑ Ⓒ Ⓓ
209. Ⓐ Ⓑ Ⓒ Ⓓ
210. Ⓐ Ⓑ Ⓒ Ⓓ
211. Ⓐ Ⓑ Ⓒ Ⓓ
212. Ⓐ Ⓑ Ⓒ Ⓓ
213. Ⓐ Ⓑ Ⓒ Ⓓ
214. Ⓐ Ⓑ Ⓒ Ⓓ
215. Ⓐ Ⓑ Ⓒ Ⓓ
216. Ⓐ Ⓑ Ⓒ Ⓓ
217. Ⓐ Ⓑ Ⓒ Ⓓ
218. Ⓐ Ⓑ Ⓒ Ⓓ
219. Ⓐ Ⓑ Ⓒ Ⓓ

WRITING SAMPLE

Part 1

TURN PAGE FOR ADDITIONAL SPACE

_____

_____

_____

_____

_____

_____

_____

_____

_____

_____

_____

_____

_____

_____

_____

_____

_____

_____

_____

_____

_____

_____

_____

END OF PART 1

WRITING SAMPLE

Part 2

_____

_____

_____

_____

_____

_____

_____

_____

_____

_____

_____

_____

_____

_____

_____

_____

_____

_____

_____

_____

_____

_____

_____

_____

_____

_____

_____

_____

_____

_____

_____

_____

_____

_____

_____

_____

_____

_____

_____

_____

_____

_____

_____

_____

TURN PAGE FOR ADDITIONAL SPACE ➤

END OF PART 2

PHYSICAL SCIENCES

Directions: This test contains 77 questions. Most of the questions consist of a descriptive passage followed by a group of questions related to the passage. For these questions, study the passage carefully and then choose the best answer to each question in the group. Some questions in this test stand alone. These questions are independent of any passage and independent of each other. For these questions, too, you must select the one best answer. Indicate all your answers by blackening the corresponding circles on your answer sheet.

A Periodic Table is provided at the beginning of this unit (page 564). You may consult it whenever you wish.

Passage I (Questions 1–8)

1. *Rationale.* An investigator sets out to determine the absorption spectrum of the $Co(NH_3)_6^{+3}$ complex, and to study the effect on the spectrum of substituting different "ligands"—groups surrounding the cobalt—for the original ammonia ligand.

The investigator hopes to gain information about the molecular orbitals in the cobalt complexes. The first step in such a process is to measure the wavelength of maximum absorption for each complex, and to interpret this wavelength in terms of a transition energy.

2. *Procedure.* The experimental setup is shown in the next column. The experimenter uses the same cell for each sample, so that the path length will not vary, and each solution is made up to be 0.01 M. By measuring the light transmitted by the sample, a photodetector at the output end of the spectrometer determines the absorbance at each wavelength and sends this information to the chart recorder. The latter displays absorbance as a function of wavelength; the investigator calculates the wavelength of maximum absorption for each compound.

Experimental Setup

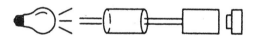

Experimental Setup

Analysis of Data. Table 1 shows ranges of wavelength and related energy.

Table 3 shows several possible series of molecular energy levels that might be used to explain the transitions in Tables 1 and 2. When

Table 1

Color of solution	clear	violet	blue/ blue-green	green	yellow	orange	red	red-purple
Color absorbed	"ultraviolet"	yellow	orange-red	purple	violet	blue	blue-green	green
λ (nm) of absorbed light	<400	400	500	530	580	610	680	700
Energy of absorbed light	>299	299	239	226	207	196	176	171

GO ON TO THE NEXT PAGE

Table 2

Complex	λ_{max} (nm)
$Co(NH_3)_6^{3+}$	430
$Co(NH_3)_5(H_2O)^{3+}$	500
$Co(NH_3)_5(CO)^+$	500
cis-$Co(NH_3)_4Cl_2^+$	560
trans-$Co(NH_3)_4Cl_2^+$	680

a photon matching the difference between two of the levels is absorbed, an electron can be promoted to a higher level.

Table 3

(energy in kJ/mol)

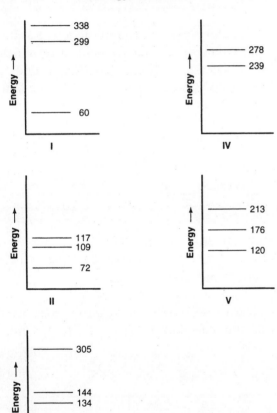

1. What is the color of a solution that absorbs light having an energy of 239 kJ/mol?

   A. orange/red
   B. blue/blue-green
   C. purple
   D. green

2. The region on the chart between 400 and 600 nm shows how many distinct, visible, solution colors?

   A. 3
   B. 4
   C. 5
   D. 6

3. The highest energy transition in Table 2 corresponds to absorption by which of the following compounds?

   A. $Co(NH_3)_6^{+3}$
   B. $Co(NH_3)_5(H_2O)^{+3}$
   C. $Co(NH_3)_5(CO)^+$
   D. *cis*-$Co(NH_3)_4Cl_2^+$

4. The replacement of one ammonia in $Co(NH_3)_6^{+3}$ by a water molecule results in a shift in absorption from

   A. indigo to blue-green.
   B. blue-green to indigo.
   C. yellow to orange-red.
   D. orange-red to yellow.

5. Using the data from Table 1, choose the expression that best describes the relationship between energy (in kJ/mol) and λ (in nm).

    A. $E = 0.75 \lambda$
    B. $E = (1.12 \times 10^5)/\lambda$
    C. $E = (\lambda - 101)$
    D. $E = 0.50\lambda + 99$

6. Which of the diagrams in Table 3 could be used to explain the absorption of $cis\text{-}Co(NH_3)_4Cl_2{}^+$?

    A. I
    B. II
    C. III
    D. IV

7. Which of the diagrams in Table 3 explains the absorption of the complexes that appear to be blue solutions?

    A. I
    B. II
    C. IV
    D. V

8. Which of the diagrams in Table 3 predicts one or more possible transitions in the ultraviolet region of the spectrum?

    A. I
    B. III
    C. IV
    D. None of the above.

Passage II (Questions 9–14)

An experimenter wishes to test the hypothesis that a concentration difference alone can produce a voltage in an electrochemical cell. In order to test her hypothesis, she constructs the cell shown below, where both sides of the cell contain $AgNO_3$, with concentrations shown in the diagram. She will use the voltmeter shown to determine what voltage, if any, exits across the electrodes at different times after the circuit is closed.

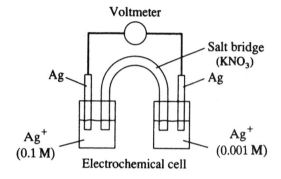

The table that follows shows the voltage in the cell as a function of the time that current has been allowed to flow in the circuit. It also displays the concentration of silver ion on each side of the cell.

t(s)	V (volts)	$[Ag^+]$ on left (mol/L)	$[Ag^+]$ on right (mol/L)
0	0.1180	0.1000	0.0010
10	0.0721	0.0953	0.0057
20	0.0567	0.0910	0.0100
30	0.0472	0.0872	0.0138
40	0.0404	0.0837	0.0173
50	0.0351	0.0805	0.0205
•			
•			
•			
1000	0.0000	0.0505	0.0505

GO ON TO THE NEXT PAGE

9. The purpose of the salt bridge in the experiment is to

   A. conduct Ag^+ ions from left to right.
   B. conduct Ag^+ ions from right to left.
   C. allow K^+ and NO_3^- ions to flow from one half cell to another in order to keep the solution electrically neutral.
   D. allow electrons to flow from left to right.

10. The reduction potential for Ag^+, $E°$, is 0.799 volts. For the net reaction that occurs in the overall cell, what is $E°_{cell}$ in v?

    A. 0
    B. 0.799
    C. −0.799
    D. 0.009

11. For how many time values listed in the chart does the value of V change by more than 0.010 v from the previous time?

    A. 1
    B. 2
    C. 3
    D. 4

12. If the apparatus were modified so that the solutions on each side could mix through a horizontal connecting tube, the measured voltages would

    A. be unchanged from those given in the table.
    B. drop rapidly to zero.
    C. increase from those shown in the table.
    D. take a longer time to reach zero.

13. Which of the following best describes the relationship among the voltage and the concentrations on each side?

    A. As time passes, electrons flow through the salt bridge from left to right, causing the ions to equilibrate and the voltage to drop.
    B. As time passes, Ag^+ ions flow through the salt bridge from left to right, causing the voltage to drop.
    C. As time passes, electrons flow through the wire from left to right, causing the ions to equilibrate and the voltage to drop.
    D. As time passes, electrons flow through the wire from right to left, causing the concentration gradient to decrease and the voltage to drop.

14. Suppose that C_1 represents the concentration of silver ion on the left of the cell, while C_2 represents the concentration on the right. Which of the following best describes the relation between C_1 and C_2?

    A. $C_1 - C_2$ is constant, owing to conservation of charge.
    B. $C_1 - C_2$ is constant, owing to conservation of Ag^+ ion.
    C. $C_1 + C_2$ is constant, owing to conservation of charge.
    D. $C_1 + C_2$ is constant, owing to conservation of Ag^+ ion.

Reaction	1st Component	2nd Component	Major Products
1	0.1 mol Ag^+	0.1 mol Cl^-	0.1 mol AgCl(s)
2	0.1 mol H^+	?	0.05 mol H^+
3	0.1 mol acetic acid	0.1 mol OH^-	?
4	0.05 mol acetate	?	0.025 mol acetic acid, 0.025 mol acetate
5	1 mol CO_3^{2-}	?	1 mol H_2CO_3
6	1 mol HCl	1 mol formic acid	?

Passage III (Questions 15–22)

Applications of equilibrium constants to real-life problems often confront a student with a reaction and ask what the products and their concentrations will be. These problems often seem to lie outside the examples frequently provided in texts. Our advice is to determine, however roughly, what the equilibrium constant is for a given reaction, and then either solve assuming total reaction (if $K_{eq} >> 1$), or, if the reaction is seen not to proceed very far, to calculate equilibrium concentrations.

The following problems combine questions about solubility with those concerning strong and weak acids.

15. Which of the following best explains the result of reaction 1?

    A. Cl^- is a weak base.
    B. K_{sp} for AgCl $>> 1$.
    C. K_{sp} for AgCl $<< 1$.
    D. Most chloride salts are soluble.

16. Which of the following could have been the second component in reaction 2?

    A. 0.05 mol H^+
    B. 0.05 mol OH^-
    C. 0.1 mol H^+
    D. 0.1 mol OH^-

17. Which of the following could be the second component in reaction 4?

    A. 0.05 mol of acetic acid
    B. 0.05 mol of HCl
    C. 0.025 mol acetic acid
    D. 0.025 mol HCl

18. The pH of the resulting solution in reaction 3 is closest to which of the following?

    A. 1
    B. 4
    C. 7
    D. 9

19. Which of the following could be the second component in reaction 5?

    A. 1 mol H^+
    B. 1 mol OH^-
    C. 2 mol H^+
    D. 2 mol OH^-

20. An investigator wishes to predict the result when 1 mole of ammonium chloride is mixed with an equal amount of strong base. Which reaction from the chart most closely resembles this reaction?

    A. Reaction 2
    B. Reaction 3
    C. Reaction 4
    D. Reaction 5

21. The final product of which reaction would make a useful buffer?

    A. 2
    B. 3
    C. 4
    D. 5

22. After reaction 6, the original formic acid has

    A. not appreciably changed.
    B. changed about 50 percent to formate.
    C. largely changed to formate.
    D. been neutralized.

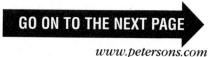

GO ON TO THE NEXT PAGE

Cell	Half-Cell 1	Polarity	Half-Cell 2	Polarity	Voltage
A	Ni^{2+}/Ni	−	Pb^{2+}/Pb	+	0.131
B	Zn^{2+}/Zn	−	Fe^{3+}/Fe^{2+}	+	1.53
C	Ni^{2+}/Ni	+	Zn^{2+}/Zn	−	0.505

Passage IV (Questions 23–31)

Several students measure the voltages in three different cells, each made from two half-cells as indicated in the table above. The concentration of each of the ions in solution is 1.0 M. The average values of the measurements, as well as the relative polarities, are shown in the table above.

By combining the results in the table above, the students derive the following chart showing reduction potential:

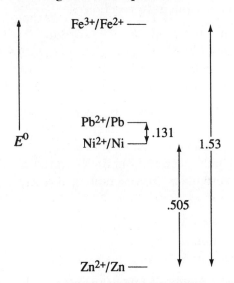

23. Based on the table above, when the circuit is closed in cell A, in which direction do electrons flow through the voltmeter?

A. Toward the Ni electrode
B. Toward the Pb electrode
C. Neither direction since they are equally attracted to both electrodes
D. Cannot be determined

24. Based on the table above, at which electrode does reduction occur in cell B?

A. Positive
B. Negative
C. Neither
D. Cannot be determined

25. By studying cells B and C, the students can determine that

A. Zn^{2+} is reduced by Fe^{2+}.
B. Zn is oxidized by both Fe^{+3} and Ni^{2+}.
C. Zn is oxidized by Fe^{3+} and is reduced by Ni.
D. Zn is reduced by Fe^{3+} and is oxidized by Ni.

26. By studying cells A and C, the students can determine that which of the following statements are true?

A. Pb is more readily oxidized than Ni. Zn is more readily oxidized than Ni.
B. Pb is less readily oxidized than Ni. Zn is more readily oxidized than Ni.
C. Pb is more readily oxidized than Ni. Zn is less readily oxidized than Ni.
D. Pb is less readily oxidized than Ni. Zn is less readily oxidized than Ni.

27. By examining the result for cell A only, what can the students find the reduction potential for Pb^{2+}/Pb to be?

A. 0.131 v
B. −0.131 v
C. 0.131 v greater than for Ni^{2+}/Ni
D. 0.131 v less than for Ni^{2+}/Ni

28. By examining the results for cells A and B only, the students can find that compared to the half-cell reduction potential for Ni^{2+}, the reduction potential for Zn^{2+}/Zn

    A. is 1.40 less.
    B. is 1.40 more.
    C. is .37 less.
    D. cannot be determined.

29. According to the chart on the previous page, will Zn react spontaneously with 1 M Pb^{2+} in solution?

    A. Yes
    B. No
    C. Only in acidic solution
    D. Cannot be determined

30. If the reduction potential for Ni^{2+}/Ni is taken arbitrarily to be 1.00 v, what is the reduction potential for Pb^{2+}/Pb?

    A. -0.87 v
    B. 0.87 v
    C. -1.131 v
    D. 1.131 v

31. If "cell D" were to be made up as cells A through C were, but with Pb^{2+}/Pb and Zn^{2+}/Zn as the half-cells, what would be the voltage and polarity?

    A. 0.37 v, with Zn positive
    B. 37 v, with Pb positive
    C. 0.636 v, with Zn positive
    D. 0.636 v, with Pb positive

Passage V (Questions 32–36)

A chemist is asked to identify two solutions whose labels have peeled off. One is known to contain 1.0 formula weight of NaCl for each kg of water in which it is dissolved. The other has an identical concentration of Na_2CO_3.

32. Which chemical test might best furnish an identification?

    A. Flame test for sodium
    B. Test for chloride by adding $AgNO_3$
    C. Test for pH
    D. Titration with NaOH

33. The chemist decides instead to measure the freezing point of each solution. This method will distinguish between the two compounds because

    A. CO_3^{2-} is more effective at lowering the freezing point of a solution.
    B. Cl^- is more effective at lowering the freezing point of a solution.
    C. the freezing point is lowered more by doubly charged ions.
    D. the freezing point is lowered in proportion to the total number of ions in the solution.

34. The freezing-point depression is directly proportional to the

    A. molarity of the solution.
    B. molality of the solution.
    C. molecular weight of the solute.
    D. volume of the solution.

35. In order to distinguish between the solutions using the freezing-point depression, the chemist must assume that

    A. NaCl is much more soluble than Na_2CO_3.
    B. Na_2CO_3 is much more soluble than NaCl.
    C. each salt dissolves completely.
    D. each salt has a negligible K_{sp}.

GO ON TO THE NEXT PAGE

36. The chemist measures the freezing-point depression and finds which of the following?

   A. One solution, which she should identify as NaCl, has a freezing-point depression that is 50 percent greater than the other's.

   B. One solution, which she should identify as Na_2CO_3, has a freezing-point depression that is 50 percent greater than the other's.

   C. One solution, which she should identify as NaCl, has a freezing-point depression that is 33 percent greater than the other's.

   D. The freezing-point depressions are equal, since each solution is completely ionized.

Passage VI (Questions 37–41)

An apparatus is devised for evaluating the properties of thin lenses. It consists of a sliding mount that holds the lens and allows it to be moved forward and backward along a track. A reference object, such as an arrow, is fixed at one end of the track. The lens position is then adjusted along the track until the object is in focus.

   In one test, an arrow 0.050 meter high is fixed at point A on the track. When the center of the sample lens is 0.60 meter from the arrow, a sharp image of the arrow is formed on the opposite side of the lens at point B, which is 0.30 meter away from the center of the lens. The position of the object arrow is more than two focal lengths away from the lens.

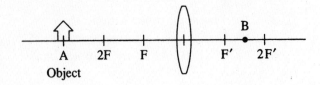

37. What is the focal length of the test lens?

   A. 0.60 m
   B. 0.30 m
   C. 0.20 m
   D. 0.15 m

38. What is the height of the image of the arrow at point B?

   A. 0.025 m
   B. 0.030 m
   C. 0.045 m
   D. 0.060 m

39. Which statement describes the image of the arrow formed at point A?

   A. The image is real and erect.
   B. The image is virtual and erect.
   C. The image is real and inverted.
   D. The image is virtual and inverted.

40. The image is formed because light from the object is

   A. polarized.
   B. reflected.
   C. refracted.
   D. diffracted.

41. Which statement describes what happens to the image as the object is moved toward the lens?

   A. The image will increase in size and move closer to the lens.
   B. The image will increase in size and move farther away from the lens.
   C. The image will decrease in size and move closer to the lens.
   D. The image will decrease in size and move farther away from the lens.

Passage VII (Questions 42–46)

A racetrack is constructed so that its opposite ends are semicircles attached to each other by long straight stretches of road. The radius of curvature of one end is 50.0 meters. The radius of curvature of the opposite end is twice that. The track is perfectly flat. A racecar with a mass of 2000 kilograms drives in a clockwise direction around the outer edge of the track at a constant speed of 20 meters per second.

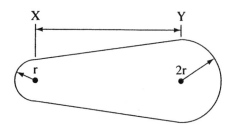

42. In comparing the centripetal acceleration acting on the car as it goes around the larger curve to the centripetal acceleration as the car goes around the smaller curve at the opposite end of the track, one finds that the centripetal acceleration around the large curve will be

   A. one-quarter the a_c associated with the small curve.
   B. half the a_c associated with the small curve.
   C. twice the a_c associated with the small curve.
   D. quadruple the a_c associated with the small curve.

43. What is the net force acting on the car as it goes around the smaller curve?

   A. 0 N
   B. 8.0×10^3 N
   C. 1.2×10^4 N
   D. 1.6×10^4 N

44. One of the two straightaways between the two curves lies between the points labeled X and Y in the diagram of the track. What is the net force acting on the car as it goes along this straightaway?

   A. 0 N
   B. 8.0×10^3N
   C. 1.2×10^4N
   D. 1.6×10^4N

45. If the car travels from point X to point Y in 20 seconds, what must be the length of this section of the straightaway?

   A. 100 m
   B. 200 m
   C. 300 m
   D. 400 m

46. The kinetic energy of the car as it goes around the larger curve is

   A. less than it is along the straightaway.
   B. greater than it is along the straightaway.
   C. exactly equal to the value along the straightaway.
   D. exactly four times greater than it is along the straightaway.

GO ON TO THE NEXT PAGE

Passage VIII (Questions 47–52)

Poiseuille's law is often used to describe blood flow rate through the circulating system. It is given by the equation

$$Q = \frac{\pi}{8\eta l}(P_1 - P_2)R^4$$

where Q = flow rate of fluid

η = coefficient of viscosity

l = length of tube through which fluid flows

R = radius of tube

P_1 and P_2 = pressures at point 1 and point 2 of tube

Poiseuille's law describes only laminar or streamline flow where layers of the fluid flow in parallel directions. If the speed of these layers increases, the flow may become turbulent where the fluid swirls and forms eddies. More pressure will then be required to maintain the flow rate because of greater frictional losses. The Reynolds number $\mathcal{R}$ is often used to determine the velocity at which laminar flow becomes turbulent.

$$\mathcal{R} = \frac{2\bar{v}Rd}{\eta}$$

where $\bar{v}$ = average speed of the fluid

d = density of the fluid

Empirical studies have shown that laminar flow occurs when $\mathcal{R}$ is less than 2000. At $\mathcal{R}$ values greater than 3000, turbulent flow occurs. Between these two values, the flow can be either laminar or turbulent.

47. A patient is given an antibiotic intravenously. According to Poiseuille's formula, which of the following will be most effective in increasing the flow rate of the antibiotic into the patient?

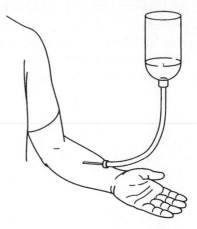

A. Raise the bag of intravenous antibiotic
B. Increase the radius of the needle
C. Dissolve the antibiotic in another solvent
D. Decrease the length of tubing

48. The radius of a person's artery decreases by 50 percent from arthereosclerosis. In order to maintain the same blood flow rate, the person's heart must

A. increase the net pressure by a factor of 32.
B. double the net pressure.
C. triple the net pressure.
D. increase the net pressure by a factor of 16.

49. The flow rate of blood at rest is about 5 L/min. If $\eta = 4.0 \times 10^{-3}$ N s/m^2 and $d = 1.030 \times 10^3$ kg/m^3, what is the Reynolds number for an artery with diameter 2.0 cm?

A. 1,365
B. 2,000
C. 6,800
D. 68

50. What is the average linear blood flow rate above which turbulence must occur for the 2.0-cm artery?

A. 2.9 m/s
B. 0.58 m/s
C. 25 L/min
D. 10 L/min

51. Poiseuille's law indicates that most of the pressure exerted by the heart is dissipated in the

A. arteries.
B. veins.
C. capillaries and arterioles that feed the capillaries.
D. heart valves.

52. For a liquid flowing through a pipe of radius R, length l, and pressure drop $(P_1 - P_2)$, a decrease in temperature most likely will

A. decrease the flow rate.
B. decrease the average speed of liquid layers.
C. increase the coefficient of viscosity.
D. All of the above.

Passage IX (Questions 53–58)

The experimental setup shown is used to determine osmotic pressure (π) of various aqueous solutions of glucose. The membrane is permeable to water.

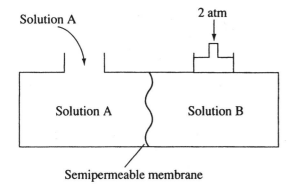

53. The diagram indicates which of the following?

A. $\pi_A > \pi_B$;
Concentration$_A$ > Concentration$_B$
B. $\pi_A < \pi_B$;
Concentration$_B$ > Concentration$_A$
C. $\pi_A > \pi_B$;
Concentration$_B$ > Concentration$_A$
D. $\pi_A < \pi_B$;
Concentration$_A$ > Concentration$_B$

54. The pressure exerted on the piston that would prevent any net flow of water from solution A to solution B is equal to

A. the osmotic pressure of solution B.
B. the osmotic pressure of solution A.
C. the difference in the osmotic pressures of the two solutions.
D. twice the osmotic pressure of solution B.

55. If solution A were replaced by water, what would happen to the pressure required to prevent net flow of water?

A. It would increase.
B. It would decrease.
C. It would remain the same.
D. The effect cannot be predicted.

56. The osmotic pressure of a red blood cell is about 7.7 atm. A red blood cell immersed in water will most likely

A. shrink in size.
B. dissolve.
C. release water.
D. burst.

57. The osmotic pressure of a 0.10 M glucose solution is

A. the same as a 0.10 M NaCl solution.
B. less than a 0.10 M NaCl solution.
C. greater than a 0.10 M NaCl solution.
D. zero.

GO ON TO THE NEXT PAGE

58. Which of the following phenomena best explains osmosis?

   A. Brownian motion
   B. Friction
   C. Capillary action
   D. Diffusion

Questions 59–77 are independent of any passage and independent of each other.

59. What is the current in a 60-W light bulb operating at 120-V household voltage?

   A. 2.0 A
   B. 1.5 A
   C. 1.0 A
   D. 0.5 A

60. A siren sounds with a frequency of 700 Hz. What frequency is heard by a driver in a car moving away from the siren with a uniform velocity of 35 m/s? (The speed of sound in air is about 350 m/s for the ambient temperature.)

   A. 720 Hz
   B. 630 Hz
   C. 540 Hz
   D. 790 Hz

61. Fluid moves with constant speed and no turbulence through a tube of uniform diameter as illustrated below. At which point is the pressure lowest?

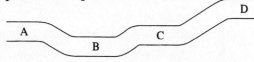

   A. A
   B. B
   C. C
   D. D

62. The threshold of hearing has an intensity of 10^{-12} W/m^2 (watts per square meter), which corresponds to a sound level β, of 0 dβ (decibels). What is the intensity of a 40-dβ sound?

   A. 40×10^{-12} W/m^2
   B. 10^{-3} W/m^2
   C. 10^{-8} W/m^2
   D. 40×10^{-3} W/m^2

63. Which of the following procedures would allow an experimenter to determine E_a for a given reaction?

   A. Measure k at 298K.
   B. Measure k at 398K.
   C. Measure k at 298K and 398K.
   D. Measure the rate for a variety of concentrations.

64. Which of the following will not change the total pressure in a closed vessel containing N_2 gas? (Assume ideal gas behavior.)

   I. Increasing the temperature.
   II. Replacing half the N_2 molecules with gaseous helium atoms.
   III. Adding an equal amount of gaseous hydrogen.

   A. I only
   B. II only
   C. III only
   D. I and II only

65. A student wishes to find the solubility of $Ba(IO_3)_2$, for which $K_{sp} = 1.6 \times 10^{-9}$. If x represents the solubility, which equation should she solve?

   A. $1.6 \times 10^{-9} = (x)(x)$
   B. $1.6 \times 10^{-9} = (x)(2x)$
   C. $1.6 \times 10^{-9} = (x)(x)^2$
   D. $1.6 \times 10^{-9} = (x)(2x)^2$

66. For which of the gas-phase reactions below would ΔS be expected to be negative?

    I. $2H_2O \rightarrow 2H_2 + O_2$
    II. $2H \rightarrow H_2$
    III. $N_2 + 3H_2 \rightarrow 2NH_3$

    A. I only
    B. II only
    C. I and II only
    D. II and III only

67. For the reaction $2NO_2(g) \rightarrow N_2O_4(g)$, which of the following is true?

    I. Removing NO_2 shifts the equilibrium to the left.
    II. Increasing the volume of the container shifts the equilibrium to the right.
    III. Adding helium gas to the container shifts the equilibrium to the right.

    A. I only
    B. II only
    C. III only
    D. I and II only

68. The pH of a solution of 0.001 M NaOH is closest to which of the following?

    A. 0.001
    B. 3
    C. 7
    D. 11

69. A student wishes to prepare a buffer whose pH is 6.3, using an acid HA with a pK_a of 6.0. Which expression below will correctly express the ratio R of HA to NaA that must be mixed in order to achieve the desired pH?

    A. $6.3 = 6.0 + \log R$
    B. $6.0 = 6.3 + \log R$
    C. $10^{-6.3} = 10^{-6.0} + \log R$
    D. $6.3 = \log 6.0 + R$

70. The period of a simple pendulum can be increased by

    A. increasing the length of the pendulum.
    B. decreasing the length of the pendulum.
    C. increasing the mass of the box.
    D. decreasing the mass of the box.

71. The depth of water in the ocean is determined by using sonar signals. Assuming that the speed of sound in water is about 1.5 km/s and it takes a total of 6 s for a sonar signal to return to the ship after being emitted, what is the estimated depth of the ocean at that point?

    A. 3.0 km
    B. 9.0 km
    C. 0.25 km
    D. 4.5 km

72. What is the work done in holding a 20-N weight at a height of 2 m above the floor for a total of 5 s?

    A. 0 J
    B. 8 J
    C. 2 J
    D. 200 J

73. Three capacitors are connected as shown to a 24-V potential voltage source

    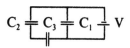

    $C_2 = C^3 = 8\mu F$
    $C_1 = 3\mu F$

    What is the total capacitance of this circuit?

    A. $4\mu F$
    B. $7\mu F$
    C. $12\mu F$
    D. $18\mu F$

GO ON TO THE NEXT PAGE

74. Pascal's principle holds that when an external pressure is applied to an enclosed fluid, the pressure

   A. is uniformly distributed undiminished to all points in the fluid.

   B. is distributed undiminished, but as a function of fluid depth.

   C. is greatest at the point of application and decreases as the distance from the application point increases.

   D. affects only the rate of flow in the fluid layers closest to the tube's walls.

75. Two point charges attract each other with a force of 3.6×10^{-6} N when they are 3 m apart. What is the force if the distance is increased to 6 m?

   A. It is tripled.

   B. It is reduced to one-ninth.

   C. It is quadrupled.

   D. It is quartered.

76. Two tuning forks vibrate so that the note produced by the first fork is exactly one octave above the note produced by the second fork. Compared to the speed of the wave produced by the first fork, the speed of the wave produced by the second fork is

   A. half as fast.

   B. twice as fast.

   C. eight times as fast.

   D. the same speed.

77. Four resistors are connected as shown.

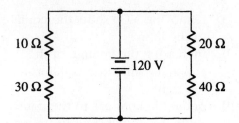

What is the current through the 40-W resistor?

   A. 1.2 A

   B. 2.0 A

   C. 3.0 A

   D. 4.0 A

END OF TEST 1.

IF YOU FINISH BEFORE THE TIME IS UP,
YOU MAY CHECK YOUR WORK ON THIS TEST ONLY.

VERBAL REASONING

TIME: 85 MINUTES   **QUESTIONS 78–142**

> **Directions:** There are nine passages in this test. Each passage is followed by questions based on its content. After reading a passage, choose the one best answer to each question and indicate your selection by blackening the corresponding circle on your answer sheet.

Passsage I (Questions 78–84)

When some 12.5 million tomato seeds returned to Earth in February 1985 after almost a year in space, several thousand American students from fifth grade through university level anxiously awaited their arrival with pots and trowels at the ready. They wanted to find out whether tomatoes grown from the tiny space travelers would be any different from their earthbound counterparts.

All 12.5 million of the seeds were carried aboard Space Shuttle Mission 41-C in April 1984 and placed in orbit inside NASA's Long Duration Exposure Facility (LDEF), a free-flying, 12-sided structure loaded with experiments designed to test results of continuous exposure to outer space. When the LDEF was recovered early in 1985, the seeds—after the first known opportunity for long-duration exposure of living tissue—were divided up in packets of fifty among hundreds of schools across America. Students in science classes were to plant them and compare their growth results with earthbound plants. Control planting of earthbound tomato seeds began in the fall of 1984. Similar plants of the "seeds from Zero G"—the space-exposed specimens—began about the fall of 1985.

There were no "cookbook" rules governing how the experiments were to be carried out or observed by the students, other than the requirement of strictly scientific methodology. At the conclusion of the experimentation, student reports describing each school's results were tabulated in a summary report by NASA headquarters and made generally available upon request. The two-year experiment, named SEEDS (Space Exposed Experiment Developed for Students), was jointly sponsored by NASA and the Park Seed Company of Greenwood, South Carolina, supplier of the seeds.

Like all great ideas, this one was born in the mind of one imaginative individual. Back in 1978, George B. Park, president of the Park Seed Company of Greenwood, S.C., was reading an article in *Scientific American* magazine about the space shuttles, called "Getaway Specials," that NASA was preparing to launch from time to time into outer space, filled with scientific experiments. His inquiries led him to the Goddard Space Flight Center's Clark Porty, administrative officer for the Getaway Specials. Porty accepted Park's idea for a two-part container as a valid experiment. One of the seed containers was to be open to vacuum exposure; the other, not.

Soon after that experiment, in the summer of 1983, Park had a visit from Bill Kinard of the Langley Research Center, Science Director for the LDEF projects. Kinard wanted to know if Park's company would be willing to enter into a joint venture with the Langley Research Center to put a large number of seeds onto the LDEF as a project involving the students of America, with part of the payload to be the company's own. Says Park, "I said 'yes' immediately, without thinking."

Control experiments back on Earth included not only the earthbound seeds planted by the students, but also a batch of similar seeds

GO ON TO THE NEXT PAGE ▶

kept in Greenwood at the seed company, and another batch in an air-conditioned area at the Kennedy Space Center at Cape Canaveral.

Park adds that one of the many benefits of the experiment for exobiologists (scientists who study possibilities of life in outer space) is knowledge gained about whether life forms could travel by passive means from one ecosystem or planet to another without a spaceship. If the seeds exposed to both vacuum and high radiation come through with little or no damage, it opens up questions (and may provide some answers) about the origins and destinations of primitive life forms. For example, scientists could extrapolate from the results of the experiment how many years organic matter might float in space and still be viable. Says Park, "If only *one* primitive life form, say a spore, or a bacterium or a virus, can live for 100,000 years, then it could get from one system to another."

But this is only one possible avenue of thought arising from the experiment. What new connections might be made by the thousands of students participating in SEEDS? Their horizons are as unlimited as outer space.

78. According to the article, an exobiologist is a scientist who studies

    A.   seeds.
    B.   the effects of space radiation on living things.
    C.   the possibility of life in outer space.
    D.   the external structures of living things.

79. The reason for sending the seeds into outer space was to test the effects on the seeds of

    A.   continuous exposure to outer space.
    B.   ultraviolet light.
    C.   weightlessness.
    D.   low-level radiation.

80. Upon their return to Earth, the seeds were distributed to

    A.   12.5 million students from fifth grade to college level.
    B.   fifty schools across America.
    C.   a laboratory jointly operated by Park Seed Company and Langley Research Center.
    D.   several thousand American students.

81. Which of the following rules were students to follow when doing their experiments?

    I.   They were to compare growth rates only.
    II.   They were to report their results honestly.
    III.   They were to follow scientific methodology.

    A.   I only
    B.   II only
    C.   III only
    D.   I and II only

82. Results of the student experiments with space-exposed seeds were

    A.   submitted to *Scientific American* magazine.
    B.   used by Park Seed Company to develop new strains of tomato plants.
    C.   tabulated in a summary report by NASA.
    D.   closely guarded until the end of the two-year experimental period.

83. According to the article, which of the following are the two most important facts to be learned from sending seeds into outer space?

   A. Some seeds are more able to survive space than others, and that seeds exposed to radiation in space are dangerous to humans.
   B. Astronauts can raise their own food in space, and such food has the same nutritional value as that grown on Earth.
   C. Life forms other than seeds can survive in space, and they can survive for an indefinite period of time.
   D. Seeds can survive the vacuum of space and the high levels of radiation in space with little or no damage.

84. Based on the article, it would be reasonable to assume that the author's attitude toward other similar projects would be

   A. strongly opposed.
   B. mildly opposed.
   C. mildly supportive.
   D. strongly supportive.

Passage II (Questions 85–91)

James Madison College of Michigan State University offers students a liberal education concentrated on public affairs. The college received support from the National Endowment for the Humanities in 1984 to bring more humanities study into the upper-level courses in social sciences.

The proposal demonstrates that a foundation for the project exists in the successful integration of the humanities and the social sciences in some parts of the Madison College curriculum. In one field of concentration, for example—justice, morality, and constitutional democracy—great books form the core of the curriculum. Students read Plato, Aristotle, Machiavelli, Hobbes, Rousseau, Hegel, and Nietzsche or Weber. By pairing faculty seminars and other faculty development activities with a revision of upper-level courses, the Madison faculty is working to increase the humanities content of other areas of the curriculum.

Faculty seminars have been conducted by Sheldon Wolin, who assigned readings by Hannah Arendt, Martin Heidegger, and Michael Oakeshott, and by philosopher Alan Bloom, who led faculty in an examination of liberal education and the study of the texts.

Although a separate, well-defined plan was presented for each activity, the proposal made clear that the project was being undertaken as an integrated effort to revitalize the college's dedication to providing a liberal arts education to its students. The proposal states, "We expect these activities to sharpen our collective understanding of the role of the humanities in the study of public affairs, contribute to faculty development, improve individual courses, and make our upper-level curricula more vital and coherent. . . . Accordingly, at the outset of the project, we emphasize those activities that deepen our common perspective and enhance our individual expertise; in the later stages, we emphasize those that are aimed at course and curricular revision." Panelists' reactions demonstrated their admiration for the strong, unified goal toward which all activities of the project were directed.

85. Which of the following is mentioned as one approach to the development of an integrated curriculum at James Madison College?

   A. Use classics in a core course.
   B. Have faculty seminars as coursework for lower-level freshmen and sophomore students.
   C. Rotate faculty members who lecture in order to revitalize the classes.
   D. Increase the public affairs content of upper-level courses.

GO ON TO THE NEXT PAGE

86. The proposal to expand humanities study for upper-division students at James Madison College of Michigan State University confirms the commitment by the college to

   A. widen students' knowledge by focusing on specific great works of literature and philosophy.

   B. further increase the core courses in the humanities through faculty involvement in curriculum and team teaching.

   C. enhance student understanding and appreciation of the curriculum with its strong emphasis on challenging readings and sensitized faculty.

   D. upgrade its standards in offering a liberal arts education.

87. It can be inferred from the article that the author

   A. does not like the integration of curriculum that is taking place at Madison College.

   B. is impressed by what is being done with the curriculum at Madison College.

   C. has no clear opinion about what is being done at Madison College.

   D. believes that despite some positive aspects to what has been done to the curriculum at Madison College, negative aspects outweigh the positive.

88. The foundation of the project described in the article is to integrate

   A. public affairs with a liberal education.

   B. English with humanities.

   C. humanities and social science.

   D. humanities and public education.

89. Which of the following are recognized as goals of the project?

   I. Increased faculty development activities

   II. Increased attention to individual student needs

   III. Extensive revision of upper-level curricula

   A. I only

   B. III only

   C. I and II only

   D. I and III only

90. The attitude of the panelists toward the integrated curriculum is best described by which of the following statements?

   A. The panelists were in favor of the integrated curriculum proposal.

   B. The panelists were opposed to the integrated curriculum proposal.

   C. The panelists supported the idea of an integrated curriculum but believed the current curriculum needed adjustment.

   D. The panelists preferred a curriculum that integrated science and humanities.

91. The article provides an example of a field of concentration in which students read works by each of the following except

   A. Spinoza and Kant.

   B. Machiavelli and Hobbes.

   C. Nietzsche and Weber.

   D. Plato and Aristotle.

Passage III (Questions 92–97)

The possibility of climate change presents a unique challenge for American electric utilities. If there is, indeed, a significant warming of the Earth's climate due to rising concentrations of greenhouse gases, utilities may be affected at three distinct levels. First, they will inevitably play an important role in any broad societal response to climate change and will have an opportunity to forge a new relationship with their customers to achieve common goals. Second, utilities recognize that their industry will be among those whose operations are most deeply affected by a changing climate, perhaps within the time frame of current planning for construction of new facilities. Finally, electric utilities are concerned that costly and potentially counterproductive regulations may be promulgated before a rational basis for policy making is achieved.

An overriding consideration in each of these three areas is the number of uncertainties that remain in the scientific understanding of the greenhouse effect and the likely effectiveness of various countermeasures. In particular, the apparent 0.6 degree C, 1 degree F rise in average global temperature over the last century lies within the long-term range of natural variability, although the recent rate of increase seems rapid. Current models suggest that a warming trend of this magnitude could result solely from the increases in atmospheric CO_2 and other greenhouse gases (e.g., nitrous oxide, methane, chlorofluorocarbons, and ozone). However, the observed rise in temperature over the last century has not been steady and has been marked by unexplained periods of cooling.

Research is needed to tell us not only when to act but also how to act. Although the focus of recent debates has been primarily on strategies to reduce emissions, it is not at all clear that the point of emissions is the best place for intervention. There is, in fact, a wide variety of options potentially available for countering the greenhouse effect:

(1) *Reducing greenhouse gas production:* Examples are reducing energy use, fuel switching from coal to natural gas, increasing the use of nonfossil sources, and reducing the rate of deforestation.

(2) *Removing greenhouse gases from effluents or the atmosphere:* Examples are removing CO_2 from power plant emissions as well as starting forestation programs.

(3) *Making countervailing modifications in climate and weather:* One example is cloud seeding; another more speculative example is changing the atmosphere's reflectivity by releasing particles in the stratosphere.

(4) *Adapting to changing climate:* Examples are heating and cooling of buildings, compensation of disadvantaged regions, and changing of agricultural practices.

Because of the large amounts of capital and time required to build generation and transmission facilities, electric utilities must plan for decades ahead. Recent studies indicate that if significant climate change occurs, some effects may be felt within the current planning horizon for utilities. The need for more air conditioning during longer, hotter summers, for example, would not only raise the annual demand for electric energy but increase demand peaks as well. Utility planners must therefore consider both the likelihood of having to build new power plants to meet higher peak demand and the probable need to purchase more fuel for increased generations.

Planners will also need to consider potential changes in energy supply resulting from climate change. Stream flows that affect the availability of hydroelectric energy, for example, depend on both the amount and timing of precipitation, which could be altered in some regions by even small changes in the average global temperature. In addition, the reliability of electricity delivery systems could be affected by

GO ON TO THE NEXT PAGE

shifts in the frequency and intensity of weather extremes, such as tornadoes, hurricanes, and severe storms. Power plant operations in some coastal regions could also be hampered by even a moderate rise in the sea level resulting from thermal expansion of the oceans and possibly increased melting of glaciers and Antarctic ice.

To meet these challenges, utilities will need to adopt more sophisticated strategies of risk management. Although many of the effects of climate change remain unpredictable, the cost of adapting will be much less if some prudent contingency plans are made well in advance.

92. According to the author, which of the following *may* be a consequence of the Greenhouse Effect on electric utilities?

A. A reduction in the need for heat
B. Institution of many useless regulations
C. Disappearance of many of the sources for producing electricity
D. Blaming the utilities themselves for the greenhouse effect

93. In planning for the future, the author suggests that utility planners take into account all of the following except

A. changes in energy supplies due to climate changes.
B. building new power plants to meet higher consumer demands.
C. encouraging future generations to decrease energy usage.
D. adopting additional sophisticated approaches for risk management.

94. The author states that over the last century, the Earth's temperature has risen

A. 1 degree C.
B. .6 degrees F.
C. .6 degrees K.
D. .6 degrees C.

95. Which one of the following is not considered a strategy for the reduction of gas emission into the air?

A. Heating and cooling buildings
B. Removing greenhouse gases from the atmosphere
C. Cloud seeding
D. Changing consumer consumption

96. Following the author's logic, it would be reasonable to assume that

A. awareness of the greenhouse effect must take the form of consumer advocacy.
B. the future of the electrical supply is in imminent danger.
C. a concerted effort between government and utility planning must be a joint venture.
D. the utility industry must gear up for intense research.

97. According to the article, which of the following are considered greenhouse gases?

I. Oxygen and hydrogen
II. Helium, radon and carbon monoxide, hydrocarbon
III. Nitrous oxide, methane, chlorofluorocarbons, and ozone

A. I only
B. II only
C. III only
D. I and II only

Passage IV (Questions 98–103)

Like so many other areas of American life, the field of aging offers opportunities to go into business for yourself. Gerontological consulting is coming into its own with the growing demand for information about older persons' spending patterns, use of leisure time, housing preferences, eating habits, and the like.

So intense is the interest in the older consumer that many of America's largest companies have launched advertising campaigns targeted at adults over 50. But their perceptions of older people leave a lot to be desired, observes David Wolfe in the July 1987 issue of *American Demographics.* "Few marketers understand older Americans," he says, "and their advertising campaigns repel the very people they're trying to attract." Age-grading of products and services intended for older people usually backfires, he warns. A marketing strategy that presents the product or service as an opportunity for personal growth is far more likely to succeed.

In an effort to link gerontologists with the business community, showing advertisers how to avoid age stereotypes, for example, the American Society on Aging has organized a Business Forum on Aging that includes representatives from Bank of America, Sandoz Corporation, American Express, Marriott Corporation, Edison Electric Institute, and others.

"Turning the hunger for information about older people into a business opportunity for gerontologists requires ingenuity and an eye for a suitable market niche," says Nancy Peppard of Peppard Associates. Taking her own advice, she organized her firm in two divisions. One advises corporations about marketing, advertising, and sensitivity training for employees; the other advises health-care facilities about setting up special units for dementia patients.

Jean Coyle, founder of the International Association of Gerontological Entrepreneurs, warns of the challenge of setting up your own firm. The most commonly mentioned issue is the tremendous amount of time it takes to set up a small business. "There's just not enough time to do it all," she says. Entrepreneurs are hard pressed to manage the business end of the operation as well as provide a professional service.

The consulting business is fiercely competitive, observes Jane Yurrow of Leo, Inc., a firm that specializes in senior housing. Her advice is to plan on putting a lot of effort into marketing. Marketing skills are important, agrees Susan Hartenbaum of Aging Information Services. Personal style is at least as important as subject expertise in bringing in business, she adds. A warm, outgoing, engaging personality helps in making calls to prospective clients in their language, says Susan. Put yourself in their shoes, she advises. Your goal as a consultant is to help clients see their situation in a new light and help them develop an appropriate solution. Imposing your own expertise is one of the pitfalls to avoid.

Private case management offers excellent opportunities for gerontological entrepreneurs with clinical expertise. Case managers assist older persons and their families for a fee, offering such help as information and referral, brokering of services, and counseling. They personalize their services, providing as much or as little assistance as the client wants. Private case managers generally have at least some graduate education in a human service discipline and substantial experience working with the elderly. More often than not, they are social workers, although nurses, psychologists, and gerontologists operate case management firms, too.

Barbara Kane, a clinical social worker in private practice with Aging Network Services in Bethesda, Maryland, ticks off the professional skills important for success in this field: counseling skills, notably the ability to develop trust and confidence; assessment skills; the ability to involve the client and facilitate decision making; the ability to resolve conflicts and negotiate agreements; and the ability to act as a liaison among clients, service providers, and families. But business skills such as bookkeeping, office management, and marketing are necessary, too, she warns.

GO ON TO THE NEXT PAGE

According to a study conducted in 1987 by the Inter-Study Center for Aging and Long-Term Care, the popularity of private case management owes much to a convergence of several trends: growth in the older population, fragmentation and complexity of the services offered, and the growing respectability of private practice in the eyes of human service professionals. Prospects should continue to be very good, considering the rapid growth projected in the number of people of advanced age and the increased willingness of many people to use social work and mental health services.

98. According to David Wolfe, a marketing strategy that works for older people is which one of the following?

A. Using older people in advertisements
B. Advertising that a product will help in personal growth
C. Making old people look young and trendy
D. Focusing on the differences between the needs of the young and the needs of the old

99. The article implies that advertisers consider the older consumer to be anyone

A. over 70.
B. between 65 and 70.
C. between 60 and 65.
D. over 50.

100. According to Barbara Kane, which skills are needed to run a successful case management firm?

A. Interactive skills and networking skills
B. Counseling skills and assessment skills
C. Communication skills and collaborative skills
D. Psychological skills and organizational skills

101. The author states that case managers come from several fields, including,

I. Psychiatry.
II. Nursing.
III. Gerontology.

A. I only
B. I and II only
C. I and III only
D. II and III only

102. The prospects in the field of case management should continue to be good because of growth in which of the following?

A. Number of professionals doing the job
B. Number of college-trained older people
C. Number of people over 85
D. Willingness of older people to use case-management services

103. The article implies that the growth and expansion of certain businesses, such as consulting firms and firms that offer private case management for the elderly, is related to

A. younger people's being less receptive to age-related products.
B. the awareness that older consumers represent an untapped market for advertising.
C. business's slow acknowledgment of the elderly as worthwhile consumers.
D. a nationwide program encouraging sensitivity toward the elderly.

Passage V (Questions 104–112)

Scientific interest in caves began in seventeenth- and eighteenth-century Europe with the development of elaborate (but erroneous) theories of the hydrogenic cycle in which cave systems were essential elements. The beginnings of a correct understanding of the geology of caves date from about 1850 in Europe and 1900 in North America. In Europe, emphasis was on karst hydrology, particularly on subterranean streams. Early biological studies emphasized faunal surveys and descriptions of the degenerate eyes of cavernicolous animals (cavernicoles); only after 1900 were a few experimental studies made.

In the early twentieth century, Racovitza and Jeannel sparked the spectacular rise of modern biospeleology in Europe. This period was, in general, an interlude for cave science in the United States, during which the only additions to knowledge about North American caves and their life were made by Europeans on field trips in North America.

Biospeleology advanced slowly in the United States from 1930 to 1950, even though this was the time of a lively debate over the origin of caves. The central point was whether caves form above or below the local water table. Davis proposed cave development deep below the water table, by random circulation of slowly percolating groundwater ("phreatic" origin). This view became textbook doctrine for many years. Other theories placed the zone of cave development at or above the local water table ("vadose" origin). This data and Davis's reputation as an authority had two stifling effects on cave studies: 1) the implied random pattern of cave development discouraged the search for specific hydrological mechanisms causative of cave system patterns, and 2) the argument over the location of the water table tended to reduce the research that was done to a sterile classification of some particular cave as having a vadose or phreatic origin.

Factors influencing reactivation of geological cave research and continued progress in biospeleology in the past decade include the amassing of a large body of descriptive data collected mainly by nonprofessional explorers and surveyors within the National Speleological Society; growing acquaintance with the large body of European literature that had been largely ignored by American theoreticians of the 1930s; near completion of a systematic description of many groups of cave organisms and their distribution, which permitted biologists to turn to ecological and physiological problems; and finally, involvement of younger researchers whose interest arose from exploration and field experience.

104. Davis said that caves developed

    A. above the water table.
    B. at the level of the water table.
    C. well below the water table.
    D. both above and below the water table.

105. According to the article, early biological studies in caves emphasized the study of

    I. Parasitic colonies found in caves that resembled coral found in the ocean.
    II. Fauna found in caves and the description of degenerate eyes of cavernicolous animals.
    III. Single-celled organisms found in caves.

    A. I only
    B. I and III only
    C. II only
    D. II and III only

106. Scientific interest in caves in Europe began in the

    A. fifteenth and sixteenth centuries.
    B. sixteenth and seventeenth centuries.
    C. seventeenth and eighteenth centuries.
    D. eighteenth and nineteenth centuries.

GO ON TO THE NEXT PAGE

107. Early scientific research on caves was based on an erroneous theory of the

A. hydrogenic cycle.
B. development of subterranean streams.
C. development of alluvial fans.
D. development of cave rock formations.

108. Davis's theory of cave development origin is referred to in the article as

A. vadose.
B. hydraulic.
C. phreatic.
D. cavernicoles.

109. According to the article, which of the following was not responsible for the resurgence of interest in geological cave research and advanced progress in biospeleology during the past decade?

A. The collection of a large body of descriptive data by nonprofessionals
B. A growing acquaintance with European literature of the 1930s
C. The contributions of European theoreticians on cave development
D. The involvement of younger researchers

110. Biospeleology is the study of

A. rock formations.
B. underground water systems.
C. the development of caves.
D. underground water tables.

111. It would be reasonable to assume that the writer believes that the discussion as to whether caves formed above the water table or below had

A. a negative effect on cave research in the United States.
B. a positive effect on cave research in the United States.
C. no discernible effect on cave research in the United States or worldwide.
D. both negative and positive effects on cave research.

112. Vadose origin refers to the development of caves

A. below the water table.
B. at or above the water table.
C. by slowly percolating groundwater.
D. in metamorphic rock.

Passage VI (Questions 113–118)

Robert Lowell is known both as a major twentieth-century American poet and as an important translator of Homer, Sappho, Aeschylus, Roman poets, and French writers. Yet, as the anniversary of his death approaches, Lowell's work remains difficult and obscure, and the critical appraisal of both his poetry and translations remains mixed.

Lowell scholar Daniel Gillis, a Haverford College classics professor—not a professor of modern literature, as most Lowell critics have been—is attempting to reform the critical view by highlighting the influence of classical literature on the poet.

"He isn't an American poet at all," Gillis explains, "but a bearer of an older, deeper tradition of European literary and poetic history, drawing on French, Italian, German, Russian, Greek, and Latin literature as nobody else can.

"I doubt it was a conscious process. Lowell knew both the Latin and Greek languages cold. He taught Greek for several years. It was second nature to him to think in terms of ancient structures and people. It didn't worry him much that some people wouldn't be able to understand everything in his poetry. At the same time, he knew he was losing his audience; maybe he was trying to raise their level. He wasn't about to abandon the Graeco-Roman legacy.

"In the poem 'My Last Afternoon with Uncle Devereux Winslow,' Lowell writes, 'Unseen and unseeing, I was Aggripina/in the Golden Halls of Nero.' This means nothing to readers—or critics—unless they know their Tacitus, know Aggripina was Nero's mother, and know this refers to Nero overthrowing her. Tacitus makes it very clear; she's walking around lost and doomed; it's a very dark reference. But if you don't know Tacitus and his history of Nero, it's just a woman walking through a house. This is the reader's problem, not Lowell's. He's saying something very clear. You have to equip yourself to deal with him."

Referring to Lowell's 1950 poem "Falling Asleep over the *Aeneid*," Gillis writes that "Anglo-American critics agree this is one of Lowell's memorable poems, but their writings tend to be limited to paraphrase. . . . Their shallow familiarity with the *Aeneid* does not serve them well." Few critics even notice that Lowell places Aeneas at a funeral the hero never actually attended.

The diminishing numbers of readers who can appreciate Lowell and scholars who can satisfactorily analyze the poet point up a disturbing trend in American education. The classical grounding in Latin and Greek language and literature that was prevalent in the nineteenth century has almost disappeared from today's schools. "We are a historyless people," Gillis quotes Arthur Schlesinger, Jr. "We wake up every morning, and for us history is born anew each day."

Also, Gillis laments, "We aren't a poetry-reading country anymore. The medium itself militates against wide readership. Around the time of Lowell's death, his new books sold about 300 copies. In general, poetry editions run about 1,000 copies."

Lowell's translations (which Gillis argues is the wrong word to use) have also been misunderstood. "He used the word *imitations*," Gillis notes. "They're much freer than literal translations. The Latin word *emulatio*, meaning 'emulations' or even 'competitions,' is more

exactly what he did. He took a poem of Horace, for instance, as raw material for a new artistic product. The Latin poets, when they adapted Greek material, did an original recasting; they were unconcerned with conveying every word literally. In that sense, Lowell was much a Roman working with Greek material. It's what Ezra Pound did, too."

Gillis's first encounter with Lowell occurred in 1979, while working on the book *Eros and Death in the Aeneid*. Gillis has found that studying Lowell's poetry and translations has deepened his understanding of the ancient works. In "Falling Asleep over the *Aeneid*," for example, Lowell, the perceptive analyst, sheds light on Virgil's eroticism, which few commentators have addressed or noted; he "brings . . . strands together with a remarkable clarity and economy of vision, suffused with warmth and an awesome sense of loss," says Gillis.

Gillis realizes that Robert Lowell's works provide an unusual opportunity. The course that the classicist is developing on Lowell and classical antiquity will be a bridge: It will address a modern poet from a fresh, rich perspective; it will serve as an entree for many students who are unfamiliar with classics and untrained in Latin and Greek; and it will give classics students a taste of modern literature while taking advantage of their academic forte.

The hope is that studying Lowell and his ties to classical antiquity will generate interest both in a poet deserving recognition and in an academic discipline in search of creative scholars.

113. Based on the article, it would be reasonable to believe that Daniel Gillis thought critics misunderstood Robert Lowell's poetry because they evaluated him as a

    A. Latin poet.
    B. Greek poet.
    C. European poet.
    D. twentieth-century American poet.

GO ON TO THE NEXT PAGE

114. Gillis strongly presents the view that Robert Lowell should be regarded as which of the following?

   A. An important translator of Roman and Greek classical literature

   B. A poet whose works were influenced by his knowledge of the classics of antiquity

   C. An avant garde poet familiar with French writers

   D. A modern poet who preferred to write only in classical Greek and Latin

115. Through his course on Lowell and classical antiquity, Gillis expects to accomplish which of the following?

   I. To generate increased interest in a deserving poet

   II. To address a modern poet from a fresh perspective

   III. To give classics students a taste of modern literature

   IV. To revive the requirement that a college education include a grounding in the classics

   A. I only

   B. I and II only

   C. I, II, and III only

   D. I, II, III, and IV

116. For a reader to understand Lowell's works, it would be necessary not only to be familiar with classic Latin and Greek literature, but also to have a background in

   A. the ancient languages of Latin and Greek.

   B. reading ancient Latin and Greek.

   C. European literary and poetic history.

   D. Greek and Roman mythology.

117. Gillis contends that the word *translations* is a misnomer for describing Lowell's translated works since they are

   I. mostly improvisational statements.

   II. commentaries about life in ancient Greece and Rome.

   III. freer renditions of classical works interpreted with perceptive clarity and depth.

   A. I and II only

   B. II only

   C. III only

   D. II and III only

118. According to Gillis, the appeal of Lowell's works to a very small number of contemporary readers and scholars is an indication of which of the following?

   A. Today's education fails to provide an adequate grounding in classical works of Latin and Greek.

   B. There is less interest in reading European literature today.

   C. Lowell's works fascinate only an eclectic group of readers.

   D. As an obscure poet and translator, Lowell is virtually unknown to the public.

Passage VII (Questions 119–126)

Of the many women who surely importuned their husbands for equal status in the new American nation, the most famous was Abigail Adams. On March 31, 1776, she wrote to her husband John, then in the Continental Congress: ". . . remember the ladies and be more generous to them than your ancestors, in the new code of laws. Do not put such unlimited power into the hands of the husbands," she warned, or women would rebel.

Although the threatened rebellion did not come about until nearly seventy-five years later, the role of women in public affairs during the colonial and post-revolutionary periods was considerably greater than their unequal political status might indicate, says Irwin Gertzog, professor of political science at Allegheny College in Meadville, Pennsylvania, who investigated the subject.

Gertzog's research shows that few women were active in politics during the colonial era, but many of them influenced religious, economic, military, and community developments. Managing taverns was an important economic function in the seventeenth and eighteenth centuries. New Jersey had more than 400 taverns, about one for every 500 residents in the state. Many women owned or managed taverns and inns. Some women were printers, crafts specialists, and merchants. During the Revolutionary War, a number of women joined the army, some in male disguise and some admitted as women. "There was a need for fighting strength," says Gertzog, "and women were prepared to provide it." Women also reported military preparations and troop movements and sabotaged British commercial and military activities.

Gertzog's work focused primarily on the political activities of women in New Jersey from 1788 to 1807, when they were the only female Americans legally eligible to participate in elections. "I wanted to discover why women were granted the vote, how many of them took advantage of it, and why it was taken away in 1807," says Gertzog.

During the Revolution, when New Jersey was breaking away from England, the provincial congress met in June of 1776 to draft a new constitution. "The British forces had landed in New Jersey at Sandy Hook," says Gertzog, "and the delegates had to work quickly. The legitimate authority of the new regime had to be established before it could raise funds, muster an army, and advise the Continental Congress that it had established a government independent of Great Britain."

The new constitution gave the vote to "all inhabitants" who were worth fifty pounds in real or personal property, thereby removing extensive real estate holdings as the sole economic test for voter eligibility. According to Gertzog, this more inclusive suffrage provision was prompted by petitions from men who were serving (or who would soon serve) in the army and supporting the war with taxes but who, without change, would not qualify to vote. Although the constitution did not explicitly grant female suffrage, neither did it say that voters had to be male. Gertzog found no evidence that women actively lobbied for the franchise.

The number of women who took advantage of the right to vote was difficult for Gertzog to estimate. The few available voting lists from the period, discovered in the archives of the New Jersey Historical Society, suggest that as many as 15 percent of the qualified women voted even though, through 1797, married women were ineligible. Under the laws governing domestic relations, a woman's property normally became her husband's as soon as they were wed. Consequently, eligible women voters were either single or widowed.

Why did women lose the vote in 1807? Gertzog is still seeking answers to this question, but some partial explanations seem evident: One is the substantial increase in competition between Republicans and Federalists after the turn of the century. Whenever a party was obliged to justify loss of a close election, it accused the opposition of fraud. Among the

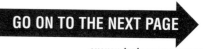

charges was that ineligible women, blacks, and aliens had been rounded up by the other party and herded to the polls.

In an 1802 legislative contest, for example, a Hunterdon County Federalist won by a single vote, and his victory resulted in an equal number of Federalists and Republicans in Trenton. Soon afterward, newspapers and leading Republicans alleged that the partisan deadlock that prevented a divided legislature from choosing a governor and U.S. senator was due to "the Federalist vote cast by an illiterate black woman."

An act disenfranchising women, free blacks, and aliens was promoted as a way of reducing election fraud by making it easier to identify ineligible voters. The act was passed later that year.

But these events in New Jersey, Gertzog notes, were a product of national as well as local forces. All states were then stripping the franchise from marginal groups—free blacks, noncitizens, native Americans, and in New Jersey, women—while at the same time removing obstacles to universal white male suffrage. Thus, New Jersey women were victims of political pressures that transcended local circumstances, and they would not be able to vote again until passage of the Nineteenth Amendment more than one hundred years later.

119. According to the article, which of the following was given as a justification for disenfranchising women in New Jersey?

A. Women were not as intellectually capable as men.
B. Women voting threatened the stability of the family.
C. Disenfranchising women would reduce voter fraud.
D. Women voted for the Federalist party, preventing the Republicans from having a majority.

120. The article implies that the political activity of women during the years preceding the passage of the Nineteenth Amendment was

A. minimal because most women were married.
B. negligible because the Constitution made no mention of women's being permitted to vote.
C. limited because women were classed alongside other powerless groups such as nonwhites and noncitizens.
D. considered unimportant by most women who believed an interest in politics to be unfeminine.

121. The reason the New Jersey constitution of 1776 was unique among the colonies was that it granted the right to vote

I. to free black men.
II. to women who owned personal or real property.
III. based on the property a person held.

A. I and II only
B. II and III only
C. II only
D. III only

122. Abigail Adams was

A. one of the first women to vote.
B. one of the first prominent women to call for women's rights.
C. the owner of a New Jersey tavern during the Revolutionary War.
D. a lookout who reported British troop movements during the Revolution.

123. According to the article, what percentage of the women who were eligible to vote did vote?

A. 15 percent
B. 25 percent
C. 40 percent
D. 50 percent

124. The New Jersey constitution of 1776 granted the right to vote to

    A. all men who had 40 pounds' worth of real property.

    B. all adults who had 40 pounds' worth of personal or real property.

    C. all men who owned real property worth more than 50 pounds.

    D. all inhabitants who had 50 pounds' worth of personal or real property.

125. After losing the vote in New Jersey, women did not regain the vote until

    A. the passage of the Bill of Rights.

    B. the passage of the Fourteenth Amendment at the end of the Civil War.

    C. a Supreme Court ruling gave all women the right to vote.

    D. the passage of the Nineteenth Amendment, a century later.

126. In which year did women in New Jersey lose the right to vote?

    A. 1788

    B. 1795

    C. 1802

    D. 1807

Passage VIII (Questions 127–134)

It was not only dark and stormy, but thirty degrees below zero in Vermont that night. I drove an hour north from my home to a small town called Wells River. When I arrived at the library, a converted storefront in the center of town, the woodstove was humming, and so was the audience. I was scheduled to give a forty-minute talk on Jean Rhys's novel *Wide Sargasso Sea,* a fictional biography of Bertha, the "mad woman in the attic" in *Jane Eyre.* My lecture was part of a series of five held over a ten-week period at the library. The audience had read the book in preparation for both the lecture and the discussion that followed, which was moderated by a discussion leader. My lectern turned out to be a shoe salesperson's slanted stool set upon a card table.

I launched into the lecture on this difficult novel, very much predicated on Brontë's long novel and narrated by three voices. The discussion reminded me again of why I loved to serve as a scholar in these programs. Talk ranged from analysis of the text to insights gained from Rhys about personal lives.

Finally, a woman at least seventy years of age rose to take issue with the interpretation I had set forth in the lecture. "Right here on page 87," she began, in a voice tremulous with excitement, "are examples that show Rochester to be more human than you have depicted him." I could see that her copy of the novel was dog-eared and underlined in several colors of ink. If only my freshmen cared this much about their reading! At the conclusion of the discussion, I had some new ideas about Jean Rhys, and these have affected my subsequent scholarship. I learned, for example, to be more subtle in my analysis of point of view.

Reading and discussion programs of this nature began just a decade ago around a kitchen table in Rutland, Vermont, across the state from Wells River. Pat Bates, then program coordinator at the Rutland Free Library and currently project director for the Howard County Library in Maryland, was a newcomer to Vermont. She had experienced the frustration of reading a good book and having no one with whom to discuss it, of saying to a friend in the grocery store, "I just read Toni Morrison's *Sula,* and it's fantastic," and drawing a complete blank.

Beginning with a reading group in her home, Bates experimented with various formats before hitting on the one that now has been successfully replicated in almost all fifty states and over one thousand libraries. Her goal was to establish a context in which a number of adults could all read the same book and later gather to discuss it. To enhance the discussion, Bates introduced the concept of opening each session with a lecture by a humanities scholar.

This scholarly component is the distinction between reading and discussion programs and other reading projects like the Great Books program. The scholar's role is not to provide a

GO ON TO THE NEXT PAGE

tidy analysis of the text, not to deliver "the answers," but rather to enrich discussion with biographical information on the author, contextual perspectives from the literary tradition or historical era, and be a catalyst for discussion by raising provocative questions about the text.

I frequently served as a scholar for Bates. I spoke about humanities texts—works by Charlotte Brontë, Mary Wilkins Freeman, Margaret Atwood, Toni Morrison—to eager audiences in small libraries, community centers, and even churches. I "got hooked" on teaching this way because the audiences were hungry—the very best *metaphor*—for the scholar's information and even hungrier for the human interaction around a text.

These audiences were diverse: adolescents and octogenarians, people with high school degrees, people with Ph.D.s, individuals from all classes and careers. Each had experienced the human need for a story. Yet they had not had their needs satisfied by the often empty calories of television. Hence, the intensity of the woman in Wells River who reacted strongly to *Wide Sargasso Sea* and needed help digesting the novel. What more could a teacher-scholar ask than for "students" who are well prepared, eager to talk, willing to argue, and replete with a wealth of life experience?

127. One of the purposes of the scholarly lecture was to provide readers with

- A. a means to participate in a cultural activity.
- B. a socializing process in isolated areas.
- C. an analysis of the text.
- D. an enriching discussion combining biographical information on the author with contextual perspectives.

128. Which of the following is a reasonable assumption based on the article?

- A. The author's college freshmen have a deeper understanding of literature than the people in these small towns.
- B. The people to whom the author speaks in these small towns have misinterpreted the literature being discussed.
- C. The author has found the talks in these small towns enriching to her own scholarly work.
- D. The people who participate in the library reading programs are culturally deprived.

129. According to the article, the presence of the humanities scholar was to

- I. provide definitive answers to all literary questions.
- II. keep an intellectual emphasis in the discussions.
- III. provide a lively, stimulating, literary ingredient to discussions.

- A. I only
- B. III only
- C. I and II only
- D. II and III only

130. The format of the discussion group that has been used successfully at over one thousand libraries is which of the following?

- A. A number of adults all read the same book, gather to discuss it, and are provided with a lecture by a humanities scholar.
- B. A number of adults select different topics to present for discussion.
- C. A number of adults read the same book and prepare open-ended discussion questions.
- D. A number of adults read the same book and select chapters to interpret and present for discussion.

131. The program discussed in this article began in

    A. Howard County, Maryland.
    B. Rutland, Vermont.
    C. Wells River, Vermont.
    D. Portland, Maine.

132. People who participated in these programs were usually

    A. scholars and academicians.
    B. young adults with a college education.
    C. older adults who were either retired or elderly.
    D. from a wide, diverse cross section of society.

133. One can infer that the author frequently lectures to reading groups because she

    A. finds the audiences well prepared and eager to discuss the book at hand.
    B. is well paid for her time.
    C. finds the participants better behaved than her students.
    D. enjoys the interacting with adults rather than students.

134. The author infers that the interest in such programs among adults was due to

    A. lack of interest in watching television.
    B. the need of adults to share reactions to books they have read through discussions.
    C. the need of adults to socialize with people of similar age and interests.
    D. a desire to read the latest novels.

Passage IX (Questions 135–142)

Two projects brought together for the first time the alumni associations from nine Big Ten universities, and a variety of other institutions, for several programs available to the public.

Under the leadership of Frank B. Jones, alumni associations from the University of Illinois, Michigan State University, University of Michigan, University of Minnesota, Northwestern University, Ohio State University, Purdue University, and the University of Wisconsin combined to co-sponsor the first project. "The Northwest Ordinance: Liberty and Justice for All" featured educational programs held on Big Ten campuses for the general public, a publishing program including articles by humanities scholars, and a two-day scholarly symposium to examine the state of current scholarship on the ordinance.

The symposium, held at the Indiana University campus, brought together a dozen scholars who were at work on the ordinance or some related aspect of American history. The Institute of Early American History and Culture in Williamsburg, Virginia, had expressed an interest in publishing the proceedings.

The alumni associations developed public education packs for distribution to libraries, historical societies, and other interested organizations. The packs contain articles commissioned by the alumni associations, a map of the Old Northwest Territory, a copy of the ordinance, a poster, a bibliography of selected reading materials, and a suggested speakers bureau of Northwest Ordinance scholars.

The second project sponsored by the Big Ten alumni associations is called "Liberty's Legacy." This traveling exhibition will bring original historical documents on the Northwest Ordinance, related ordinances, and the Constitution to the general public; to elementary, secondary, and university students; and to alumni in six states.

Among the 56 items included in the Northwest Ordinance part of the exhibition are a rare first printing of *The Definitive Treaty between Great Britain and the United States* (1783), written and printed at the instruction of

GO ON TO THE NEXT PAGE

Ambassador Benjamin Franklin in Paris; Jefferson's Ordinance of 1784, which set up a temporary government for the West; and the Land Ordinance of 1785, which established the system for the surveying and eventual sale of the new lands to settlers in the Northwest Territory. Colorful maps that illustrate the new land system will also be included, along with pages of the original Northwest Ordinance.

"These ordinances and documents rank among the most important in our early American history, both for what they accomplished and for what they inspired," says Frank Jones.

Those projects should help to engender public understanding and appreciation of the Northwest Ordinance as one of the cornerstone documents of our founding. Like any enduring cornerstone, the Northwest Ordinance has been built upon again and again. It has served as a blueprint for the nation's westward expansion. Without the ordinance, the United States could not have grown so tall or stood so long.

135. Based on the article, it would be reasonable to assume that the author believes the Northwest Ordinance was

- A. an important document that helped lead to the development of a strong America.
- B. a key component to the development of the American constitution.
- C. a building block for local governments on the frontier.
- D. a model for laws up to the present day in the United States.

136. Which of the following was not generated by the Northwest Ordinance project sponsored by the alumni associations of Big Ten universities?

- A. Exhibitions featuring original treaties related to the government and development of the Northwest Territory
- B. Scholarly research and seminars on the ordinance and related documents
- C. Increased public awareness of the document's role in American history
- D. Increased federal funding for similar historical efforts

137. According to the article, the Northwest Ordinance served as a plan that stimulated which of the following?

- A. Westward expansion among settlers
- B. Resolution of conflicts between Indian tribes in the area and incoming farmers
- C. Setting up of definite boundary lines for future states
- D. Involvement of the federal government in solving any land disputes

138. Which of the following was not one of the purposes behind the alumni associations' co-sponsoring of the Northwest Ordinance project?

- A. To promote greater cooperation among alumni associations in the future
- B. To emphasize the ordinance's historical role in American history
- C. To demonstrate the ordinance's impact on westward expansion into new territories
- D. To show the establishment of a system for surveying and selling new lands to settlers in the Northwest Territory

139. Two European countries mentioned in some capacity in relationship to the printing and publication of the Northwest Ordinance were

    A. England and France.
    B. England and Belgium.
    C. England and Spain.
    D. England and the Netherlands.

140. The land ordinance discussed in the article did which one of the following?

    A. It gave the land known as the thirteen colonies to the new government of the United States.
    B. It divided the land of the Northwest Territory.
    C. It created a system for surveying and ultimately selling land to settlers.
    D. It became the foundation of the new U.S. Constitution.

141. Among the historical documents displayed with the Northwest Ordinance exhibition were which of the following?

    I. Pages from the original Northwest Ordinance document
    II. The rare first printing of *The Definitive Treaty between Great Britain and the United States* (1783)
    III. Jefferson's Ordinance of 1784, which established the surveying and sale of lands to settlers in the Northwest Territory

    A. I only
    B. I and II only
    C. I and III only
    D. I, II, and III

142. The role of the alumni associations in the Northwest Ordinance project included

    A. hiring the Institute of Early American History and Culture to publicize the proceedings.
    B. developing public information packs for libraries, historical societies, and other interested organizations.
    C. writing scholarly articles on the Northwest Ordinance for distribution to elementary and secondary schools.
    D. selling posters and maps to raise money for future historical projects.

END OF TEST 2.

IF YOU FINISH BEFORE THE TIME IS UP,
YOU MAY CHECK YOUR WORK ON THIS TEST ONLY.

WRITING SAMPLE

TIME: 60 MINUTES   2 ESSAYS

Directions: This test consists of two parts. You will have 30 minutes to complete each part. During the first 30 minutes, you may work on Part 1 only. During the second 30 minutes, you may work on Part 2 only. You will have three pages for each essay answer, but you do not have to fill all three pages. Be sure to write legibly; illegible essays will not be scored.

Part 1

Consider this statement:

Necessity is the mother of invention.

Write a unified essay in which you perform the following tasks. Explain what you think the above statement means. Describe a specific situation in which necessity does *not* lead to invention. Discuss what you think determines when necessity is the mother of invention and when it is not.

DO NOT START THE NEXT TOPIC UNTIL THE TIME IS UP.

Part 2

Consider this statement:

> The key to failure is to try to please everyone.

Write a unified essay in which you perform the following tasks. Explain what you think the above statement means. Describe a specific situation in which the key to failure is in *not* trying to please everyone. Discuss what you think determines whether failure is accomplished when no one is pleased.

END OF TEST 3.
DO NOT RETURN TO PART 1.

BIOLOGICAL SCIENCES

Time: 100 Minutes   Questions 143–219

Directions: This test contains 77 questions. Most of the questions consist of a descriptive passage followed by a group of questions related to the passage. For these questions, study the passage carefully and then choose the best answer to each question in the group. Some questions in this test stand alone. These questions are independent of any passage and independent of each other. For these questions, too, you must select the one best answer. Indicate all your answers by blackening the corresponding circles on your answer sheet.

A Periodic Table is provided at the beginning of this unit (page 564). You may consult it whenever you wish.

Passage I (Questions 143–149)

Hemoglobin is a vital protein that transports oxygen in the red blood cells. It consists of four polypeptide chains, and at least seven different genes code for the subunits or chains of the molecule. Not all these genes are equally active throughout life.

All types of hemoglobin contain two alpha chains, but the remaining two chains of the molecule vary depending on age. At different times in the life of the individual, the proportion of hemoglobin molecules containing a particular type of chain (pair) may vary (see y-axis). The molecule found in RBCs at a particular time is designated by the types of chains present and how many of each (example: alpha$_2$beta$_2$). The figure below reflects the timing of production of the different chains during human development.

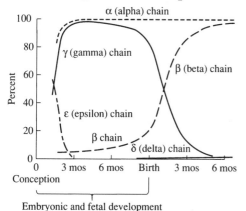

143. According to the figure, most fetal hemoglobin contains

   A. alpha and beta chains.
   B. alpha and gamma chains.
   C. alpha and epsilon chains.
   D. gamma and beta chains.

144. By extrapolating from the figure, what is the composition of most adult hemoglobin molecules?

   A. Alpha and beta chains
   B. Alpha and gamma chains
   C. Beta and delta chains
   D. Alpha and delta chains

145. The hemoglobin gene that appears to stop functioning earliest encodes the

   A. delta chain.
   B. gamma chain.
   C. epsilon chain.
   D. beta chain.

GO ON TO THE NEXT PAGE

146. At approximately what point does the beta chain start to appear in a higher proportion of hemoglobin molecules than the gamma chain?

    A. Three to six months before birth
    B. Just before birth
    C. Between birth and three months of age
    D. After six months of age

147. After determining from the figure when each type of hemoglobin is present, which types would you predict have an extremely high affinity for oxygen?

    A. $alpha_2gamma_2$ and $alpha_2delta_2$
    B. $alpha_2gamma_2$ and $gamma_2epsilon_2$
    C. $alpha_2epsilon_2$ and $gamma_2beta_2$
    D. $alpha_2gamma_2$ and $alpha_2epsilon_2$

148. Not all adult hemoglobin is of the same type. Based on information in the graph, a small proportion of adult hemoglobin is probably

    A. $alpha_2beta_2$.
    B. $alpha_2gamma_2$.
    C. $alpha_2delta_2$.
    D. $alpha_2epsilon_2$.

149. Based on information in the figure, what is the maximum percentage of hemoglobin molecules present at any one time that can be $epsilon_2delta_2$?

    A. 0 percent
    B. 55 percent–58 percent
    C. 0 percent–5 percent
    D. Cannot be determined

Passage II (Questions 150–156)

A set of experiments designed to investigate possible mechanisms of hormone action was carried out. One experiment examined the action of epinephrine, a hormone that is an amino acid derivative. The second experiment utilized the steroid hormones estrogen and progesterone.

Experiment 1

It is known that epinephrine stimulates the cytoplasmic enzyme glycogen phosphorylase to hydrolyze glycogen into sugar in cells of the liver and skeletal muscles. However, when epinephrine was added to a test-tube mixture containing the enzyme and glycogen, no hydrolysis occurred. Similarly, injecting epinephrine directly into the cells did not result in the hydrolysis of glycogen either. The effects of epinephrine were observable only if the hormone was added to the extracellular solution surrounding intact cells.

Experiment 2

It is known that estrogen and progesterone are necessary for the normal development and proper functioning of the reproductive system in mammals. In an experiment using rats and monkeys as subjects, target tissues along the reproductive tract and inside the brain were examined to detect the presence of these hormones. Results showed that the hormones were not only inside target cells, but inside the nucleus of these cells. In addition, they were found in association with special protein receptor molecules. When cells that are not normally affected by these hormones (spleen cells) were examined in a similar way, no trace of the hormones was found.

150. Based on the experimental observations, which hormone is least likely to have a *direct* effect on the genes?

A. Estrogen
B. Progesterone
C. Epinephrine
D. Both A and B

151. What is the probable reason that the steroid hormones could be found inside their target cells?

A. They are lipid soluble and can normally pass through cell membranes.
B. They are water soluble and can normally pass through cell membranes.
C. They are lipid soluble and carrier molecules transport them across cell membranes.
D. They are water soluble and carrier molecules transport them across cell membranes.

152. If steroids can enter cells, what is a reasonable hypothesis as to why there was no trace of the hormones in non-target cells such as the spleen?

A. They passed in and passed out again.
B. No special protein receptor molecule was present.
C. Both A and B.
D. Neither A nor B.

153. Which statement is compatible with the observations in Experiment 1?

A. Epinephrine stimulates glycogen phosphorylase by contact inside cells.
B. Epinephrine stimulates glycogen phosphorylase by contact outside cells.
C. Epinephrine stimulates glycogen phosphorylase when the hormone is outside and the enzyme is inside a cell.
D. All of the above.

154. Which conclusion is implied by the observations made in Experiment 1?

A. Epinephrine interacts with the membrane of its target cells.
B. Epinephrine does not interact with the membrane of nontarget cells.
C. Epinephrine interacts with the membrane of liver cells and skeletal muscle cells.
D. All of the above.

155. It is now known that most peptide hormones and hormones that are derivatives of amino acids bind to specific protein receptors in the membrane, which then activate a "second messenger" responsible for affecting activities inside the cell. What might be a major difference between a target cell and nontarget cell with respect to a particular hormone of this type?

A. Nontarget cells do not have the appropriate membrane receptors.
B. Nontarget cells have the membrane receptors but do not have the "second messenger."
C. Nontarget cells have the same "second messenger" as target cells, but may have membrane receptors for a different hormone.
D. Both A and C.

156. It has been stated that the surface of a target cell has approximately 10,000 protein receptor molecules. Yet this accounts for only 1/10,000 of the total number of proteins that help make up the cell's membrane structure. Based on this estimate, approximately how many proteins are on a typical cell membrane?

A. 10^7
B. 10^8
C. 10^9
D. 10^{10}

GO ON TO THE NEXT PAGE

Passage III (Questions 157–163)

There are three major "fluid compartments" of the human body. The regions of fluid are found inside the cells (intracellular fluid), outside or in between the cells (interstitial fluid), and in the blood (plasma). The two latter regions make up the extracellular fluid. Although the three compartments may contain many of the same materials in solution, each contains a different combination of concentrations. These differences in solute concentration contribute to the functioning of living systems, and must be maintained in order to ensure that normal cellular activities proceed. The figure below compares some of the dissolved constituents of the three fluid regions.

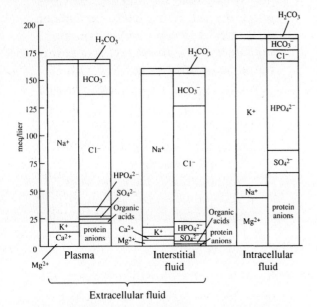

Key to symbols

Na^+	Sodium	Mg^{2+}	Magnesium	HPO_4^{2-}	Phosphate
K^+	Potassium	HCO_3^-	Bicarbonate	SO_4^{2-}	Sulfate
Ca^{2+}	Calcium	Cl^-	Chloride	H_2CO_3	Carbonic Acid

157. An important difference between extra-cellular fluids and intracellular fluid is that outside the cells, there is

A. more sodium.
B. more chloride.
C. less potassium.
D. all of the above.

158. The charge difference that exists between the inside and outside of cellular membranes (especially obvious in the resting potential of nerve and muscle cells) is due, in part, to the concentration differences noted in Question 157. A major factor shown in the figure that contributes to the final charge difference is:

A. the higher magnesium concentrations inside the cells.
B. the higher bicarbonate concentrations outside the cells.
C. the higher phosphate and protein concentrations inside the cells.
D. the similarities in carbonic acid concentrations.

159. Magnesium is an important intracellular electrolyte that is essential for the proper functioning of the sodium-potassium pump. Based on this information, which symptom would most likely result from a magnesium deficiency?

A. Endocrine gland malfunctions
B. Neuromuscular irritability
C. Lowered body temperature
D. Low blood sugar

160. Movement of fluid between the plasma and interstitial compartment takes place across the capillaries. Since blood hydrostatic pressure is higher than blood colloid osmotic pressure at the arteriole end of the capillaries, fluid (water and small proteins) leaks out. Most, but not all, returns at the venule end. Fluid not reabsorbed into the capillaries is eventually returned by the

A. urinary system.
B. liver.
C. spleen.
D. lymphatic system.

161. Homeostatic regulation of electrolytes such as sodium, potassium, calcium, and phosphate is monitored and controlled by the

    A. liver.
    B. endocrine system.
    C. brain.
    D. None of the above.

162. If an individual drinks seawater, the blood plasma becomes hypertonic. What will be the primary effect of this change on the intracellular fluid?

    A. Water will move from cells to blood.
    B. Water will move from blood to cells.
    C. Solutes will move from blood to cells.
    D. Solutes will move from cells to blood.

163. The bicarbonate ion is an important component of the blood buffer system. Buffers, the respiratory system, and the urinary system work together to help maintain homeostatic levels of

    A. glucose.
    B. water.
    C. gases.
    D. pH.

Passage IV (Questions 164–169)

Meiosis is the basis by which chromosome number is reduced by half and gametes are formed. Because sexual reproduction involves the union of two such haploid gametes, genetic variability is maintained.

An immense source of variability during meiosis is the process whereby linked genes (genes at different loci on the same chromosome) undergo crossing over. Homologous chromosomes break and exchange equivalent segments, forming chromosomes with brand-new combinations of genes to be passed on in the gametes (recombinant gametes) to prospective offspring. The appearance of recombinant offspring provides evidence that a chromosome break and crossing over has taken place between linked loci, and the frequency of such recombinant offspring suggests how often the chromosome breaks occurred. By monitoring new combinations of traits that result from crossover events, one can ultimately estimate the distance between the gene loci controlling those traits (the further apart two loci are on a chromosome, the more frequently breaks can occur between them).

In the fruit fly, *Drosophila melanogaster*, gray body and normal wings are two linked dominant traits. The recessive alleles for these genes are black body and vestigial wings, respectively. Flies homozygous for gray body and normal wings were crossed with flies having black bodies and vestigial wings, The F_1 offspring were then crossed with individuals having both recessive phenotypes with the following results in the F_2:

gray body, normal wings:	335
black body, vestigial wings:	305
gray body, vestigial wings:	75
black body, normal wings:	85

GO ON TO THE NEXT PAGE

164. Between which loci did crossing over occur?

   A. Gray body and black body
   B. Normal wings and vestigial wings
   C. Body color and wing type
   D. Both A and B

165. How many map units apart are the two gene loci?

   A. Less than 10
   B. Between 10 and 11
   C. 20
   D. 25

166. In fruit flies, the genes for normal bristles and normal eye color have been mapped to be about 20 units apart on the same chromosome. In a cross between heterozygotes for both traits and recessive individuals, how many offspring (out of 600) would be expected to have recombinant phenotypes?

   A. 100
   B. 120
   C. 30
   D. 150

167. The crossover frequency between linked genes A and B is 40 percent, between B and C is 65 percent, and between A and C is 25 percent. What is the sequence of genes on the chromosome?

   A. A-B-C
   B. C-A-B
   C. A-C-B
   D. C-B-A

168. If all the chromosomes are to be mapped, how many linkage groups should there be in an organism with 64 chromosomes per somatic cell?

   A. 64
   B. 32
   C. 16
   D. 48

169. In a cross between a heterozygote for the linked genes A, B, and D and a partner with the recessive phenotype for all three traits, what would be the phenotypes of the *double-crossover* recombinant offspring, if the map order of the loci is A-D-B?

   A. A-D-B and a-d-b
   B. A-D-b and a-d-B
   C. A-d-B and a-D-b
   D. A-d-b and a-D-B

Passage V (Questions 170–175)

Clotting or coagulation is part of a larger process called hemostasis (stoppage of bleeding) and occurs to close wounds that would otherwise cause blood loss. The clot itself, a network of insoluble fibers (fibrin), is the end result of a multistep sequence of events involving numerous coagulation factors, most of which are present in the plasma (plasma proteins and other factors designated by roman numerals) or are released by blood platelets (Pf_{1-4}).

Two parallel clotting systems are present. Both the *extrinsic system* and *intrinsic system* share a number of the same coagulation factors, even though each pathway is initiated by a different mechanism. The extrinsic system is triggered when a blood vessel is ruptured. The surrounding damaged tissues release tissue thromboplastin, and a series of reactions involving plasma coagulation factors eventually leads to the production of extrinsic thromboplastin (Stage 1). The intrinsic system (all components are present in the blood itself) is triggered when the rough surface of a ruptured vessel contacts platelets, causing them to release various platelet factors that eventually lead to the formation of intrinsic thromboplastin (Stage 1).

Steps involved in both systems are outlined in the following figure.

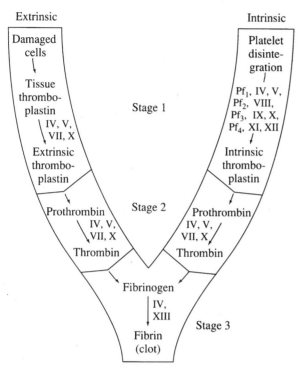

170. Based on information presented in the figure, which statement is correct about the two clotting systems?

    A.   Differences are seen only in Stage 1.
    B.   Both types of thromboplastin lead to the conversion of prothrombin to thrombin.
    C.   Plasma factor IV (calcium) is used in all steps of each system.
    D.   All of the above.

171. Most plasma coagulation factors in the figure are made in the

    A.   blood vessel walls.
    B.   liver.
    C.   spleen.
    D.   bone marrow.

172. Heparin is a substance produced by basophils (a type of white blood cell) and mast cells (a connective tissue cell). It interferes with the formation of thromboplastin and fibrin. The correct term for such a compound is

    A.   agglutinin.
    B.   agglutinogen.
    C.   antigenic.
    D.   anticoagulant.

173. Hemophilia is a sex-linked group of heredity disorders in which affected individuals lack one of the coagulation factors. If a normal woman whose father was a hemophiliac marries a normal man, what is the probability of producing a hemophiliac child (regardless of sex)?

    A.   100 percent
    B.   75 percent
    C.   50 percent
    D.   25 percent

174. Vitamin K is required for the synthesis of numerous coagulation factors. The pharmaceutical *dicumarol* acts as an antagonist to vitamin K. For which condition might this compound be recommended?

    A.   A patient with slow clotting time
    B.   A patient with excess heparin production
    C.   A patient prone to forming thromboses (clots in unbroken blood vessels)
    D.   A patient with internal hemorrhaging

175. A secondary effect of thrombin (besides converting fibrinogen to fibrin) is to cause platelets to adhere to each other and disintegrate. This added effect

    A.   feeds back and reinforces the intrinsic system.
    B.   feeds back and reinforces the extrinsic system.
    C.   both A and B.
    D.   neither A nor B.

GO ON TO THE NEXT PAGE

Table 1.

Protein and Peptide Levels of "Pepsin" Samples Maintained in Different Environments.

Temperature	pH		
	2–4	4–6	6–8
22°C	moderate protein moderate peptide	high protein no peptide	high protein no peptide
37°C	low protein high peptide	high protein no peptide	high protein no peptide
62°C	high protein no peptide	high protein no peptide	high protein no peptide

Passage VI (Questions 176–181)

An experiment designed concurrently to examine many variables was carried out. The goal of the experiment was to determine the appropriate environment for the proper functioning of two protein-digesting enzymes, pepsin (an enzyme that converts proteins to peptides in the stomach), and chymotrypsin (a pancreatic enzyme that converts proteins to peptides in the small intestine).

The Experiment

Each enzyme was placed separately in nine beakers containing identical mixtures of food proteins. To each beaker, a solution of buffering agents was added so that the activity of the enzymes could be compared at three different pH levels (pH: 2-4, 4-6, 6-8). *Three replicates* of the three pH environments were established for each enzyme.

One replicate beaker of each pH environment was then maintained in a water bath at each of three different temperature settings (temperatures: 22°C, 37°C, 62°C). At regular time intervals, samples identical in size were removed from each beaker to monitor the amounts of intact protein and peptides present.

Results are shown in Tables 1 and 2.

176. The most appropriate environment for chymotrypsin activity is

    A. 37°C, pH: 4-6
    B. 22°C, pH: 6-8
    C. 37°C, pH: 6-8
    D. 22°C, pH: 4-6

Table 2.

Protein and Peptide Levels of "Chymotrypsin" Samples Maintained in Different Environments.

Temperature	pH		
	2–4	4–6	6–8
22°C	high protein no peptide	high protein no peptide	moderate peptide moderate protein
37°C	high protein no peptide	moderate protein moderate peptide	low protein high peptide
62°C	high protein no peptide	high protein no peptide	high protein no peptide

177. Which statement most correctly reflects the data in Tables 1 and 2?

A. Both enzymes have some pH flexibility, but no temperature flexibility.
B. Both enzymes have some temperature flexibility, but no pH flexibility.
C. Both enzymes have some pH flexibility, but only pepsin has temperature flexibility.
D. Both enzymes have some temperature flexibility, but only chymotrypsin has pH flexibility.

178. Which environment appears to be incompatible with both enzymes?

A. pH: 4–6
B. pH: 2–4
C. 22°
D. 62°

179. Pepsin digests proteins in the specific environment of the stomach. What is the most reasonable explanation for why pepsin does not digest the proteins that make up part of the stomach's own walls?

A. The environment of the entire stomach is highly acidic.
B. The wall of the stomach is maintained at approximately 62°C.
C. Food proteins are surrounded by an acidic environment, while mucous secretions keep the walls alkaline.
D. Food proteins are surrounded by an alkaline environment, while mucous secretions keep the walls acidic.

180. The soupy material (chyme) released from the stomach into the small intestine is highly acidic. What occurs to ensure that digestion of proteins by pancreatic enzymes continues in the intestinal environment?

A. The pancreas releases different enzymes with different pH ranges for digesting proteins.
B. The pancreas delays its release of enzymes until alkaline food arrives in the intestine.
C. The pancreas sends sodium bicarbonate to adjust intestinal pH.
D. The small intestine passes the acidic chyme to the large intestine while retaining undigested food molecules.

181. After both pepsin and chymotrypsin successfully digest proteins to peptides, what takes place in the small intestine that allows body tissues to benefit from these nutrients?

A. The peptides are absorbed into the blood.
B. The peptides are combined to form polypeptides for more efficient protein synthesis by cells.
C. The peptides are digested further into amino acids.
D. All of the above.

GO ON TO THE NEXT PAGE

Table 3.

Chemical Constituents in Plasma; Filtered and Reabsorbed in 24 Hrs.

Chemical	Plasma	Filtrate Immediately after Glomerular Capsule	Reabsorbed from Filtrate
Water	180,000 mL	180,000 mL	178,000–179,000 mL
Proteins	7,000–9,000	10–20	10–20
Chloride (Cl^-)	630	630	625
Sodium (Na^+)	540	540	537
Bicarbonate (HCO_3^-)	300	300	299.7
Glucose	180	180	180
Urea	53	53	28
Potassium (K^+)	28	28	24
Uric acid	8.5	8.5	7.7
Creatinine	1.5	1.5	0

Passage VII (Questions 182–187)

The kidneys help remove metabolic waste products from the blood. They further contribute to the maintenance of homeostasis by regulating the volume, composition, and pH of the blood. The nephrons of the kidney carry out these various roles through the processes of filtration, reabsorption, and secretion. Filtration takes place from glomerular capillaries into Bowman's capsule. Materials forced out of the blood this way make up the resulting fluid, the filtrate. Substances in the filtrate include waste products, water, nutrients, and electrolytes. Vital substances needed by the body are reabsorbed from filtrate to peritubular capillaries, while wastes and materials not needed continue in the filtrate and are excreted in the urine. Additional changes can be made by transporting materials from peritubular capillaries to filtrate (secretion).

Table 3 shows some of the chemical constituents of the plasma, as well as how much of each chemical is filtered and reabsorbed in the nephron in one day (all values, except for water, are expressed in grams).

182. In a single day, approximately what percentage of water filtered from the plasma leaves the body as urine?

   A. 0.05 percent–0.1 percent
   B. 0.5 percent–1 percent
   C. 1.5 percent–2 percent
   D. 5 percent–10 percent

183. According to information in the table, all plasma constituents are filtered completely except

   A. chloride ions.
   B. sodium ions.
   C. urea.
   D. proteins.

184. The afferent arteriole leading into the glomerulus has a wider diameter than the efferent arteriole, which carries blood away to the peritubular capillaries. This arrangement

A. increases the efficiency of reabsorption.
B. represents a countercurrent mechanism.
C. increases pressure in the glomerulus.
D. allows red blood cells to pass into the filtrate.

185. Normally, glucose from the plasma is filtered into Bowman's capsule and then completely reabsorbed by active transport in the proximal convoluted tubules. Which of the following is a probable reason that diabetics have high glucose levels in the urine?

A. The level of glucose that is filtered is higher than normal.
B. The number of glucose carrier molecules is limited.
C. Both A and B.
D. Neither A nor B.

186. The kidney helps maintain pH balance with a variety of urinary adjustments. If an individual's blood pH is too high, which of the following would be an appropriate urinary system response?

A. Secrete bicarbonate ions
B. Reabsorb additional bicarbonate ions in the distal convoluted tubules
C. Filter additional acidic proteins
D. Allow the larger alkaline proteins through the glomerulus

187. The kidney can increase red blood cell production by releasing the hormone erythropoietin. It can also cause additional reabsorption of sodium ions through the renin-angiotensin system's stimulatory effects on aldosterone production. Why do both of these actions help raise blood pressure?

A. Both lead to a decrease in plasma water content.
B. Both lead to vasodilation of blood vessels.
C. Both lead to an increase in blood volume.
D. Both lead to an increase in secretion at the collecting tubules.

GO ON TO THE NEXT PAGE

Passage VIII (Questions 188–192)

An organic chemistry student heats benzil with a strong base to form the benzilate anion.

When methoxide ion in methanol is used instead of base, the methyl ester of benzilic acid is formed. Two mechanisms are considered

Mechanism A.

Mechanism B.

786

188. Both mechanisms involve a(n)

    A. reversible step.
    B. molecular rearrangement.
    C. nucleophilic substitution.
    D. electrophilic substitution.

189. If the methoxide ion in methanol is substituted for OH^-/H_2O, step (1) of Mechanism A will most likely yield which of the following?

A.
$$C_6H_5-\underset{|}{\overset{\overset{OCH_3}{|}}{C}}=O$$
$$C_6H_5-\underset{\overset{|}{OCH_3}}{C}=O$$

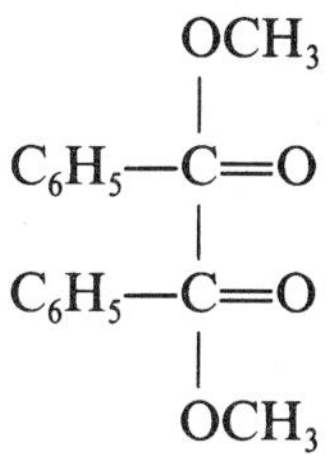

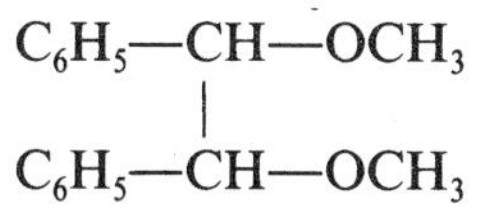

B.
$$C_6H_5-\underset{|}{CH}-OCH_3$$
$$C_6H_5-CH-OCH_3$$

C.
$$C_6H_5-\underset{\overset{|}{C_6H_5-C=O}}{\overset{\overset{O^-}{|}}{C}}-OCH_3$$

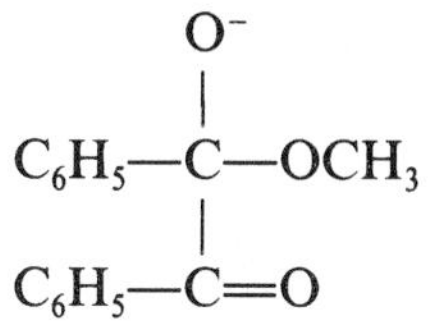

D.
$$C_6H_5-\underset{|}{\overset{\overset{OCH_3}{|}}{C}}=O$$
$$C_6H_5-C=O$$

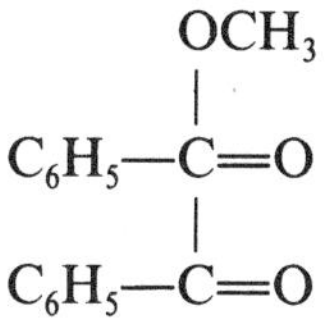

190. Which of the following studies can be used to help determine the correct mechanism?

    A. Carry out the same reaction using O^{18}-labeled water.
    B. Measure the rate of formation of benzilate anion for different initial concentrations of benzil.
    C. Measure the rate of formation of benzilate anion for different pH values.
    D. Carry out the same reaction using a deuterated phenyl group.

191. Aliphatic diketones like $CH_3-\overset{\overset{O}{\|}}{C}-\overset{\overset{O}{\|}}{C}-CH_3$ do not undergo similar reactions in alkaline solution because

    A. they never undergo nucleophilic addition reactions.
    B. they do not react with bases.
    C. they undergo condensation reactions due to the presence of α-hydrogen atoms.
    D. the central carbon-carbon bond undergoes cleavage in alkaline solution.

192. Which of the following reactions is unlikely?

    A. benzilic acid + $CH_3NH_2 \rightarrow$ amide formation
    B. benzilic acid + $CH_3OH \rightarrow$ esterification
    C. benzilic acid + $CH_3COOH \rightarrow$ acylation of alcohol group
    D. benzilic acid + HCN $\rightarrow$ substitution of OH^- by CN^-

Passage IX (Questions 193–197)

The reactivity of carbon-carbon double bonds toward nucleophilic addition is increased by the presence of an electron-withdrawing substituent. Thus α, β-unsaturated ketones, acids, esters, and nitriles undergo nucleophilic addition reactions that simple alkenes do not undergo. On the other hand, electron-withdrawing substituents deactivate the carbon-carbon double bond toward electrophilic addition as well as determine the orientation of the addition. (See reaction 1 below.) The following reactions are known to occur:

Reaction 1

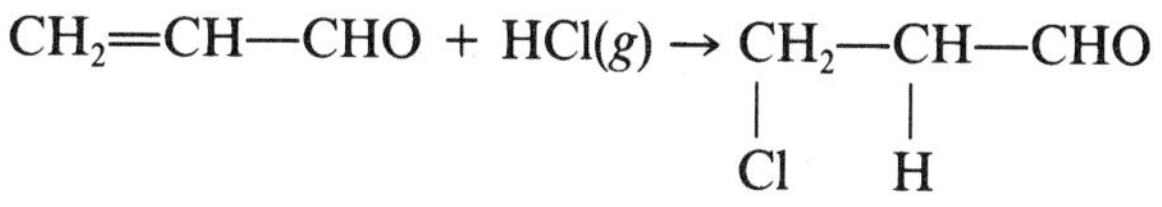

$$CH_2=CH-CHO + HCl(g) \rightarrow CH_2-CH-CHO$$
$$\underset{Cl}{|} \quad \underset{H}{|}$$

GO ON TO THE NEXT PAGE

Reaction 2

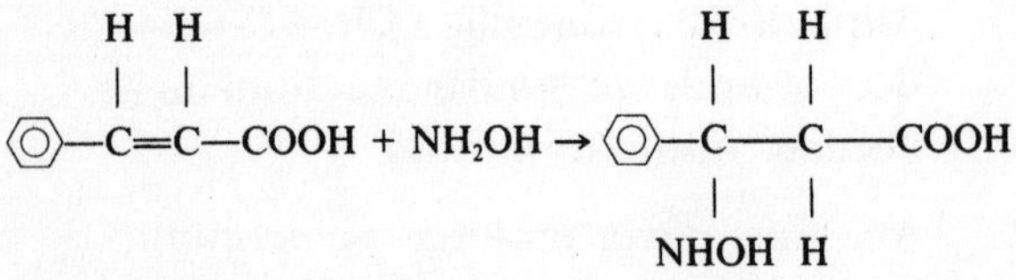

$$\text{\textcircled{O}}-\underset{\underset{H}{|}}{C}=\underset{\underset{H}{|}}{C}-COOH + NH_2OH \rightarrow \text{\textcircled{O}}-\underset{\underset{NHOH}{|}}{C}-\underset{\underset{H}{|}}{C}-COOH$$

193. From the above reactions, it appears that a basic molecule or ion adds to α, β-unsaturated carbonyl compounds in the

   A. α position.
   B. β position.
   C. carbonyl oxygen.
   D. carbonyl carbon.

194. An H^+ ion will most likely attack the α, β-unsaturated carbonyl compound at the

   A. α carbon.
   B. β carbon.
   C. carbonyl oxygen.
   D. carbonyl carbon.

195. What product(s) will be formed from the following reaction?

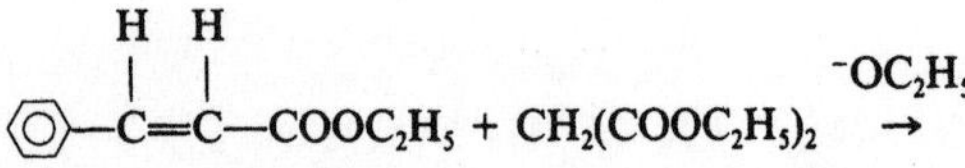

$$\text{\textcircled{O}}-\underset{\underset{H}{|}}{C}=\underset{\underset{H}{|}}{C}-COOC_2H_5 + CH_2(COOC_2H_5)_2 \xrightarrow{\ ^-OC_2H_5\ }$$

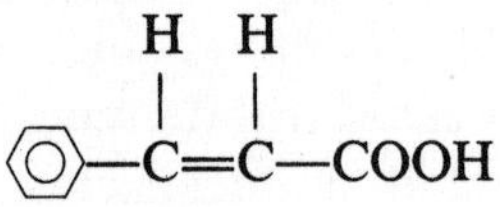

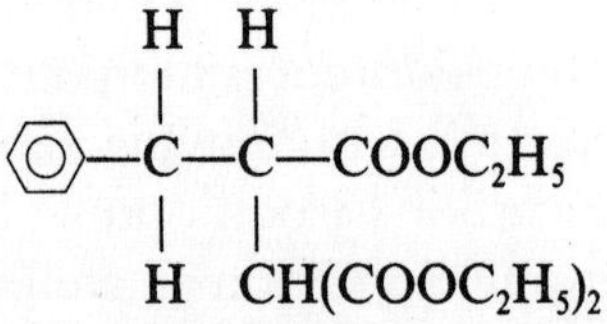

   A.
$$\text{\textcircled{O}}-\underset{\underset{H}{|}}{C}=\underset{\underset{H}{|}}{C}-COOH$$

   B.
$$\text{\textcircled{O}}-\underset{\underset{H}{|}}{C}-\underset{\underset{CH(COOC_2H_5)_2}{|}}{C}-COOC_2H_5$$

   C.
$$\text{\textcircled{O}}-\underset{\underset{H}{|}}{C}=\underset{\underset{H}{|}}{C}-\underset{\underset{OC_2H_5}{|}}{CH}$$
(with OH above)

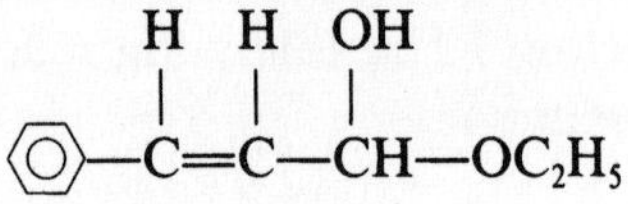

   D.
$$\text{\textcircled{O}}-\underset{\underset{H}{|}}{C}-\underset{\underset{CH(COOC_2H_5)_2}{\underset{|}{H}}}{C}-COOC_2H_5$$

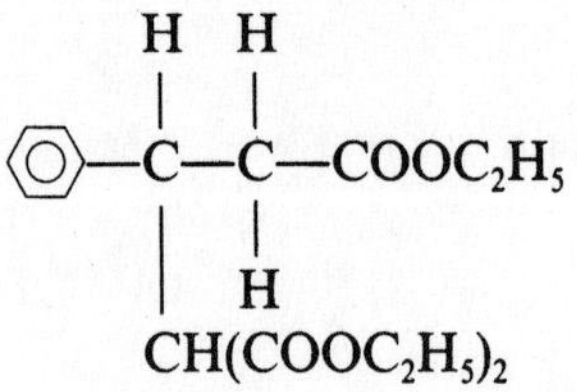

196. A plausible explanation for the fact that electron-withdrawing groups activate nucleophilic addition is that they

   A. stabilize an anionic intermediate by dispersing the negative charge.
   B. increase the negative charge on the carbon atoms of the double bond, increasing their susceptibility to attack by nucleophiles.
   C. destabilize the transition state.
   D. stabilize an anionic intermediate by dispersing the negative charge through inductive effects only.

197. Given compounds A, B, and C below, rank them in order of increasing reactivity toward $CN^\ominus$.

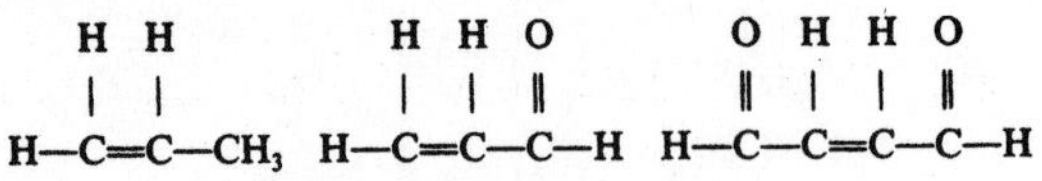

$$\underset{A}{H-\underset{\underset{H}{|}}{C}=\underset{\underset{H}{|}}{C}-CH_3} \quad \underset{B}{H-\underset{\underset{H}{|}}{C}=\underset{\underset{H}{|}}{C}-\underset{\underset{}{\|}}{\overset{O}{C}}-H} \quad \underset{C}{H-\overset{O}{\underset{\underset{H}{|}}{\overset{\|}{C}}}-\underset{\underset{H}{|}}{C}=\underset{\underset{H}{|}}{C}-\overset{O}{\overset{\|}{C}}-H}$$

   A. A < C < B
   B. B < C < A
   C. A < B < C
   D. C < B < A

Passage X (Questions 198–202)

An organic chemist is interested in studying free radical addition to conjugated dienes. The following reactions are performed:

Experiment 1

Step (1) Peroxide decomposes to form a free radical peroxide → R•

Step (2) The free radical abstracts bromine from $BrCCl_3$ R• + $BrCCl_3$ → R—Br + •CCl_3

Step (3) The •CCl_3 adds to the conjugated system
$$•CCl_3 + CH_2\!=\!CH\!-\!CH\!=\!CH_2 \rightarrow \text{allylic free radical}$$

Step (4) $BrCCl_3$
allylic free → $Cl_3C\!-\!CH_2\!-\!\underset{\underset{Br}{|}}{CH}\!-\!CH\!=\!CH_2$ +

$Cl_3C\!-\!CH_2\!-\!CH\!=\!CH\!-\!CH_2\!-\!Br$

Experiment 2

BrCCl$_3$ is also reacted with a 50:50 mixture of 1,3-butadiene and 1-octene. BrCCl$_3$ reacts mostly with 1,3-butadiene.

198. Based on the above reactions, which of the following statements is false?

   A. Conjugated dienes undergo addition by free radicals.

   B. Alkenes undergo addition by free radicals.

   C. Simple alkenes undergo free radical addition reactions faster than conjugated dienes.

   D. Conjugated dienes undergo free radical addition reactions faster than simple alkenes.

199. Which radicals are formed by the addition of •CCl$_3$ to 1,3-butadiene?

   A. Cl$_3$C—CH$_2$—CH—CH=CH$_2$ •

       Cl$_3$C—CH$_2$—CH=CH—CH$_2$ •

   B. Cl$_3$C—CH—CH$_2$—CH=CH$_2$ •

       Cl$_3$C—CH$_2$—CH—CH=CH$_2$ •

   C. Cl$_3$C—CH$_2$—CH=CH—CH$_2$ •

       Cl$_3$C—CH—CH$_2$—CH=CH$_2$ •

   D. Cl$_3$C—CH$_2$—CH—CH=CH$_2$ •

       Cl$_3$C—CH—CH=CH—CH$_3$ •

200. Which statement is supported by Experiment 2?

   A. The transition state of the diene is more stable than the transition state of the simple alkene.

   B. The diene is more stable than the simple alkene.

   C. The activation energy for the diene is lower than the activation energy for the simple alkene.

   D. The activation energy for the diene is higher than the activation energy for the simple alkene.

201. Both alkenes and dienes undergo free radical polymerization. Polymers formed from dienes, however, differ from polymers of alkenes in that polymers formed from dienes

   A. contain double bonds.

   B. are saturated.

   C. require an initiator to begin the polymerization.

   D. are all substituted.

202. Dienes like simple alkenes undergo electrophilic addition. Butadiene when treated with bromine forms which of the following?

   A. 3,4-dibromo-1-butene only

   B. 1,4-dibromo-2-butene only

   C. 3,4-dibromo-1-butene and 1,4-dibromo-2-butene

   D. 1-bromo-2-butene only

Questions 203–219 are independent of any passage and independent of each other.

203. The α and β forms of D-glucose are

   A. enantiomers.

   B. epimers.

   C. meso structures.

   D. anomers.

204. Chromatography can be used to

   A. separate nonvolatile liquids.

   B. separate volatile liquids.

   C. separate a nonvolatile liquid from a volatile liquid.

   D. All of the above.

GO ON TO THE NEXT PAGE

205. Human blood types are most often examined in reference to the ABO gene locus. The I^A and I^B alleles are both dominant to the i^O allele. If blood from a type AB individual were donated to three individuals who were, respectively, types A, B, and O, which of the recipients' blood would agglutinate?

A. The recipients with blood types A and B
B. The recipient with blood type O
C. None of the recipients
D. All of the recipients

206. The conversion of threonine to isoleucine is a five-step enzymatic pathway. The end product, isoleucine, fits into the allosteric site of the enzyme at step 1, preventing its normal function. This is an example of

A. enzyme specificity.
B. competitive inhibition.
C. enzyme enhancement.
D. feedback inhibition.

207. The cerebellum is the part of the brain that helps coordinate skeletal muscles and helps maintain posture and balance. To perform this complex function, the cerebellum must receive input from

A. the cerebrum and proprioceptors.
B. the cerebrum and the inner ear.
C. proprioceptors and the inner ear.
D. the cerebrum, proprioceptors, and the inner ear.

208.

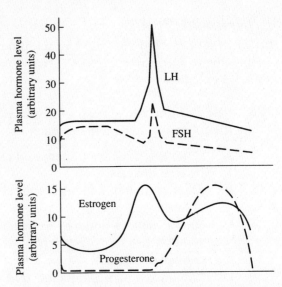

The figure above shows relative hormone concentrations during the menstrual cycle. As estrogen levels go up, Follicle Stimulating Hormone (FSH) is inhibited. Luteinizing Hormone (LH), after stimulating ovulation, also stimulates the corpus luteum to produce high levels of progesterone. Progesterone helps maintain the preparedness of the uterus in case fertilization takes place. As LH levels decrease, corpus luteum activity slows down and progesterone levels rapidly drop. This causes a disintegration of uterine tissues, resulting in the menstrual flow. If fertilization occurs, Human Chorionic Gonadotropin (HCG) is produced by embryonic cells. This hormone maintains the corpus luteum and the pregnancy proceeds. HCG seems to mimic the actions of

A. estrogen.
B. FSH.
C. LH.
D. progesterone.

209. Chromosome puffs can be observed along giant polytene chromosomes in the salivary gland cells of insect larvae. They appear to be regions of DNA that uncoil or decondense. The locations of puffs change at different times during larval development in response to hormonal signals. This phenomenon is an example of

A. gene regulation at the transcriptional level.
B. a polygenic trait.
C. posttranscriptional RNA processing.
D. gene expression at the translational level.

210. Curare is a chemical used in arrow poisons as well as in pharmaceutical compounds. It competes with acetylcholine for receptor sites along the motor end plate. The immediate physiological effects of high doses of curare can include

A. decreased ability to relax muscles.
B. inability to contract muscles and paralysis.
C. inability to repolarize muscles.
D. abnormal heat production in the affected muscle cells.

211. Arrector pili muscles are smooth muscles associated with hair follicles in the skin. When contracted, the muscles pull the hairs erect and "goose bumps" appear as the skin around the hair shafts slightly elevates. What stimulates the arrector pili muscles to contract?

A. Somatic motor neurons
B. Autonomic motor neurons
C. Exocrine secretions
D. Endocrine secretions

212. A variety of organs with similar functions among the vertebrates are thin, moist, highly vascular, and cover a relatively large surface area. These are necessary characteristics for an efficient

A. heart.
B. blood-brain barrier.
C. neuromuscular interface.
D. respiratory membrane.

213. If a muscle cell is stimulated a second time before it has time to relax completely, a stronger contraction results. What is this phenomenon called?

A. Tetany
B. Partial (incomplete) tetany
C. Summation
D. Threshold stimulation

214. The inflammatory response results from the release of histamine by mast cells or basophils. The redness, heat, pain, and swelling associated with inflammation are due to which physiological effects of histamine?

A. Dilation of local blood vessels/less fluid leakage from capillaries
B. Dilation of local blood vessels/more fluid leakage from capillaries
C. Constriction of local blood vessels/ less fluid leakage from capillaries
D. Constriction of local blood vessels/ more fluid leakage from capillaries

215. Toluene will show peaks in its

A. IR spectrum only.
B. UV and IR spectrum only.
C. IR, UV, and NMR spectrum.
D. UV spectrum only.

GO ON TO THE NEXT PAGE

216. Acetone and acetaldehyde in the presence of a strong base will yield which of the following?

    A.   Two different β-hydroxyaldehydes

    B.   Four different β-hydroxycarbonyl compounds

    C.   Two different β-hydroxyketones

    D.   Three different β-hydroxycarbonyl compounds

217. Which of the following compounds will not react with acetyl chloride?

    A. NH_3

    B. CH_3NH_2

    C. $(CH_3)_2NH$

    D. $(CH_3)_4N^+Cl^-$

218. Aldehydes react with alcohols in acidic solution to form

    A.   hemiacetals and acetals.

    B.   hemiacetals only.

    C.   ketals only.

    D.   hemiketals only.

219. Basic hydrolysis of the dipeptide

Ala-Gly:

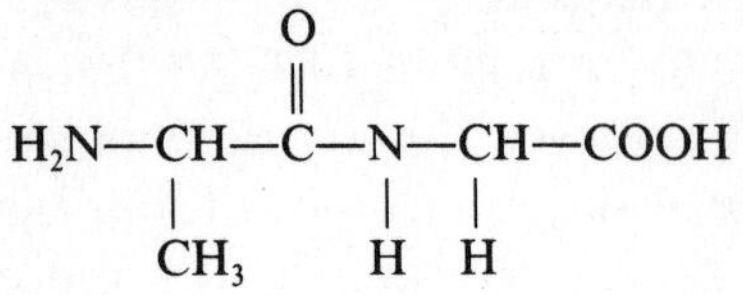

$$H_2N-\underset{\underset{CH_3}{|}}{CH}-\underset{\overset{\|}{O}}{C}-\underset{\underset{H}{|}}{N}-\underset{\underset{H}{|}}{CH}-COOH$$

gives

A. $H_3\overset{+}{N}-\underset{\underset{CH_3}{|}}{CH}-\underset{\overset{\|}{O}}{C}-O^- + H_3\overset{+}{N}-CH_2-COO^-$

B. $H_2N-\underset{\underset{CH_3}{|}}{CH}-COOH + H_3\overset{+}{N}-CH_2-COO^-$

C. $H_2N-\underset{\underset{CH_3}{|}}{CH}-COO^- + H_2N-CH_2-COO^-$

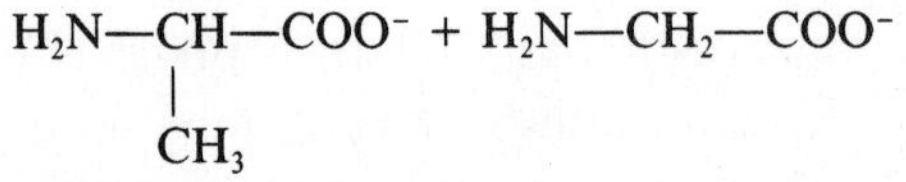

D. $H_2N-\underset{\underset{CH_3}{|}}{CH}-COOH + H_2N-CH_2-COOH$

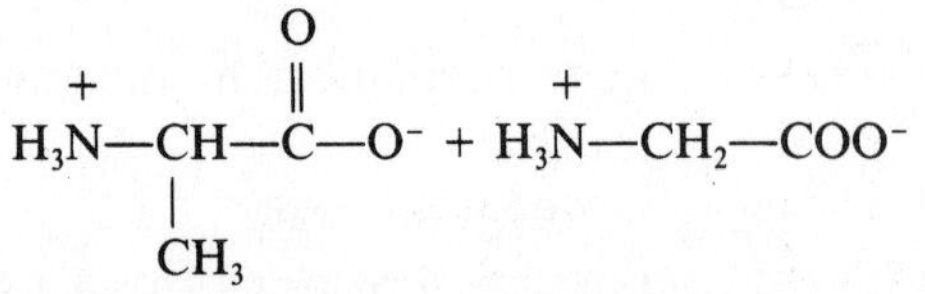

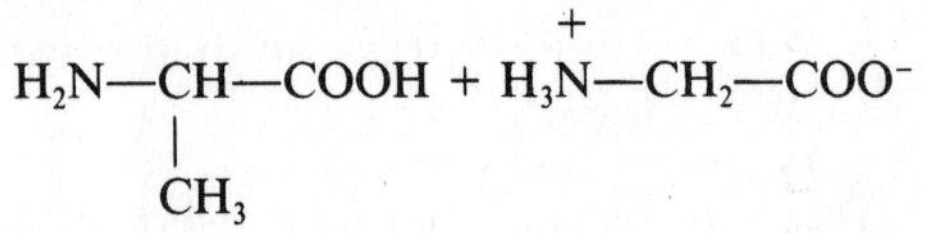

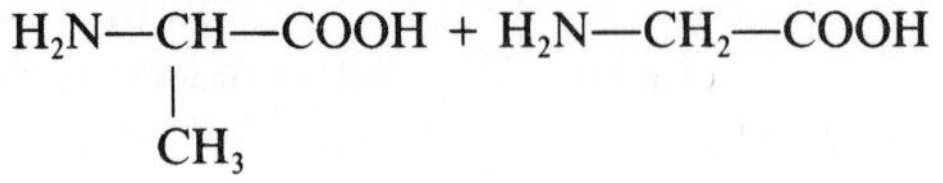

END OF TEST 4.

IF YOU FINISH BEFORE THE TIME IS UP,

YOU MAY CHECK YOUR WORK ON THIS TEST ONLY.

ANSWER KEY

Physical Sciences		Verbal Reasoning		Biological Sciences	
1. B	40. C	78. C	111. A	143. B	182. B
2. C	41. B	79. A	112. B	144. A	183. D
3. A	42. B	80. D	113. D	145. C	184. C
4. C	43. D	81. C	114. B	146. C	185. C
5. C	44. A	82. C	115. C	147. D	186. A
6. C	45. D	83. D	116. A	148. C	187. C
7. A	46. C	84. D	117. C	149. A	188. B
8. D	47. B	85. A	118. A	150. C	189. C
9. C	48. D	86. D	119. C	151. A	190. A
10. A	49. A	87. B	120. C	152. C	191. C
11. B	50. B	88. C	121. C	153. C	192. D
12. B	51. C	89. D	122. B	154. D	193. B
13. D	52. D	90. A	123. A	155. D	194. C
14. D	53. B	91. A	124. D	156. B	195. D
15. C	54. C	92. B	125. D	157. D	196. A
16. B	55. A	93. C	126. D	158. C	197. C
17. D	56. D	94. D	127. D	159. B	198. C
18. D	57. B	95. D	128. C	160. D	199. A
19. C	58. D	96. D	129. B	161. B	200. C
20. B	59. D	97. C	130. A	162. A	201. A
21. C	60. B	98. B	131. B	163. D	202. C
22. A	61. D	99. D	132. D	164. C	203. D
23. B	62. C	100. B	133. A	165. C	204. D
24. A	63. C	101. D	134. B	166. B	205. D
25. B	64. B	102. D	135. A	167. B	206. D
26. B	65. D	103. B	136. D	168. B	207. D
27. C	66. D	104. C	137. A	169. C	208. C
28. D	67. A	105. C	138. A	170. D	209. A
29. A	68. D	106. C	139. A	171. B	210. B
30. D	69. B	107. A	140. C	172. D	211. B
31. D	70. A	108. C	141. B	173. D	212. D
32. C	71. D	109. C	142. B	174. C	213. C
33. D	72. A	110. C		175. A	214. B
34. B	73. B			176. C	215. C
35. C	74. A			177. D	216. B
36. B	75. D			178. D	217. D
37. C	76. D			179. C	218. A
38. A	77. B			180. C	219. C
39. C				181. C	

ANSWERS AND EXPLANATIONS

PHYSICAL SCIENCES

1. **The correct answer is (B).** Note that one scale measures color observed in solution, while the other measures color absorbed—the complement of the first.

2. **The correct answer is (C).** Violet, blue, blue-green, green, yellow.

3. **The correct answer is (A).** The hexamminecobalt (III) complex ion has the shortest wavelength of maximum absorption, hence the greatest transition energy.

4. **The correct answer is (C).** The absorbed wavelength shifts from 430 nm to 500 nm. The *absorption* colors shift from yellow to orange-red.

5. **The correct answer is (C).** You can first narrow the choices to those with an inverse relationship between energy and wavelength. To pinpoint, try plugging in values for one energy and wavelength.

6. **The correct answer is (C).** The absorption at 560 nm corresponds to an energy gap slightly *higher* than that at 580 nm, or about 211 kJ/mol. Such a gap is found between the top and bottom levels of III.

7. **The correct answer is (A).** A blue solution absorbs light in the orange-red region, around 239 kJ/mol. The gap between the middle and bottom levels shown in (I) could produce this absorption.

8. **The correct answer is (D).** None of the pairs of levels shown could lead to an energy gap greater than 25,000 cm^{-1}, which is needed for the onset of ultraviolet light.

9. **The correct answer is (C).** Sodium and nitrate ions (not silver ions or electrons) flow through the bridge.

10. **The correct answer is (A).** $E^{\circ}_{cell} = E^{\circ}_{RED} + E^{\circ}_{OXID}$
$$= 0.799 \text{ v} + (-0.799 \text{ v})$$
$$= 0$$

11. **The correct answer is (B).** The second and third time values recorded show a voltage drop of more than 0.010 v.

12. **The correct answer is (B).** As shown, a potential develops owing to the difference in concentration between the two sides; current flows so as to diminish this difference by oxidation on one side and reduction on the other. Physical mixing allows the concentration difference to be eliminated without the need for a flow of electrons between the cells.

13. **The correct answer is (D).** The salt bridge does not allow electrons to pass; the wire does. The electrons go from right to left, since in that way oxidation occurs at the dilute solution, increasing the silver ion concentration. Simultaneously, reduction occurs at the concentrated side, lowering the silver ion concentration.

14. **The correct answer is (D).** Any silver ion that appears on the right due to oxidation is balanced by a like amount that disappears on the left due to reduction.

15. **The correct answer is (C).** Since K_{sp} is small, and since K_{eq} for the reaction describing the combination of the two ions is $1/K_{sp}$, the reaction goes essentially to completion.

16. **The correct answer is (B).** The second reactant must have been a strong base, since some of the H^+ is used up and there is no other major product.

17. **The correct answer is (D).** You start with a weak base, and need to convert half of its original amount to its conjugate acid. You'll need 0.025 moles of a strong acid to do this.

18. **The correct answer is (D).** The solution is mostly sodium acetate, which is slightly basic owing to hydrolysis of the acetate ion.

19. **The correct answer is (C).** Each mole of carbonate requires 2 moles of H^+ to convert it to carbonic acid.

20. **The correct answer is (B).** Weak acid with strong base.

21. **The correct answer is (C).** This reaction results in an equal mixture of a weak acid with its conjugate base; such a solution is a buffer.

22. **The correct answer is (A).** Its slight dissociation before the HCl was added will be decreased owing to the excess of hydrogen ion.

23. **The correct answer is (B).** Electrons flow through the circuit toward the *positively* charged electrode.

24. **The correct answer is (A).** Electrons flow spontaneously toward the positive electrode, combining with and reducing Fe^{3+} ions at the electrode surface.

25. **The correct answer is (B).** Zn is the negative electrode, thus electrons flow from it and it is the anode in cells B and C.

26. **The correct answer is (B).** Nickel is the negative electrode, hence more readily oxidized in cell A; similarly, it is more readily reduced in cell C.

27. **The correct answer is (C).** The data give no indication of *absolute* potential, so choices A and B cannot be correct. Since the Pb electrode is positive, it must be reduced, with a potential that is 0.131 v greater than that for the reduction of Ni^{2+}.

28. **The correct answer is (D).** Cell A has no half-reaction in common with cell B, so no comparison can be made.

29. **The correct answer is (A).** The chart shows that the half-reaction for Pb^{2+}/Pb has the greater reduction potential, so Pb^{2+} will be reduced while Zn will be oxidized.

30. **The correct answer is (D).** 1.00 v + 0.131 v = 1.131 v.

31. **The correct answer is (D).** According to the chart, Pb^{2+} is more readily reduced than Zn^{2+} by 0.505 + 0.131 = 0.636 v.

32. **The correct answer is (C).** Since $CO_3{}^{2-}$ is a weak base, the solution of sodium carbonate should have a pH above 7, while that of NaCl should be 7. The chloride test using silver ion would be inconclusive, since Ag_2CO_3 would also precipitate. Titration with a strong base would give no reaction with either negative ion.

33. **The correct answer is (D).** Although each solution has the same number of formula weights of salt per weight of solvent, each Na_2CO_3 entity furnishes 3 ions when it dissolves, while each NaCl furnishes only 2.

34. **The correct answer is (B).** Freezing-point depression and boiling-point elevation represent one of the few uses of molality generally encountered in introductory chemistry.

35. **The correct answer is (C).** Use of the freezing-point depression to distinguish the solutions will assume that each salt dissociates completely, as sodium salts generally do.

36. **The correct answer is (B).** Since freezing-point depression is proportional to total molality of ions, the depression for the sodium carbonate will be 1.5 times larger than that for sodium chloride.

37. **The correct answer is (C).** The reciprocal of the focal length is equal to the sum of the reciprocals of the object and image distances.

    $1/F = 1/d_{object} + 1/d_{image}$
    $= 1/0.60 \text{ m} + 1/0.30 \text{ m} = 3/0.60 \text{ m}$
    $F = 0.20 \text{ meters}$

38. **The correct answer is (A).** The ratio of the object to image size is equal to the ratio of the object to image distance.

    $S_{object}/S_{image} = d_{object}/d_{image}$
    $S_{image} = (0.050 \text{ m})(.30 \text{ m})/(.60 \text{ m})$
    $= .025 \text{ m}$

39. **The correct answer is (C).** Since the surface on both sides of the lens is convex, the lens is a converging lens. For any converging lens, an object that is more than two focal lengths away from the lens will produce an image that is real, inverted, and smaller than the object.

40. **The correct answer is (C).** Light is bent or refracted when it passes from one medium (air) into another (the material of the lens).

41. **The correct answer is (B).** For a converging lens: 1) If the object is more than two focal lengths away, the image will be smaller than the object and appear on the opposite side of the lens at a distance between one and two focal lengths from the lens. 2) If the object is two focal lengths away, the image on the opposite side of the lens will be the same size as the object and appear at a distance of two focal lengths from the lens. The net effect of moving the object toward the lens is to increase the size of the image on the opposite side of the lens and to increase its distance from the lens.

42. **The correct answer is (B).** Centripetal acceleration is inversely proportional to the radius of the curve: $a_c = v^2/r$. Since the radius of the larger curve is twice that of the smaller curve, the centripetal acceleration at the larger curve will be half as great as that at the smaller curve.

43. **The correct answer is (D).** The force is given by Newton's second law, where

    $F = ma_c = mv^2/r$
    $= (2000 \text{ kg})(20 \text{ m/s})^2/50.0 \text{ m}$
    $= 1.6 \times 10^4 \text{ N}$

44. **The correct answer is (A).** Along the straightaway, the car travels at a constant speed, so there is no acceleration and therefore no force acting on the car. In the turns, although the speed is still constant, the direction of the car is changing so that the presence of a force is required.

45. **The correct answer is (D).** The distance is the product of the velocity and the time required to cover the distance.

    $d = vt = (20 \text{ m/s})(20 \text{ s}) = 400 \text{ m}$

46. **The correct answer is (C).** Kinetic energy is $\frac{1}{2}mv^2$ or $\frac{mv^2}{2}$. Since the mass of the car is constant and its velocity is constant, its kinetic energy must be the same along the straightaway as it is going around the curves.

47. **The correct answer is (B).** Poiseuille's formula shows an R^4 dependence of the flow rate. Thus, increasing the bore of the needle (R) will have the most marked effect on the flow rate.

48. **The correct answer is (D).** $Q \sim \Delta P \times R^4$. If the radius is halved, then $\left(\frac{1}{2}\right)^4 = 1/16$. To maintain Q, ΔP must increase by a factor of 16.

49. **The correct answer is (A).** 5L/min $= 5000$ cm^3/min
$$= 8.333 \times 10^{-5}\ \text{m}^3/\text{s};$$
$$Q = \bar{v}A \text{ and } \bar{v} = Q/A$$
$$= 8.333 \times 10^{-5}/3.14 \times (1.0 \times 10^{-2})^2$$
$$= 0.265\ \text{m/s};$$
$$= 2\bar{v}Rd/\eta$$
$$= \frac{2 \times 0.265 \times 0.010 \times 1030}{0.0040}$$
$$= 1{,}365$$

50. **The correct answer is (B).** $\bar{v} = \eta\mathcal{R}/2Rd$
$$= (0.0040)(3000)/2(0.010)(1030)$$
$$= 0.58\ \text{m/s}$$

51. **The correct answer is (C).** Because the flow rate must necessarily be the same in the arteries, veins, and capillaries, Poiseuille's formula shows the pressure drop will increase with decreasing R.

52. **The correct answer is (D).** A decrease in temperature usually increases friction between fluid layers, thus increasing the viscosity coefficient. As $\eta \uparrow$, $\bar{v} \downarrow$, and $Q \downarrow$.

53. **The correct answer is (B).** Because a pressure of 2.0 atm must be exerted on the piston to prevent water from entering solution B, $\pi_B > \pi_A$ and the concentration of solution B is more concentrated than solution A: $\pi = $ molarity $\times RT$ ($T = $ temperature; $R = $ universal gas constant).

54. **The correct answer is (C).** See Question 53.

55. **The correct answer is (A).** Osmotic pressure difference would increase, requiring more pressure on the piston to prevent water from entering solution B.

56. **The correct answer is (D).** Water will enter the RBC causing hemolysis (bursting).

57. **The correct answer is (B).** Osmotic pressure is a colligative property, meaning it depends on the moles of particles. A 1.0 M solution of NaCl contains more particles in solution than 1.0 M glucose solution.

$$NaCl(s) \rightarrow Na^+(aq) + Cl^-(aq)$$

58. **The correct answer is (D).** Osmosis results from the diffusion that occurs across a membrane. Diffusion is the spreading of molecules from high concentration to low concentration due to random collisions. More water molecules per unit volume are in the dilute solution than in the more concentrated solution. Thus, more water molecules of the dilute solution will collide with the membrane per unit time, causing a net flow of water molecules from the dilute to the concentrated solution.

59. **The correct answer is (D).** 60 W represents the power usage of the bulb. Power is the product of current and voltage. Thus,

$$I = P/V = \frac{60W}{120V} = 0.5A$$

60. **The correct answer is (B).** The Doppler effect is given by

$$v = v_i \frac{(v - v_0)}{(v)}$$

where v_i is the actual frequency and v is the frequency perceived; v is the velocity of sound in air, and v_0 is the velocity of the observer.

$$v = 700 \text{ Hz} \frac{(350 - 35)}{(350)} = 700 \text{ Hz}(0.90) = 630 \text{ Hz}$$

Choices A and D can be eliminated immediately because as the source and observer move apart, the frequency drops.

61. **The correct answer is (D).** For fluids Bernoulli's equation relates the pressure, P, the kinetic energy (speed), $\rho v^2/2$, and the potential energy (elevation), ρgh, for any point in the fluid as follows:

$$P + \rho v^2/2 + \rho gh = \text{constant} \qquad \text{where } \rho \text{ is the density of the fluid}$$

Since the velocity is constant, $\rho v^2/2$ is constant and P will vary with the elevation only. The greater the elevation, the greater the value of ρgh and the lower the value of P.

62. **The correct answer is (C).** Use the relation $d\beta = 10 \log_{10}(I/I_0)$ where $I_0 = 10^{-12} \text{W/m}^2$

Then,

$$40 \ d\beta = 10 \log_{10} (I/10^{-12}\text{W/m}^2)$$
$$4 = \log_{10} (I/10^{-12})$$

Taking the antilog (exponential) of both sides gives $10^4 = I/10^{-12}$.

$$I = 10^4 \times 10^{-12} \text{ W/m}^2 = 10^{-8} \text{ W/m}^2$$

63. **The correct answer is (C).** To use $k = A \exp(-E_a/RT)$, where neither k nor A is known, requires two equations, obtained by measuring different values of k at two different temperatures.

64. **The correct answer is (B).** The pressure exerted by a gas depends on the total number of molecules, not on its molecular weight or the number of atoms per molecule. Changes in T, however, *will* affect the pressure.

65. **The correct answer is (D).** If "x" equals the solubility of $Ba(IO_3)_2$, then $[Ba^{2+}] = x$ and $[IO_3^-] = 2x$.

66. **The correct answer is (D).** In each of II and III, the number of moles of gaseous products is less than that of gaseous reactants; thus, "disorder" decreases.

67. **The correct answer is (A).** The reaction shifts to the left in response to the loss of NO_2. Increasing the volume has the reverse effect from that stated in II—there's more room for the more numerous NO_2's. Adding an inert gas raises the *total* pressure, but only partial pressures of reactants and products figure into the equilibrium expression, so the equilibrium will not shift in III.

68. **The correct answer is (D).** pH $= 14 - $ pOH $= 14 - 3 = 11$; alternatively, find $[H^+]$ using $[H^+] = K_w/[OH^-] = 1 \times 10^{-14}/(0.001) = 1 \times 10^{-11}$; pH $= 11$

69. **The correct answer is (B).** Rearrange this expression to get the familiar Henderson-Hasselbalch equation; the trick is that the H—H equation uses the ratio of conjugate base to conjugate acid, the reciprocal of R as defined here. So,

    $6.3 = 6.0 + \log (1/R)$

    $6.0 = 6.3 - \log (1/R)$

    $6.0 = 6.3 + \log R$

    If you do not notice this, you'll probably choose A.

70. **The correct answer is (A).** The period T is equal to:

    $$T = 2\pi\sqrt{L/g}$$

    Thus, the period is directly proportional to the square root of the length. Any increase in L will produce an increase in T. The mass of the box does not influence the period.

71. **The correct answer is (D).** Six seconds represent the round-trip time of the sonar signal. Therefore, it takes 3 s for a signal traveling at 1.5 km/s to reach the ocean floor. Since distance equals speed times time,

    $$\left(1.5\frac{km}{s}\right)(3 \text{ s}) = 4.5 \text{ km}$$

72. **The correct answer is (A).** Work is force times distance moved. A body held at a given height is not in motion, so work is no longer being performed on it.

73. **The correct answer is (B).** Capacitors C_2 and C_3 are connected in series and can be replaced by a single equivalent capacitor of

    $$\frac{1}{C_{eq}} = \frac{1}{C_2} + \frac{1}{C_3} = \frac{1}{4}$$

    So $C_{eq} = 4 \mu\mathscr{F}$. The equivalent capacitor and C_1 are connected in parallel and can be replaced by a single equivalent capacitor given by

    $$C_{EQ} = C_{eq} + C_1 = 4 \mu\mathscr{F} + 3 \mu\mathscr{F} = 7 \mu\mathscr{F}$$

74. **The correct answer is (A).** This is the definition of Pascal's Principle.

75. **The correct answer is (D).** The force is inversely proportional to the square of the distance between the point charges. Since the distance is doubled, the force must be quartered.

76. **The correct answer is (D).** The speed of sound in air is constant at any given temperature regardless of the frequency of the sound.

77. **The correct answer is (B).** This is a parallel circuit diagram. The voltage drop is the same across both branches, but the current is divided between them. The resistors on each branch are connected in series. The equivalent resistance in the right-hand branch is 60 Ω. The current through that loop and through each R in that loop is

$$I = V/R = \frac{120V}{60\Omega} = 2.0 \text{ amperes}$$

VERBAL REASONING

78. **The correct answer is (C).** The answer to this question is based on the following statement in paragraph 7: "Park adds that one of the many benefits of the experiment for exobiologists (scientists who study possibilities of life in outer space) is knowledge gained about whether life forms could travel . . . ."

79. **The correct answer is (A).** The answer to this question is based on the following statement made in paragraph 2: "All 12.5 million of the seeds were carried aboard Space Shuttle Mission 41-C . . . and placed in orbit inside . . . (LDEF), a free-flying, 12-sided structure loaded with experiments designed to test results of continuous exposure to outer space."

80. **The correct answer is (D).** The answer to this question is based on the following statement in paragraph 1: "When some 12.5 million tomato seeds returned to Earth in February 1985 after almost a year in space, several thousand American students . . . anxiously awaited their arrival . . ." and on this statement from paragraph 2: "the seeds . . . were divided up . . . among hundreds of schools."

81. **The correct answer is (C).** The answer to this question is based on the following statement made in paragraph 3: "There are no 'cookbook' rules governing how the experiments are to be conducted other than the requirement of strictly scientific methodology."

82. **The correct answer is (C).** The answer to this question is based on the following statement in paragraph 3: "At the conclusion of the experimentation, student reports . . . are to be tabulated in a summary report by NASA headquarters and made generally available upon request."

83. **The correct answer is (D).** The answer to this question is based on paragraph 7: ". . . one of the many benefits of the experiment . . . is knowledge gained about whether life forms could travel by passive means from one ecosystem or planet to another without a spaceship. If the seeds exposed to both vacuum and high radiation come through with little or no damage, it opens up questions . . . about the origins and destinations of primitive life forms."

84. **The correct answer is (D).** The answer to this question can be inferred from the following statements found in paragraphs 4 and 8 and the generally positive tone of the article: "Like all great ideas, this one was born in the mind of an imaginative individual." (paragraph 4) "What new connections might be made by the thousands of students participating in SEEDS? Their horizons are as unlimited as outer space." (paragraph 8)

85. **The correct answer is (A).** The answer to this question is based on the following statement in paragraph 2: "In one field of concentration, for example—justice, morality, and constitutional democracy—great books form the core of the curriculum. Students read Plato, Aristotle, Machiavelli, Hobbes, Rousseau, Hegel, and Nietzsche or Weber."

86. **The correct answer is (D).** The answer is based on the statement in paragraph 4: ". . . the proposal made clear that the project was being undertaken as an integrated effort to revitalize the college's dedication to providing a liberal arts education to its students."

87. **The correct answer is (B).** The answer to this question can be inferred from the fact that the author does not include any criticism of the program in the article, but does quote a number of positive statements such as this one from paragraph 4: "Panelists' reactions demonstrated their admiration for the strong, unified goal toward which all activities of the project were directed."

88. **The correct answer is (C).** The answer to this question is based on a statement in paragraph 2: "The proposal demonstrates that a foundation for the project exists in the successful integration of the humanities and the social sciences in some parts of the Madison College curriculum."

89. **The correct answer is (D).** The answer to this question is based on the following statement in paragraph 4: "We expect these activities to . . . contribute to faculty development, improve individual courses, and make our upper-level curricula more vital . . . ." There is no mention of individual student needs.

90. **The correct answer is (A).** The answer to this question is supported by the following statement in paragraph 4: "Panelists' reactions demonstrated their admiration for the strong, unified goal toward which all activities of the project were directed."

91. **The correct answer is (A).** The answer to this question is based on a statement from paragraph 2: "Students read Plato, Aristotle, Machiavelli, Hobbes, Rousseau, Hegel, and Nietzsche or Weber."

92. **The correct answer is (B).** The answer to this question is found in the following statement from paragraph 1: "Finally, electric utilities are concerned that costly and potentially counterproductive regulations may he promulgated before a rational basis for policy making is achieved."

93. **The correct answer is (C).** The answer to this question can be chosen by ruling out choices A, B, and D, all of which are referred to in the article. That leaves choice C as the only possible answer. Choice A is referred to in paragraph 5: "Planners will need to consider potential changes in energy supply resulting from climate change." Choice B is referred to in paragraph 4: "Utility planners must therefore consider both the likelihood of having to build new power plants to meet higher peak demand and the probable need to purchase more fuel for increased generation." Choice D is referred to in a statement in paragraph 6: "To meet these challenges, utilities will need to adopt more sophisticated strategies of risk management."

94. **The correct answer is (D).** The answer to this question is based on the following statement in paragraph 2: "In particular, the apparent 0.6 degree C, 1 degree F rise in average global temperature over the last century lies within the long-term range of natural variability, although the recent rate of increase seems rapid."

95. **The correct answer is (D).** The answer to this question can be chosen on the basis of ruling out A, B, and C, leaving D as the answer. Choice A is referred to in paragraph 4 (point 4): "Adapting to changing climate: Examples are heating and cooling of buildings, compensation of disadvantaged regions, and changing of agricultural practices." Choice B is referred to in paragraph 4 (point 2): "Removing greenhouse gases from effluents or the atmosphere: Examples are removing CO_2 from power plant emissions as well as starting forestation programs." Choice C is referred to in paragraph 4 (point 3): "Making countervailing modifications in climate and weather: One example is cloud seeding; another more speculative example is changing the atmosphere's reflectivity by releasing particles in the stratosphere."

96. **The correct answer is (D).** The answer to this question is based on the following statement in paragraph 3 and by the constant references in the article for the need for better understanding of the greenhouse effect: "Research is needed to tell us not only when to act but also how to act."

97. **The correct answer is (C).** The answer to this question is supported by this statement in paragraph 2: "Current models suggest that a warming trend of this magnitude could result solely from the increases in atmospheric CO_2 and other greenhouse gases (e.g., nitrous oxide, methane, chlorofluorocarbons, and ozone)."

98. **The correct answer is (B).** The answer to this question is based on the following statement in paragraph 2: "A marketing strategy that presents the product or service as an opportunity for personal growth is far more likely to succeed."

99. **The correct answer is (D).** The answer to this question is based on the following statement in paragraph 2: "So intense is the interest in the older consumer that many of America's largest companies have launched advertising campaigns targeted at adults over 50."

100. **The correct answer is (B).** The answer to this question is based on the following statement in paragraph 8: "Barbara Kane . . . ticks off the professional skills important for success in this field: counseling skills . . . (and) assessment skills."

101. **The correct answer is (D).** The answer to this question is based on the following statement in paragraph 7: "More often than not, they are social workers; although nurses, psychologists, and gerontologists operate case management firms, too."

102. **The correct answer is (D).** The answer to this question can be inferred from the following statement in paragraph 9: "Prospects should continue to be very good, considering the rapid growth in the number of people of advanced age and the increased willingness of many people to use social work and mental health services."

103. **The correct answer is (B).** The second paragraph discusses the emergence of an increasing elderly market and the need for advertising targeting that market. It also notes the poor perception of advertisers of just how to appeal to the elderly and the need for marketing consultants to advise them.

104. **The correct answer is (C).** The answer to this question can be found in the following statement in paragraph 3: "Davis proposed cave development deep below the water table . . ."

105. **The correct answer is (C).** The answer to this question is supported by the following statement in paragraph 1: "Early biological studies emphasized faunal surveys and descriptions of the degenerate eyes of cavernicolous animals (cavernicoles) . . ."

106. **The correct answer is (C).** The answer to this question is based on the following statement in paragraph 1: "Scientific interest in caves began in seventeenth- and eighteenth-century Europe . . ."

107. **The correct answer is (A).** The answer to this question is contained in the following statement from paragraph 1: ". . . with the development of elaborate (but erroneous) theories of the hydrogenic cycle in which cave systems were essential elements."

108. **The correct answer is (C).** The answer to this question is supported by the following statement from paragraph 3: "Davis proposed cave development deep below the water table, by random circulation of slowly percolating groundwater ('phreatic' origin)."

109. **The correct answer is (C).** The answer to this question is based on ruling out A, B, and D, which are supported by statements in the article, leaving C, which is not supported by any statement. In paragraph 4 are the following statements, which support A, B, and D: "Factors influencing reactivation of geological cave research and continued progress in biospeleology in the past decade include amassment of a large body of descriptive data collected mainly by nonprofessional explorers and surveyors (A) . . . growing acquaintance with the large body of European literature that had been largely ignored by American theoreticians of the 1930s (B) . . . and finally, involvement of younger researchers whose interest arose from exploration and field experience (D)."

110. **The correct answer is (C).** The answer to this question is based on the following statement in paragraph 3: "Biospeleology advanced slowly in the United States from 1930 to 1950, even though this was the time of a lively debate over the origin of caves."

111. **The correct answer is (A).** The answer is clear from the statement: "The argument over location of the water table tended to reduce the research that was done to a sterile classification of some particular cave as having vadose or phreatic origin."

112. **The correct answer is (B).** The answer to this question is supported by the following statement from paragraph 3: "Other theories place the zone of cave development at or above the local water table ('vadose' origin)."

113. **The correct answer is (D).** The answer to this question can be inferred from several statements in paragraph 1 and a statement in paragraph 3. "Robert Lowell is known both as a major twentieth-century American poet and as an important translator" and "Lowell's work remains difficult and obscure" are from paragraph 1. Another statement that implies the answer is in paragraph 3: " 'He isn't an American poet at all,' Gillis explains, 'but a bearer of an older, deeper tradition of European literary and poetic history . . .' "

114. **The correct answer is (B).** The answer to this statement can be inferred from several statements in paragraph 2: "Lowell scholar Daniel Gillis . . . is attempting to reform the critical view (of Lowell) by highlighting the influence of classical literature on the poet." Paragraph 3 points out that Lowell is a "bearer of an older, deeper tradition of European literary and poetic history . . . and Latin literature. . . ."

115. **The correct answer is (C).** The answer to this question is based on the following statements from paragraphs 11 and 12: "The course . . . will address a modern poet from a fresh, rich perspective; . . . it will give the classics students a taste of modern literature while taking advantage of their academic forte." (paragraph 11) "The hope is that studying Lowell and his ties to classical antiquity will generate interest both in a poet deserving recognition and in an academic discipline in search of creative scholars." (paragraph 12) While the author laments the lack of a classical grounding in today's education, he does not expect his course to change this fact.

116. **The correct answer is (A).** The answer to this question can be inferred from the following statement found in paragraph 7: "The diminishing numbers of readers who can appreciate Lowell and scholars who can satisfactorily analyze the poet point up a disturbing trend in American education. The classical grounding in Latin and Greek language and literature that was prevalent in the nineteenth century has almost disappeared from today's schools."

117. **The correct answer is (C).** The answer to this question is based on the following statement made in paragraph 9: "Lowell's translations (which Gillis argues is the wrong word to use) have also been misunderstood. 'He used the word *imitations*,' Gillis notes. 'They're much freer than literal translations.' "

118. **The correct answer is (A).** The answer to this question is based on the statement from paragraph 7 which was cited as the answer to Question 116.

119. **The correct answer is (C).** The answer to this question is based on the following statement from paragraph 10: "An act disenfranchising women, free blacks, and aliens was promoted as a way of reducing election fraud by making it easier to identify ineligible voters."

120. **The correct answer is (C).** The answer is in the last paragraph. "All states were then stripping the franchise from marginal groups—free blacks, noncitizens, native Americans, and in New Jersey, women—while at the same time removing obstacles to universal white male suffrage."

121. **The correct answer is (C).** The answer to this question is based on the following statement in paragraph 6: "The new constitution gave the vote to 'all inhabitants' who were worth fifty pounds in real or personal property, thereby removing extensive real estate holdings as the sole economic test for voter eligibility."

122. **The correct answer is (B).** The answer to this question is based on several statements in paragraph 1: "Of the many women who surely importuned their husbands for equal status in the new American nation, the most famous was Abigail Adams . . . (who) wrote to her husband John to '. . . remember the ladies and be more generous to them than your ancestors, in the new code of laws. Do not put such unlimited power into the hands of the husbands. . . .' "

123. **The correct answer is (A).** The answer to this question is supported by the following statement in paragraph 7: "The few available voting lists from the period . . . suggest that as many as 15 percent of the qualified women voted . . ."

124. **The correct answer is (D).** The answer to this question is based on the following statement in paragraph 6: "The new constitution gave the vote to 'all inhabitants' who were worth fifty pounds in real or personal property. . . ."

125. **The correct answer is (D).** The answer to this question is based on the following statement in paragraph 11: "Thus, New Jersey women were victims of political pressures that transcended local circumstances, and they would not be able to vote again until the passage of the Nineteenth Amendment more than one hundred years later."

126. **The correct answer is (D).** The answer to this question is supported by the following statement in paragraph 8: "Why did women lose the vote in 1807?"

127. **The correct answer is (D).** The answer to this question is based on the following statement in paragraph 6: "The scholar's role is not to provide a tidy analysis of the text, not to deliver 'the answers,' but rather to enrich discussion with biographical information on the author, with contextual perspectives from the literary tradition or historical era . . ."

128. **The correct answer is (C).** The answer to this question is based on several statements from paragraphs 2 and 3. In paragraph 2 are the following statements: "The discussion reminded me again of why I loved to serve as a scholar in these programs. Talk ranged from analysis of the text to insights gained from Rhys about personal lives." In paragraph 3 are these statements: "If only my freshmen cared this much about their reading! At the conclusion of the discussion, I had some new ideas about Jean Rhys, and these have affected my subsequent scholarship. I learned, for example, to be more subtle in my analysis of point of view."

129. **The correct answer is (B).** The answer to this question can be inferred from several statements. In paragraph 5 is this statement: "To enhance the discussion, Bates introduced the concept of opening each session with a lecture by a humanities scholar." In paragraph 6 is the statement: "The scholar's role is . . . to enrich discussion with biographical information on the author . . . and to be a catalyst for discussion by raising provocative questions about the text."

130. **The correct answer is (A).** The answer to this question is supported by the following statements in paragraph 5: "Her goal was to establish a context in which a number of adults could all read the same book and later gather to discuss it. To enhance the discussion, Bates introduced the concept of opening each session with a lecture by a humanities scholar."

131. **The correct answer is (B).** The answer to this question is based on the following statement in paragraph 4: "Reading and discussion programs of this nature began just a decade ago around a kitchen table in Rutland, Vermont, across the state from Wells River."

132. **The correct answer is (D).** The answer to this question is based on the following statement in paragraph 8: "These audiences were diverse: adolescents and octogenarians, people with high school degrees, people with Ph.D.s, individuals from all classes and careers."

133. **The correct answer is (A).** The answer to this question can be inferred from statements in paragraphs 7 and 8. In paragraph 7 is the statement: "I spoke about humanities texts . . . to eager audiences . . . (who) were hungry . . . for the scholar's information and even hungrier for the human interaction around a text." In paragraph 8 is the statement: "What more could a teacher-scholar ask than for 'students' who are well prepared, eager to talk, willing to argue, and replete with a wealth of life experience?"

134. **The correct answer is (B).** The answer to this question is supported by a number of statements. In paragraph 4, we learn that the program grew out of the "frustration of reading a good book and having no one with whom to discuss it." In paragraph 7, the author states, "I spoke about humanities texts . . . to eager audiences in small libraries, community centers, and even churches . . . because the audiences were hungry . . . for the scholar's information and even hungrier for the human interaction around a text."

135. **The correct answer is (A).** The answer to this question is supported by the following statements in paragraph 8: "These projects should help to engender public understanding . . . of the Northwest Ordinance as one of the cornerstone documents of our founding. Like any enduring cornerstone, the Northwest Ordinance has been built upon again and again. It has served as a blueprint for the nation's westward expansion."

136. **The correct answer is (D).** The answer to this question is based on ruling out A, B, and C, as they are supported by statements in the article, leaving D as the remaining answer. A is supported by the following statement in paragraph 6: "Among the items included . . . are a rare first printing of *The Definitive Treaty between Great Britain and the United States* (1783); . . . Jefferson's Ordinance of 1784, which set up a temporary government for the West; and the Land Ordinance of 1785, which established the system for surveying and eventual sale of the new lands." B is supported by the following statement in paragraph 2: " 'The Northwest Ordinance: Liberty and Justice for All' (project) featured . . . a two-day scholarly symposium to examine the state of current scholarship on the ordinance." It is also supported by the following statement in paragraph 3: "The symposium . . . brought together a dozen scholars who were at work on the ordinance or some related aspect of American history." C is inferred by the following statements found in paragraphs 1, 2, and 4. From paragraph 1 is the statement: "Two projects brought together for the first time the alumni associations from nine Big Ten universities, and a variety of other institutions, for several programs available to the public." From paragraph 2 comes the following statement: "[the first project entitled] Northwest Ordinance . . . featured education programs . . . for the general public." The statement, "The alumni associations developed public educational packs for distribution . . ." is from paragraph 4.

137. **The correct answer is (A).** The answer to this question is supported by the following statement in paragraph 8: "[The Northwest Ordinance] has served as a blueprint for the nation's westward expansion . . ."

138. **The correct answer is (A).** The answer is based on ruling out B, C, and D. They are supported by statements in the article, leaving A the remaining answer, as it is not supported by any statements. From paragraph 7 is the following statement that supports B: "These ordinances and documents rank among the most important in our early American history, both for what they accomplish and for what they inspired. . . ." C is supported by the following statements from paragraph 8: "Like any enduring cornerstone, the Northwest Ordinance has been built upon again and again. It has served as a blueprint for the nation's westward expansion." From paragraph 6 is the following sentence that supports D: "Among the 56 items included in the Northwest Ordinance part of the exhibition [is] . . . the Land Ordinance of 1785, which established the system for surveying and eventual sale of the new lands to settlers in the Northwest Territory."

139. **The correct answer is (A).** The answer to this question can be inferred from paragraph 6: "Among the 56 items included in the Northwest Ordinance part of the exhibition are a rare first printing of *The Definitive Treaty between Great Britain and the United States* (1783), written and printed at the instruction of Ambassador Benjamin Franklin in Paris. . . ."

140. **The correct answer is (C).** The answer to this question is based on the following statement in paragraph 6: ". . . the Land Ordinance of 1785, which established the system for the surveying and eventual sale of the new lands to settlers in the Northwest Territory."

141. **The correct answer is (B).** The answer to this question is based on the following statements in paragraph 6: "[Included are] a rare first printing of *The Definitive Treaty between Great Britain and the United States* (1783)" and ". . . along with pages of the original Northwest Ordinance."

142. **The correct answer is (B).** The answer to this question is based on the following statement in paragraph 4: "The alumni associations developed public education packs for distribution to libraries, historical societies, and other interested organizations."

BIOLOGICAL SCIENCES

143. **The correct answer is (B).** The fetal stage begins in the third month of pregnancy. The graph shows that starting at that time and through birth, 90–100 percent of all hemoglobin molecules contain the alpha and gamma chains.

144. **The correct answer is (A).** If extended beyond the graph, only the alpha, beta, and delta chains could possibly continue to adulthood. Clearly, the alpha and beta chains would predominate.

145. **The correct answer is (C).** The epsilon chain is produced in the first trimester only. It no longer is made after the embryo reaches three months (after conception).

146. **The correct answer is (C).** The graphic lines representing the beta and gamma chains cross each other between birth and three months of age. Hereafter, the gamma chain decreases in percentage while the beta chain increases in the percentage of hemoglobin molecules in which it is found.

147. **The correct answer is (D).** Although the alpha and beta chains are present in the adult (and adults need efficient oxygen transport), the gamma and epsilon chains are those present prior to birth when the embryo and fetus must have hemoglobin with an extremely high oxygen affinity in order to be able to draw oxygen from the mother's blood supply.

148. **The correct answer is (C).** Again, as described in Question 144, the delta chain can be extrapolated to extend (although at a very low percentage) beyond birth toward adulthood.

149. **The correct answer is (A).** Since the epsilon chain is no longer produced after the first three months of pregnancy, and the delta chain is not produced *until* at least four to five months later, no hemoglobin molecule can contain both types of chain at the same time.

150. **The correct answer is (C).** None of the three hormones actually has a *direct* effect on the genes. However, since the two steroid hormones can freely enter cells and eventually reach the nucleus, while the water-soluble epinephrine cannot even cross the cell membrane, the latter is the LEAST likely to affect the genes *directly*.

151. **The correct answer is (A).** Steroids are lipids that can freely cross the cell membrane without the need for carrier molecules to help them.

152. **The correct answer is (C).** Since steroid hormones can freely cross cell membranes, they should be able to enter all cells (as well as leave all cells). The description of Experiment 2 states that in target cells, these hormones were bound to receptor proteins inside. Why aren't such hormones found in nontarget cells of the spleen? They entered, there was no receptor to bind with them, and they passed out freely!

153. **The correct answer is (C).** Injecting epinephrine into the cells has no effect. Epinephrine and glycogen phosphorylase in contact in a beaker has no effect. Only choice C is a reasonable answer.

154. **The correct answer is (D).** The description of Experiment 1 indicates that epinephrine has an effect only when in *solution surrounding* intact cells (see explanation for Question 153). This suggests a form of membrane interaction. Thus, all three conclusions make logical sense.

155. **The correct answer is (D).** Receptors on the cell membrane can make target cells "noticed" by insoluble hormones passing by in the blood, whereas nontarget cells would lack such a recognition site (therefore, A is a correct answer). However, the question states in a very general way that after a hormone binds to a cell's membrane, the "second messenger" is responsible for "affecting activities inside a cell." This suggests a more general mechanism of action (other hormones bind to special membrane receptors, leading to the same "second messenger" carrying out the next steps). Thus, C is a reasonable answer as well. Choice B makes no sense (Why bind with the hormone if you don't have the next ingredient in the chain?).

156. **The correct answer is (B).** This question simply requires a familiarity with scientific notation (exponents). $10,000 = 10^4$. If $10^4 = 1/10^4$ of the total number of proteins, then $10^4 = X/10^4$, and $X = 10^8$.

157. **The correct answer is (D).** "Outside" the cell includes both the plasma and the interstitial fluids. Simply examining the bar graphs reveals that all three statements are true.

158. **The correct answer is (C).** One has to know that the *resting potential* of nerve and muscle cells reflects concentration differences between the inside and outside of the cell. These concentration differences result in a more *negatively charged* environment *inside* the cells compared to outside. An anion is a negatively charged substance attracted to the positively charged anode. Thus, C is the reasonable choice since it involves higher levels of two groups of negatively charged substances inside.

159. **The correct answer is (B).** Knowledge about the role of the sodium–potassium pump is crucial to answering this question correctly. It should be understood that this pump helps repolarize nerve and muscle cells. Without it, such tissues would not be able to restore their resting states, and as a result, would depolarize inappropriately (a form of irritability).

160. **The correct answer is (D).** Basic knowledge about the function of the lymphatic system is required.

161. **The correct answer is (B).** Various hormones of the endocrine system regulate the substances mentioned in the question (sodium and potassium: aldosterone; calcium and phosphate; calcitonin and parathyroid hormone). If one chose D as the answer with the urinary system in mind, it should be understood that kidney activities with respect to most of these ions are in response to hormonal signals.

162. **The correct answer is (A).** An understanding of osmotic principles as well as of the selective permeability of the cell membrane is required. Only the water will move freely from one fluid compartment to the other. Since the blood is hypertonic (more solute), it has less water. Thus, water moves from where there is more of it, to where there is less of it (cell to blood).

163. **The correct answer is (D).** Basic knowledge about the role of buffers in acid-base balance is required.

164. **The correct answer is (C).** Crossing over can only take place between two separate loci on the same chromosome (different loci for different traits). Gray and black body (as well as normal and vestigial wings) are *two alleles for the same trait at the same locus!*

165. **The correct answer is (C).** The distance between loci can be reflected by how often random breaks in the chromosome occur between them. Evidence that a break occurred is the appearance of a phenotype that could only have come about if a crossover event took place. The F_1 parent that is heterozygous has one chromosome with gray body together with normal wings, and the other chromosome with black body and vestigial wings together. The double recessive parent can only contribute a chromosome with black body and vestigial wings. The only way an offspring can have gray body with vestigial wings, or black body with normal wings, is if a crossover event took place in the heterozygous parent during gamete formation. 160 offspring are "recombinants" (75 + 85) out of a total of 800 (suggesting that 160 crossover events took place). 160/800 = 20 percent = 20 map units.

166. **The correct answer is (B).** 20 map units represents 20 percent recombinants out of 600. 20% × 600 = 120.

167. **The correct answer is (B).** If A and B are 40 units apart, and A and C are 25 units apart, C could be between A and B or on the outer side of A. The key information is that the distance between B and C is 65 units. C must be on the outer side of A. (If C were between A and B, it would have to be 15 units from B.)

168. **The correct answer is (B).** A linkage group is a group of genes with loci on the same chromosome. The number of linkage groups is the same as the haploid number of the species (since crossing over occurs between *homologous pairs* during meiosis). If there are 64 chromosomes in a somatic cell, then 64 is the diploid number and 32 is the haploid number.

169. **The correct answer is (C).** A double-crossover involves breaks at two different loci at the same time. If the map order of the loci is A-D-B, the heterozygous parent will have one A-D-B chromosome and one a-d-b chromosome. One break will be between the A-D loci, and the other break will be between the B-D loci.

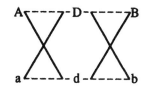

With two breaks involved, A will join with d, and d with B. Similarly, a will join with D.

170. **The correct answer is (D).** Examination of the flow chart figure reveals that all statements are correct.

171. **The correct answer is (B).** Basic knowledge about the various functions of the liver is required; specifically, the synthesis of prothrombin, fibrinogen, and numerous other blood proteins and clotting factors.

172. **The correct answer is (D).** Knowledge of blood topic terminology is needed. Since heparin interferes with the formation of two vital clotting factors (coagulation factors), it is referred to as an anticoagulant. An agglutinogen is another term for antigen, while agglutinin is synonymous with blood antibody.

173. **The correct answer is (D).** Knowledge of Mendelian genetics and the uniqueness of sex-linked traits is essential. If the normal woman's father was a hemophiliac, she must be a carrier for the trait ($X^H X^h$). The normal man has the normal allele on his only X chromosome ($X^H Y$). Their offspring have an equal chance of being any of the following genotypes:

$X^H X^H$	$X^H X^h$	$X^H Y$	$X^h Y$
normal female	normal female	normal male	hemophiliac male

174. **The correct answer is (C).** If vitamin K is needed to make clotting factors, dicumarol indirectly acts as an "anticoagulant." This "anticoagulant" characteristic is helpful in preventing unwanted clots like thromboses.

175. **The correct answer is (A).** A look at the flow chart reveals that platelet disintegration leads to the release of platelet clotting factors, which is a repetition of the first step of the intrinsic system.

176. **The correct answer is (C).** Enzyme activity is reflected by proteins being digested to peptides (low protein, high peptide). Table 2 reveals that chymotrypsin is most active at 37°C (body temperature) and pH 6–8 (which is the approximate pH of the small intestine where the enzyme is at work).

177. **The correct answer is (D).** Both enzymes show activity at two temperatures (37°C and 22°C), but only chymotrypsin shows activity at two pH ranges (pH 6–8 and 4–6). Pepsin shows activity only at pH 2–4 (the pH of the stomach).

178. **The correct answer is (D).** Neither enzyme shows any activity at structure of the molecules. The other two categories of temperature and all three pH ranges show at least moderate activity by at least one of the enzymes.

179. **The correct answer is (C).** Basic knowledge of the characteristics of the stomach is helpful but not necessary. The mucous secretions of the stomach are highly alkaline. This inactivates pepsin (which is only active in a highly acidic environment) when it comes in contact with the inner walls. Table 1 shows the acidic pH required for pepsin activity. Thus, choices A and D make no sense (pepsin *would* digest the stomach if these choices were correct). Additionally, since 62°C is far too high above the body's homeostatic temperature range, choice B is ruled out.

180. **The correct answer is (C).** Basic knowledge of pancreatic and intestinal function is helpful. The small intestine releases the hormone secretin, which signals the pancreas to secrete sodium bicarbonate. This helps neutralize the acidic chyme and allows all pancreatic and intestinal enzymes to work properly. Choice A cannot be correct because any enzyme released by the pancreas through the pancreatic duct would have to work at the pH range maintained in the small intestine. Choice B cannot be correct, because food arriving is always a part of the acidic soup from the stomach. Choice D seems to stretch the imagination a bit too far!

181. **The correct answer is (C).** An understanding of digestive and absorptive processes is necessary. Protein material must be digested into amino acids before absorption can occur. Cells cannot synthesize proteins unless they first receive amino acids (the polypeptides in B will be of no use since they have no way of getting to the cells).

182. **The correct answer is (B).** Data from the table indicates that out of 180 liters of water that are filtered from the plasma, 178-179 are reabsorbed. Thus, 1-2 liters leave in the urine. $\frac{1}{180} = .006; \frac{2}{180} = .011$. These figures are read as slightly more than one-half of one percent and slightly more than one percent, respectively.

183. **The correct answer is (D).** An examination of the first two columns shows all constituents except proteins have every gram (or mL) that is present in the plasma filtered into the filtrate.

184. **The correct answer is (C).** Any situation in which a wide vessel (or pipe) feeds fluids into an area that is drained by a narrower vessel will have fluid accumulate and pressure build up between them. Having red blood cells in the filtrate is not a usual situation, since they are too large normally to pass through the glomerulus. The countercurrent mechanism of the kidney refers to the directional flow of salts around the Loop of Henle.

185. **The correct answer is (C).** Without proper insulin function, plasma glucose levels are high in diabetics. Therefore, higher than normal quantities will be filtered into the nephrons. However, there are only the "normal" numbers of carrier molecules to reabsorb glucose into the peritubular capillaries, and the excess glucose continues through the kidney and leaves in the urine.

186. **The correct answer is (A).** If an individual's blood pH is too high (too alkaline), the urinary system can adjust by either retaining additional sources of H^+ or by allowing additional alkaline substances out in the urine. HCO_3^- is such a basic ion. Reabsorption of HCO_3^- or filtering acidic substances will only increase pH further. "Larger alkaline proteins" do not normally get filtered through the glomerulus.

187. **The correct answer is (C).** Knowledge of the variables that influence blood pressure, and the role of the adrenal cortex hormone aldosterone (increasing reabsorption of Na^+), are essential. An understanding of osmotic relationships is also required. For example, increased levels of cells and solutes in the blood will osmotically attract additional water. This will raise blood volume, which in turn raises blood pressure (vasodilation lowers blood pressure).

188. **The correct answer is (B).** Step 2 of both mechanisms involves transfer of an aryl group with its bonding electrons to the adjacent carbon atom (carbanion rearrangement).

189. **The correct answer is (C).** $^{\ominus}OCH_3$ will add to one carbonyl group forming

$$\begin{array}{c} O^- \\ | \\ C_6H_5{-}C{-}OCH_3 \\ | \\ C_6H_5{-}C{=\!=}O \end{array}$$ according to Mechanism A.

190. **The correct answer is (A).** Oxygen exchange with O^{18}-labeled water will indicate that step 1 is reversible (and faster than step 2).

191. **The correct answer is (C).** The aliphatic analogs undergo aldol condensations in alkaline solution.

192.   **The correct answer is (D).** Reactions include acylation of the alcohol group and reaction of the carboxyl group (amide formation, esterification).

193.   **The correct answer is (B).** In reaction 1, Cl^- adds, while in reaction 2, the neutral base :NH_2OH attacks the β carbon. Attack at the β position produces the intermediate

$$\left[\begin{array}{c} \underset{\underset{\text{Nu}}{|}}{-C}-\overset{H}{\underset{|}{C}}=\overset{H}{\underset{|}{C}}-\overline{O}| \end{array} \ominus \leftrightarrow \begin{array}{c} \underset{\underset{\text{Nu}}{|}}{-C}-\overset{H}{\underset{|}{C}}-\overset{H}{\underset{|}{C}}=O \end{array} \ominus \right]$$

which is resonance-stabilized. By adding to an end of the conjugated system, the electronegative oxygen can carry the negative charge.

194.   **The correct answer is (C).** Addition to oxygen yields the carbocation

$$\left[-\overset{|}{C} \cdots \overset{|}{C} \cdots \overset{|}{C}-OH \right]^{+}$$

in which the positive charge is shared among three carbon atoms. Addition to carbon would give the intermediate $-\overset{|}{\underset{\underset{H}{|}}{C}}-\overset{|}{C}\cdots\overset{|}{C}\cdots O$ which is less stable.

195.   **The correct answer is (D).** This is a nucleophilic addition of a carbanion to an α, β-unsaturated, carbonyl compound. Again, attack occurs at the end of the conjugated system.

196.   **The correct answer is (A).**

197.   **The correct answer is (C).** The carbonyl group activates the carbon-carbon double bond toward electron-rich reactants.

198.   **The correct answer is (C).** Experiment 2 shows that 1,3-butadiene reacts more rapidly than 1-octene.

199.   **The correct answer is (A).** These two structures account for the 1,2- and 1,4- addition products shown in step (4).

200.   **The correct answer is (C).** The magnitude of the activation energy determines the rate of the reaction. Activation energy is the *difference* in energy between the reactant(s) and the transition state.

201.   **The correct answer is (A).** Free Radical • $CH_2\!=\!CH\!-\!CH\!=\!CH_2$
$$CH_2\!=\!CH\!-\!CH\!=\!CH_2 \nearrow$$
$$[-CH_2\!-\!CH\!=\!CH\!-\!CH_2\!-\!]_n$$
polybutadiene

202.   **The correct answer is (C).** As with free radical addition, the 1,2- and 1,4- addition products are formed.

203.   **The correct answer is (D).** The glucose anomers are diastereomers that differ in configuration about C—1.

204.   **The correct answer is (D).**

205. **The correct answer is (D).** This question requires an understanding of Mendelian genetics and antigen-antibody relationships. The A and B antigens on the RBCs donated from the Type AB donor will be agglutinated by anti-B in the plasma of the Type A recipient, anti-A (in the Type B recipient), and both anti-A and anti-B (in the Type O recipient).

206. **The correct answer is (D).** A basic understanding of enzyme function is needed. When the product of an enzymatic pathway inhibits any of the previous steps in the pathway, this is referred to as feedback inhibition. Enzyme specificity refers to the conditions appropriate for an enzyme to work (substrate, pH, temperature, etc.). Competitive inhibition occurs when a substance occupies the active site that normally binds to the substrate involved in the reaction. The question states that isoleucine fits into the allosteric site.

207. **The correct answer is (D).** Knowledge of the basic functions of brain structures is necessary, as well as an understanding of the various sources of sensory and CNS information needed to coordinate movement, posture, and balance. The movement of skeletal muscles is initiated in the cerebrum. Posture and balance are influenced, in part, from sensory signals originating in the joints, tendons, and muscles themselves (proprioception), as well as from the utricle, saccule, and semicircular canals in the inner ear.

208. **The correct answer is (C).** The ability to interpret the figure showing hormonal changes during the menstrual cycle is helpful, but not essential. The paragraph contains the information needed to answer this question. HCG maintains the corpus luteum. Earlier in the paragraph, it is stated that "As LH levels decrease, corpus luteum activity slows down. . . ." Thus, HCG mimics LH.

209. **The correct answer is (A).** A basic understanding of the processes of transcription and translation is needed. If chromosome puffs represent uncoiled or decondensed regions of DNA, this suggests that the DNA sequence has to be "read," either for DNA replication (mitosis) or protein synthesis. Since the insect larva is undergoing different developmental changes in response to hormones, the synthesis of various proteins needed during each subsequent stage seems most probable. The hormone appears to be "activating" genes along the DNA so that transcription of these DNA sequences can occur.

210. **The correct answer is (B).** General knowledge of neuromuscular relationships is needed. If curare competes with acetylcholine along the motor end plate (at the neuromuscular junction), ACh cannot perform its function. ACh normally causes skeletal muscles to depolarize and contract. If this is blocked, B is clearly the correct choice. Choices A and C refer to events after depolarization has already taken place. Heat production results from contraction (muscle activity), which requires ACh in the first place.

211. **The correct answer is (B).** Broad knowledge of the functions of the nervous and endocrine systems is helpful. The main point is that the arrector pili muscles are described as "smooth muscles." These are involuntary muscles that are under the direct control of the autonomic nervous system.

212. **The correct answer is (D).** Basic knowledge about vertebrate biology is helpful. The characteristics described are shared by structures including gills, lungs, and even the skin of frogs (which can serve as an extra respiratory organ underwater).

213. **The correct answer is (C).** Knowledge of basic concepts in muscle physiology is helpful. Since the described phenomenon involves only a second contraction, summation is the appropriate answer. If the situation involved multiple stimuli (20–30) in rapid succession, partial tetany would be correct. Tetany occurs when multiple stimuli occur so rapidly that there is no time to relax at all. Threshold refers to the level of stimulation required to initiate any response by the muscle cell.

214. **The correct answer is (B).** An understanding of the effects of histamine and the inflammatory response are helpful, but not essential. Logical thinking will come through here as well. The symptoms described—e.g., redness and heat—would result from *more* red, warm blood in the area (dilation of blood vessels). Similarly, swelling and pain would result from *additional fluids* in the area stimulating pain receptors (more fluid leakage from capillaries).

215. **The correct answer is (C).** Aromatic systems show strong absorptions in the UV region of the system. C—C and C—H bonds will absorb in the IR region. The NMR will show the inequivalent hydrogens.

216. **The correct answer is (B).** Because both reactants contain acidic α-H's, two different carbanions will form and attack the carbonyl groups in condensation reactions.

217. **The correct answer is (D).** Quaternary nitrogen atoms cannot react to form an amide because it already has four bonds.

$$R'-C{=}O + ROH \rightleftharpoons \underset{\substack{|\\OH}}{\overset{\substack{H\\|}}{R'-C-OR}} \rightleftharpoons \underset{\substack{|\\OR}}{\overset{\substack{H\\|}}{R'-C-OR}}$$

hemiacetal   acetal

218. **The correct answer is (A).**

219. **The correct answer is (C).** Hydrolysis breaks the amide linkage to form the amino acid residues alanine and glycine. Because the acids are in basic solution, their dibasic form predominates.

Appendices

APPENDIX A

Typical Interview Questions

1. Why did you attend _____ College?

2. What extracurricular activities do you participate in?

3. Why do you want to become a physician?

4. What newspapers do you read?

5. How have you spent your summer vacations since you entered college?

6. How will you finance your medical education?

7. What other schools have you applied to?

8. Why did you apply to this medical school?

9. Are you interested in a particular medical specialty? If so, why?

10. Why did you get a poor grade in _____ ?

11. Which medical school is your first choice?

12. Please discuss your social life.

13. Describe your schedule in college.

14. What were your favorite courses? Why?

15. Did you do any special science project? If yes, discuss.

16. Will your religious convictions interfere in your studies or practice of medicine?

17. What was the greatest strength of the college where you did your undergraduate work?

18. What was the greatest weakness of the college where you did your undergraduate work?

19. Do you feel you should have gone to a different college to do your undergraduate course work? Why/why not?

20. Have you done any research? Please discuss.

21. Have you done any volunteer work? Please discuss.

22. How do you think HMO's are affecting the medical profession?

23. What do you do in your spare time?

24. Tell me about yourself and your family.

25. What are your long-term objectives?

26. Do you have any hobbies? What are they?

27. What do you enjoy about your hobbies?

28. Was there a particular experience that led you to your career choice? Please discuss.

29. What are your plans for marriage and having a family?

30. Why isn't this medical school your first choice?

31. Describe the characteristics of a good physician.

32. Why do you think you are better suited for admission than your classmates?

33. What is the status of the MD in modern society?

34. What has been your most significant accomplishment to date?

35. If you had great willpower, how would you change yourself?

36. What are the characteristics of a mature person?

37. What do you think can be determined about an applicant at an interview?

38. What books have you recently read? Please discuss what you liked about a recent book you read.

39. Would you perform an abortion? Why? Why not?

40. What do you think is the most important ethical issue facing medicine today?

41. What is your opinion on _____ (major current event issues)?

42. Discuss the ethical questions concerning cloning of humans.

43. How do you cope with frustrating situations?

44. What will you do if you are not accepted to medical school?

45. How do you rank among the pre-professional students at your school?

46. Have you ever worked with people, and, if so, in what capacity?

47. Who has had the greatest influence on your life and why?

48. How do you spend your spare time?

49. Should drugs like marijuana and heroin, if they are shown to have medicinal value, be available to patients with prescriptions? Why/why not?

50. If you couldn't be a doctor, what other profession would interest you? Why?

51. How do you think medicine will be different 20 years from now?

52. What is your greatest strength?

53. What is your greatest weakness?

54. Given your strong grades, why didn't you receive a stronger MCAT score?

55. Give an example of a stressful situation that you have been in and how you were able to successfully deal with the situation.

56. Where do you think you will practice and why?

57. Are any members of your family doctors?

58. What is your opinion of euthanasia of humans?

59. Do you have any questions?

60. (For D.O. candidates only) Why do you want to be a doctor of Osteopathic Medicine?

61. (For D.O. candidates only) Please discuss what makes Osteopathic Medicine different from allopathic medicine.

62. (For D.O. candidates only) Do you know an Osteopathic Doctor?

APPENDIX B

What to Expect in Medical School and Beyond*

MEDICAL SCHOOL

Once you've passed the MCAT and have been accepted to medical school, you might start asking yourself, "What have I gotten myself into?" Although the answer varies among schools, most institutions provide a similar four-year format of instruction.

During the first two years you will receive the basic science portion of your medical training. Most students find these years to be the most rigorous and demanding of their lives.

THE BASIC SCIENCES

FRESHMAN YEAR

Freshman year of medical school typically involves courses in gross anatomy, histology, embryology, neuroanatomy, genetics, biochemistry, physiology, and behavioral science. Courses in medical ethics and legal medicine are often included in the first-year curriculum. As a rule, you will be in class from 8 A.M. to 5 P.M., Monday through Friday. The following gives a fairly accurate picture of what lies ahead.

Gross Anatomy

Gross anatomy is the study of the structures of the human body. Traditionally it is taught through lectures and dissection of a human cadaver. Every month you will study a new area of the body. The anatomy course is often divided into sections: head and neck, arms, legs, thorax, abdomen, back, perineum, and pelvis. Lectures usually last one or two hours, three to five times a week, for one or two semesters. Afternoons will be spent dissecting body parts covered in the lectures. Most students find gross anatomy their most interesting and most challenging course.

Histology

Histology might better be called "microanatomy." It is the study of the cells that make up the human body.

You will learn the location, type, and function of cells that are found throughout the body. Histology is usually taught three to five times a week in one-hour lectures and lasts one semester. At least one afternoon a week is spent in a histology lab looking at slides of body organs and tissue.

Embryology

Embryology is the study of developmental anatomy. The course traces human cellular development from the sperm and ovum stage to the infant. Every structure of the human body comes from specialized cellular tissues, which develop into functional body parts. Often included in embryology are lectures on the drugs and diseases that can adversely affect embryo growth. You will learn what body part or organ system develops during each phase of the nine-month developmental process. Lectures will also cover attempts at preventing fertilization through the use of birth control devices. Lectures are given three to five times per week, usually for one semester.

Neuroanatomy

Neuroanatomy, the study of the central and peripheral nervous systems, is the bane of many a medical student. Because of the many intricate nerve pathways that must be learned, most students find this one of their most challenging courses. It is usually a one-semester course that meets three to five times a week. A brain and spinal cord dissection lab also meets once a week.

Genetics

Genetics is usually a one-semester course. Classes typically meet once or twice a week for an hour. Much of the course is spent learning to identify key features of children with genetic disorders. The class studies the many diseases caused by gene crosses and the consequences for the fetus.

Biochemistry

Biochemistry is one of the "big three" courses taught to most freshman medical students, the other two being gross anatomy and physiology. Biochemistry is the study of chemical reactions that occur in the human body, examined on a cellular level. The ways in

* Adapted from *Getting into Medical School: Strategies for the '90s*, by Scott H. Plantz, M.D., with Nicholas Y. Lorenzo, M.D., and Jesse A. Cole, M.D. (ARCO, 1993).

which these chemicals react to make organ systems function is also part of the course. The class often meets five times a week, one to two hours per day, for one or two semesters.

Physiology

Physiology is the study of the interaction of cellular systems and how they make the human body function. Topics covered include respiratory, kidney, cardiovascular (heart), and gastrointestinal functions. The course meets one or two hours a day, five days per week for one or two semesters.

Behavioral Science

Behavioral science is the study of how humans think and feel. Topics addressed might include how different races deal with pain, death, or birth. This class is usually limited, meeting one or two hours a week for one semester.

Ethics

Some schools require students to complete an ethics course and a legal medicine course. Ethics usually concentrates on such issues as euthanasia and abortion. Legal medicine covers the laws that affect the practice of medicine, such as malpractice laws. These courses usually meet one or two hours a week for one semester.

If the first-year curriculum seems as if it involves a lot of class time, it does. Medical school courses, in general, are not intellectually difficult, but the volume of material covered can be overwhelming. Most students consider themselves lucky to read textbooks once and notes twice before exams. Those students with the sharpest memorization and retainment skills quickly rise to the top of any medical school class. Students with science backgrounds who have covered some or all of these courses also have an advantage. It is possible, however, to do well simply by studying a great deal, that is, six to ten hours a day, seven days a week.

SOPHOMORE YEAR

Most students find the second year of medical school more interesting, as schools concentrate on classes in understanding, diagnosis, evaluation, and treatment of disease. Courses typically include pathology, clinical pathology, microbiology, pharmacology, and diagnostic examination and evaluation. Many schools allow students to see patients and do practice histories and physicals.

Pathology

Pathology, by definition, is the study of suffering. It examines why diseases arise and how they affect tissue change or growth in the human body. Topics covered in pathology courses include immunology, infectious diseases, environmentally induced diseases, heart and blood vessel diseases, respiratory system diseases, and organ systems such as the liver, pancreas, kidney, urinary tract, gastrointestinal tract, spleen, genitals, skin, breasts, nervous system, and musculoskeletal system. Pathology is usually considered the most important class in the second year. It involves two hours of lecture time, five days a week, for the entire year. Additional time may be spent in the afternoons studying specimens of diseased tissue.

Clinical Pathology

An extension of pathology is clinical pathology. The course covers clinical interpretation of laboratory tests. Some schools offer this as part of pathology; others separate the two.

Microbiology

A close cousin of pathology, microbiology covers many topics studied in pathology. A typical microbiology course studies bacterial, parasitic, and viral infectious diseases—some already well known to you, such as strep throat. You will learn about the many varieties of strep throat and the complications that can occur as a result of the disease. You will also study the bacteria that cause such diseases as meningitis (brain and spinal cord infection) and cellulitis (skin infection). In addition, you will discover that having a "worm" infection means you have one of hundreds of parasites that infect the human body. A final aspect of the course covers viruses, which cause illnesses ranging from the common cold to AIDS. This class will study how viruses reproduce, infect, and transmit the diseases they induce.

You will also study some of the basics of treatment of these diseases. Microbiology meets at least one hour a day, five days a week, for the entire year. Afternoon labs are spent studying these little beasties under both light and electron microscopes.

Pharmacology

Pharmacology is the study of how drugs function and interact, and how they are used in the treatment of disease. This is one of the most practical courses you will take during your second year. It meets one or two hours per day for the entire year; most schools do not offer labs.

Clinical Diagnosis

Most schools offer this course in the second year. Typically it teaches students to do histories and physicals (H & P), and to recognize many of the physical findings of disease. Often, students will work with a physician who will have them practice physical exam techniques on the physician's patients. The course usually meets one or two hours a day. Lab time is spent with the doctor learning history and physical exam skills.

Boards Part I

At the completion of the second year, most institutions require students to take National Boards Part I, a comprehensive exam covering the course work studied in the first two years of medical school. In many schools you must pass this exam to continue into the third year. Many residency programs will also look at these scores in evaluating applicants. If you thought the MCAT was tough, wait till you see this one. You will be reviewing 10,000 pages of graduate-level texts in the two to three weeks you will be given to prepare for this exam.

THE CLINICAL SCIENCES

The final two years of medical school are spent on clinical rotations in several specialties. This is when you first begin to experience the "art and science" of medicine. Two to three months into your senior year, you will have to choose one of these clinical specialties as part of your long-term career plans. Although many doctors eventually change specialties, the first years of internship and residency were often decided upon early in their senior year of medical school.

JUNIOR YEAR

The light at the end of the tunnel grows bright as you start your third year of medical school. After this point, it would be unusual not to complete your medical degree. The third year generally consists of five two-month rotations in surgery, obstetrics and gynecology, pediatrics, internal medicine, and psychiatry. The other two months are often devoted to electives and vacation time.

Surgery

Surgical rotation usually consists of two months of general surgery. A general surgeon does operations on the abdomen and may also operate on other areas of the body such as the arms, legs, chest, breasts, and neck. While in surgery you will be responsible for doing histories and physicals on patients admitted to the hospital, writing daily orders for maintaining the patients' diets, and, most important, assisting the surgeons in the operating room.

At the student level you will soon learn to think of yourself as a "human retractor." As a surgical assistant you will be asked to hold retractors and pull organs and body fat out of the way, so the surgeon can dissect, remove, or revise whatever organ on which he or she is working. Not a particularly glamorous job, and a privilege for which you will be paying!

While the operation is going on, you will be reviewing anatomy. Most surgeons enjoy quizzing medical students on obscure body parts that have long since escaped the students' memory banks. Besides the daily quiz sessions, you will spend every third or fourth night "on call" in the hospital. This means you will be awakened by the nurse every hour or so, all

night long, to check an oozing wound, prescribe a sleeping pill, or renew an IV order that happens to run out at 3 A.M. You will also admit new patients who arrive at the hospital for next-morning surgery.

Despite your lack of sleep, the next day you will be expected to stay awake in the operating room holding clamps and answering questions. And, despite chronic sleep deprivation, you will spend most of your "free" time reading surgical texts so you can pass the surgery exam at the end of the rotation. You will spend two to three afternoons a week in surgery clinic, seeing new patients or following up on patients recovering from surgery.

Most students either love or hate surgery. The time demands are intense, but many students and doctors find the rewards of interesting and challenging surgery worth the mental and physical rigors.

Obstetrics and Gynecology

Obstetrics and gynecology is often divided into two one-month rotations. You will spend one month doing gynecologic surgery, the other in obstetrics, delivering babies. The month in gynecology will be similar to your time in general surgery. You will be expected to assist in patient management, do admission histories and physicals, and help the surgeon in operations. Gynecologic operations include removal of the uterus and ovaries, operations on the vagina and bladder in elderly women who develop difficulty controlling urination, and the removal of tumors involving the reproductive organs. You will also assist in many dilations and curettages (D and C's), a common operation to remove abnormal tissue lining the uterus.

Your month of obstetrics will involve assisting in the delivery of babies by either normal vaginal delivery or c-section. In vaginal delivery your responsibilities will be to check the mother for progression of labor, get the surgical tray ready in case special instruments such as forceps are needed, and awaken the obstetrician in time to deliver the baby. Just before the baby emerges, the surgeon will often make a small cut called an episiotomy to widen the cervix. After the baby is delivered, the mother will need the episiotomy sewn shut. As you get to know the surgeons you work with, they will let you do more and more of the delivery, including sewing the episiotomy closed. During c-section deliveries, you will again be the surgical assistant and hold clamps while the surgeon performs the operation to remove the infant. Near the end of your rotation in Ob/Gyn, you may be allowed to assist in closing the layers of fat, muscle, and skin of the c-section incision. During both of these months, in-hospital call will be every third or fourth night.

Pediatrics

At most institutions, pediatrics is two months devoted to taking care of sick children in the hospital. Some schools allow time to see children in a clinic, perhaps one or two days per week. While on the pediatric service, you will be on call every third or fourth night. Your responsibility will be to assist the intern or resident in admitting sick children to the hospital throughout the night. This often involves doing a history and physical and sometimes procedures such as a spinal tap to check for meningitis as a cause of the child's illness. While awake you will spend your free time reading about your patients' problems and developing plans for helping patients get over their illnesses. You will also help to care for patients who develop problems during the night.

In the morning you will make rounds on your patients with the intern, resident, and attending pediatrician. During rounds you will present your new patients to the attending doctor by giving him or her a brief summary of the key features of the H & P. You will be quizzed about your workup of each child's problem and your treatment plan. In your free time, you will prepare for your pediatric exam at the end of the rotation. If you like children, you will probably find this rotation interesting.

Internal Medicine

For many students, the months of internal medicine will be some of the most intense of their medical training. This is the field of medicine that deals with medical problems in adults. Usually these problems occur in elderly patients with multiple medical conditions. Each day will begin early, usually around 6 A.M. You will start by making rounds on your patients, charting their progress, checking vital signs, ensuring their medicine orders are up to date, checking their IV fluids, and making sure that no complications occurred during the night.

Your rounds will be followed by rounds with the intern assigned to cover your patients, who will recheck them and make any adjustments he or she finds necessary. These rounds are followed by rounds with the senior medical resident. These are often quick rounds in which only the key features of each patient's problems are addressed. Finally the patient's doctor appears and attending rounds begin.

The doctor will question you about your treatment of the patients and check their progress. He or she will also indicate physical exam findings you may have missed. Rounds usually last most of the morning. When they are complete, you will spend the afternoon looking up lab values, performing procedures on your patients, and making sure all diagnostic tests are complete. You may also have to attend a medicine clinic and see outpatients one or two afternoons per week. Assuming all is well, you can now go home for the day.

You will be on call every third or fourth night. You will be responsible, along with the intern and the chief resident, for admitting patients to the hospital. As a new patient arrives, you will complete a history and physical, and develop a treatment plan, which will be reviewed by the intern and resident. You rarely get to sleep, as new patients are always arriving and your patients already in the hospital will require supervision as new problems develop. In your few minutes of free time, you will be reading your medicine text in preparation for morning rounds.

The next day, your attending physician will have you present the histories and physicals of the patients you admitted the previous night. Internists are obsessive-compulsive people, and they will expect to have no facts missed. You will have to know the reason each patient is currently being hospitalized, the patient's medical history, all drugs the patient is now taking, allergies, social history, family history, and surgical history, and to have made a detailed and complete physical exam. You will outline the possible causes of the patient's problems, how you plan to evaluate them, any test results available, and your treatment plan. As you make this presentation, you will frequently be interrupted with questions about the items you are outlining. Keep in mind that you have been up all night, admitted at least five patients, and probably will have a difficult time remembering these new patients, to say nothing of being able to answer questions about your management of their problems.

Psychiatry

Psychiatry is usually a more laid-back rotation than most of the others in your third year of medical school. As with the others, you will be on call every third or fourth night. Each day and call night you will be responsible for doing histories and physicals, and psych evaluations, specialized exams that assist in the diagnosis of psychiatric disease. Generally, the next day you will present your patients to your attending psychiatrist and resident. With them you will develop a treatment plan and monitor your patients' progresses. You may also spend a few afternoons a week seeing outpatient clinic patients to monitor their home therapy and progress.

Senior Year
Electives

The fourth year of medical school is generally all electives. That is, you may do additional rotations in the specialties already covered or do electives in many other specialty fields of medicine, including aerospace medicine, allergy and immunology, anesthesiology, pathology, cardiology, neurology, child psychiatry, critical care, preventive medicine, dermatology, radiology, emergency medicine, endocrinology, family practice, gastroenterology, geriatrics, hematology, infectious disease, oncology, neonatology, nephrology, neurosurgery, nuclear medicine, occupational medicine, ophthalmology, orthopedic surgery, otolaryngology, plastic surgery, pulmonology, radiation oncology, rheumatology, thoracic surgery, urology, and vascular surgery. Each of these specialties will be discussed in detail in the following section on your residency.

Matching

By September of your senior year, you will have determined the specialty you plan to pursue. You will begin to fill in applications for residency training programs. Starting in October and ending in February, you will take days off to travel across the United States interviewing for positions. In February you will send a list of the residency training programs that interest you, ranked in order of preference, to a national computer matching service. At the same time, the residency programs will turn in a list of candidates in which they are interested, also ranked in order of preference. In March or April a computer will match you with the residency program that ranked you the highest and the one you ranked the highest. In other words, both you and the hospital training program will get your top mutual choice, your destiny being decided by a method similar to a computer dating service.

Boards Part II

Near the end of your fourth year, you will take Part II of the National Boards. This exam covers surgery, internal medicine, pediatrics, psychiatry, and obstetrics and gynecology. Some schools require passing this exam to graduate from medical school. Boards Part III is taken near the end of your internship. It covers clinical management of patients in the hospital.

Federal Licensing Exam (F.L.E.X.)

Some schools will not require you to take boards. In these cases, you may elect to take the F.L.E.X. exam, a comprehensive board exam that covers all the material in Boards Parts I–III. This test is taken at the conclusion of medical school.

Virtually all states require you to pass either Boards Part I–III or F.L.E.X. to obtain a medical license in the state. Residency programs also often use these tests to monitor your achievement.

GRADUATION

At the end of your senior year of medical school, you may be inclined to breathe a long sigh of relief. The medical degree you have received means little, however, until you have completed your internship, residency, and possibly a fellowship. Besides these, you will have to pass specialty board exams. Although you may now be called "Doctor," you must still devote a lot of time and effort to your education.

RESIDENCY

Medical school provides the foundation of knowledge on which a physician builds his or her career, but it is in the subsequent years of internship and residency that the doctor learns the skills necessary to practice medicine. Residency training is spent at teaching hospitals throughout the United States and is comparable to an apprenticeship—although you may feel more like an indentured servant. You will be paid approximately $25,000 a year and will put in a 60- to 120-hour work week. Most interns and residents work seven days a week with rare weekends off.

You will also be on call every second, third, or fourth night, depending on your selected training program. For example, every third night on call means that you work from 6 A.M. Monday to about 6 P.M. Tuesday; Wednesday you work from 6 A.M. to 6 P.M.; Thursday from 6 A.M. to Friday at 6 P.M.; Saturday from 6 A.M. to 6 P.M.; and Sunday from 6 A.M. to Monday at 6 P.M. This cycle can continue for your entire three to seven years of training, depending on your specialty.

Every second night on call is a 126-hour work week; every third night on call is 114 hours; and every fourth night is 108 hours! Keep in mind that when another resident is sick or on vacation, you are often on call every second night.

INTERNSHIP

During your first year of training after medical school, you are called a "first-year resident" or "intern." Virtually all specialties require an internship. Some require a "rotating" internship or "transitional" year. This is similar to your third year of medical school; you will spend one to two months each doing surgery, internal medicine, pediatrics, obstetrics and gynecology, psychiatry, and one elective. You will also have three or four weeks of vacation time.

Other specialties will require your internship year to be more closely focused. For example, a first-year general surgery residency training program may require its first-year residents to spend six months doing general surgery and six months at assigned rotations in urologic surgery, thoracic surgery, plastic surgery, vascular surgery, and trauma surgery.

An internal-medicine residency training program may require six months of general medicine caring for moderately sick patients in the medical intensive care unit, two months assigned to patients in the cardiac intensive care unit, and two months of electives such as neurology, hematology, cardiology, and oncology.

Generally, your first year of training demands the most time. Most residency training programs decrease the time commitment with each year of training; a few demand every third night on call for the entire training period. The average program requires interns to spend every third night in the hospital on call. This means being up all night admitting patients to the hospital, doing histories and physicals, writing admitting orders, teaching medical students, and taking care of patients' problems, which always seem to develop around 3 A.M. You will also be expected to work a full day after your on-call night.

After the internship year, you are a "resident" and no longer the low man on the totem pole. In some programs, you may continue every second, third, or fourth night on call; in others, your call can decrease to a few nights a month. Some specialties require training in clinics or elective surgery during the day and do not involve treating patients who arrive during the night. Other residencies, such as radiology, have little or no direct patient care and will require only one resident in the hospital at night. Most radiologists' work is done during the day. Thus, if a hospital has twelve radiology residents, you may have to take call only every twelfth night, when your job may be to interpret the relatively few X-rays done at night.

Some residencies have home call. Dermatology emergencies are rare, so dermatology residents may take call from home or carry beepers and have to come in only a few times during their training. The majority of specialties, however, have patients in the hospital who develop complications at night or admit new patients during the night and require residents on the spot. A neurosurgery (brain surgery) resident's typical night may be spent attending several patients in a neuro intensive care unit, and when such a resident does get to bed at 2 A.M., he or she may be awakened by a call from the emergency-room physician. It seems another drunken motorcyclist has crashed and must be rushed to the operating room to have blood drained from his skull before the brain tissue is crushed and the patient dies.

As an intern or resident, you are never completely alone. Most hospitals have a hierarchy. For instance, every third night four pediatric interns may be on call. With them is one second- or third-year pediatric resident who now takes call every fifth or sixth night. If a problem develops beyond the latter's capacities, the patient's attending (fully trained) pediatrician may be called at home to assist in solving the problem. Sometimes the attending pediatrician may come in from home to look at the patient and help decide on treatment. In more difficult cases, he or she may ask that a specialist be consulted to assist in diagnosis and treatment. For instance, if a child came in with a new heart murmur and the heart was no longer operating effectively, you might be asked to call in a pediatric cardiologist (heart specialist).

Medicine has many specialties. Some require several years of initial training in internal medicine, surgery, pediatrics, or psychiatry, followed by a fellowship in a more focused area. For instance, an oncologist is a doctor specializing in the treatment of cancer. This specialist does a three-year residency in internal medicine or pediatrics followed by a three-year fellowship in oncology. Other specialties require an internship followed by two to three years of training. An emergency physician generally does a one-year rotating internship followed by three years of residency training in the emergency room. An anesthesiologist does an internship and three years of an anesthesiology residency.

The following details most of the residencies and fellowships available.

Anesthesiology

Internship plus three years of residency training. These doctors are responsible for putting patients to sleep during operations. Other than emergency surgery, they have no patient-care responsibilities at night. Call after the first year is infrequent, perhaps every fifth night. Fellowships are available in pediatric anesthesiology and critical care, each lasting one to three additional years.

Dermatology

Internship plus three years of residency training. These doctors diagnose and treat skin conditions. Their patient-care responsibilities at night are minimal and call is often taken from home. Fellowships are available in dermatopathology, which requires one or two more years.

Radiology

Internship plus three years of residency training. Radiologists interpret X-rays and perform specialized tests using radiographic equipment. They have little patient care at night. Call is usually in hospital but as infrequently as three or four times a month. One- to two-year fellowships are available in ultrasound, CAT scan, MRI scan, nuclear medicine, and invasive radiology.

Emergency Medicine

Internship plus two or three years of residency training. These doctors specialize in treating emergencies in the emergency room. Rather than taking call, they work a set number of 8- to 12-hour shifts each month. One- to two-year fellowships are available in toxicology, pediatrics, emergency medical systems, and research.

Family Practice

Three years of residency training. Considered general practitioners, these doctors spend their years of training doing rotations in internal medicine, pediatrics, surgery, obstetrics and gynecology, psychiatry, radiology, orthopedics, critical care, and other electives. They learn to treat a wide spectrum of diseases and refer patients to specialists when their condition warrants it. Call is usually every third to fourth night during internship and may decrease to every fifth or sixth night in the second and third years of training. One- to two-year fellowships are available in geriatric medicine (treating older patients), sports medicine, and obstetrics.

Internal Medicine

Three years of residency. These doctors specialize in the diagnosis and treatment of adult diseases. Because elderly adults tend to have more medical problems requiring hospitalization, many internists devote a significant part of their time to taking care of patients in the hospital in addition to busy office practices. Call is usually every third to fourth night for interns, decreasing to every fifth or sixth night in the final two years of training.

Many fellowships are available after three years of internal-medicine training. They generally last three to four years, with part of the time devoted to research. Cardiology fellows study patients with heart problems and do procedures such as echocardiograms and heart catheterizations. Critical-care fellows spend their training in medical intensive-care units. Endocrinology fellows learn specialized care of difficult-to-manage endocrine diseases such as diabetes. Gastroenterologists learn to treat diseases of the intestinal tract and learn specialized procedures, such as those in which fiber-optic scopes are used via mouth and rectum to examine the gastrointestinal tract. Fellows in geriatric medicine learn special skills needed to care for elderly patients. A hematology fellow studies the specialized care of patients with blood diseases such as hemophilia and cancers of the blood such as leukemia. Infectious disease fellows assist with the treatment of such complicated diseases as AIDS, tuberculosis, and meningitis. Nephrology fellows study patients with kidney problems and learn to manage patients undergoing dialysis. Oncologists take extra training in the treatment of cancers with chemotherapy. Fellows in pulmonary medicine specialize in diseases that infect the lungs, learning a special procedure in which a scope is put into the lungs through the mouth to take tissue specimens for diagnosis. Doctors learning to treat diseases that cause bone and joint breakdown do fellowships in rheumatology.

Thus, in addition to three years of demanding generalized internal medicine training, specialists devote additional years of training, taking call and working long days at relatively low pay, to develop the skills necessary to handle a narrow spectrum of patient problems.

Neurosurgery

Considered to be one of the most demanding surgical specialties, residency training in neurosurgery is typically six to seven years including internship. These doctors take call as often as every second to third night for seven years. Because of the delicacy of the operations performed, most being on the brain and spinal cord, the training is particularly rigorous. Residents attend neurosurgical emergencies such as bleeding inside the skull from trauma and remove tumors and aneurysms in brain tissue. There are no fellowships in neurosurgery.

Obstetrics and Gynecology

Ob/Gyn training begins with a one-year internship followed by a three-year residency. Call is every third to fourth night for most of the four years. These doctors learn to deliver babies, do caesarean sections, and perform gynecologic surgery, such as removal of the uterus and ovaries, and tubal ligations. Fellowships are available in high-risk obstetrics, fertility, genetics, and oncology.

Ophthalmology

Ophthalmologists complete an internship followed by three years of surgical training. Eye emergencies are relatively few, so call is minimal after the internship and may usually be taken at home by carrying a beeper. These doctors do surgery on the eyes and prescribe eyeglasses. Fellowships are available in areas such as retinal repair and oncology.

Orthopedic Surgery

Orthopedic surgeons are "bone doctors" whose training consists of a general surgery internship followed by three to four years of orthopedic surgery. Orthopedists are frequently involved in the care of trauma victims and typically have a demanding call schedule of every third to fourth night for their four years of training. These specialists set bones, put on casts, and perform surgeries such as prosthetic hip replacements. Many also do an extra one or two years of fellowship training in specialties such as the hand, spine, oncology, sports medicine, and pediatrics.

Otolaryngology

Otolaryngologists are also known as ear, nose, and throat surgeons. Training consists of at least one year of general surgery followed by four years of ENT surgery. Call is generally every third to fourth night for five years. These doctors repair injuries to the ear, nose, and throat, as well as remove tumors, do sinus-draining procedures, and revise congenital abnormalities such as repairing a child's deformed lip or mouth. Fellowships are available in areas such as pediatrics and oncology.

Pathology

Pathologists study diseased tissue by viewing microscopic tissue specimens removed during surgery or autopsy. They are also responsible for all the laboratory tests hospital lab technicians perform. Pathologists usually follow a one-year internship with four years of pathology training. After the first year, few pathology programs require in-hospital call. Many pathologists do fellowships and a number of one- to two-year fellowships are available.

Blood bank pathologists study blood used in transfusions. Chemical pathologists study tests evaluating chemical exposure to drugs and hazardous chemicals, and become expert in laboratory tests. Dermatopathologists study diseases affecting the skin. Forensic pathologists do autopsies and assist police departments in looking for clues in the bodies of homicide victims. Hematologists study diseases affecting the blood, such as leukemia and sickle cell anemia. Immunopathologists study diseases of the immune system. Pathologists in microbiology learn about infectious diseases and their effect on human tissue. Radioisotopic pathologists study laboratory tests that use isotopes in diagnosing disease.

Pediatrics

Pediatricians treat children. Training involves a three-year residency and call is every third or fourth night. Pediatricians may do a number of two-year fellowships in areas such as cardiology, where they learn to treat children with heart problems. Pediatric endocrinologists treat children with diseases such as diabetes. Pediatric hematologists and oncologists treat children with blood diseases and cancer. Nephrologists treat children with diseases affecting the kidneys. Pediatric geneticists diagnose children with genetic diseases. Pediatricians in emergency medicine fellowships work in pediatric emergency rooms.

Physical Medicine and Rehabilitation

Training in physical medicine and rehabilitation usually lasts four years—one year of internship and three years of residency. Call may be every third to fourth night. These doctors care for patients recovering from accidents or debilitating diseases such as strokes. They also often assist in directing physical therapists in devising exercises for patients.

Plastic Surgery

Training in plastic surgery occurs in one of two ways. Most plastic surgeons complete a five- to six-year residency in general surgery, followed by a two-year residency in plastic surgery. A few programs allow residents to complete two years of general surgery followed by three years of plastic surgery. Plastic surgeons generally take call every third or fourth night for most of their training. These doctors perform many kinds of operations, including scar revision, breast enlargement and reduction, and face lifts. They may do fellowships in specialties such as hand surgery and microvascular surgery.

Preventive Medicine

Physicians in this field spend their careers in intervention in health and disease processes in communities and defined population groups. They work to increase behaviors that prevent disease and injury, and aim at early diagnosis and treatment. Training lasts two to three years including a one-year internship. Subspecialization is available within preventive medicine in fields such as aerospace medicine, occupational medicine, and public health.

Psychiatry

Psychiatrists care for the mentally ill and patients suffering from diseases such as depression, schizophre-nia, and manic-depression. Training includes a one-year internship followed by a four-year residency. Call usually decreases to a few times a month as residents progress. A two- to three-year fellowship may be completed in child psychiatry. Also available is a fellowship in forensic psychiatry, which trains psychiatrists to care for patients deemed criminally insane.

Radiation Oncology

Radiation oncology requires a one-year internship followed by a four-year residency. Very few medical emergencies require the immediate attention of a radiation oncologist, and these doctors typically take call from home. They treat cancer patients with radiation, in some cases attempting to cure the patient; in others, simply to slow down the disease's progression and decrease pain. Radiation oncology has few fellowships, and most involve extra training in research.

Surgery

Training in general surgery is demanding; residency usually requires five to seven years. Call may be every second to fifth night for all those years. These doctors do many surgical procedures on the abdomen, breasts, and extremities, and are trained to care for trauma victims. Many fellowships, usually lasting two to four years, are available after general surgery training. Colon and rectal surgery fellowships train doctors to do the more challenging operations on the lower bowel. Hand surgery fellowships develop skills in repairing hand injuries. Pediatric fellowships offer training in operating on small children. Plastic surgery fellowships supply training in specialized plastic surgery techniques. A thoracic surgeon may be trained to repair heart valves and do heart bypasses. Fellowships are also available in treating burn victims.

General surgeons may also do fellowships to become transplant surgeons of the pancreas, liver, and kidneys. Vascular surgeons receive training in operating on blood vessels and do procedures such as repairing abdominal aortic aneurysms. Surgeons may become critical-care specialists who take care of very sick surgery patients in intensive care units. Many basic general surgery skills can be acquired in the first five to six years of residency, but the advanced skills, which allow doctors to do difficult, highly specialized operations, require additional training time.

Urology

A urologist operates on the urethra, penis, testicles, bladder, and kidneys. They perform operations to remove tumors and to repair traumatic injuries and dysfunctional organs. Training includes two years of general surgery followed by three years of urologic surgery. Fellowship training is available in pediatrics and oncology.

CONCLUSION

As you can see, the road to becoming a fully trained physician is long and arduous. Being on call several times a week is hard on you and your family. Spouses and children may find it difficult to accept the demands on your time from the hospital and your fatigue when you are at home. Additionally, most of your free time must be spent reading and studying textbooks and journal articles that help you learn the skills required of a specialist. Despite the great sacrifices, in the end, most doctors feel the reward of their work is the accomplishment of a lifelong dream.